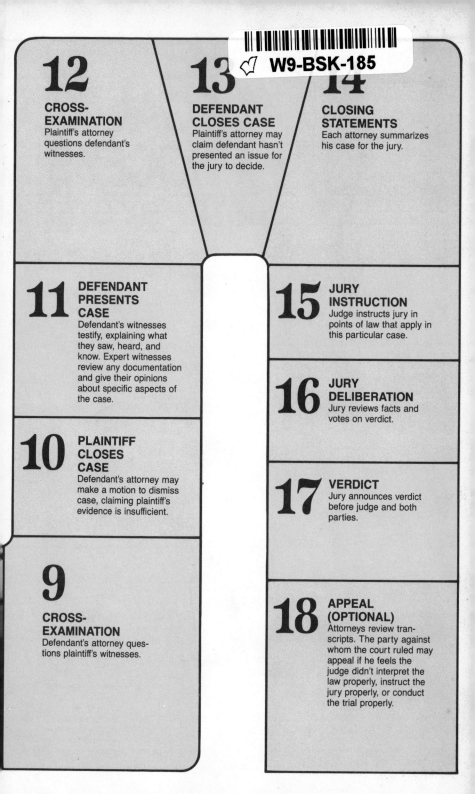

**12**

**CROSS-EXAMINATION**
Plaintiff's attorney questions defendant's witnesses.

**13**

**DEFENDANT CLOSES CASE**
Plaintiff's attorney may claim defendant hasn't presented an issue for the jury to decide.

**14**

**CLOSING STATEMENTS**
Each attorney summarizes his case for the jury.

**11**

**DEFENDANT PRESENTS CASE**
Defendant's witnesses testify, explaining what they saw, heard, and know. Expert witnesses review any documentation and give their opinions about specific aspects of the case.

**10**

**PLAINTIFF CLOSES CASE**
Defendant's attorney may make a motion to dismiss case, claiming plaintiff's evidence is insufficient.

**9**

**CROSS-EXAMINATION**
Defendant's attorney questions plaintiff's witnesses.

**15**

**JURY INSTRUCTION**
Judge instructs jury in points of law that apply in this particular case.

**16**

**JURY DELIBERATION**
Jury reviews facts and votes on verdict.

**17**

**VERDICT**
Jury announces verdict before judge and both parties.

**18**

**APPEAL (OPTIONAL)**
Attorneys review transcripts. The party against whom the court ruled may appeal if he feels the judge didn't interpret the law properly, instruct the jury properly, or conduct the trial properly.

# NURSE'S REFERENCE LIBRARY®

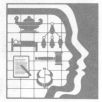

# Practices

*Nursing84* Books™
Springhouse Corporation
Springhouse, Pennsylvania

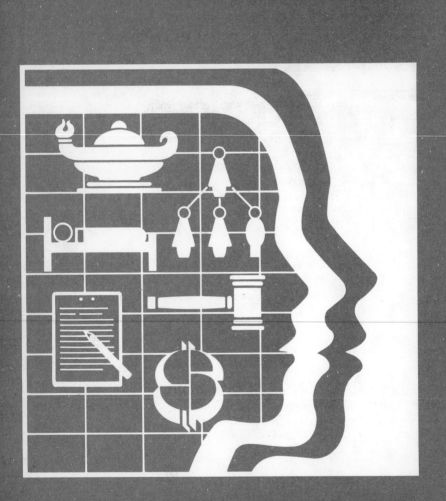

# NURSE'S REFERENCE LIBRARY®

# Practices

*Nursing84* Books™
Springhouse Corporation
Springhouse, Pennsylvania

NURSING84
BOOKS™

## Springhouse Corporation Book Division

**CHAIRMAN**
Eugene W. Jackson

**PRESIDENT**
Daniel L. Cheney

**VICE-PRESIDENT AND DIRECTOR**
Timothy B. King

**VICE-PRESIDENT, BOOK OPERATIONS**
Thomas A. Temple

**VICE-PRESIDENT, PRODUCTION AND PURCHASING**
Bacil Guiley

**RESEARCH DIRECTOR**
Elizabeth O'Brien

**Library of Congress Cataloging in Publication Data**
Main entry under title:

Practices.

    (Nurse's reference library)
    "Nursing84 books."
    Includes bibliographies and index.
    1. Nursing—Practice. I. Series.   [DNLM:
1. Ethics, Nursing.   2. Nursing.   3. Nurse-
Patient relations.
4. Legislation, Nursing.   WY 16 P895]
RT86.7.P7   1983   610.73   83-12879
ISBN 0-916730-41-7

# NURSE'S REFERENCE LIBRARY®

# Staff for this volume

**EDITORIAL DIRECTOR**
Diana Odell Potter

**CLINICAL DIRECTOR**
Minnie Bowen Rose, RN, BSN, MEd

**ART DIRECTOR**
Sonja Douglas

**Editorial Manager:** Richard Samuel West
**Senior Clinical Editor:** Regina Daley Ford, RN, BSN, MA
**Acquisitions Editor:** Elizabeth J. Cobbs
**Clinical Editor:** Judith A. Schilling McCann, RN, BSN
**Contributing Clinical Editors:** Helen Hahler D'Angelo, RN, MSN; Karen Dyer Vance, RN, BSN; Kathleen E. Viall Gallagher, RN, MSN; Mary Gyetvan, RN, BSEd; Ramon Lavandero, RN, BSN, MA, MSN; Patricia Schull, RN, BS; Barbara Gorham Slaymaker, RN, BSN, CRNP
**Drug Information Manager:** Larry N. Gever, RPh, PharmD
**Senior Editor:** Matthew T. Corso
**Associate Editors:** June F. Gomez, William J. Kelly
**Assistant Editor:** Holly Ann Burdick
**Contributing Editors:** Marylou Ambrose, Jeff Heller, Judith McDevitt, Elizabeth McNulty, Frederick Nohl, Loy Wiley
**Copy Chief:** Jill Lasker
**Copy Supervisor:** David R. Moreau
**Copy Editors:** Timothy Gaul, Sharyl Wolf
**Contributing Copy Editors:** Dario Bernardini, Max A. Fogel, Linda Johnson, David Jones, Diane M. Labus, Jeff Schein, J.A. Simoneau, Jr., Adam Tait III, William J. Wright
**Production Coordinators:** Jacqueline S. Miles, Rebecca S. Van Dine
**Associate Designer:** Carol Cameron-Sears
**Assistant Designers:** Jacalyn Bove Facciolo, Christopher Laird
**Contributing Designers:** Darcy Feralio, Lynn Foulk
**Illustrators:** Marion Banks, Dimitrios Bastas, Jack Freas, Robert Jackson, Robert Jones, Dennis Schofield
**Art Production Manager:** Robert Perry
**Art Assistants:** Diane Fox, Don Knauss, Sandy Sanders, Louise Stamper, Thom Staudenmayer
**Typography Manager:** David C. Kosten
**Typography Assistants:** Janice Haber, Ethel Halle, Debra Lee Judy, Diane Paluba, Nancy Wirs
**Production Manager:** Wilbur D. Davidson
**Quality Control Manager:** Robert L. Dean
**Editorial Assistants:** Maree E. DeRosa, Bernadette M. Glenn
**Indexer:** Gloria R. Hamilton
**Researcher:** Vonda Heller

Special thanks to H. Nancy Holmes, Daniel H. O'Connell, Esq., Jerome Rubin, and Anne Marie Brennan, who assisted in the preparation of this volume.

# Contents

 **The Law and Nursing Practice**

## Patients' Rights

# 3 Your Legal Risks in Nursing Practice

**Entry**

# 4 Your Legal Risks While Off Duty

**Entry**

# 5 Documentation

**Entry**

# 6 Malpractice: Understand It, Avoid It

# 7 Contracts and Collective Bargaining

# 8 Your Choices in Nursing Education

# 9 Your Choices about Your Job

**Entry**

# 10 Working Toward Job Satisfaction

**Entry**

# 11 Ethical Problems

**Entry**

# 12 Relating with Patients and Their Families
**Entry**

# 13 Understanding and Working with Doctors
**Entry**

# 14 Working with Other Professionals

NURSING84
BOOKS™

# NURSE'S REFERENCE LIBRARY®

This volume is part of a series conceived by the publishers of *Nursing84*®
magazine and written by hundreds of nursing and medical specialists. This
series, the NURSE'S REFERENCE LIBRARY, is the most comprehensive
reference set ever created exclusively for the nursing profession. Each
volume brings together the most up-to-date clinical information and related
nursing practice. Each volume informs, explains, alerts, guides, educates.
Taken together, the NURSE'S REFERENCE LIBRARY provides today's
nurse with the knowledge and the skills that she needs to be effective in her
daily practice and to advance in her career.

## *Other volumes in the series:*

| | | |
|---|---|---|
| Diseases | Drugs | Procedures |
| Diagnostics | Assessment | Definitions |

## *Other publications:*

**NEW NURSING SKILLBOOK™ SERIES**

Giving Emergency Care Competently      Coping with Neurologic Problems Proficiently
Assessing Vital Functions Accurately      Combatting Cardiovascular Diseases Skillfully
Reading EKGs Correctly      Monitoring Fluid and Electrolytes Precisely

**NURSING PHOTOBOOK™ SERIES**

Providing Respiratory Care      Controlling Infection
Managing I.V. Therapy      Ensuring Intensive Care
Dealing with Emergencies      Coping with Neurologic Disorders
Giving Medications      Caring for Surgical Patients
Assessing Your Patients      Working with Orthopedic Patients
Using Monitors      Nursing Pediatric Patients
Providing Early Mobility      Helping Geriatric Patients
Giving Cardiac Care      Attending Ob/Gyn Patients
Performing GI Procedures      Aiding Ambulatory Patients
Implementing Urologic Procedures      Carrying Out Special Procedures

**NURSING NOW™**
Shock
Hypertension

**NURSE'S CLINICAL LIBRARY™**
Cardiovascular Disorders
Respiratory Disorders

***Nursing84* DRUG HANDBOOK™**

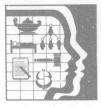

# Advisory Board

*At the time of publication, the advisors, contributors, and clinical and legal consultants held the following positions:*

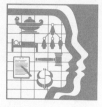

# Contributors

**Roberta S. Abruzzese, RN, FAAN, EdD,** Director of Continuing Education, Adelphi University School of Nursing, Garden City, N.Y.

**Dolores M. Alford, RN, MSN, FAAN,** Gerontological Nursing Consultant, Nursing Associates, Dallas

**Madalon O'Rawe Amenta, RN, MPH, DrPH,** Hospice Consultant, Pittsburgh

**Judith A. Baron, RN, MSN,** Corporate Consultant, Health Care Services, Burroughs Corporation, Chicago

**Arleen Behling, RN,** Associate Director of Nursing, Mount Sinai Medical Center, Milwaukee

**H. Michael Bennett, JD,** Attorney, Nashville, Tenn.

**Jo Anne Bennett, RN, MA,** Assistant Director of Nursing, Long Island College Hospital, Brooklyn, N.Y.; Adjunct Instructor, Lienhard School of Nursing, Pace University Graduate Division, Pleasantville, N.Y.

**Michelle Brandhandler, RN, BA,** Student, John Marshall Law School, Chicago

**Anne E. Braun, RNC, MSN,** Staff Nurse, Surgical Intensive Care Unit, Wilmington (Del.) Medical Center

**Nancy J. Brent, RN, MS, JD,** Attorney, Chicago

**Dona L. Bruton, RN, BA,** Assistant Administrator, Patient Care Services, Eskaton American River Hospital, Carmichael, Calif.

**Debra Szabo Bubba, RN, MSN,** Administrative Assistant, Nursing Administration, Lehigh Valley Hospital Center, Allentown, Pa.

**Betsy Jessup Caine, RN, BSN,** Manager, Nurse Recruitment and Retention, Georgetown University Medical Center, Washington, D.C.

**Patricia J. Canders, RN, BSN,** Charge Nurse, Mt. Diablo Hospital Medical Center, Concord, Calif.

**Verna J. Carson, RN, MSN,** Assistant Professor, University of Maryland School of Nursing, Baltimore

**Robin Chagares, RN, MA, MS,** Surgical Clinical Nurse Specialist, Montefiore Hospital, Bronx, N.Y.

**Sarah D. Cohn, RN, MSN, CNM, JD,** Associate Editor, *Law, Medicine and Health Care,* Boston

**Carmelle Pellerin Cournoyer, RN, MA, JD,** Attorney, Health Law Educator and Consultant, Manchester, N.H.

**Leah Curtin, RN, MA, MS, FAAN,** Editor, *Nursing Management,* Cincinnati

**George F. Dale, JD,** Attorney, Philadelphia

**Amy Burcham de Vasquez, BA,** Public Relations Director, Skilled Nursing Inc., Springhouse, Pa.

**Lillian DeYoung, RN, PhD,** Dean and Professor of Nursing, University of Akron (Ohio) College of Nursing

**Judy Donlen, RNC, MSN,** Instructor, University of Pennsylvania School of Nursing, Philadelphia

**Gloria Ferraro Donnelly, RN, MSN, FAAN,** Director, Department of Nursing, LaSalle College, Philadelphia

Debra Ann Edwards, RN, BSN, MSN, Clinical Nursing Supervisor, Northwestern Memorial Hospital, Chicago

John S. Fehir, RN, BSN, MA, Clinical Instructor, New York University Division of Nursing, New York

Eleanor R. Fine, RN, BSN, MA, JD, Attorney, Tacoma, Wash.

Carole A. Gassert, RN, MN, Clinical Instructor, University of Virginia School of Nursing, Charlottesville

Denise Bonenfant Gaunya, RN, MSN, Director, Cardiac Rehabilitation, Alexandria (Va.) Hospital

Carol Ann Gramse, RN, PhD, Assistant Professor of Nursing, Hunter College–Bellevue School of Nursing, New York

J. Gregory Hannigan, JD, Attorney, Hagerstown, Md.

Lovena L. Haumann, RN, MA, Instructor, Trenton (N.J.) State College School of Nursing

Arlene Nash Hayne, RN, MSN, Director, Critical Care Division of Nursing, Baptist Medical Center–Montclair, Birmingham, Ala.

Joanne V. Hickey, RN, MSN, MA, CNRN, Associate Professor of Nursing, Community College of Rhode Island, Warwick

Sharon E. Hoffman, RN, PhD, Associate Dean for Graduate Nursing Program, School of Nursing, University of Texas Health Science Center, San Antonio

Nancy M. Holloway, RN, MSN, CCRN, CEN, Consultant, Critical Care and

Emergency Nursing Director, Nancy Holloway & Associates, Berkeley, Calif.

Dorothy Ann Holveck, RN, CNA, Charge Nurse, ICU-CCU, Saudi Arabian National Guard Hospital, Riyadh, Saudi Arabia

Patricia Ann Horner, RN, MSN, Former Home Care Coordinator, Mercy Catholic Medical Center–Misericordia Division, Philadelphia

Judith Moore Johnson, RN, BA, Program Director, Continuing Education, University of Minnesota School of Nursing; Senior Consultant, Health Management Systems Associates, Minneapolis

Lynne Jungman, RN, MSN, Clinician, Psychiatric Nurse, Lake County Mental Health, Waukegan, Ill.

Beatrice J. Kalisch, RN, EdD, FAAN, Shirley C. Titus Distinguished Professor of Nursing, and Chairperson, Parent-Child Nursing, University of Michigan, Ann Arbor

Kenneth W. Kirkpatrick, RN, MS, CNA, Assistant Administrator, Director of Nursing Services, Barberton (Ohio) Citizens Hospital

Judith A. Kopper, RN, MS, Assistant Professor, Winona State University, Rochester, Minn.

Michael J. Korolishin, JD, Attorney, Philadelphia

Linda J. Lalor, RN, MSN, Clinical Specialist, Thoracic-Cardiovascular Surgery, University of Virginia Medical Center, Charlottesville

Linda Armstrong Lazure, RN, MSN, Assistant Professor, Department of Continuing Education, Creighton University School of Nursing, Omaha

**Carrie B. Lenburg, RN, EdD, FAAN,** Coordinator, Regents External Degrees in Nursing Program, University of the State of New York, Albany

**Lori J. Lustig, RN, BSN, JD,** Attorney, Health-Care Consultant, Alexandria, Va.

**Edwina A. McConnell, RN, MS,** Consultant, Medical Surgical Nursing; Staff Nurse, Madison General Hospital, Madison, Wis.

**Belva Chang McDavid, RN, BSN, MN, JD,** Free-lance Lecturer, Consultant, Wakarusa, Kan.

**Paul Mainardi, JD,** Attorney, Haddonfield, N.J.

**Cynthia M. Maleski, JD,** General Counsel, Mercy Hospital of Pittsburgh

**Gail A. Mallory, RN, MS,** Psychiatric Liaison Practitioner, Medical Nursing Teacher, Rush–Presbyterian–St. Luke's Medical Center, Chicago

**Catherine Malloy, RN, DrPH,** Associate Dean, Associate Professor, Duquesne University School of Nursing, Pittsburgh

**Carolyn G. Smith Marker, RN, MSN, CNA,** Faculty Consultant, Critical Care Continuing Education, Resource Applications, Inc., Baltimore

**Ann Marriner, RN, PhD,** Professor, Associate Dean, Indiana University School of Nursing, Indianapolis

**Judith E. Meissner, RN, MSN,** Senior Associate Professor, Bucks County Community College, Newtown, Pa.

**Margaret Miller, RN, BSN, MSEd,** Coordinator, Department of Continuing Education, Creighton University School of Nursing, Omaha

**Martha Jean Minniti, RN, BS, CCRN,** President/Administrator, Skilled Nursing, Inc., Springhouse, Pa.

**Anne Moraca-Sawicki, RN, BSN, MSN,** Clinical Nurse Specialist, Mt. St. Mary's Hospital, Lewiston, N.Y.

**Ellen K. Murphy, RN, MS, JD,** Assistant Professor, University of Wisconsin, Milwaukee

**Lois M. Murphy, RN, MS,** Executive Director, New Hampshire Nurses' Association, Concord

**Mary Duffin Naylor, RN, PhD,** Chairman, Department of Baccalaureate Nursing, Thomas Jefferson University, Philadelphia

**Claire C. Obade, RN, BA, JD,** Attorney, Philadelphia

**Robin Adair Burkart Peeples, RN, BSN, MS,** Instructor, University of Maryland, Baltimore

**Marlys E. Peterson, RN, MS,** Vice-President, Nursing, Methodist Hospital, Madison, Wis.

**Deborah M. Peyton, RN, BSN,** Assistant Director, Risk Management, St. Joseph Hospital, Inc., Towson, Md.

**Patricia M. Pierce, RN, PhD, CFNP,** Associate Director, REACH Project, University of Florida College of Nursing, Gainesville

**Elizabeth Price, RN, BSN, MS, JD,** Attorney Advisor, Department of Health and Human Services, Office of the General Counsel, Rockville, Md.; Staff Nurse, Temporary Nursing Agencies, Maryland

**Jean Rabinow, JD,** Attorney, New Haven, Conn.

**Peggy J. Reiley, RN, MS,** Charge Nurse, Beth Israel Hospital, Boston

**Erline A. Reilly, RN, BA, JD,** Attorney, Concord, N.H.

**Pamela Reinert, RN, MSN,** Director

of Patient Care, St. Luke's Hospital, Denver

**Paula Laros Rich, RN, MSN,** Nurse Consultant, Professional Nursing Development, Philadelphia

**Joan Kelly Richards, RN, MSN,** Director of Clinical Nursing, Crozer-Chester Medical Center, Chester, Pa.

**Susan K. Riesch, MSN, DNSc,** Associate Professor of Nursing, University of Wisconsin, Milwaukee

**Mary Margaret Rock, RN, BSN,** RN Manager, Mercy Care Center Division of Bergan Mercy Hospital, Omaha

**Linda Faith Rosen, RN, MA, JD,** Attorney, Philadelphia

**Thomas E. Rubbert, JD,** Attorney, Los Angeles

**Jean M. Scheideman, CRN, MA,** Clinical Supervisor, Out-Patient Services, Mental Health North, Seattle

**Anna Marie Seroka, RN, BSN, CCRN, MEd,** Staff Development Instructor II, University of Colorado Health Sciences Center, Denver

**Harold H. Simpson II, JD,** Attorney, Little Rock, Ark.

**Suzanne Marr Skinner, RN, MS,** Lecturer, University of Maryland School of Nursing, Baltimore

**Carol E. Smith, RN, MSN,** Assistant Professor, Winona State University, Rochester Center, Rochester, Minn.

**Mary L. Smith, RN, BSN, MA,** Instructor, Psychiatric and Medical Nursing, Indian Hills Community College, Ottumwa, Iowa

**Maryann R. Sparks, RN, MEd,** Assistant Professor, Associate Degree Nursing Program, School of Allied Health Professions, Hahnemann University, Philadelphia.

**Frances J. Storlie, RN, PhD, ANP,** Adult Nurse Practitioner, Vancouver, Wash.

**Marlene Thompson, RN, MSN, CCRN,** Clinical Director, Medical Special Care Nursing, St. John Medical Center, Tulsa, Okla.

**Pat Thompson, RN, BSN, MSPH,** Assistant Professor, Winona State University, Winona, Minn.

**Virgie M. Vakil, RN, BA, JD,** Attorney, Media, Pa.

**Claudette Varricchio, RN, DNS,** Assistant Dean and Undergraduate Program Director, Marcella Niehoff School of Nursing, Loyola University, Chicago

**Betty A. Velthouse, RN, BSN, MSN,** Visiting Assistant Professor, University of West Florida, Pensacola

**Katherine W. Vestal, RN, BSN, MSN, PhD,** Associate Executive Director, Hermann Hospital, Houston

**Barbara J. Virnig, RN, CHN, BSN, MSN,** Community Health Nurse Team Leader, Olmsted County Health Department; Nurse Educator, Winona State University, Rochester, Minn.

**Joanne F. White, RN, BSN, MNEd,** Assistant Dean, Duquesne University School of Nursing, Pittsburgh

**Leslie Wilson, RN, MSN,** Instructor, University of Maryland School of Nursing, Baltimore

**Janice W. Wise, BS, MA, JD,** Assistant Director, Economic and General Welfare Program, Ohio Nurses Association, Columbus

**Pat S. Yoder Wise, RN, MSN,** Associate Dean and Associate Professor, Texas Tech University Health Sciences Center School of Nursing, Lubbock

**Lynn M. Worley, RN, JD,** Assistant State's Attorney, Health Division, Cook County State's Attorney's Office, Chicago

**Barbara J. Youngberg, RN, BSN, MICN, MSW, JD,** Medical/Legal Consultant; Staff Nurse, Emergency Department, Illinois Masonic Medical Center, Chicago

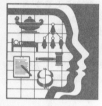

# Clinical and Legal Consultants

**Glenn M. Barnes, BSc, MHA, LLB,** Barrister and Solicitor, Ottawa

**Judith Renzi Brown, RN, JD,** Director of Risk Management, Assistant Counsel for Claims, Pennsylvania Medical Society Liability Insurance Company, Lemoyne, Pa.

**Glynis Smith Chadwick, RN, BSN,** Former Coordinator, Division of Clinical Nursing Education, Anne Arundel General Hospital, Annapolis, Md.

**Carmelle Pellerin Cournoyer, RN, MA, JD,** Attorney, Health Law Educator and Consultant, Manchester, N.H.

**Bonnie W. Duldt, RN, PhD,** Professor and Director of Graduate Studies, College of Nursing, University of North Dakota, Grand Forks

**Kate M. Fenner, RN, PhD,** Vice-President for Institutional Advancement, Lewis University, Romeoville, Ill.

**Tanya I. Hanger, RN, BSN, MA,** Assistant Director of Nursing, Staffing and Recruiting, New York University Medical Center–University Hospital, New York

**JoAnn Shafer Jamann, RN, MSN, EdD,** Dean and Professor, Columbia University School of Nursing, New York

**Marguerite C. McKelvey, RN, BSN, MSN,** Director, Economic and General Welfare, Pennsylvania Nurses Association, Harrisburg, Pa.

**Margaret Miller, RN, MSN,** Chairperson, Associate Degree Nurse Program, Bellarmine College, Louisville, Ky.

**Barbara A. Mlynczak, RN, CCRN,** Coordinator, Division of Nursing Education, Anne Arundel General Hospital, Annapolis, Md.

**Kathleen M. Nokes, RN, MA,** Community Health Nurse, Group Health Incorporated, New York University, New York

**Claire C. Obade, RN, BA, JD,** Attorney, Philadelphia

**LaVerne Rodgers Rocereto, RN, PhD,** Associate Professor, School of Nursing, University of Pittsburgh

**Ann Romberg, RN, BSN,** Staff Nurse, St. Elizabeth Medical Center, Yakima, Wash.

**Mary Patricia Ryan, RN, PhD,** Associate Professor, Marcella Niehoff School of Nursing, Loyola University of Chicago

**Corinne L. Sklar, BSN, MSN, JD,** Attorney, Imperial Life Assurance Company of America, Toronto

**Christine B. Spak, BSN, JD,** Attorney, Public Health Hearing Officer, Department of Health Services, Hartford, Conn.

**Patricia Valoon, RN, MS,** Director of Nursing, Assistant Administrator, University Hospital, New York

**Pat S. Yoder Wise, RN, MSN,** Associate Dean/Associate Professor, Texas Tech University Health Sciences Center School of Nursing, Lubbock

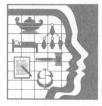

# Foreword

As nurses, we work long and hard to achieve greater respect for our education and for our skill as health-care providers. We can be proud of our expanded roles in all aspects of health care today, and of the increasingly complex and important functions we fulfill. We must remember, however, that the ever-broadening scope of nursing practice, which makes contemporary nursing so exciting and rewarding, has also complicated our work. Yes, nursing has emerged as a challenging profession requiring a high level of education, knowledge, skill, and decision-making capabilities. Nurses today have a lot more responsibility than they used to. But with increased clinical responsibility comes increased risk of liability. As a nurse today, you owe it to yourself and your patients to keep abreast of changes in the laws and regulations that define your professional responsibilities. You also need to come to terms with the difficult ethical and professional dilemmas that modern society and science have created for the health team (for example, the dilemma of whether or not to keep a brain-dead patient alive with life-support equipment). These issues create a paradoxical situation for you: they require a lot of thought before you can be sure of your feelings about them, but often they arise in patient-care circumstances where you're required to act quickly as well as conscientiously.

So you can see that keeping up with the development and application of new nursing interventions isn't enough to help you chart the specific nursing career path that's best suited to your skills and values. Nor can the clinical skills you apply in your everyday work help you when you're not sure how to proceed legally, or when you feel your ethics are being compromised. PRACTICES, the newest volume in the Nurse's Reference Library, has been published to give you this kind of help. Its contributors and editors have sorted through our complicated legal system, tuned in to our lengthy and ongoing ethical de\

and selected those portions relevant to you as a nurse. They've also considered such important topics as employment contracts, benefits, education, and career advancement. They've organized this specialized information into succinct and comprehensive chapters and entries that present the information in a readily understandable and accessible form.

Chapters 1 through 6 of PRACTICES deal with the interaction between nursing and the law. Because your nursing responsibilities are expanding so rapidly, the laws defining them can't always keep up. This means you must be thoroughly familiar with the legal boundaries and duties of nursing practice in your state, so you know when you're on solid legal ground and when you should get legal or administrative advice before proceeding. These chapters comprehensively describe your legal risks and responsibilities in traditional and alternative practice settings, on and off duty. You'll find in-depth coverage of documenting and of strategies for preventing malpractice charges—even for coping with a lawsuit. You'll also find a full chapter on patients' legal rights in the hospital—a topic of great interest to nurses, who do so much to safeguard patients' rights.

Chapters 7 through 11 deal with *your* rights and options as a health-care employee. Here you'll discover vital information on employment contracts, collective bargaining, grievance procedures, career planning and job satisfaction, finding the job you want, negotiating the best possible salary and benefits, and even coping effectively with job termination. These chapters include a thorough discussion of the entry-into-practice issue and of nursing education programs available—including specialization and continuing education. These chapters also deal with a topic that's vitally involved in job satisfaction but that generally isn't discussed in relation to it—the burgeoning area of health-care ethics. Besides outlining your legal responsibilities, the entries on this topic will help you clarify your own ethical stance concerning abortion, transplants, life support for brain-dead patients, no-code and slow-code orders, and occasions when you're asked to cover up a colleague's errors or incompetence.

The remaining chapters pointedly discuss the interpersonal and political skills so vital to your success on the job. Starting with thoughtful probing of the nurse-patient-family relationship, entries tell you how you can provide emotional support to patients and their families, how you can gain the respect of your health-care colleagues, and even how you can use conflict in the unit in constructive ways that strengthen your professional relationships. You'll also learn how to analyze the power structure within your institution so you know the proper channels for getting answers to your questions and for pursuing concerns you're unable to resolve directly with your colleagues.

Each of PRACTICES' 16 chapters begins with a clear and concise introduction. Within each chapter, a short glossary of key terms accompanies every entry. In the chapters that have a legal focus, every effort has been made to relate "the law" directly to your circumstances as a practicing nurse. Here you'll find no abstract theories or vague generalizations. Instead, you'll find illustrative court cases, boxed questions and answers about legal problems that every nurse faces, charts that describe state-by-state variations in nursing law, and many other ways in which the contributors and editors of PRACTICES have made understanding nursing law easy for you. These chapters also provide guidance for professional advancement and for managing staff once you've been promoted. For nurses on both sides of the administrative "fence," PRACTICES is an indispensable handbook for day-to-day practice.

But PRACTICES doesn't stop here. Following its 16 chapters, you'll find a detailed and most interesting Fact-finder section containing charts, lists, and other information to supplement what you've learned in PRACTICES' pages. You'll consult this section often for help in managing legal and professional problems on the job. Throughout the book, you'll discover finely drawn illustrations that will enhance your enjoyment of the text.

Both in content and format, PRACTICES is a clearly written and exhaustively detailed reference that will quickly become indispensable. A handbook like PRACTICES is a must if you're a nurse who wants to protect and advance her career to the fullest extent. PRACTICES can help you achieve true satisfaction on the job—the satisfaction of knowing that, within the limits of the law, you're reaping the full potential of your capabilities and your ambitions.

BEATRICE J. KALISCH, RN, EdD, FAAN

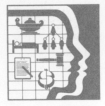

# Professional Overview

This book's time is *now*. As nurses, most of us have struggled for a long time with unanswered—sometimes unrecognized—questions about our practice. We've read about nurses' being sued for the "practice of medicine," for example, and wondered how they got into such predicaments. Could this happen to *us?* And we remember the courageous nurse who put her career on the line by questioning a doctor's order. We wonder—would *we* have the courage? We've espoused patients' rights, even fought for them, without necessarily asking, "What does *patients' rights* mean?" Finally, we've warned—and been warned—about the dangers of divisiveness in our profession. Yet we've sometimes unquestioningly watched economic forces—and others seemingly beyond our control—divide us even further. This book, PRACTICES, has been written to give nurses in *today's* nursing environment, with its evolving professional challenges and increased legal risks, some answers to questions like these.

Over the years, I (and many others) have written about "the role of the nurse in a changing society." And for many years, too, this topic has been professional nursing organizations' chief concern—indeed, their passion. But today, I believe that the way nurses practice that role resembles less and less what's being *written* about practicing it. A nurse who's educated to believe that her nursing role will be the way it's described in the literature may well find, once she starts working, that her expectations are in conflict with reality. This nurse may well ask herself: "Why didn't I get a hint of these kinds of career problems when I was in school?"

"These kinds of problems," the *real-life* problems you face every day of your nursing career, are just what PRACTICES is all about. Here are some examples you're sure to recognize:

- when you "know" that your college degree will get you the next head nurse position that opens up—but your employer, faced with budget cutbacks, hires a lower-salaried A.D. graduate instead.

- when you're asked to take an assignment your training didn't prepare you for.
- when you're asked to alter a patient's chart to show that the doctor responded immediately, even though he didn't.
- when you're told not to respond to a patient's or his family's questions about his illness.

In these situations and so many more, you need to know your legal rights and responsibilities and how to handle yourself so your actions don't jeopardize your career. But you can't expect to resolve these situations by quoting nursing theories or by citing textbook references. Now that you own PRACTICES, you have the *one* source you need for down-to-earth advice and guidance you can apply directly to your day-to-day nursing activities.

But PRACTICES delivers more. In its pages you'll find many instances where differing viewpoints on important nursing issues, including ethical issues, are contrasted and compared. This isn't a book that takes its own stand, without respecting its readers' capacity to make choices. I've observed over the years—not without some anger!—that many nursing publications seem to be trying to force us into a consensus on important issues. I consider this to be intellectual robbery. As a nurse, I want to know what others believe about key issues, and why. And I think that nursing students, in particular, need this. For them, nursing's legal, ethical, and professional issues may otherwise translate into bewildering reality.

Perhaps, in the long run, PRACTICES' endorsement of nurses' taking action to control their careers and their profession will have the greatest impact on its readers. The gravest dangers to our profession may well be apathy and noninvolvement. Nurses must be at the bedside, sure—but this isn't enough. They must be in legislatures, at the polling places, and in the administrative offices of every health-care institution, *helping to make policy.*

Some 10 or 12 years ago, Elizabeth Rambousek wrote *There Used To Be Nurses,* a treatise in which she pointed out the risks of nonnursing personnel's usurping our authority. She foresaw deterioration of nursing's role, through apathy. When I first read this treatise, I didn't agree with it. Well, the picture it painted then seems dreadfully real to me now. We must realize that nursing's future depends upon our survival in a society that "appreciates" the altruism of service professions while trying to keep them powerless. When nurses finally realize that their collective know-how has both practical and political clout, they'll find that their practice is something *they* can control.

PRACTICES is a milestone on that long road.

FRANCES J. STORLIE, RN, PhD, ANP

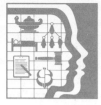

# Legal Overview

What is "the law"?

Basically, laws help us define our personal and professional relationships. Laws tell us what we may and may not do, alone and to and with each other. But "the law" isn't as clear-cut as this definition is. It isn't a static body of knowledge, something you can learn once that's valid forever. The law has movement and momentum; it can expand or contract. Parts of it can even die off—like the laws that prevented women from inheriting property and the laws that sanctioned slavery.

Nursing law is changing, too, as our profession matures toward the goals of increased autonomy and independent responsibility for patient care. Nursing law doesn't exist as a separate entity, apart from the general laws, rules, and regulations that society uses to govern itself. Instead, the term *nursing law* describes specific areas of federal and state constitutional, civil, criminal, and administrative law. These areas of law directly influence the professional relationships so essential to nursing practice.

Both you and your patient benefit when you practice your profession within appropriate legal limits. Your patient benefits because your care protects him from unnecessary harm. You benefit by protecting yourself from lawsuits, from damage to your professional reputation, and from possible financial hardship if you must pay damages to a patient who wins his case against you.

So nursing law isn't, as some nurses believe, an array of narrow, confusing ultimatums designed to contain and constrain the nursing profession. Instead, the effect of the law on nursing is like the many veins that run through a leaf: it provides definition, strength, and integrity.

To understand nurses' legal relationships, you need to understand the various types of laws that create rights and responsibilities for nurses.

*Public law* determines your relationship to the

federal government and the states. It consists of constitutional law, administrative law, and criminal law. *Private law* (also called civil law) determines your relationship to other individuals. It consists of contract law and tort law.

*Constitutional law* is the type of public law that considers your rights and responsibilities under the federal and state constitutions, as the U.S. and state supreme courts interpret them. Patients' right to life, right to die, and right to self-determination in refusing treatment, and your rights to life, liberty, and religious freedom, are all founded in constitutional law. This is an area of intimate issues, where law and ethics are closely intertwined.

*Administrative law* is the type of public law that concerns the administrative agencies, boards, and commissions legislated by Congress or the state legislatures. For nurses, the most important administrative agency is the state board of nursing, created under the provisions of each state's nurse practice act. This agency has the power to regulate nursing practice and nursing education, and it's the supreme authority on nursing practice issues in the state. No other agency may legally institute a nursing policy that contradicts a state board of nursing ruling. However, if a nurse is censured in a board action, she may appeal the board's decision to a state court.

*Criminal law* is public law concerning each state's criminal statutes, which define criminal actions such as murder, manslaughter, criminal negligence, theft, and illegal possession of drugs. Nurses risk violating criminal laws when they become involved in such actions as removing life-support systems, carrying out no-code orders, administering high doses of pain-killing medication to terminally ill patients, failing to nourish or medicate deformed newborns, and obviously criminal acts such as stealing medications or narcotics. Nurses also may be involved in criminal court proceedings as witnesses, if they care for victims of rape, shootings, and other violent crimes.

*Contract law* is private law involving agreements (contracts) between two or more parties to do something, for some type of remuneration—a "bargained-for exchange." In essence, a contract is a promissory agreement between two or more persons that creates, modifies, or destroys a legal relationship. In many situations, an oral agreement is also legally binding. Many nurses have individual oral or written contracts detailing their work schedules and job descriptions, as well as the personnel policies they're expected to follow. Similar contracts exist for unionized nurses, private-duty nurses, and others. If it can be said that job satisfaction begins with a clear understanding of your rights and responsibilities and those of your employer, then a written contract is an effective starting point on the road to that goal.

*Tort law* is private law concerning reparation of a wrong or injury inflicted by one person on another. This is the area of law that nurses are most familiar with. Why? Because it specifically addresses the nurse-patient relationship. Tort law is particularly concerned with the way you practice your profession and with your ability to prove that your care meets the required legal standard. Common causes of tort law action include malpractice, assault and battery, invasion of privacy, false imprisonment, and defamation.

The area of professional malpractice is very broad, encompassing any professional misconduct including negligence, betrayal of patients' trust and confidence, and other illegal or immoral actions. Of these, negligence is the most common charge against nurses. A charge of negligence against a nurse focuses on the standard of care: the patient attempts to prove that a certain standard was required in his care, that the defendant-nurse breached that standard, and that harm directly resulted. The defendant-nurse, of course, must attempt to disprove these charges. In this critical situation, the nursing process, properly documented, is every nurse's best defense.

No one has to tell you that the practice of nursing has become increasingly complex—and that nurses' risk of liability has increased proportionately. To make sure your care consistently meets appropriate legal and professional standards, you need sound knowledge of the relationship between the law and nursing practice. PRACTICES can answer your questions and help you provide high-quality care at minimal legal risk. With the information PRACTICES provides, you'll also be better prepared to identify and promote legal reforms for advancing our profession—and, by extension, your own career as a nurse.

CARMELLE P. COURNOYER, RN, MA, JD

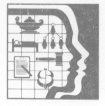

# Point of View: Developing Political and Economic Savvy

"For what they actually do, nurses are overpaid... For what they can do or should do and want to do, nurses are underpaid." So says Peter F. Drucker in *Hospital Management Quarterly*. Drucker goes on to note, "Years ago, nurses made about 40 or 50 percent of what physicians did. Today, the take-home pay of nurses is about 20 or 25 percent of the median income of the physicians...In economic terms, nurses have gotten a very short end of the stick..."

Over the years, nursing salaries have not increased proportionally with nursing-care responsibilities. In the future, as health-care dollars become increasingly scarce, your only hope of achieving parity in the health industry is by learning the art of health-care politics and the science of health-care economics.

### Political skills
If people are to work together at all, then someone must practice politics—and the more astute you are, the more likely your efforts at practicing politics will meet with success. The art of politics consists of three functions: persuasion, negotiation, and compromise. *Persuasion* is the art of getting people to share the same perception of the truth so that they will work together to achieve the same goal. *Negotiation* is the art of coordinating different perceptions of the truth so that people will work together to achieve common goals. *Compromise* is the art of accommodating different perceptions of the truth so that people will work together to achieve a solution that encompasses *disparate* goals.

### Economic skills
Even the most skilled politician will meet with failure unless he knows the economics involved in any project—and understands them from a variety of viewpoints. Nurses must learn the language of money, develop the skill of interpreting financial

statements, and prepare themselves to present their goals—and justify them—in fiscal terms. Most nurses (and women) were taught that the golden rule is "Do unto others as you would have them do unto you." However, in business, the golden rule is "He who has the gold, rules." You don't need to abandon the objective of the old rule to learn how to manipulate the new one. Unfortunately, most hospital administrators and fiscal managers view nurses (and the services they provide) solely in terms of expense—money spent—rather than income generated. For example, nursing units almost universally are designated as "cost centers." Yet people are admitted to hospitals because they need a special kind of skilled care: observation, monitoring, and treatment. And the American Hospital Association itself claims that over 90 percent of the care people receive in hospitals is given by nurses. In short, the *care givers* are the *revenue producers*. If administrators and fiscal managers can be brought to understand that nurses really are their prime revenue producers, the relative power of nurses in the health industry will increase considerably. To bring about this happy state of affairs, you must learn to present patients' care needs in fiscal language and to analyze finances so you can demonstrate that nursing generates more revenue than it expends.

From the beginning of recorded time, economics and politics have figured largely in human affairs. Now's the time for nurses to learn and use the arts and skills involved in both. Neither is terribly difficult, and both are necessary for nurses and nursing to achieve their rightful places in the health-care system.

LEAH CURTIN, RN, FAAN, MS, MA

# How to Use This Book

PRACTICES is designed to give you instant access to its wealth of legal, ethical, and professional nursing information. Foremost among the book's many features is its *numbered-entry format*. The individual entries, each covering a single important topic, are easy to locate because the entry numbers are large— they catch your eye as you quickly skim through PRACTICES' pages. Whether you use PRACTICES as a quick, on-the-job reference for legal and professional advice, as a learning or teaching tool, or as a resource for reviewing your knowledge of law and ethics as they relate to nursing practice, the numbered entries will help you find information quickly and easily.

**Special features**
In every entry, a boxed "Key Terms" feature concisely explains legal and professional terms used in the entry. (You'll also find a comprehensive glossary of legal, ethical, and professional terms in the back of the book.) At the end of each chapter, a *list of selected references* shows you where to look for further information.

Within the entries, important points are highlighted in *charts, text pieces, and graphs*. To help you locate these supplemental pieces easily, you'll find cross-references to many of them in the main text.

**Important reference section**
Consult the *Fact-Finder section*, following Chapter 16, for valuable legal and professional reference information. Here you'll find comprehensive charts, lists, and text pieces describing grounds for license denial, revocation, and suspension; guidelines for negotiating an individual employment contract; and qualifications for Medicare reimbursement, including an explanation of Diagnostic-Related Groups (DRGs). You'll also discover state-by-state definitions of

nursing practice, position statements on entry into practice from the major nursing organizations, a state-by-state listing of child abuse statutes, and much more.

## Legal coverage

Whenever possible, legal points are illustrated by *summaries of actual court cases*. (Note: When the outcome of a court case isn't discussed, either the outcome wasn't reported or the outcome isn't the focus of what the case illustrates in the text.)

You probably know that *court-case citations* are complicated amalgams of numbers, letters, and abbreviations. You'll find that cases in PRACTICES' text are cited simply by title and year, for easy reading. However, you'll find an indexed list of full court-case citations in the back of the book. Refer to this list—and to "How to Interpret Legal Citations," in the Fact-Finder section—when you want to look up more information on a case.

When you read and consult PRACTICES, remember that laws affecting nurses vary from state to state in the United States and from province to province in Canada. (Differing nurse practice acts are excellent examples of this.) For your best protection, keep up to date on nursing-related court decisions that are made in your state or province. And for advice on specific legal matters, always consult your own attorney.

As you use PRACTICES day after day, you'll find it provides you with complete, accurate, and up-to-date information. You can't afford to be without it as you daily confront the legal, ethical, and professional problems of modern nursing practice.

**ENTRIES IN THIS CHAPTER**

# The Law and Nursing Practice

## Introduction

PRACTICES offers you, as a nurse, a thorough understanding of nursing's relationships to the law. You know that law is the body of rules and regulations that govern all of society—protecting the health, safety, and welfare of its citizens. And, of course, you also know that any departure from the law spells trouble.

The federal government and the states hold constitutional authority to enact laws. As you might expect, this means the health-care field abounds with federal and state legislation that directly shapes and influences the practice of nursing. But the laws aren't rigid and unyielding. Instead, they're dynamic, responsive—like the nursing profession they serve. As nursing changes, laws change, too. The laws must have this flexibility so that nurses can care for patients in a variety of clinical situations, while still remaining within the legal scope of nursing practice.

Why should you concern yourself with the law? Because you've worked hard to earn entry into the nursing profession. You've spent time, effort, and money to graduate from an accredited school of nursing. And you've demonstrated your nursing knowledge and skill by successfully completing your state board examination or (after 1981) the National Council Licensure Examination (NCLEX). Your nursing license was the beginning of a lifelong commitment to a challenging and rewarding career. Now, like other professionals, you want opportunities for personal advancement, increased economic benefits, and a guarantee that your profession will have the means to keep pace with the latest technologic advancements. These are worthy goals for the nursing profession. But they can only be realized if you're willing to accept the professional and legal responsibilities involved. And remember, ignorance of the law isn't a valid defense in any type of legal proceeding. As a nurse, you're expected to know and understand the laws that directly and indirectly affect your practice. Chapter 1 explores these and other timely issues. Each entry will provide you with accurate, comprehensive legal information that you need every day as you care for patients.

### A history of nursing law

By the early 1900s, nursing practice had developed and matured to the point where laws and regulations became necessary to establish minimum standards for entry into the profession.

The first such laws were nurse registration acts. These acts were *permissive*, meaning that anyone could practice nursing but only those regis-

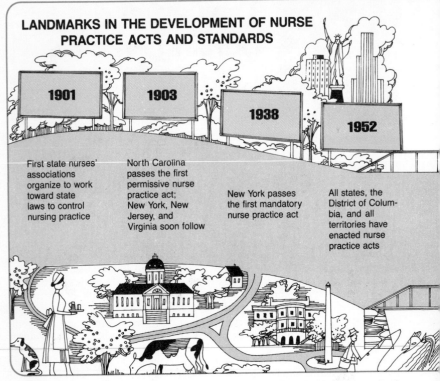

## LANDMARKS IN THE DEVELOPMENT OF NURSE PRACTICE ACTS AND STANDARDS

**1901**
First state nurses' associations organize to work toward state laws to control nursing practice

**1903**
North Carolina passes the first permissive nurse practice act; New York, New Jersey, and Virginia soon follow

**1938**
New York passes the first mandatory nurse practice act

**1952**
All states, the District of Columbia, and all territories have enacted nurse practice acts

tered could use the initials "RN." The first nurse registration act was made law in North Carolina in March 1903. It stated that anyone who paid a fee to be listed in the state register could practice nursing. (Unregistered persons could still practice nursing, whether or not they'd completed nursing training.) By 1923, every state had some type of nurse registration law. In 1938, New York State passed the first *mandatory* nurse practice act, a law that established two levels of nursing: licensed registered nurse and licensed practical nurse. This practice act mandated that *only* professionals licensed under the act could practice nursing. Other states followed with similar laws. By 1952, all the states, the District of Columbia, and all U.S. territories had enacted nurse practice acts.

Since those early years of legislative activity, numerous significant changes have occurred, including changes in the definition of nursing practice and (recently, in a few states) recognition of the nurse's modern role, which allows nurses to make nursing diagnoses. In 1970, the American Nurses' Association (ANA) amended the wording of its 1955 model definition of nursing to eliminate the prohibition on nursing diagnosis. By 1977, 24 states had enacted new or additional amendments to their nurse practice acts, generally eliminating the prohibition on nursing diagnosis. Some states also legally recognized the nurse's expanded role. In 1979, the ANA further amended its definition of nursing to encompass the broad scope of nursing in today's practice settings. To date, only New York and California have enacted adaptations of the 1979 ANA definition into law.

Other areas of nursing concern, however, have received only selective

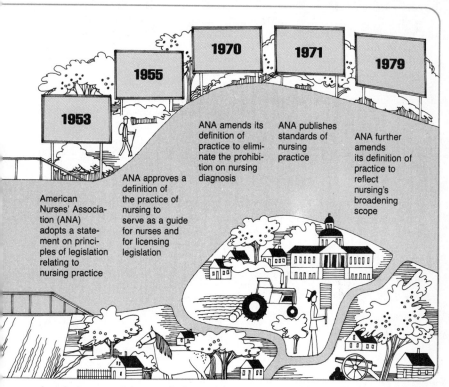

**1953**

American Nurses' Association (ANA) adopts a statement on principles of legislation relating to nursing practice

**1955**

ANA approves a definition of the practice of nursing to serve as a guide for nurses and for licensing legislation

**1970**

ANA amends its definition of practice to eliminate the prohibition on nursing diagnosis

**1971**

ANA publishes standards of nursing practice

**1979**

ANA further amends its definition of practice to reflect nursing's broadening scope

legislative attention or verbal support. Two such areas are standards of patient care and standards of nursing practice.

## Standards of patient care

The purpose of all health law and regulation is to protect the public from the uninformed, the unprepared, and the unscrupulous health-care practitioner. However, some consumers and legislators—and even some health-care professionals—argue that only minimal regulation is necessary to safeguard health-care consumers. In these persons' view, the proliferation of health-care providers and subsequent regulation is a costly impediment to optimum delivery of health-care services.

The law has responded to such arguments in a limited way—for example, by establishing standards of care for patients in government-sponsored health-care programs. Medicare and Medicaid regulations, which cover elderly (and some disabled) patients in hospitals and nursing homes, specify which conditions can be treated and, in some instances, minimum treatment requirements. Patients' rights legislation protects the rights of all patients, including those in nursing homes and mental hospitals. And so-called right-to-die legislation recognizes health-care professionals' ethical as well as professional responsibilities when using life-sustaining technology. These laws preserve the patient's right to choose the direction of his care in life-or-death situations.

In some states, standards for care of hospital patients have been incorporated into state law by a process that accepts or adapts the accreditation of the Joint Commission on Accreditation of Hospitals. This incorporation into law has resulted in broadly applicable standards of patient care. These standards are increasingly used in preference to local standards when courts seek to determine applicable standards of care and admit expert-witness testimony in malpractice lawsuits. National patient-care standards will help develop uniform expectations of nursing care and eliminate regional differences in evaluating that care.

## Nursing practice standards

Nursing practice standards are established by state boards of nursing. Some states refer to standards in their nurse practice acts. Unless they're specifically cited in nurse practice acts, professional standards aren't laws—they're guidelines for sound nursing practice. Until 1971, individual hos-

---

*"Basically, the registered nurse is responsible for developing and managing patient care."*

---

pitals determined nursing practice standards according to local standards. But in 1971 the ANA published its nursing standards, which has since gained widespread acceptance.

Nursing standards may or may not be in written form (see Entry 2, where the ANA standards of nursing practice are reproduced). Nevertheless, courts decide nursing malpractice lawsuits largely on whether defendant-nurses meet applicable standards of nursing care. So, although they aren't laws themselves, standards have important legal significance for nurses.

## RN and LPN/LVN practice: legal differences

As you know, two levels of nursing practice currently exist—the registered nurse (RN) and the licensed practical/vocational nurse (LPN/LVN). RNs complete a longer and more intensive educational program for entry into practice than LPNs/LVNs do. Once li-

censed, the RN is responsible for developing and managing patient care. She must also make professional nursing judgments based on the nursing process—including patient assessment, nursing diagnosis, treatment, and evaluation.

Definitions of the RN's role vary somewhat among states, but her basic responsibilities include observing patients' signs and symptoms, recording her observations, carrying out doctors' orders for patient treatments, and appropriately delegating responsibilities for patient care.

The LPN/LVN is often referred to as the "bedside nurse" because her role has traditionally centered on the patient's basic physical needs for hygiene and comfort. Many state nurse practice acts define LPN/LVN practice as the performance of duties that assist the professional nurse in a team relationship. In some states, the duties of LPNs/LVNs are more clearly defined in terms of scope of practice. For example, Washington State's nurse practice act prohibits LPNs/LVNs from administering medications and injections.

## Nursing practice in Canada

Canada permits licensure of registered nurses, registered nursing assistants, and—in some provinces—practical or vocational nurses. In recent years, some Canadian nursing associations have recognized clinical nurse specialists (who generally have master's or doctoral degrees in specific specialties).

In most of Canada's 10 provinces, professional nurses' associations set requirements for graduation from an approved school of nursing, for licensing, for nurses' professional behavior, and for registration fees.

The Canadian registered nurse may receive her education in a diploma school (such as a hospital school of nursing), in a community college, or in a bachelor's program. The licensing examination she must take varies by province—some use NCLEX and some compile their own (thus complicating

U.S.-Canadian nurse licensure reciprocity). Requirements for becoming a registered nursing assistant usually consist of a 10-month program and, in some provinces, a licensure examination.

Entry 1, "Why you need to understand your nurse practice act," explains how nurse practice acts, which are the basis of all nursing practice, define nursing and establish guidelines and minimum requirements for nursing education and licensing within each state.

Entry 2, "How standards of nursing care affect you legally," describes how standards may be used as evidence in a malpractice lawsuit against a nurse.

Entry 3, "The value of your nursing license," examines the privileges and responsibilities that your nursing license represents.

Entry 4, "Safeguarding your nursing license," deals with the reasons why a nurse's license may be denied, suspended, or revoked.

Entry 5, "How nursing practice compares legally with medical practice," studies the legal relationship between medicine and nursing. This subject has become increasingly important as the boundaries of authority in some areas of nursing and medical practice have become blurred.

Entry 6, "Working as a nurse practitioner," discusses the nurse's recently recognized abilities to function in an expanded role, assessing patients and making nursing diagnoses. Some nurse practitioners function independently, others collaborate with doctors. Nursing in the expanded role has also fostered the development of more nurse partnerships and nurse corporations. As these trends continue, changes in nursing legislation in some states or provinces (Canada) may follow.

Entry 7, "Working as a private-duty nurse," explores the law's view of private-duty nurses as independent contractors who are individually liable and solely responsible to the patient for their nursing practice.

Entry 8, "Working in geriatric facilities," takes an in-depth look at the fastest-growing area in health care today. Elderly and disabled persons receive care in facilities where about 70% of the personnel may be nurse's aides— a staffing pattern sanctioned by regulations for Medicare and Medicaid reimbursement. The changing ratio of RNs to LPNs/LVNs to aides in many nursing homes (along with the generally changing ratio of health-care staff to patients needing nursing care) has resulted in a shift of traditional nursing roles and responsibilities. This shift may have important professional and legal consequences.

Entry 9, "Working in alternative settings," and Entry 10, "Working for an agency," deal with the special legal and professional concerns of nurses who work in doctors' offices, private homes, schools, industry, and other nontraditional settings.

### What's ahead for nursing?

Surveys predict many challenges for the nursing profession in the 1990s, such as deciding on requirements for entry-level education, establishing greater responsibilities for clinical nursing specialists, resolving conflicts between nursing and medicine, improving the nurse's status as an independent health-care provider, securing increased economic advantages for nurses, and retaining control of the profession. These challenges may seem diverse at first glance, but they're united by their relationship with the law and its effect on nursing practice.

# 1 Why you need to understand your nurse practice act

Every nurse practice act is designed to protect the public by broadly defining the legal scope of nursing practice. Ev-

GLOSSARY

## KEY TERMS IN THIS ENTRY

**liability** • Legal responsibility for *failure to act,* and so causing harm to another person, or for *actions* that fail to meet standards of care and so cause another person harm.

**malpractice** • A professional person's wrongful conduct, improper discharge of professional duties, or failure to meet standards of care—any such actions that result in harm to another person.

**scope of practice** • In nursing, the professional nursing activities defined under state or provincial law in each state's (or Canadian province's) nurse practice act.

**statutory law** • A law passed by a federal or state legislature.

ery nurse can thus be expected to care for patients within *defined practice limits;* if she gives care beyond those limits, she becomes vulnerable to charges of violating her state nurse practice act. Of course, nurse practice acts also serve to exclude untrained or unlicensed persons from practicing nursing.

Your state nurse practice act is the most important law affecting your nursing practice. In every state and Canadian province, the nurse practice act creates a state or provincial board of nursing, authorized to formulate and enforce rules and regulations concerning the nursing profession. The board of nursing is bound by the provisions of the nurse practice act that created it. The nurse practice act is the *law;* the board of nursing can't grant exemptions to it or waive any of its provisions. Only the state or provincial legislature can change the law. For example, if the nurse practice act specifies that, to be licensed, a nurse must have graduated from an approved school of nursing, then the board of nursing must deny a license to anyone

who hasn't. This holds true even for applicants who can provide evidence of equivalency and competence (*Richardson v. Brunelle,* 1979).

In many states and provinces, the board of nursing may grant exemptions and waivers to the rules and regulations (which are not laws) it has formulated. For example, if a regulation says that all nursing faculty must have master's degrees, the board may waive this requirement temporarily for a faculty member who's in the process of obtaining one.

A state legislature can change or expand the state's nurse practice act, but it must also repeal sections that conflict with its changes. For example, if a state legislature decides to adopt the board of nursing's recommendation for a newly broadened definition of nursing, it must repeal the old definition in the state nurse practice act before it can enact the new definition into law.

### A short history

In 1938, the New York State legislature passed the first mandatory nurse practice act (see Introduction). This law, requiring nurses to obtain licenses to practice, raised the question, "Exactly what should a nursing license permit a nurse to do?" The answer was specified in nurse practice acts on a state-by-state basis until 1955, when the American Nurses' Association developed a model definition of nursing practice. Eventually, many states incorporated this model definition, and its 1970 amendments, into their state nurse practice acts. (See *State-by-State Definitions of Nursing Practice* in the appendices.)

### How your nurse practice act defines nursing practice

Nurse practice acts generally begin by defining important terms, including *the practice of registered nursing* and *the practice of licensed practical/vocational nursing.* These definitions are very important because they differentiate between RNs and LPNs/LVNs according to their specific scopes of practice and their educational requirements.

(Note: Some states have separate nurse practice acts for registered and practical/vocational nurses.)

Early nurse practice acts contained statements prohibiting nurses from performing tasks considered to be within the scope of medical practice. Nurses could not diagnose any patient problem or treat a patient without instructions from a doctor. More recently, however, interdisciplinary committees (consisting of nurses, doctors, pharmacists, dentists, and hospital representatives) have helped ease this restriction on nursing practice. After reviewing some medical procedures that nurses commonly perform, these committees have issued *joint statements* recommending that nurses be legally permitted to do these procedures in specified circumstances. (Note that such joint statements have no force of law—unless state legislatures amend their nurse practice acts to include them.) Some joint statements have recommended that nurses be allowed to perform venipunctures, cardiopulmonary resuscitation, and cardiac defibrillation. Still other joint statements (as well as *interpretative statements,* issued by state boards of nursing and nursing organizations) recommend that nurses be permitted to perform such functions as nursing assessment and nursing diagnosis. Some state legislatures have responded by incorporating these tasks and functions into nurse practice acts, thus legally expanding the scope of nursing practice.

In addition to specifying the conditions for RN and LPN/LVN licensure (see Entry 3 for details), your nurse practice act may also specify the rules and regulations for licensure (usually termed *certification)* in special areas of nursing practice. (See Entry 53.) Your nurse practice act also establishes your state nursing board's authority to administer and enforce the act's provisions (see *Your State Board of Nursing Is People Like You,* page 14) and specifies the makeup of the board—the number of members as well as their educational and professional requirements. (In most states, the governor appoints board members.) In some states, the nurse practice act requires two nursing boards—one for RNs and one for LPNs/LVNs.

Your practice act also lists violations that can result in disciplinary action against a nurse (see Entry 4). Depending on the nature of the violation, a nurse may face not only state board disciplinary action but also liability for her actions.

## Interpreting your nurse practice act

Nurse practice acts tend to be broadly worded, and their wording varies from state to state. Your nurse practice act's general provisions help you stay within the legal scope of nursing practice in your state. But you should be aware of problems in interpreting nurse practice acts. For example, one problem stems from the simple fact that nurse practice acts are statutory laws. Any amendment to a nurse practice act, then, must be accomplished via the inevitably slow legislative process. Because of the time involved in pondering, drafting, and enacting laws, amendments to nurse practice acts usually lag well behind the progress of changes in nursing. What does this mean to you? For one thing, you may be expected to perform tasks that seem to be within the accepted scope of nursing but, in fact, violate your nurse practice act.

Maybe that seems unlikely to you. After all, who would knowingly break a law and put herself in legal jeopardy? Well, consider that some nurses now regularly make nursing diagnoses although their state nurse practice acts don't spell out whether they legally may do so.

Unfortunately, some nurse practice acts that *do* permit nursing diagnosis

## STATE NURSE PRACTICE ACTS: QUALIFICATIONS FOR LICENSURE

| STATE AND STATUTE TITLE | Alabama Title 46, Section 189 | Alaska Title 8, Section 08.68 | Arizona Title 32, Section 32 | Arkansas Title 72, Section 72 | California Business and Professions Code | Colorado Chapter 12, Section 12-70 | Connecticut Title 19, Section 19-4M | |
|---|---|---|---|---|---|---|---|---|
| Frequency of license renewal (annual or biennial) | b | b | a | a | b | b | a | |
| **RNs** | | | | | | | | |
| Good moral character | • | | • | • | • | | | |
| Good physical and mental health | | | • | | | | | |
| High school graduation (or equivalent) | • | • | • | • | | | | |
| Completion of basic professional nursing education program | • | • | • | • | • | • | • | |
| No drug/alcohol addiction | | | | | | • | | |
| Minimum age | | | | | | | | |
| U.S. citizen or registered resident alien | | | | | | | | |
| Fluency in English | | | | | | | | |
| **LPNs/LVNs** | | | | | | | | |
| Good moral character | • | | • | • | • | | | |
| Good physical and mental health | | | • | | | | | |
| High school graduation (or equivalent) | • | 10th grade | 10th grade | • | | | | |
| Completion of basic professional nursing education program | • | • | • | • | • | • | • | |
| No drug/alcohol addiction | | | | | | • | | |
| Minimum age | | 18 | | | | | | |
| U.S. citizen or registered resident alien | | | | | | | | |
| Fluency in English | | | | | | | | |

To become licensed to practice nursing in your state, you not only have to pass the required examination, you have to meet certain other qualifications as well. For information on these requirements, check your state's listing below. For additional information about licensure, such as grounds for denial, suspension and revocation, and misdemeanors subject to penalty, consult the Fact Finder section.

| | Delaware Title 24 | District of Columbia Title 2, Section 2-1701 | Florida Chapter 464 | Georgia Section 84-1008 | Hawaii Title 25, Section 457-2 | Idaho Title 54-1401 | Illinois Chapter 3, Par. 3401 | Indiana Section 25 | Iowa Title 8, Section 147.1 | Kansas Section 17-2707 |
|---|---|---|---|---|---|---|---|---|---|---|
| | a | a | b | b | b | b | b | b | b | b |
| | | | | | | | | | | |
| | • | • | • | | | | • | • | | • |
| | • | • | | | | • | | | | |
| | • | • | | | • | | • | • | • | • |
| | • | • | • | • | • | • | • | • | • | • |
| | | | | | | | | | | |
| | | | | | | 18 | | | | |
| | | | | | | | | | | |
| | | | | | | | | | | |
| | | | | | | | | | | |
| | • | • | • | | | | • | • | | • |
| | • | • | | | | • | | | | |
| | | 10th grade | | • | | | • | • | • | • |
| | • | • | • | | • | • | • | • | • | • |
| | | | | | | | | | | |
| | | 18 | | | | | 18 | | | |
| | | | | | | | | | | |
| | | | • | | | | | | | |

(continued)

**STATE NURSE PRACTICE ACTS: QUALIFICATIONS FOR LICENSURE** (continued)

| STATE AND STATUTE TITLE | Kentucky Title 26, Section 311-376 | Louisiana Title 37, Section 914 | Maine Title 32, Section 320.1 | Maryland Section 7 | Massachusetts Chapter 13, Section 13 | Michigan Chapter 325, Section 333.16101 | Minnesota Part I, Section 15-0424 | |
|---|---|---|---|---|---|---|---|---|
| Frequency of license renewal (annual or biennial) | a | a | a | b | b | a | b | |
| **RNs** | | | | | | | | |
| Good moral character | | • | • | | • | | | |
| Good physical and mental health | • | | | | | | | |
| High school graduation (or equivalent) | • | | • | • | | • | • | |
| Completion of basic professional nursing education program | • | • | • | • | • | • | • | |
| No drug/alcohol addiction | | | | | | | | |
| Minimum age | | | | | | | | |
| U.S. citizen or registered resident alien | | • | | | | | | |
| Fluency in English | | | | | | | | |
| **LPNs/LVNs** | | | | | | | | |
| Good moral character | | • | • | | • | | | |
| Good physical and mental health | • | | • | | | | | |
| High school graduation (or equivalent) | • | | • | • | | • | • | |
| Completion of basic professional nursing education program | • | • | • | • | • | • | • | |
| No drug/alcohol addiction | | | | | | | | |
| Minimum age | | | | | | | | |
| U.S. citizen or registered resident alien | | • | | | | | | |
| Fluency in English | | | | | | | | |

| | Mississippi Title 73-15-1 | Missouri Title 22, Section 161.252 | Montana Title 62, Section 2-15-1844 | Nebraska Chapter 33, Section 33-150 | Nevada Title 54, Section 632.010 | New Hampshire Title 30 | New Jersey Section 45:1-2-3 | New Mexico Chapter 61, Section 61-1-1 | New York Section 6500 | North Carolina Division 12, Section 90-160.2 |
|---|---|---|---|---|---|---|---|---|---|---|
| | b | a | a | a | b | b | a | b | b | b |
| | | | | | | | | | | |
| | • | • | | • | • | • | • | | | • |
| | | • | | | | | | | | |
| | | • | • | • | • | • | • | • | • | • |
| | • | • | • | • | • | • | • | • | • | • |
| | | | | | | | • | | | |
| | | 19 | | | 18 | | 18 | | 18 | |
| | | | | | | | | | | |
| | • | | | | | | | | | |
| | | | | | | | | | | |
| | • | • | | • | • | • | • | | | • |
| | | • | | | | | | | | |
| | • | • | • | • | • | • | 10th grade | • | • | 9th grade |
| | • | • | • | • | • | • | • | • | • | • |
| | | | | | | | | | | |
| | | 19 | | | 18 | | 18 | | 17 | |
| | | | | | | | | | | |
| | • | | | | | | | | | |

(continued)

**STATE NURSE PRACTICE ACTS: QUALIFICATIONS
FOR LICENSURE** (continued)

| | North Dakota Chapter 43-12-03 | Ohio Title 47, Section 4723.01 | Oklahoma Title 59, Section 492 | Oregon Title 52, Section 678.800 | Pennsylvania Title 35, Section 780-111 | Rhode Island Chapter 5-34 | South Carolina Section 40-33-10 | |
|---|---|---|---|---|---|---|---|---|
| Frequency of license renewal (annual or biennial) | a | b | b | b | b | a | a | |
| **RNs** | | | | | | | | |
| Good moral character | | ● | ● | | ● | ● | ● | |
| Good physical and mental health | | | | ● | | ● | ● | |
| High school graduation (or equivalent) | | ● | ● | | ● | ● | ● | |
| Completion of basic professional nursing education program | ● | ● | ● | ● | ● | ● | ● | |
| No drug/alcohol addiction | | | | | | | | |
| Minimum age | | | | | 18 | | 18 | |
| U.S. citizen or registered resident alien | | | | | | | | |
| Fluency in English | | | | | | | | |
| **LPNs/LVNs** | | | | | | | | |
| Good moral character | | ● | ● | | ● | ● | ● | |
| Good physical and mental health | | | | ● | | ● | ● | |
| High school graduation (or equivalent) | | | 10th grade | | ● | * | 10th grade | |
| Completion of basic professional nursing education program | ● | ● | ● | ● | ● | ● | ● | |
| No drug/alcohol addiction | | | | | | | | |
| Minimum age | | 18 | | | 18 | | 18 | |
| U.S. citizen or registered resident alien | | | | | | | | |
| Fluency in English | | | | | | | | |

* Determined by Board

| South Dakota Title 36, Section 36 | Tennessee Section 63-1-107 | Texas Article 4520 | Utah Title 58, Section 58-3-5 | Vermont Title 26, Section 1581 | Virginia | Washington Chapter 18.88 RCW | West Virginia Chapter 30, Article 7A, Section 7, Doc. #21053 | Wisconsin Title 3, Section 15.405 | Wyoming Title 33, Section 33-21-102 |
|---|---|---|---|---|---|---|---|---|---|
| a | b | b | b | b | a | a | a | b | a |
|  |  |  |  |  |  |  |  |  |  |
|  |  |  | • |  | • |  | • | • |  |
|  | • |  | • |  |  |  |  |  |  |
| • | • |  |  |  | • |  | • | • |  |
| • | • | • | • | • | • | • | • | • | • |
|  |  |  |  |  |  |  |  |  |  |
|  |  |  |  |  |  |  |  |  |  |
| • |  |  |  |  |  |  |  | • |  |
|  |  |  |  |  |  |  |  |  |  |
| • |  |  | • |  | • |  | • | • |  |
|  | • |  | • |  |  |  |  |  |  |
| • | 10th grade |  |  |  | 10th grade |  | • | 10th grade |  |
| • | • | • | • | • | • | • | • | • | • |
|  |  |  |  |  |  |  |  |  |  |
|  |  |  |  |  |  |  |  |  |  |
| • |  |  |  |  |  |  |  | • |  |
|  |  |  |  |  |  |  |  |  |  |

fail to define what they mean by the term. For instance, the Pennsylvania Nurse Practice Act defines the practice of professional nursing as *"diagnosing and treating* human responses to actual (or potential) health problems through such services as case finding, health teaching, health counseling, and provision of care supportive to or restorative of life and well-being, and executing medical regimens as prescribed by a licensed physician or dentist. The foregoing shall not be deemed to include acts of medical diagnosis or prescription of medical therapeutic or corrective measures, except as may be authorized by rules and regulations jointly promulgated by the [Medical Board] and the [State] Board [of Nurse Examiners]." This definition and others like it don't distinguish clearly between medical and nursing diagnoses.

What does this mean to you? Essentially, it means that the law can't be all things to all nurses. Your state nurse practice act isn't a word-for-word checklist on how you should do your work. You must rely on your own education, training, and knowledge of your hospital's policies and procedures. For example, you know that a nursing diagnosis is part of your

## YOUR STATE BOARD OF NURSING IS PEOPLE LIKE YOU

In most states, the board of nursing (often called the state board of nursing examiners) consists of nurses like you—experienced, currently licensed, and practicing. Many boards also include LPNs/LVNs, hospital administrators, and consumers—usually financial or legal experts. The state legislature decides on the board's mix; in almost every state, the governor appoints members from a list of nominees submitted by the state nursing association. One state, North Carolina, recently replaced this appointment process with an elective one—allowing licensed nurses to elect their own board members.

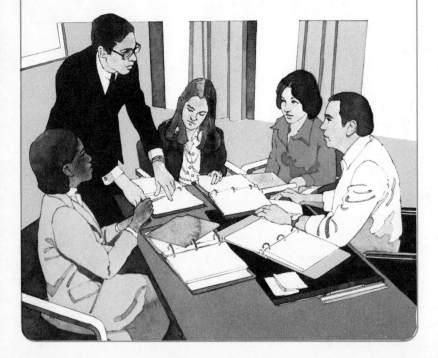

nursing assessment. It's your professional evaluation of the patient's progress, his responses to treatment, and his nursing care needs. You perform this evaluation so you can carry out your nursing care plan. And you know that nursing diagnosis is not a judgment about a patient's medical disorder. So, if your state nurse practice act permits you to make nursing diagnoses, your sound judgment in applying its provisions should help you avoid legal consequences. If your state practice act doesn't permit nursing diagnoses, or its wording permitting nursing diagnoses is unclear, request an official interpretation from your state board of nursing.

Obviously, making nursing diagnoses can be risky under a law that permits them without clearly defining them. (See *When Your Practice Exceeds the Law*, page 16.) Because the language of nurse practice acts is so broad, in many instances a decision on whether certain nursing conduct is a violation must be based on analysis of whether that conduct was intended to be included within conduct permitted by the act.

Most nurse practice acts also pose another problem: They state that you have a legal duty to carry out a doctor's or a dentist's orders. Yet, as a licensed professional, you also have an ethical and legal duty to use your own judgment when providing patient care.

In an effort to deal with this problem, some nurse practice acts give guidance on how to obey orders and still act independently. For example, the Delaware Nurse Practice Act says a nurse must administer "medications and treatments as prescribed by a licensed physician or dentist" while using "substantial specialized judgment and skill . . . based on knowledge and application of the principles of biological, physical and social science." This wording may be interpreted to mean that a nurse practicing in Delaware is required to follow a doctor's or dentist's orders, unless those orders are clearly wrong or he's unqualified to give them. When you feel an order is clearly wrong, tell the doctor. If you're confused about an order, ask the doctor to clarify it. If he fails to correct the error or to answer your questions, inform your head nurse or supervisor of your doubts.

A related problem arises when you deal with physician assistants (PAs). Nurse practice acts in some states say you may only follow orders given by doctors or dentists—but those states' medical practice acts may allow PAs to give orders to nurses. Washington and Florida, for example, have decided that a PA is a doctor's agent and may legally give orders to nurses (*Washington State Nurses Ass'n. v. Board of Medical Examiners,* 1980, and 1977 *Fla. Att'y. Gen. Ann. Rep.).* Find out if your hospital policy allows PAs to give you orders. If it doesn't, you should *not* follow such orders. If hospital policy *does* permit PAs to give you orders, check if such orders must be verified or countersigned by the doctor. (This same question of verification may arise over a

---

*"Making nursing diagnoses can be risky under a law that permits them without defining them."*

---

nurse practitioner's orders written in a patient's chart.) For further clarification, check with your state board of nursing.

You may be asking, how come nurse practice acts and hospital policies don't always agree? Hospital licensing laws require each hospital to establish policies and procedures for its operation. So the nursing service department develops detailed policies and procedures for staff nurses. Usually these policies and procedures specify the allowable scope of nursing practice within the

## WHEN YOUR PRACTICE EXCEEDS THE LAW

Here's a simple but important legal tip: Be sure you're familiar with the legally permissible scope of your nursing practice, as it's defined in your state's nurse practice act, and never exceed its limits. If you do, you're inviting legal problems.

*Here's an example.* Pennsylvania's Nurse Practice Act forbids a nurse to give an anesthetic unless the patient's doctor is present. The case of *McCarl v. State Board of Nurse Examiners* (1979) involved a hospital nurse who administered an anesthetic to a patient whose doctor was *not* present. The Pennsylvania Board of Nurse Examiners received a complaint about the incident and conducted a hearing. The nurse admitted to knowing about the law's requirement but argued that the requirement was satisfied by the presence of another doctor—although this doctor wasn't supervising the nurse during the procedure. The board ruled that the nurse had willfully violated a section of the Pennsylvania Nurse Practice Act and issued a reprimand. The nurse appealed the reprimand, but the court upheld it.

hospital. The scope may be narrower than the scope described in your nurse practice act, but it can't be broader. Remember, your employer *can't* legally expand the scope of your practice to include tasks prohibited by your nurse practice act. You have a legal obligation to practice within your nurse practice act's limits. Except in a life-threatening emergency, you can't exceed these limits without risking disciplinary action. To protect yourself, compare your hospital policies and your nurse practice act.

You may have concluded, by now, that most nurse practice acts aren't what they say, but what they *don't* say. Most don't specify your day-to-day legal responsibilities with respect to specific procedures and functions. For instance, along with nursing diagnosis, many nurse practice acts don't specify such things as your responsibility for patient teaching or the legal limitations on nurse-patient discussions about treatment. Yet, in a recent case in Idaho (*Tuma v. Board of Nursing*, 1979), a state board of nursing took disciplinary action against a nurse who discussed, at a patient's request, the possibility of using Laetrile as alternative therapy. The board suspended her license on the grounds of unprofessional conduct.

However, the Supreme Court of Idaho revoked the suspension and ordered the board to reinstate the nurse's license. Why? Because the Idaho Nurse Practice Act contained no provision stating that such a nurse-patient discussion would constitute a violation.

## Keeping nurse practice acts up to date

To align nurse practice acts with current nursing practice, professional nursing organizations and state boards of nursing have lobbied for two types of legislation affecting the acts: amendments and redefinitions.

An *amendment* may be used to add to a nurse practice act or to its regulations, specifically giving nurses legal permission to perform certain procedures or functions that have become part of accepted nursing practice. These amendments have the same legal force as the original act.

Compared to redefinition, though, amendments do have a disadvantage: They represent a piecemeal approach that may allow an outdated nurse practice act to remain in effect.

*Redefinition*, on the other hand, is a rewriting of the fundamental provision of a nurse practice act—the definition of nursing practice. This approach changes the basic premise of the entire act without the necessity to amend or repeal it. Redefinition might be used, for example, to reverse a definition of nursing practice that prohibits diagnosis. How? By clarifying the term *diagnosis* to allow nurses to make nursing diagnoses. This type of change helps nurses understand exactly what is and isn't prohibited.

### A final word

To help protect yourself legally, you need to understand your nurse practice act thoroughly and keep up with any changes in it. Be sure you're up to date on your hospital's policies and procedures, too. Only when you know the legal limits of your responsibilities, can you practice your profession safely.

# 2 How standards of nursing care affect you legally

Are standards of nursing care merely pie-in-the-sky ideals that have little bearing on the tasks you perform daily? Absolutely not. You're expected to meet standards of nursing care for every nursing task you perform. And any time your care falls below standard, you're risking malpractice liability.

### What are standards of nursing care?

Standards of nursing care set minimum criteria for your proficiency on the job, enabling you—and others—to judge the quality of care you and your nursing colleagues provide.

For example, if you're a medical-surgical staff nurse, minimal standards require that you develop a nursing care plan for your patient based on the nursing process—assessment, planning, intervention, and evaluation—including nursing diagnosis, nursing goals, and nursing actions for

implementing the care plan. Standards also call for documentation, in the patient's record, of your completion and evaluation of the plan. When you document your patient care, you're really writing a record of how well you've met these standards.

Before 1950, nurses had only Florence Nightingale's early treatments, plus reports of court cases, to use as standards. But as nursing gradually became recognized as an independent profession, nursing organizations stressed the importance of having recognized standards for all nurses. Then, in 1950, the American Nurses' Association (ANA) published the "Code of Ethics for Nursing," a general mandate stating that nurses should offer nursing care without prejudice and in a confidential and safe manner. The code wasn't very specific, but it was the beginning of written nursing standards. In 1973, the ANA Congress for Nursing Practice established the first generic standards for the profession—standards that could be applied to all nurses in all settings. (See *The American Nurses' Association Standards of*

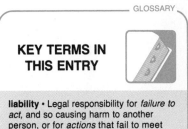

GLOSSARY

## KEY TERMS IN THIS ENTRY

**liability** • Legal responsibility for *failure to act*, and so causing harm to another person, or for *actions* that fail to meet standards of care and so cause another person harm.

**malpractice** • A professional person's wrongful conduct, improper discharge of professional duties, or failure to meet standards of care—any such actions that result in harm to another person.

**standards of care** • In a malpractice lawsuit, those acts performed or omitted that an ordinary, prudent person, in the defendant's position, would have done or not done; a measure by which the defendant's alleged wrongful conduct is compared.

## WHAT THE COURTS USE TO JUDGE NURSING CARE

How would a court judge the appropriateness of the care you give your patients? One important way involves measuring your care against recognized national and local standards. Usually a court draws on several applicable standards to make a decision. Exactly which standards a court uses depends on the nature of the case.

   National standards include those of the professional organizations—such as the American Nurses' Association and the American Association of Critical-Care Nurses—and those of the Joint Commission on Accreditation of Hospitals.

   Local standards would include those established by the hospital where you work, by testimony of expert witnesses—professionals with training and work experience similar to yours—and by previous court rulings (common law standards).

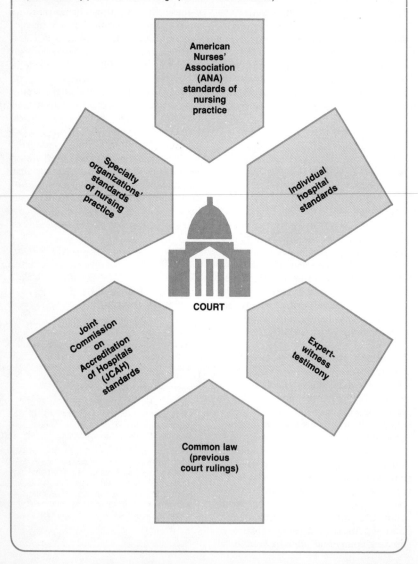

*Nursing Practice,* pages 20 to 23.) The Canadian Nurses Association (CNA) has established similar nursing standards.

By 1974, each of the ANA divisions of nursing practice (Community Health, Geriatrics, Maternal-Child, Mental Health, and Medical-Surgical), had established distinct standards for its specialty. The ANA Congress called these *specialty standards.* State nursing associations also helped develop specialty nursing standards.

ANA specialty standards are really national in nature because they can apply wherever nurses practice. But the courts may also use local standards—reflecting a community's accepted, common nursing practices—to judge the quality of nursing care. Use of local standards is becoming less common, however, as national standards receive increasing endorsement.

As you may know, local standards are established in two ways: by individual hospitals, through their policies and procedures, and by expert witnesses who testify in court cases involving nurses. Every hospital establishes standards to fit its own community's needs. An expert witness interprets local standards by testifying about how nursing is commonly practiced in her community.

You can see that a number of nursing institutions and organizations have contributed to the development of nursing standards. The ANA and the CNA established standards for nurses and recommended that state and provincial boards of nursing endorse them for incorporation into nurse practice acts. The Joint Commission on Accreditation of Hospitals also has developed nursing standards to be used in hospital audit systems. And state nursing associations and the specialty-nursing organizations actively work with hospital nursing administrators for adoption of standards.

Federal regulations for staffing Medicare and Medicaid services influence the development of standards, especially nursing home standards. By suggesting ethical approaches to nursing practice, ethics codes written by the ANA, the CNA, and the International Council of Nurses also influence how nursing care standards are developed.

Nursing standards will change as technology advances and nurses' responsibilities expand. Hospital audit committees and professional nursing associations continually monitor nursing standards to be sure they're up to date.

## How courts apply nursing standards in malpractice lawsuits

The allegation that a nurse failed to meet appropriate standards of care is the basic premise of every nursing malpractice lawsuit (see Chapter 6). During the trial, the court will measure the defendant-nurse's action against the answers it obtains to the following question: *What would a reasonably prudent nurse, with like training and experience, do under similar conditions in the same community?* To answer this question, the plaintiff-patient, through his attorney, must determine that certain standards of care exist that the defendant-nurse should have applied to him, prove the appropriateness of those standards, and show how the nurse failed to meet them—and so caused him injury—in giving her nursing care.

When local standards are at issue, usually the plaintiff-patient uses expert-witness testimony to support his claims. This is known as the *locality rule.* The defendant-nurse and her attorney, of course, will also arrange for expert-witness testimony—in support of her claim that her actions did *not* fall below accepted standards of care and that she acted in a reasonable and prudent manner.

The court can also draw on sources of written standards in examining the standards of care involved in a nursing malpractice lawsuit. The court will seek information about all the national

# THE AMERICAN NURSES' ASSOCIATION'S STANDARDS OF NURSING PRACTICE

The American Nurses' Association developed the following standards of nursing practice in 1971 to give the courts, hospitals, nurses, and patients guidelines for determining quality nursing care. The standards are based on the steps of the nursing process: assessment, planning, implementation, and evaluation. Each standard is followed by a rationale— explaining the standard—and assessment factors for use in determining if the standard has been met.

### AMERICAN NURSES' ASSOCIATION
## Standards of Nursing Practice

**STANDARD I**
  THE COLLECTION OF DATA ABOUT THE HEALTH STATUS OF THE CLIENT/ PATIENT IS SYSTEMATIC AND CONTINUOUS. THE DATA ARE ACCESSIBLE, COMMUNICATED, AND RECORDED.

**Rationale**
  Comprehensive care requires complete and ongoing collection of data about the client/patient to determine the nursing care needs of the client/patient. All health status data about the client/patient must be available for all members of the health-care team.

**Assessment Factors**
  - Health status data include:
    —Growth and development
    —Biophysical status
    —Emotional status
    —Cultural, religious, socioeconomic background
    —Performance of activities of daily living
    —Patterns of coping
    —Interaction patterns
    —Client's/patient's perception of and satisfaction with his health status
    —Client/patient health goals
    —Environment (physical, social, emotional, ecological)
    —Available and accessible human and material resources
  - Data are collected from:
    —Client/patient, family, significant others
    —Health-care personnel
    —Individuals within the immediate environment and/or the community
  - Data are obtained by:
    —Interview
    —Examination
    —Observation
    —Reading records, reports, etc.
  - There is a format for the collection of data which:
    —Provides for a systematic collection of data
    —Facilitates the completeness of data collection
  - Continuous collection of data is evident by:
    —Frequent updating
    —Recording of changes in health status
  - The data are:
    —Accessible on the client/patient records
    —Retrievable from record-keeping systems
    —Confidential when appropriate

**STANDARD II**
NURSING DIAGNOSES ARE DERIVED FROM HEALTH STATUS DATA.

**Rationale**
The health status of the client/patient is the basis for determining the nursing care needs. The data are analyzed and compared to norms when possible.

**Assessment Factors**
- The client's/patient's health status is compared to the norm in order to determine if there is a deviation from the norm and the degree and direction of deviation.
- The client's/patient's capabilities and limitations are identified.
- The nursing diagnoses are related to and congruent with the diagnoses of all other professionals caring for the client/patient.

**STANDARD III**
THE PLAN OF NURSING CARE INCLUDES GOALS DERIVED FROM THE NURSING DIAGNOSES.

**Rationale**
The determination of the results to be achieved is an essential part of planning care.

**Assessment Factors**
- Goals are mutually set with the client/patient and pertinent others:
  —They are congruent with other planned therapies.
  —They are stated in realistic and measurable terms.
  —They are assigned a time period for achievement.
- Goals are established to maximize functional capabilities and are congruent with:
  —Growth and development
  —Biophysical status
  —Behavioral patterns
  —Human and material resources

**STANDARD IV**
THE PLAN OF NURSING CARE INCLUDES PRIORITIES AND THE PRE-SCRIBED NURSING APPROACHES OR MEASURES TO ACHIEVE THE GOALS DERIVED FROM THE NURSING DIAGNOSES.

**Rationale**
Nursing actions are planned to promote, maintain and restore the client's/patient's well-being.

**Assessment Factors**
- Physiological measures are planned to manage (prevent or control) specific patient problems and are related to the nursing diagnoses and goals of care, e.g. ADL, use of self-help devices, etc.

*(continued)*

**THE AMERICAN NURSES' ASSOCIATION'S STANDARDS OF NURSING PRACTICE** *(continued)*

- Psychosocial measures are specific to the client's/patient's nursing care problem and to the nursing care goals, e.g. techniques to control aggression, motivation.
- Teaching-learning principles are incorporated into the plan of care and objectives for learning stated in behavioral terms, e.g. specification of content for learner's level, reinforcement, readiness, etc.
- Approaches are planned to provide for a therapeutic environment:
  —Physical environmental factors are used to influence the therapeutic environment, e.g. control of noise, control of temperature, etc.
  —Psychosocial measures are used to structure the environment for therapeutic ends, e.g. paternal participation in all phases of the maternity experience.
  —Group behaviors are used to structure interaction and influence the therapeutic environment, e.g. comformity, ethos, territorial rights, locomotion, etc.
- Approaches are specified for orientation of the client/patient to:
  —New roles and relationships
  —Relevant health (human and material) resources
  —Modifications in plan of nursing care
  —Relationship of modifications in nursing care plan to the total care plan
- The plan of nursing care includes the utilization of available and appropriate resources:
  —Human resources (other health personnel)
  —Material resources
  —Community
- The plan includes an ordered sequence of nursing actions.
- Nursing approaches are planned on the basis of current scientific knowledge.

## STANDARD V
NURSING ACTIONS PROVIDE FOR CLIENT/PATIENT PARTICIPATION IN HEALTH PROMOTION, MAINTENANCE AND RESTORATION.

### Rationale
The client/patient and family are continually involved in nursing care.

### Assessment Factors
- The client/patient and family are kept informed about:
  —Current health status
  —Changes in health status
  —Total health-care plan
  —Nursing care plan
  —Roles of health-care personnel
  —Health-care resources
- The client/patient and family are provided with the information needed to make decisions and choices about:
  —Promoting, maintaining and restoring health
  —Seeking and utilizing appropriate health-care personnel
  —Maintaining and using health-care resources

## STANDARD VI
NURSING ACTIONS ASSIST THE CLIENT/PATIENT TO MAXIMIZE HIS HEALTH CAPABILITIES.

**Rationale**
Nursing actions are designed to promote, maintain and restore health.

**Assessment Factors**
- Nursing actions:
  —Are consistent with the plan of care.
  —Are based on scientific principles.
  —Are individualized to the specific situation.
  —Are used to provide a safe and therapeutic environment.
  —Employ teaching-learning opportunities for the client/patient.
  —Include utilization of appropriate resources.
- Nursing actions are directed by the client's/patient's physical, physiological, psychological and social behavior associated with:
  —Ingestion of food, fluid and nutrients
  —Elimination of body wastes and excesses in fluid
  —Locomotion and exercise
  —Regulatory mechanisms — body heat, metabolism
  —Relating to others
  —Self-actualization

## STANDARD VII
THE CLIENT'S/PATIENT'S PROGRESS OR LACK OF PROGRESS TOWARD GOAL ACHIEVEMENT IS DETERMINED BY THE CLIENT/PATIENT AND THE NURSE.

**Rationale**
The quality of nursing care depends upon comprehensive and intelligent determination of nursing's impact upon the health status of the client/patient. The client/patient is an essential part of this determination.

**Assessment Factors**
- Current data about the client/patient are used to measure his progress toward goal achievement.
- Nursing actions are analyzed for their effectiveness in the goal achievement of the client/patient.
- The client/patient evaluates nursing actions and goal achievement.
- Provision is made for nursing follow-up of a particular client/patient to determine the long-term effects of nursing care.

## STANDARD VIII
THE CLIENT'S/PATIENT'S PROGRESS OR LACK OF PROGRESS TOWARD GOAL ACHIEVEMENT DIRECTS REASSESSMENT, REORDERING OF PRIORITIES, NEW GOAL SETTING AND REVISION OF THE PLAN OF NURSING CARE.

**Rationale**
The nursing process remains the same, but the input of new information may dictate new or revised approaches.

**Assessment Factors**
- Reassessment is directed by goal achievement or lack of goal achievement.
- New priorities and goals are determined and additional nursing approaches are prescribed appropriately.
- New nursing actions are accurately and appropriately initiated.

and state standards applicable to the defendant-nurse's actions. The court may also seek applicable information about the policies of the defendant-nurse's employer.

What if state and national standards contradict each other? When that happens, the court must decide which standards apply in the case, often giving state standards top priority. But sometimes courts favor the national standards. Why? Because two trends—toward uniform nursing educational requirements and standardized medical treatment regimens—are making national standards widely applicable. This court bias has made the ANA's standards more influential than local standards or the standards of other organizations.

The court may also allow nonnursing professionals, including doctors, to speak as expert witnesses about nursing practice. This has happened in several key cases. For example, in *Hiatt v. Groce* (1974), a patient sued an obstetric nurse for failing to notify a doctor when the patient was about to deliver a baby. The court permitted a

> *"The trend toward national standards has made the ANA's standards more influential than local standards."*

doctor to testify about the adequacy of the nurse's care. In *Gugino v. Harvard Community Health Plan* (1980), the court allowed a doctor to testify about the standards for a nurse practitioner.

The case of *Pisel v. Stamford Community Hospital* (1980) provides a good example of how courts consider local, state, and national standards in nursing malpractice lawsuits. In this case, nurses at a mental health hospital

left a young psychotic patient unattended in a locked seclusion room. The patient forcibly wedged her head between the bed frame and side rail, suffering permanent neurologic damage. The patient's relatives sued the nurses and the hospital for malpractice. In the absence of hospital policies that might have applied to this case, the court relied on expert-witness testimony, ANA standards, and federal regulations to judge the nurses' care. The court found the nurses and the hospital guilty of violating applicable standards of care according to the following evidence:

• failure to remove a steel bed from a seclusion room
• failure to constantly observe the patient
• failure to completely assess the patient's status
• failure to notify the attending psychiatrist of the patient's acutely psychotic condition
• failure to implement medical orders.

As further evidence against the hospital, testimony revealed that the nursing notes describing the incident had been destroyed and that new notes had been written. This falsified record was considered evidence that the hospital was conscious of its negligence. (For detailed information on the legal risks involved in falsifying medical records, see Entry 37.)

Nurses may also be judged by standards of care that ordinarily aren't considered nursing standards. For example, in the California case of *Fein v. Permanente Medical Group* (1981), a patient who went to a medical clinic complaining of chest pain sued the clinic and the nurse practitioner who attended him for failing to diagnose his myocardial infarction. Although diagnosis is normally considered a medical rather than a nursing function, the court found the nurse negligent. The reasoning? In directing the jury, the judge stated, "I instruct you that the standard of care required of a nurse practitioner is that of a physician and surgeon duly licensed to practice med-

# UNDERSTANDING THE JCAH

The public wants to know that the health-care institutions that treat them have high professional standards. That's where the Joint Commission on Accreditation of Hospitals (JCAH) comes in. It sets voluntary standards of operation for hospitals and other health-care institutions and accredits those which meet JCAH standards. The JCAH grants accreditation for 3 years, requiring the health-care institution to conduct its own survey, 18 months after it receives accreditation, and to report the results to the JCAH. The American College of Physicians, the American College of Surgeons, and the American Hospital Association sponsor the JCAH. Representatives from each of these organizations make up the JCAH board of commissioners.

To receive JCAH accreditation, a hospital must:

The JCAH recommends (but doesn't require for accreditation) that health-care institutions do the following to maintain high-quality care:

• maintain a safe, clean facility and exercise continuous infection control

• maintain a staff of doctors

• maintain a pharmacy that's staffed by a registered pharmacist

• publish rules and regulations for the medical staff

• provide supervision for nursing staff and other nursing services

• provide diagnostic X-ray services for patients

• publish the procedure doctors can follow to apply for medical staff memberships

• maintain a governing body that's responsible for all hospital functions, headed by a chief executive responsible for hospital administration

• provide clinical laboratory services

• form medical staff committees to review the quality of medical care given by its members

• maintain a room suitable for surgery

icine in the state of California when the nurse practitioner is examining a patient or making a diagnosis." In other words, the nurse practitioner could be presumed to have the knowledge and skills to make a diagnosis.

This court decision was appealed. The higher court examining the case on appeal noted that although the roles of a nurse practitioner and a doctor differ, the plaintiff was entitled to the same standard of care a doctor would give when the plaintiff went to the clinic with his complaint of chest pain. So the higher court sustained the lower court's decision.

In another case, *Jones v. Hawkes Hospital* (1964), the court ruled against a nurse's request to have expert testimony used to judge her action. The nurse was sued for malpractice when she left a sedated patient, who was in labor, to assist a doctor with another patient in labor. She did this because the hospital had a rule that no doctor could attend a woman in labor unless a nurse was present. Left alone, the plaintiff-patient got out of her bed, fell, and suffered serious injuries. The nurse wanted the court to allow expert testimony to establish the standard of care that should have been applied. But the court ruled that any reasonably prudent person could determine this case on the basis of ordinary experience and knowledge, so the jurors could decide on their own whether the defendant-nurse's nontechnical nursing tasks met reasonable standards of care. The jury found the nurse negligent.

A similar case was *Larrimore v. Homeopathic Hospital Association* (1962) in which a nurse was found liable for failing to read a new order or for reading it negligently. The court stated that the jury could apply ordinary common sense, without an expert witness, to establish the applicable standard of care.

A nurse who administers medication when the prescribing doctor isn't present is legally responsible for clarifying the doctor's instructions. What amount of medication should she give? How should she give it—by what route? In the Louisiana case *Norton v. Argonaut Insurance Co.* (1962), a doctor left an incomplete order for administration of 3 cc of digoxin to a young patient. A nurse supervisor, helping out on the pediatric floor, picked up the order. Unsure of the amount of digoxin the doctor had prescribed, she asked two other doctors (who were on the ward) if 3 cc was an excessive dose. These two doctors, believing the nurse was describing an *oral* dose, told her 3 cc was correct. The nurse gave the patient 3 cc of digoxin *by injection,* and the young patient died.

In a subsequent malpractice lawsuit against the nurse, the court ruled that she breached her duty and violated a standard, which holds that each nurse has the duty to make absolutely certain that the dose and route of administration of every medication she administers are correct. The court made this decision based on the following evidence:

• The nurse attempted to administer a medication with which she wasn't familiar.

• The nurse failed to call the attending doctor for clarification of his orders.

(For more information on your legal risks when administering medications, see Entry 23.)

## A final word

Without standards of care, nursing couldn't claim to be a profession. Why? Because standards, by establishing minimum levels of quality for performing nursing tasks, provide the criteria for placing nursing practice on a professional level. Your profession and the courts have taken a firm position regarding standards of nursing care. Both have insisted that your practice be held up to—and when necessary judged by—specific standards. Meeting these standards will protect you legally, ensure that your patients receive quality care, and strengthen the standing of your profession.

# 3 The value of your nursing license

Your nursing license entitles you to practice as a professionally qualified nurse. But as with most privileges, your nursing license imposes certain responsibilities on you. As a licensed professional—registered nurse (RN) or licensed practical/vocational nurse (LPN/LVN), in the United States or Canada—you're responsible for providing quality care to your patients. To do this, *and* to protect your right to practice, you need to know the professional and legal meaning of your nursing license.

## What do licensing laws do?

Licensing laws are contained within each nurse practice act. They establish qualifications for obtaining and maintaining a nursing license. They also broadly define the legally permissible scope of nursing practice. (All but six states have general definitions of nursing in their nurse practice acts.)

Licensing laws, which vary somewhat from state to state, generally specify the following:
• the qualifications a nurse needs in order to be granted a license
• license-application procedures for new licenses and reciprocal (state-to-state) licensing arrangements
• application fees
• authorization to grant use of the title *registered nurse* or *licensed practical/vocational nurse* to applicants who receive their licenses
• grounds for license denial, revocation, or suspension
• license-renewal procedures.

Licensing laws generally do not prohibit nursing students, a patient's friends, or members of his family from caring for him (as long as no fee is involved), nor do the laws prohibit a nurse licensed in one state from caring for a patient traveling with her through another state. The laws also usually permit a newly graduated nurse to practice for a specified period while her license application is being processed, and they allow unlicensed persons to give care in an emergency. According to state and federal constitutional requirements, state laws *must* exempt the following types of nurses from state licensure requirements:
• nurses working in federal institutions
• nurses practicing in accordance with their religious beliefs
• nurses traveling with patients from one state to another.

## How licensing laws work for you

By defining the scope of your professional nursing practice, licensing laws help you avoid the civil and criminal liabilities that can result if you practice beyond the limits specified by your nursing license.

If you're named in a malpractice lawsuit (see Entry 44), your state licensing laws will be used as partial

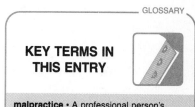

GLOSSARY

**KEY TERMS IN THIS ENTRY**

**malpractice** • A professional person's wrongful conduct, improper discharge of professional duties, or failure to meet standards of care—any such actions that result in harm to another person.

**respondeat superior** • "Let the master answer." A legal doctrine that makes an employer liable for the consequences of his employee's wrongful conduct while the employee is acting within the scope of his employment.

**standards of care** • In a malpractice lawsuit, those acts performed or omitted that an ordinary, prudent person in the defendant's position would have done or not done; a measure by which the defendant's alleged wrongful conduct is compared.

# REQUIREMENTS FOR LICENSURE BY ENDORSEMENT IN THE UNITED STATES AND CANADA

Are you considering moving to another state or to (or from) Canada? This chart tells you the states' and provinces' requirements for a nursing license by endorsement. Almost every state and province requires the National Council Licensure Examination (NCLEX); about half the states accept the Canadian Nursing Association Testing Services (CNATS); some states require foreign nurses to take the Commission on Graduates of Foreign Nursing Schools (CGFNS) Examination. Other requirements vary. Because these requirements can change with new legislation, ask the board of nursing in the state you're interested in for the most current information.

| | | NCLEX REQUIRED | CNATS ACCEPTED | CURRENT LICENSE REQUIRED | NURSING SCHOOL DIPLOMA or DEGREE REQUIRED |
|---|---|:---:|:---:|:---:|:---:|
| Alabama | | | ● | | ● |
| Alaska | | ● | ● | | ● |
| Arizona | | ● | ● | | ● |
| Arkansas | | ● | ● | | ● |
| California | RN | ● | ● | | |
| | LVN | | | ● | |
| Colorado | | ● | | ● | ● |
| Connecticut | | ● | | ● | |
| Delaware | | ● | ● | | ● |
| District of Columbia | | ● | | ● | ● |
| Florida | | ● | | | ● |
| Georgia | RN | | | | |
| | LPN | ● | ● | ● | ● |
| Hawaii | | ● | | | |
| Idaho | | ● | ● | ● | |
| Illinois | | ● | | | |
| Indiana | | ● | | | ● |
| Iowa | | ● | | | ● |
| Kansas | | ● | | ● | ● |

| RECENT-EMPLOYMENT REQUIREMENTS | SPECIAL REQUIREMENTS |
|---|---|
| None | |
| Employed within last 5 years | Four professional references |
| None | |
| None | |
| None | California educational requirements |
| None | California educational requirements |
| None | |
| None | |
| Employed within last 5 years or completed a refresher course | |
| None | Three references |
| None | Personnel record free of disciplinary actions |
| Employed 1 year in last 5 years or completed a refresher course | |
| None | Certification in good standing in current state and verified eligibility from employer |
| None | |
| Employed within last 3 years | |
| None | Any other requirements in effect in Illinois at time of licensure |
| None | CGFNS examination for Canadians |
| None | |
| None | |

*(continued)*

## REQUIREMENTS FOR LICENSURE BY ENDORSEMENT IN THE UNITED STATES AND CANADA (continued)

| | | NCLEX REQUIRED | CNATS ACCEPTED | CURRENT LICENSE REQUIRED | NURSING SCHOOL DIPLOMA or DEGREE REQUIRED |
|---|---|:---:|:---:|:---:|:---:|
| Kentucky | | ● | ● | ● | |
| Louisiana | RN | ● | ● | | ● |
| | LPN | ● | | | ● |
| Maine | | ● | ● | ● | |
| Maryland | | ● | | | ● |
| Massachusetts | | ● | | ● | |
| Michigan | | ● | | ● | |
| Minnesota | RN | ● | | | |
| | LPN | ● | | | |
| Mississippi | | ● | ● | | ● |
| Missouri | | ● | ● | ● | |
| Montana | | ● | | ● | |
| Nebraska | | ● | | | ● |
| New Hampshire | | ● | | ● | ● |
| New Jersey | | ● | | ● | |
| New Mexico | | ● | ● (Taken after 1970) | ● | |
| New York | | ● | | ● | |
| North Carolina | | ● | | | |
| North Dakota | | | ● | ● | ● |
| Ohio | | ● | ● | | ● |
| Oklahoma | | | | | ● |

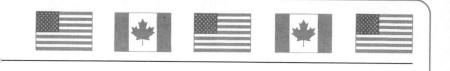

| RECENT-<br>EMPLOYMENT<br>REQUIREMENTS | SPECIAL<br>REQUIREMENTS |
|---|---|
| Employed 1 year in last 5 years or completed a refresher course | |
| None | |
| None | |
| None | |
| None | |
| None | |
| None | |
| Employed within last 2 years or completed a refresher course | |
| Employed within last 5 years or completed a refresher course | |
| None | |
| None | |
| None | CGFNS examination for Canadians |
| None | |
| Employed within last 5 years or completed a refresher course | |
| None | |
| Employed 1,000 hours within last 5 years if 5 years since receiving license | |
| None | If examination taken after 5/31/1974, must have taken the same examination on the same day it was given in New York or must retake the examination |
| None | |
| None | |
| None | Proof of current license |
| None | Any other requirements in effect in Oklahoma at time of registration |

*(continued)*

**REQUIREMENTS FOR LICENSURE BY ENDORSEMENT IN
THE UNITED STATES AND CANADA** *(continued)*

| | | NCLEX REQUIRED | CNATS ACCEPTED | CURRENT LICENSE REQUIRED | NURSING SCHOOL DIPLOMA or DEGREE REQUIRED |
|---|---|---|---|---|---|
| Oregon | | ● | | ● | |
| Pennsylvania | | ● | ● | | ● |
| Rhode Island | | ● | ● | ● | ● |
| South Carolina | | ● | | ● | |
| South Dakota | | ● | | | ● |
| Tennessee | | ● | ● | ● | |
| Texas | RN | ● | | | ● |
| | LVN | ● | | | ● |
| Utah | | ● | ● | | |
| Vermont | | | | | ● |
| Virginia | | | | ● | |
| Washington | RN | ● | | | ● |
| | LPN | ● | | | |
| West Virginia | RN | ● | | | ● |
| | LPN | ● | | | ● |
| Wisconsin | | ● | ● | | ● |
| Wyoming | | ● | | | ● |
| **CANADA** | | | | | |
| Alberta | RN | ● | ● | ● | |
| | LNA | | ● | | ● |
| British Columbia | RN | ● | ● | | ● |
| | LPN | | ● | | |

| RECENT-EMPLOYMENT REQUIREMENTS | SPECIAL REQUIREMENTS |
|---|---|
| Employed 960 hours within last 5 years if license isn't current | |
| None | |
| None | |
| None | |
| None | CGFNS examination for Canadians |
| None | |
| None | |
| Employed within last 5 years or an accredited nursing school graduate | Current license from another state for Canadians |
| Employed 200 hours in last 5 years | |
| Employed in the last 5 years | |
| None | Educational requirements equivalent to those in Virginia |
| None | CGFNS examination for Canadians |
| None | CGFNS examination for Canadians |
| None | |
| None | |
| None | Official nursing transcript |
| None | Individual review of Canadian applications |
| Employed 150 days, graduated, or completed refresher course in last 5 years | Professional reference; employment in Alberta before endorsement is completed |
| None | Alberta examination for U.S. nurses |
| None | Some hospitals do not require B.C. registration for employment |
| Employed, graduated, or completed refresher course in last 5 years | Fluency in English; British Columbia educational requirements or equivalent |

*(continued)*

**REQUIREMENTS FOR LICENSURE BY ENDORSEMENT IN THE UNITED STATES AND CANADA** *(continued)*

| | | NCLEX REQUIRED | CNATS ACCEPTED | CURRENT LICENSE REQUIRED | NURSING SCHOOL DIPLOMA or DEGREE REQUIRED |
|---|---|---|---|---|---|
| Manitoba | RN | ● | ● | | |
| | LPN | ● | ● | | |
| New Brunswick | RN | | ● | | |
| | RNA | ● | ● | | ● |
| Newfoundland | RN | ● | ● | | ● |
| | LNA | | | | |
| Northwest Territories | | | | | |
| Nova Scotia | RN | | | ● | ● |
| | LNA | ● | ● | | ● |
| Ontario | | | | | ● |
| Prince Edward Island | RN | | | ● | ● |
| | LNA | ● | ● | | |
| Quebec | RN | | ● | | |
| | LNA | | | | |
| Saskatchewan | | ● | ● | | |
| Yukon | | | | | |

| RECENT-EMPLOYMENT REQUIREMENTS | SPECIAL REQUIREMENTS |
|---|---|
| Employed 60 days in last 3 years | |
| None | Manitoba educational requirements |
| Employed in last 4 years | Canadian nursing school degree and professional reference |
| None | |
| Employed 150 days in last 5 years or 60 days in last 2 years | Proof of registration |
| None | No examination or fees; completion of nursing program accepted by the Newfoundland Department of Health |
| None | Good professional reputation; registration or qualifications sufficient for registration in another province |
| None | NCLEX for U.S. nurses |
| None | Working knowledge of English |
| Employed 6 months in last 5 years | Registration in province where educated; CNATS for U.S. RNs and LPNs/LVNs licensed after 7/1/80 |
| None | Record of employment; NCLEX for U.S. nurses |
| Employed 60 shifts in last 5 years, or 30 consecutive shifts in last 2 years, or completed a refresher course | Canadian citizenship; Prince Edward Island educational requirements |
| None | Canadian education |
| None | No fees, examination, or license requirements |
| Employed 60 days in last 5 years | Birth certificate; if married, marriage certificate |
| None | Canadian government employs most nurses in province; nurses wanting to work in Yukon should be registered in another province |

evidence in determining if you acted within the legally permissible scope of nursing practice.

Consider *Vassey v. Burch* (1980), in which a patient sued an emergency department nurse for failing to recognize his signs and symptoms of appendicitis. The court reviewed the state licensing law and determined that the nurse had not violated the applicable standard of nursing care. The court ruled that the nurse had acted properly by notifying the attending doctor of the patient's signs and symptoms, and that she was under no obligation to diagnose a patient's condition.

In *Barber v. Reinking* (1966), the court used the licensing laws in the Washington State nurse practice act to rule against the defendant-nurse. In this case, a boy age 2 was taken to a doctor's office for a polio booster shot. The doctor (who was also named in the suit) delegated this task to the LPN who worked in his office. While the nurse was administering the shot, the child moved suddenly and the needle broke off in his buttock. Despite attempts to remove it surgically and with a magnet, the needle remained lodged in the child's buttock for 9 months.

During the lawsuit that followed, the licensing law for practical nurses became the controlling factor in the court's decision. According to the Washington State nurse practice act, a practical nurse can't legally give an injection. The court declared that the nurse had violated the nurse practice act by performing services beyond the legal limit of her practice. The nurse's attorney attempted to introduce as evidence the "fact" that LPNs/LVNs commonly gave injections in the town where she practiced. This contention wasn't allowed as evidence, however. Instead, the judge instructed the jury to consider the violation of the nurse practice act along with other evidence in the case, including the doctor's liability under the *respondeat superior* doctrine, to determine if the nurse was negligent.

## Canadian licensing laws

Nursing practice in Canada is regulated within each province. Each province has its own nurse practice act, so the laws vary somewhat from province to province. Licensing laws in all provinces except Prince Edward Island and Ontario require nurses to join provincial nursing associations in order to obtain their licenses.

In all provinces, Canadian licensing laws establish the following:
• qualifications for membership in the provincial nursing association
• examination requirements
• applicable fees
• conditions for reciprocal licensure
• penalties for practicing without a license
• grounds for denial, suspension, or revocation of a nurse's license.

Within those provinces that license practical nurses, licensing laws for LPNs/LVNs are similar to those for RNs.

## Keeping your license current

When you begin a new job, your employer is responsible for checking your credentials and confirming that you're properly licensed. Make sure that your nursing license is always current, and be prepared to furnish proof that you've renewed your license in the past, when necessary, in order to keep it current.

If you fail to renew your license, you can no longer legally practice nursing. In the United States and Canada, you can be prosecuted and fined for practicing without a license. Fines vary from state to state. For example, section 223 of the Professional Nursing Law of Pennsylvania stipulates a $300 fine for nurses who violate the licensing law or practice nursing without a license; if a nurse doesn't pay the fine, she faces a 90-day prison term. In the United States and Canada, fines generally range from as little as $5 to as much as $2,000.

The courts have occasionally addressed the question of failure to renew a nursing license, usually for an appeal proceeding concerning a state board of nursing's disciplinary action (see Entry 4). In some cases, the courts have disagreed with boards' decisions. *Kansas State Board of Nursing v. Burkman* (1975) is one such case. A registered nurse failed to renew her license and continued to practice nursing. No evidence showed that she had intentionally failed to renew her license or knowingly practiced without it. Ruling that her failure to apply for renewal was a violation of state licensing laws, the state board of nursing suspended her license for 6 months. After several appeals, a high court ruled that the board of nursing had erred in suspending the nurse's license and instructed the board to renew it.

In *Oliff v. Florida State Board of Nursing* (1979), the court again disagreed with the state board of nursing and ruled in favor of the nurse. In this case, the board of nursing refused to

---

*"Your license may be revoked or suspended for cause in most states and Canadian provinces."*

---

renew an LPN's certificate because it had not received her application by a particular date. Evidence indicated that the nurse had mailed her application before the date specified by the state board of nursing. The court ruled that the date adopted by the board was a deadline for applications to be mailed, not received.

If you discover that you've forgotten to renew your license, several simple measures will help you avoid serious legal consequences. First, notify your employer. Then, find your original license application and immediately notify the state board of nursing of your oversight. Ask them for a temporary license or for authorization to continue nursing until you receive your license. If you can't find your license application, write to the state board of nursing

for a renewal application and instructions on how to proceed. Then, follow the board's instructions exactly.

## License suspension and revocation

Your nursing license may be revoked or suspended for cause in most states and Canadian provinces. Grounds for suspension or revocation include inability to function competently because of alcohol intake or drug addiction, lack of mental or physical well-being, and failure to abide by the standards and requirements of the nurse practice act of the particular state or province. (For a complete discussion, see Entry 4.)

## Moving? Make sure your license remains valid

Before the American Nurses' Association and the National League for Nursing established a national standardized examination for nursing licensure (the National Council Licensure Examination, or NCLEX), qualifications for entry into nursing practice were not consistent from state to state. As a result, a nurse had a difficult time arranging for a license in one state on the basis of her license in another state. NCLEX established standard qualifications for entry into nursing throughout the country, so nurses now are able to move more freely to new jobs in other states.

When you move to another state to practice nursing, you must obtain a license or temporary practice permit from that state before you can legally practice nursing there.

Most state boards of nursing will license you if you're currently licensed to practice nursing in another state or territory or in Canada, if your education fulfills the issuing state's requirements. This is called *endorsement*. (See *Requirements for Licensure by Endorsement in the United States and Canada*, pages 28 to 35.) Many state boards waive reexamination if you're licensed in Canada and wish to practice in the United States. The same usually applies

## INSTITUTIONAL LICENSURE: YES OR NO?

Just the mention of institutional licensure triggers emotional responses from advocates and opponents of the process. Here's why:

As you know, the vast majority of nurses today practice under professional licensure. State law gives a nurse legal permission to engage in a profession that involves public health and safety. With this permission come practice guidelines designed to protect the public.

Institutional licensure means an institution, such as a hospital, is licensed and granted the authority to regulate its staff members' practice directly. Its professional employees don't have their own licenses. The institution's self-regulation is overseen, but not controlled, by an independent monitoring agency (such as the state agency charged with licensing institutions) or a national organization (such as the Joint Commission on Accreditation of Hospitals).

Suppose staff nurse Mary Owens and hospital administrator Ellen Gardiner find themselves discussing this issue over lunch one day. Mary is a staunch defender of professional licensure; Ellen thinks institutional licensure might work. Here's their conversation:

**MARY**  Ellen, look at licensure in a historical perspective! The whole thrust of the nursing movement in this century has been to ensure the quality of patient care. Institutional licensure would throw us back to the days when anyone could practice as a registered nurse—just by saying she *was* one.

**ELLEN**  Why do you say that? Institutional licensure doesn't let just anyone walk in off the street and start giving nursing care. We're talking about an elaborate system of accountabilities. Each hospital will go overboard to protect its license. I can assure you, administrators won't leave one stone unturned when they're checking out prospective employees. And do you think a hospital would be crazy enough not to monitor its staff's performances very carefully? After all, it'd be the hospital that would lose its license if any of its staff violated the terms. I can tell you, Mary, not a hospital in the country would want that to happen.

**MARY**  The way you describe it, institutional licensure sounds safe, theoretically. But *are* all hospitals concerned enough about patients to provide more than minimal care? And remember, all those checks and reviews would cost the hospitals a bundle.

**ELLEN**  Well, first of all, no system could cost as much as individual licensure, with its state boards of nursing and elaborate testing and licensing procedures. Besides that, every hospital already has a credential review system set up and working. Institutional licensure would just mean expanding that system.

**MARY**  Wait a minute, Ellen. First of all, quality health care is worth whatever it costs—within reason, of course! And I've got my doubts about how useful credential reviews would be for institutional licensure—are those reviewers qualified to judge nursing practice?

**ELLEN**  Mary, quality care isn't the question. Everyone agrees about that. The question is, how do we *get* quality care? We need more freedom to *pursue* quality care. Imagine how much more innovative we could be if we didn't have so many outside boards on our backs.

**MARY**  I was waiting for that. "Innovation" could mean that maintaining minimum qualifications to practice nursing would go out the window. To save money, the hospital could theoretically use *anyone* to do *any* tasks, instead of paying qualified nurses. I wouldn't want to be a patient in *that* hospital!

**ELLEN**  If we misused our staff by putting them in positions they couldn't fill, we'd be putting our own necks on the block. That just doesn't make any sense, and I don't think it'd happen.

**MARY**  Well, we do have a precedent, you know. What do you think hospitals all over the country have done

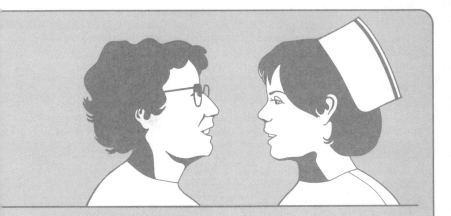

with associate degree nurses? That's a classic case of the way hospitals take people trained for one position and force them into other positions with only on-the-job training.

**ELLEN**  Come on, Mary. That's a poor example. You know as well as I do that the distinctions between nursing degree programs are all on paper, not in practice. Associate degree programs all over the country teach students things that technically aren't part of an associate degree. What do you expect us to do? Ignore skills an employee has because she's not *supposed* to have them?

**MARY**  That's not how it happened. Administrators plugged nurses into holes, period. They never considered their qualifications. What's the issue? It's that a nurse is licensed to perform her job in a professional way. You take away that licensure and you open the door to misuse of staff *and* abuse of patients. We're not talking about hospital convenience. We're talking about ensuring safe care and protecting the public.

**ELLEN**  That's the hospital's goal, too! I think institutional licensure will promote safe care not only because the hospital's license is on the line but also—and more importantly—because employees will have incentives and fewer restrictions on broadening their skills. The health-care profession has been dominated too long by this "I don't do windows" mentality. Break through that thinking and people will want to learn more. Mary,

I'm not saying the hospital will give an inexperienced nurse a scalpel and point her toward surgery. We're talking about easing restrictions, making limits on practice more flexible, letting employees learn and use what they learn. All medicine is based on testing skills. And give people more credit! They're not going to perform tasks they know nothing about. With institutional licensure, instead of saying, "My license won't permit me to do that," a nurse can honestly say, "I'm sorry. I don't know how to do that. Could you show me?"

**MARY**  You're saying that licensing restrictions are why there hasn't been teamwork in hospitals? Even doctors would laugh at that one. Mark my word, if you take away licensure guidelines, you're going to create a *more* defensive atmosphere. People are going to guard what they consider to be their prerogatives as if they were gold.

**ELLEN**  You've got a point there, Mary. I suppose that could happen. But I still think the benefits would outweigh the costs. Just look at it personally. Wouldn't you prefer a system that's more responsive to you—that rewards you directly for your achievements and has room for you to grow to your potential? Basically, institutional licensure introduces a free marketplace for talent in the hospital.

**MARY**  I'm just not sure, Ellen. I guess I'd rather take my chances with other nurses, instead of administrators, controlling my practice.

if you hold a U.S. license and wish to move to a Canadian province.

If you must move to another state before its board of nursing has had time to approve your application, you'll probably be granted a temporary license. Be sure to check both the time limit of the temporary license and the specific nursing functions it authorizes.

Remember, if you must travel with a patient from one state to another, your license is valid for the duration of the trip in most states (and Canadian provinces). For example, you might be assigned to care for a patient who's being transferred to a medical facility in another state or province.

If the state board finds that you don't have the necessary qualifications to practice nursing in that state, it may reject your application or require that you complete a written examination—regardless of your education or the laws of the state where you presently live.
In *Richardson v. Brunelle* (1979), a licensed practical nurse who'd practiced in Massachusetts for 15 years brought suit because she was refused a license to practice in New Hampshire. In her New Hampshire application, she requested a decree of educational equivalency. (Although she'd originally taken and passed a Massachusetts state licensing examination, she'd never graduated from an approved school of practical nursing.) At that time, only nursing-school graduates were permitted to practice in New Hampshire, so her request was denied. Her lawsuit was unsuccessful in reversing the New Hampshire decision, and subsequent appeals upheld the original ruling.

*Snelson v. Culton* (1949) is a similar case involving Maine's licensing requirements, which also specify that an applicant must be a graduate of a state-approved school of nursing.

## How federal laws affect your nursing license

In some instances, federal laws can affect nursing licensure (although no federal law has jurisdiction over state boards of nursing). For example, if you're a nurse in the armed forces who is often subject to transfer, you're required by federal law to hold a current state license—but not necessarily in the state to which you are assigned.

And a recently enacted federal public health code requires all state boards that license health-care professionals to develop systems for verifying those professionals' continued competence. (See Entries 55 and 56.)

## Foreign licensure

If you move to a foreign country, your U.S. nursing license will be reviewed by the appropriate authority, which will either reject or endorse (accept) it (possibly with conditions). If you're a nurse in the American armed forces working in an American installation, you're exempt from this review.

In a non-English-speaking country, the licensing authority may require you to complete a language-proficiency examination.

If you're an RN or an LPN/LVN licensed in a foreign country, you can't practice nursing in any state, territory, or Canadian province until the appropriate licensing authority has approved your application and issued a nursing license to you. When you're granted licensure in the United States or Canada, you function at the same legal status, depending on your level of expertise, as a U.S.- or Canadian-educated RN or LPN/LVN. You're also equally accountable for your professional nursing actions.

Many states are beginning to require that foreign nurses take and pass the examination prepared by the Commission on Graduates of Foreign Nursing Schools (the so-called CGFN examination). If a foreign nurse successfully completes this examination—which includes an English-proficiency segment—she may then take the NCLEX examination. If she passes that, she qualifies for licensure (and for a visa that allows her to work).

### A final word

Your nursing license guarantees that you've satisfied your state's minimum requirements for entry into nursing practice. It also provides proof of your nursing qualifications and protects the public by allowing *only* qualified persons to enter the nursing profession. Be sure to keep your license in a safe place at all times—and keep it current.

# 4 Safeguarding your nursing license

Your state board of nursing can take disciplinary action against a nurse for any violation of your state's nurse practice act. In all states and all Canadian provinces, the board of nursing has authority to discipline a nurse if she endangers a patient's health, safety, or welfare.

Depending on how severe a nurse's violation is, a state board may formally reprimand her, place her on probation, refuse to renew her license, suspend her license, or even revoke her license. The list of possible violations varies from state to state. The most common are:

● conviction of a crime involving moral turpitude, if the offense bears directly on whether the individual is fit to be licensed
● use of fraud or deceit in obtaining or attempting to obtain a nursing license
● incompetence because of negligence or because of physical or psychological impairments
● habitual use of, or addiction to, drugs or alcohol
● unprofessional conduct, including (but not limited to) falsifying, inaccurately recording, or improperly altering patient records; negligently administering medications or treatments; performing tasks beyond the limits of the state's nurse practice act; failing to take appropriate action to safeguard the patient from incompetent health care; violating the patient's confidentiality; taking on nursing duties that require skills and education beyond one's competence; violating the patient's dignity and human rights by basing nursing care on prejudice; abandoning a patient; and abusing a patient verbally or physically.

Here's how a state board of nursing typically investigates when a nurse is accused of professional misconduct: It conducts an *administrative review*.

You probably know that your state board of nursing is an administrative body that wields broad discretionary powers. But do you know that it can't issue a *final* decision? This is because it doesn't have legal authority, although court proceedings—and possibly legal penalties—may result from the board's administrative-review findings. And a state board's decision to reprimand a nurse or suspend or revoke her license isn't final. She always has the right to appeal, through the court system, for reversal of the nursing board's decision. (See *Disciplinary Proceedings for Nurse Misconduct: Typical Steps,* page 43.)

### Understanding the administrative review process

In most states and Canadian provinces, the nurse practice act specifies the steps

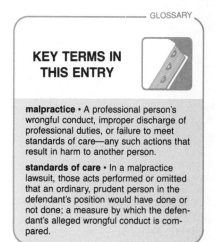

GLOSSARY

## KEY TERMS IN THIS ENTRY

**malpractice** • A professional person's wrongful conduct, improper discharge of professional duties, or failure to meet standards of care—any such actions that result in harm to another person.

**standards of care** • In a malpractice lawsuit, those acts performed or omitted that an ordinary, prudent person in the defendant's position would have done or not done; a measure by which the defendant's alleged wrongful conduct is compared.

the board of nursing must follow during an administrative review. In some states, however, a general administrative procedure act (separate from the nurse practice act) specifies the steps; in still other states, the board of nursing decides them.

In Canada, the process for administrative review of complaints against nurses is similar to the U.S. process. In some Canadian provinces, a complaints committee of the provincial nursing board hears the complaint first and either dismisses or endorses it. If the complaints committee endorses it, the complaint is sent along to a discipline committee for a full hearing. In other provinces, only a discipline committee hears the complaint.

As you may know, an administrative review begins when a person, a healthcare facility (the nurse's employer), or a professional organization files a signed complaint against a nurse with the state board of nursing—or when the board itself initiates such action. The board then reviews the complaint to decide if the nurse's action appears to violate the state's nurse practice act.

If it decides the nurse's action does appear to violate the act, the board prepares for a formal hearing, including subpoenaing witnesses. When these preparations begin, the accused nurse's due-process rights include the right to receive timely notice of both the charge against her and the hearing date. At the hearing, these are her rights under due process:

• to have an attorney represent her
• to present evidence and cross-examine witnesses
• to appeal the board's decision to a court.

In many Canadian provinces, an employer (except a patient) who terminates a nurse's employment for incompetence, misconduct, or incapacity must report the termination to the board of nursing in writing. If the employer fails to do this, the board may impose a fine.

At the formal hearing, an impartial attorney may act as a hearing officer (in lieu of a judge), or the board itself may hear the case. A court reporter documents the entire proceeding, or it may be taped. Members of the board are present, acting as the plaintiffs bringing the claim against the defendant-nurse. Witnesses—including co-workers—testify for the board and the nurse. If the board or hearing officer finds her guilty, she may be fined or reprimanded or have her license suspended or revoked.

## Understanding the judicial review process
In every state, as you know, nurses have the right to challenge the boards' disciplinary decisions by the process of appeal through the courts. This basic right cannot be revoked by any means. In many states, the nurse practice act guarantees this right. But even when it isn't spelled out, this right is guaranteed to every nurse.

Of course, each state and court jurisdiction sets its own rules on how to file this type of appeal. In some jurisdictions, the nurse (through her attorney) must appeal to a special court that only handles cases from state agencies. In other states, she must appeal to the lowest-level court.

In an appeal, the court is reviewing the legality of the state board's original decision against the nurse—not the nurse's allegedly improper conduct. The court should only attempt to determine whether the board of nursing exceeded its legal powers or conducted the hearing improperly. It decides if the state board's decision is unlawful, arbitrary, or unreasonable according to law, or whether it constitutes "abuse of discretion" (meaning the board didn't have enough evidence to determine unprofessional conduct, and so made a decision without proper foundation). The court may also review the original evidence before deciding whether to sustain or reverse the board's decision.

The court may also allow a *trial de*

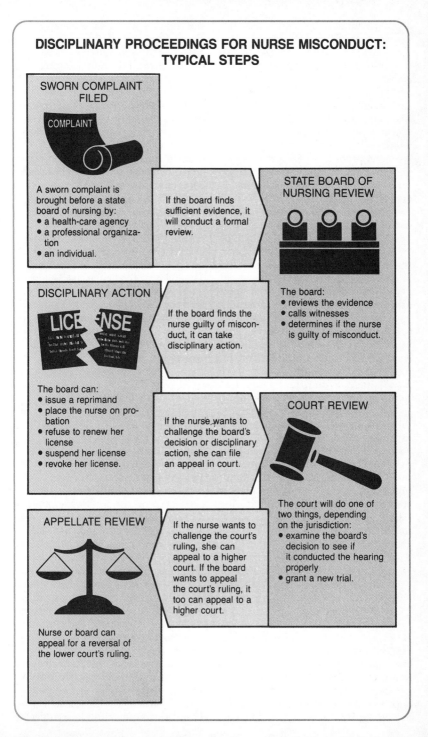

## DISCIPLINARY PROCEEDINGS FOR NURSE MISCONDUCT: TYPICAL STEPS

### SWORN COMPLAINT FILED

COMPLAINT

A sworn complaint is brought before a state board of nursing by:
- a health-care agency
- a professional organization
- an individual.

If the board finds sufficient evidence, it will conduct a formal review.

### STATE BOARD OF NURSING REVIEW

The board:
- reviews the evidence
- calls witnesses
- determines if the nurse is guilty of misconduct.

### DISCIPLINARY ACTION

LICENSE

If the board finds the nurse guilty of misconduct, it can take disciplinary action.

The board can:
- issue a reprimand
- place the nurse on probation
- refuse to renew her license
- suspend her license
- revoke her license.

If the nurse wants to challenge the board's decision or disciplinary action, she can file an appeal in court.

### COURT REVIEW

The court will do one of two things, depending on the jurisdiction:
- examine the board's decision to see if it conducted the hearing properly
- grant a new trial.

### APPELLATE REVIEW

If the nurse wants to challenge the court's ruling, she can appeal to a higher court. If the board wants to appeal the court's ruling, it too can appeal to a higher court.

Nurse or board can appeal for a reversal of the lower court's ruling.

*novo,* in which the appellate court hears the board's complete case against the nurse, as though the administrative review had never happened. New evidence, if it exists, may be introduced by the plaintiff (the board) or the defendant-nurse, through her attorney. The court hears the case and then either sustains or reverses the board's original decision.

You're probably aware that if the defendant-nurse loses this appeal, she may—depending on the jurisdiction— appeal to a higher court. (Of course, if the nurse wins, the board of nursing can appeal to a higher court, too.) To begin her new appeal, the nurse's attorney must file it with the lower court that ruled against her; this court will send the trial transcript and the appeal to the higher court. (Note that all states have rules and regulations governing appeals, and abiding by them is an attorney's legal responsibility.) The higher court then decides whether to hear the case, based on the merits of the grounds for appeal. Usually, these must establish that the lower court made an error of law in admitting (or not admitting) certain evidence. If the appeal doesn't establish this, the higher court may dismiss it. The higher court will *not* hear the case again, but the defendant-nurse and her attorney may continue to appeal through all higher courts up to the state's highest court. (Only exceptional cases can be heard by the United States Supreme Court.)

## Two illustrative cases
Now, let's look at two actual cases that went through the administrative and judicial review processes.

In *Leib v. Board of Examiners for Nursing of the State of Connecticut* (1979), a nurse was accused of conduct that failed to meet accepted standards of the nursing profession (see Entry 2). Her conduct? Charting the administration of meperidine hydrochloride to her patient, but using the drug herself. After voluntarily admitting to this action,

she testified on her own behalf at the board hearing. The board issued an order revoking her nursing license. The nurse appealed the revocation order to the court of common pleas. When this court dismissed her appeal, she appealed to the Supreme Court of Connecticut. This higher court also ruled that the evidence supported the board's findings of unprofessional conduct. The nurse's license was revoked. Other cases in which courts upheld boards' decisions include *Tighe v. Commonwealth of Pennsylvania, State Board of Nurse Examiners* (1979) and *Ullo v. Commonwealth of Pennsylvania, State Board of Nurse Examiners* (1979).

In *Colorado State Board of Nurse Examiners v. Hohu* (1954), a doctor filed a complaint of incompetence against a nurse, claiming that her failure to admit a patient quickly and to contact the doctor caused the patient's injury. The board of nursing ordered the nurse's license revoked. But when the nurse appealed, the court reversed the board's revocation order. This court ruled that the board of nursing had abused its discretionary powers because the evidence did not support the doctor's charges.

## License reinstatement
License revocation, if sustained despite all appeal efforts, is usually permanent. (Check to see if your state's nurse practice act provides for revoked-license reinstatement.) A nurse whose license is suspended usually may petition for reinstatement. Every nurse practice act contains a provision allowing reinstatement of a suspended license, and some license-suspension orders specify a date when the nurse may apply. In most states, after a suspension has been in effect for more than a year, the board of nursing will consider reinstating the license.

If *your* license were suspended, would you know how to get it back? Your first step would probably be to petition the board for reinstatement. Then the board would have to decide whether you're qualified to practice nursing again. (In some states, you have the right to another hearing before the board makes this decision.) After weighing the evidence, the board would issue its ruling.

The board will usually base its decision on current evidence of the nurse's fitness to practice. (For example, in a drug violation case, the board may consider whether a nurse has successfully completed a drug rehabilitation program.)

### A final word

As you know, you can't stop someone from accusing you of unprofessional behavior or of practicing beyond the scope of your nursing license. A state board of nursing must consider every such complaint it receives. Your best defense against having this happen to you, of course, is prevention—practicing nursing according to the appropriate care standards and the provisions of your state nurse practice act. If you ever *do* have to defend yourself against a complaint about your nursing care, be sure you know your legal rights, so you can use them to defend yourself.

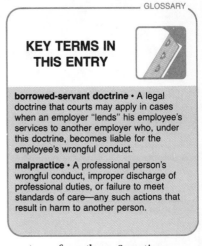

---

# 5 How nursing practice compares legally with medical practice

Could you describe, in a simple sentence, how nursing practice and medical practice relate to each other? Don't try. You probably know that each state's (and Canadian province's) nurse practice act and medical practice act are intended to distinguish the two professions. But in fact—as you probably also know—social, professional, and judicial forces have blurred the distinction. More and more, the public expects you to perform many tasks formerly reserved for doctors. And the law allows

you to perform them. Sometimes.

Because nursing practice and medical practice have blurred into each other in some areas, you need to know the legal risks involved in *not* knowing where your practice begins and where it ends. One key to this is knowing where the two practice acts differ and where they overlap—keeping in mind the lack of specific detail that characterizes most such acts (see Entry 1).

When state legislatures began writing medical and nursing practice acts, a doctor could legally perform any task a nurse performed. That remains true, although doctors today are likely to be unfamiliar with some nursing practices. Legislatures also reserved certain tasks exclusively for doctors. In theory, as a nurse, you perform such actions at your own legal peril. However, the blurring of nursing and medical responsibilities has forced corresponding changes in the law. Some of the causes for this are:

• patients' expectations of which health-care tasks nurses should perform

• hospitals' and doctors' increased inclination to delegate medical tasks to nurses.

How have patients forced nursing to broaden? By increasingly filing (and winning) lawsuits that express their expectation that you provide expanded

# PRACTICING MEDICINE WITHOUT A LICENSE?

### Doctor's orders, but not nurse's job

*For 5 years, I've been office nurse to a very fine doctor. Professionally, he's taught me many new things—including suturing.*

*He now has me cover for him when he's called out, and on these occasions I've often done minor suturing.*

*At a recent nursing seminar, the lecturer was an attorney. In his discussion, he described my job situation to a "T". Then he said that any nurse doing such suturing was leaving herself wide open for a lawsuit!*

*I reported this to the doctor I work for. He said that as long as he's taught me to suture correctly and I do it in his office, I have nothing to worry about because he'll be responsible for me. I'd appreciate another opinion, though.—RN, Mo.*

Suturing is not ordinarily an accepted nursing procedure, and nurses ordinarily may not do it. However, a nurse *may* suture under certain circumstances—for example, if the nurse is a nurse clinician practicing in a state whose statutes permit her to suture; or if the nurse is a particular part of a health-care delivery team (say, an operating room nurse) who works under the immediate direction, control, and supervision of a doctor.

Since you're not working in either of these circumstances, you're in legal jeopardy and subject to disciplinary action by your licensing board—to say nothing of what the outcome could be if you were sued by a patient claiming injury because of your suturing. In such a situation, losing the case would seem bad enough—but you might also find that your professional liability insurance doesn't cover your legal fees or the damages assessed against you.

### Who may read lab values?

*A question about laboratory values came up at a recent nursing standards meeting. Some of our nurses think nurses should read a patient's lab values and act on them. Other nurses say that's a medical responsibility—and too much to ask of nurses. What do you say?—RN, Ariz.*

Reading laboratory values *used to be* strictly the doctor's responsibility. Today, though, most nurses consider lab values an essential part of the nursing assessment, particularly when the test results are obviously going to affect treatment. For example, if a doctor orders hematocrit and hemoglobin tests for a GI bleeder, the nurse caring for that patient should make sure the tests are done and notify the doctor if the results warrant it.

In some hospitals, the charge nurse takes responsibility for laboratory tests, but more often staff nurses are responsible. Since most laboratories list normal values next to the patient's actual value, you needn't memorize all the numbers.

patient care, including some forms of medical diagnosis, treatment, and referral. The law traditionally reserves diagnosis and treatment for doctors, but this is changing. (See *Charting the Boundaries of Nursing Practice,* page 48.)

In *Fein v. Permanente Medical Group* (1981), the court agreed with a patient's claim that a nurse erred when she failed to diagnose the patient's myocardial infarction—even though doctors reserve the professional duty to diagnose. (See Entry 2 for a discussion of this case.)

Hospitals and doctors have delegated more authority to nurses—for example, in intensive-care units (ICU) and critical-care units (CCU). Nursing in those units today includes diagnosis (reading EKGs) and treatment (performing cardiopulmonary resuscitation).

Reductions in health-care funding have also led to increased responsibilities for nurses, whose lower salaries make them less expensive than doctors.

In many Canadian provinces, the boards of nursing and medicine jointly determine which medical tasks may be delegated to nurses and specify the requirements for appropriate delegation.

**Standing orders for the school nurse**

*I'm a school nurse for a small private college. Once a month, a doctor comes on campus to teach a class and see patients. He leaves standing orders for me to follow when he's not here. The orders generally involve only routine prescription medications, because our dispensary doesn't stock any controlled substances.*

*I enjoy my work but sometimes wonder if I'm not really diagnosing and prescribing by using these standing orders. The doctor almost never sees any of the patients. And although I can and do talk to the doctor frequently by phone, I can't send patients to his office—150 miles (240 km) away. I do, of course, refer any patients I'm in doubt about to local doctors.*

*Several doctors have assured me that what I'm doing is perfectly legal and standard procedure for small schools, but I'd appreciate your opinion.—*RN, Calif.

Unfortunately, in medicine, a long distance call *isn't* "the next best thing to being there." By adapting the doctor's standing orders for patients he "almost never sees," you *are* diagnosing and prescribing.

True, standing orders have been routine procedure in many small schools. But lately these orders have been disappearing from college campuses. However, doesn't common sense tell us that even a small school should have a doctor on campus at least twice a week, if only for an hour?

If you were to misdiagnose a student's condition and treat it with a medication—even if it's what you call a "routine prescription medication"—the student could sue you and the college if he has an adverse reaction.

Although most institutions *say* they'll stand behind a nurse unless she errs grossly, you can't afford to take this for granted. When confronted with an actual lawsuit, the school could claim you're responsible for *any* error. You should definitely have your own professional liability insurance.

Check with college personnel to find out exactly what the doctor's contract calls for and whether he is or isn't living up to his full obligation. If he isn't, take the matter up with the proper college authority. If he *is* doing exactly what his contract calls for, insist that the college hire someone closer to the campus who can give more hours to the health service.

In the meantime, protect yourself: Refer students to a doctor in the area. If the students are miffed at the unexpected expense and inconvenience, that may help to light a small fire under the college authorities and move them to make better arrangements for the students' health care. And get that professional liability insurance!

These letters were taken from the files of *Nursing* magazine.

## Defining medical practice

Medical practice acts may be divided into two types: those that define medical practice and those that don't. Both types forbid non-MDs from practicing medicine. (No Canadian law related to medical practice defines it.)

When a state's medical practice act includes a definition, it typically defines medicine as any act of diagnosis, prescription, surgery, or treatment. Not every definition includes all four elements, and some states' definitions add other elements.

Whether or not a state's medical practice act defines medical practice, the courts are regularly called upon to decide if a specific action constitutes medical practice. In the past, one area of considerable overlap between nursing and medicine was midwifery; the courts usually decided that delivering babies was a medical rather than nursing function. For example, in *Commonwealth of Massachusetts v. Porn* (1907) a state court upheld the conviction of a nurse-midwife for practicing medicine without a license. The legislature could have created a midwifery practice act, the court said, but hadn't done so. Obstetrics was therefore reserved for doctors.

## CHARTING THE BOUNDARIES OF NURSING PRACTICE

You can characterize your state's nurse practice act (NPA) as traditional, transitional, or modern, depending on how it defines the boundaries of nursing practice.

States with *traditional* NPAs allow only the most conventional nursing roles. These states—Idaho, for example—limit registered nursing activities to traditional patient care, disease prevention, and health maintenance.

States with *transitional* NPAs have broader boundaries, often including a "laundry list" of permitted nursing functions. For example, Maine's act lists six specific registered nursing activities: traditional patient care, collaboration with other health professionals in planning care, diagnosis and prescription delegated by doctors, delegation of tasks to LPNs/LVNs and aides, supervision and teaching, and carrying out doctors' orders. This list of duties—particularly the expanded duties of diagnosis and prescription—make Maine a state edging toward a modern type of nurse practice act. Other states with transitional acts broaden nurses' roles by including an additional-acts clause. For example, Massachusetts' clause gives RNs the legal permission to diagnose and evaluate patients—but not to treat them.

States with *modern* NPAs—New York, for example—allow registered nurses to diagnose and treat health problems as well as provide traditional nursing care. New York's definition of registered nursing is so broad it encompasses not only what nurses in the state do today but also much of what they're likely to do in the future.

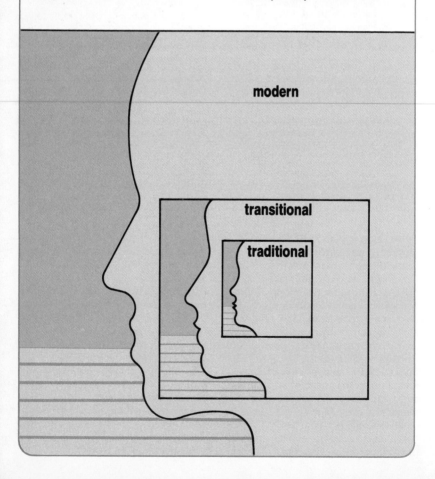

modern

transitional

traditional

## How state legislatures deal with nursing-medical overlap

Some states have solved the problem of overlap between the nursing and medical professions by passing laws making some functions common to both. New York's law, for example, allows both registered nurses and doctors to diagnose and treat patients—with the proviso that a nursing diagnosis should not alter a patient's medical regimen. And, as you probably know, almost all states permit you to perform any patient care a doctor requests, as long as a written or oral order exists. Some court decisions have concluded that a doctor's presence during patient care isn't necessary once he's delegated a task to a nurse. These decisions have also been interpreted as meaning that a nurse may perform some medical tasks on the basis of standing orders and nursing protocols, as well as on the basis of doctors' written and oral orders. This means that a nurse's scope of actions, when working under standing orders or nursing protocols, can be very broad in certain practice settings, no matter how restrictive her state nurse practice act may seem. Orders such as these form the basis for ICU/CCU practice, I.V. team practice, and similar practice circumstances in all states where the nurse practice acts don't grant nurses clear-cut independent authority to treat patients.

Some state medical practice acts limit doctors' rights to delegate tasks. For example, Texas' medical practice act permits doctors to delegate tasks only to "any qualified and properly trained person or persons," and then only if doing so is "reasonable and prudent," and then only if the delegating doesn't violate any other state laws. Most state courts would probably interpret their state medical practice acts similarly, even if this restriction isn't written into the acts. Texas makes these limits explicit.

Remember, you can perform tasks that involve overlap of nursing and medical practices—such as ICU func-tions—even if your nurse practice act doesn't state that you can, through standing orders and through nursing protocols.

## How the courts deal with nursing-medical overlap

In recent years, the two most common areas of nursing practice/medical practice overlap concern anesthesia treatment and emergency-department diagnosis. Interestingly, courts rarely give more than a passing reference to their state practice acts when dealing with these problems.

In *Mohr v. Jenkins* (1980), the patient sued a nurse anesthetist, claiming she incorrectly injected Valium into his arm and so caused phlebitis. The court dismissed the suit, saying the nurse "performed the procedure correctly and conformed to accepted medical practice." The patient appealed, but the appellate court affirmed that the standard for "specialists in similar circumstances" is "accepted medical practice," and that the defendant nurse had met the appropriate standards.

A similar result occurred in *Whitney v. Day* (1980): In this case, a Michigan court said—without reference to the practice acts—that nurse anesthetists are professionals with expertise in an area akin to medical practice. As such, the court said, they can be held to the same practice standards—those of the "similar specialist."

In a North Carolina case that involved a question of licensure, *Maloney v. Wake Hospital Systems* (1980), the court refused to let a nurse testify as an expert witness, on a patient's behalf, about the correct practice in I.V. potassium chloride administration. The court said the nurse wasn't qualified to testify because the action in question belonged to medical practice. But an appellate court reversed the ruling because the nurse, although not a doctor, had acquired skills that qualified her to form an opinion. The appellate court decided that the nurse's "expertise is different from, but no less exalted than, that of the physician."

In *McKinney v. Tromly* (1964), a family sued their son's surgeon because the nurse anesthetist administered ether while the surgeon used an electrical surgical instrument, causing an explosion. The boy died from the burns that resulted. The Texas court said: "The administration of an anaesthetic . . . constitutes the practice of medicine. Although the nurse could not practice medicine, . . . she was trained . . . and knew how to administer an anaesthetic." The court also found that the administration of anesthesia by nurses was common practice in that locality. Based on these facts, the court ruled that the case be tried solely on the basis of whether the nurse was practicing as a hospital employee or as the surgeon's "borrowed servant." Thus, the issue of whether she was practicing medicine without a license became irrelevant.

In some situations, of course, you have no alternative to practicing medicine without a license, and the courts

---

### "In general, the courts will tend to interpret the law in ways most likely to protect patients."

---

expect you to do so when a patient requires treatment. (See Entries 31 and 34.) In *Cooper v. National Motor Bearing Co.* (1955), a California nurse was accused of failing to make a medical diagnosis of cancer in one of her patients. The nurse defended herself by arguing that state law at that time prohibited her from making diagnoses of any sort. The court ruled against her, finding that nurses were supposed to have sufficient training to tell whether a patient had signs or symptoms of a disease that would require a doctor's attention.

A federal court in Illinois reached a similar conclusion when a nurse failed to recognize that her patient's complaint resulted from a subdural hematoma rather than drunkenness. In *Stahlin v. Hilton Hotels Corp.* (1973), the court said the nurse "failed to exercise the degree of care required" even though doing so could be considered medical diagnosis—a task the Illinois nurse practice act forbids.

Can you safely assume, then, that courts will generally ignore the difference between medical practice and expanded nursing roles—for example, a nurse practitioner's role? Unfortunately, no. A case in point is *Hernicz v. State Dept. of Professional Regulation* (1980), which involved a registered nurse practitioner who examined and treated two patients without doctors' orders. The state board of nursing suspended his license, and the court decision upheld the suspension.

In general, the courts will tend to interpret the law in ways most likely to protect patients. If protecting patients means not strictly interpreting nursing and medical practice acts, the courts will usually follow that course.

### A final word

You should have a keen interest in how your state defines nursing practice, and in how your practice overlaps with medical practice. Why? Because you'll improve your chances of avoiding a malpractice lawsuit. And if you know your nurse practice act, you can help your state's nursing association to lobby for any needed changes.

Legislatures tend to resist amending nurse practice acts to reflect expanded roles. You can overcome that tendency through united professional activity—working together with hospital administrators, nursing home operators, and doctors to convince legislators to pass practice acts that incorporate present practices and future needs. Then you can concentrate on the key questions: What should we be doing for this patient? And who can do it best?

# 6 Working as a nurse practitioner

If you're a nurse practitioner, you regularly perform functions that formerly were doctors' exclusive responsibilities. You're an RN who's specially trained to make independent judgments about a patient's condition (under a doctor's direction or order)—for example, forming a diagnosis and prescribing treatment.

Or maybe you're not a nurse practitioner—but you're interested in what's required to become one. You know that this expanded role offers nurses exciting new challenges. For example, besides diagnosing, prescribing, and treating, nurse practitioners evaluate patients' therapeutic procedures, assess changes in their health status, and manage their medical-care regimens. (Of course, nurse practitioners also perform many tasks that hospital staff nurses perform.) And becoming a nurse practitioner means choosing a specialty. You could choose to become certified in such important nursing specialties as mental health, critical care, emergency care, neonatal care, family planning, rural health, and many others.

## How the nurse practitioner's role developed
In 1965, Loretta Ford, RN, Ed.D., and Henry Silver, MD, began a program at the University of Colorado that taught expanded nursing roles—roles that would place nurses into new practice settings and increase their traditional patient-care responsibilities. (Viewing shortages of doctors around the country, some health-care experts saw nurse practitioners as a means of providing medical care in places where doctors were scarce, such as extremely rural areas and inner-city neighborhoods.) That program provided a model for subsequent nurse practitioner programs around the country. In 1970, the American Nurses' Association (ANA) amended its definition of nursing to include nurses' right to take on expanded roles, with the proper preparation.

During the 1970s, many states amended their nurse practice acts to recognize nurse practitioners. By 1973, nurse practitioners were numerous enough to organize their first national convention. And by 1980, all 50 states had certification programs for nurse practitioners.

In 1973, Canadian nurses and doctors also endorsed nurses' expanded roles. In a joint statement, associations for both professions declared that expanding the nurse's role would improve Canadian health care.

Today, nurse practitioners work in a variety of settings including nursing homes, hospital emergency departments, industrial medical offices, rural

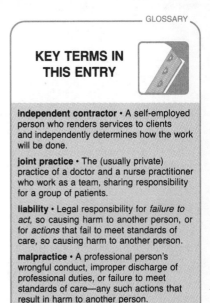

GLOSSARY

## KEY TERMS IN THIS ENTRY

**independent contractor** • A self-employed person who renders services to clients and independently determines how the work will be done.

**joint practice** • The (usually private) practice of a doctor and a nurse practitioner who work as a team, sharing responsibility for a group of patients.

**liability** • Legal responsibility for *failure to act*, so causing harm to another person, or for *actions* that fail to meet standards of care, so causing harm to another person.

**malpractice** • A professional person's wrongful conduct, improper discharge of professional duties, or failure to meet standards of care—any such actions that result in harm to another person.

**respondeat superior** • "Let the master answer." A legal doctrine that makes an employer liable for the consequences of his employee's wrongful conduct while the employee is acting within the scope of his employment.

## SHOULD YOU PRACTICE AS AN INDEPENDENT CONTRACTOR?

Thousands of nurses in the United States, including nurse practitioners and private-duty nurses, have chosen to become independent contractors. They work directly for patients (or patients' families) and bill their patients (or third-party insurers) on a fee-for-service basis. If you're considering practicing on an independent-contractor basis, you'll want to weigh the pros and cons.

| PROs | CONs |
| --- | --- |
| • You can schedule your work hours to suit your life-style.<br>• You can put your nursing philosophy into practice by independently planning each patient's nursing care.<br>• You'll be relatively free from institutional politics and bureaucracy.<br>• You can negotiate your own contract with each patient and set your own fee for nursing services.<br>• You may improve your working relationship with other professionals because you'll assume a more prestigious role in the health-care community.<br>• You'll keep more of the money you make, because tax laws favor self-employment.<br>• You can tailor your benefits package to your own personal needs.<br>• You can become more involved in the total care of your patient. | • You'll lose the security that continuous employment provides.<br>• You may experience strained working relationships with professionals who feel threatened by your autonomy and status.<br>• You'll have to compete for work with other nurses working as independent contractors.<br>• Your patients may sometimes be admitted to hospitals (or other health-care institutions) where you don't have privileges.<br>• You'll have to deal with unclear legal definitions of your practice.<br>• You'll have to educate yourself about the financial and legal aspects of running a business.<br>• You'll have to deal with getting patients to pay their bills. |

clinics, and in remote and sparsely populated areas. Some nurse educators even work part-time as nurse practitioners.

Once the value of nurse practitioners' services was demonstrated, state legislatures took steps to legalize this expanded role. They amended their nursing and medical practice acts to allow nurses to perform nurse practitioner tasks, and they expanded the formerly limited right of doctors to delegate medical tasks to nurses. The amended nurse practice acts gave nurse practitioners the rights to diagnose, to prescribe (with a doctor's co-signature), and to treat their patients. Some states—such as Idaho, Indiana, Alaska, Pennsylvania, and Florida—set up guidelines for joint nursing-medical practices. (See Entry 1.)

### Becoming a nurse practitioner

What's involved in becoming a nurse practitioner? Because certification requirements vary, the ANA has begun a move to establish national qualifications. But for now, you'll need to check your state's certification program. Remember, you must meet all of a state's certification requirements before you may practice there. However, this may cause problems when you move to a different state. State boards of nursing can give you details about their nurse practitioner certification programs.

Among the most common certifica-

tion requirements, you must:
- be a registered nurse
- have a college or university degree
- have at least 2 years of experience working as a nurse
- choose a nursing specialty.

Many certification programs also require that you obtain approval from a hospital's medical board if you want to work in that hospital.

Here's another requirement in many states: If you work in a nursing home or clinic, you must meet with the facility's administrator and doctors at least once a year. The reason? To review procedures, standing orders, and documentation regulations concerning your job.

### Interpreting the limits of nurse practitioner practice

Because expanded roles for nurses are fairly new, few questions about a nurse practitioner's role and liability yield clear-cut answers. So complaints settled both in and out of court are important right now in defining the limits of the nurse practitioner's expanded role—and they will continue to be important in the future.

So far, complaints and lawsuits involving nurse practitioners have usually been based on alleged unauthorized medical practice. For example, the New Jersey Board of Medical Examiners reviewed the complaints of two patients who charged two nurse practitioners in a health maintenance organization with prescribing drugs and making a medical diagnosis. The ANA supported the nurses, stating that they were acting well within the nurse practice act. Although the parties settled out of court, the board cited the complaints as the basis for issuing stricter definitions of doctors' and nurse practitioners' responsibilities.

In another New Jersey complaint, the Board of Medical Examiners inquired about four school nurse practitioners said to be performing physical assessments of students. Even though the nurse practitioners were trained to do

physical assessments, they agreed to stop when the school district's medical director gave them a written order, at their request, to do so.

In Missouri, doctors on the Board of Registration of Healing Arts accused two nurse practitioners, who provided family planning services, of practicing medicine. And two consulting doctors were accused of contributing to the nurses' alleged illegal practice by delegating medical tasks to them. The tasks included performing pelvic examinations and pap smears, treating vaginitis, counseling, providing contraceptives, and inserting intrauterine devices. The nurses claimed that their tasks were valid under protocols signed by their consulting doctors.

Remember: When disputes about nurse practitioner practice arise, your nurse practice act probably won't be enough help. You'll find that court decisions on medical or nursing board rulings provide more current and descriptive legal clarifications of the nurse practitioner's role.

### Assessing the legal risks

Many states' nurse practice acts now legally permit nursing in an expanded role, but you should be aware that serious legal concerns exist for nurse practitioners. One legal concern is simply the fact that some states have not amended their practice acts to recognize nurse practitioners. In those states, functioning as a nurse practitioner is illegal. A nurse practitioner's responsibility to practice only under a doctor's direction or with his orders also has legal significance. Without a doctor's order, she can perform only traditional nursing tasks.

You may already know about another legal concern of nurse practitioners—the fact that their liability depends on whether they provide their services:
- as an employee of an institution, such as a hospital or public health agency
- as an employee of a doctor; sometimes as part of a joint practice
- as an independent contractor.

If you work for an institution or a doctor and you're sued for malpractice (and lose), the court will apply the traditional nurse-employer doctrine—respondeat superior—to determine liability. The doctrine doesn't necessarily relieve you of professional liability.

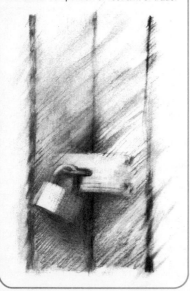

## GAINING HOSPITAL PRIVILEGES

As a nurse practitioner, you know how important hospital privileges are. Fortunately, you'll find that most hospitals are cooperative. But what if one of your patients is admitted to a hospital that won't grant you privileges?

You can appeal the hospital's decision through the hospital's nursing department committee, depending on your state laws. The hospital has a legal responsibility to tell you how its appeal process works. By appealing the hospital's decision, you can learn the reason why your request for privileges was denied—whether it was because the privilege requested isn't in the scope of your nursing practice, or for some other reason. If the denial is found to be baseless, designed to limit competition with medical staff, or obliged by an exclusive contract between the hospital and another practitioner, then you have grounds for charging the hospital with unfair competition or restraint of trade.

But if you were working within the scope of your employment, application of the doctrine makes your employer responsible for all damages a court may award to the plaintiff.

If you're sued for malpractice while working as an independent contractor, however, you carry the full responsibility for your liability. That means you'll have to pay the entire cost of any cash damages the plaintiff may be awarded. (See *Should You Practice As an Independent Contractor?* page 52.)

You can see that the circumstances of your employment as a nurse practitioner are important in determining the type and amount of professional liability insurance you'll need.

### How can you protect yourself legally when working as a nurse practitioner?

You now know that a number of state nurse practice acts have expanded-role provisions that give a nurse practitioner legal protection. You should also be aware of other forms of protection. For example, a *written contract* can offer some protection. In any practice setting, have an attorney draw up a contract before you begin caring for patients. Be sure it defines such important conditions as what services you're expected to perform, your fees, how and when you'll be paid, the amount of professional liability insurance (if any) your employer will carry, and how disputes will be handled. To be valid, the contract must have a legal purpose and the willing consent of both parties (see Entry 46).

Professional liability insurance is important, but you can't beat the protection that comes with maintaining the highest competence in your practice. You may even want to take advanced courses and classes to improve your professional credentials and to strengthen your defense if you're sued.

### Financial concerns you should consider

Nurse practitioners have to consider

some possible financial problems. For example, you may know that many third-party insurance carriers won't provide reimbursement for a nurse practitioner's services, even though state and professional nurse organizations have lobbied to persuade carriers to do so. If you're a nurse practitioner, or if you become one, always have your patient check that his health insurance covers your services. If it doesn't, he may not want your services after all—or you may have difficulty collecting your fee.

Remember that if you work as an independent contractor, no employer withholds taxes (federal, state, or local), unemployment compensation, or social security payments. You're solely responsible for keeping track of these obligations and making payments on schedule.

If you have your own office, you'll also need property liability insurance. This will protect you if someone's injured on your property. Also, establish contact with an accountant who's familiar with business-finance regulations. And consider asking an attorney to help set up your business along sound legal lines.

### Professional concerns to keep in mind

A nurse practitioner's professional concerns differ from a staff nurse's. For example, to be most effective as a nurse practitioner, you'll need a certain degree of cooperation and acceptance from the community you choose to practice in. Some communities will oppose your practice because people feel uncomfortable with your increased responsibilities.

If you work as a nurse practitioner on an independent-contractor basis, you'll have to get local hospitals and health-care institutions to grant you patient-care privileges. (For some tips on doing this, see *Gaining Hospital Privileges.*)

Remember, you may face opposition from staff nurses who are concerned

that your expanded role could implicate them in a malpractice lawsuit. You'll have to work at winning their trust and confidence.

### A final word

You may wonder whether more job opportunities will exist for nurse practitioners in the future. No one can say for sure, although some believe that a surplus of doctors may have a significant impact. And although the nurse practitioner's expanded role appeals to many nurses, they must examine their willingness to deal with the special legal, financial, and professional concerns nurse practitioners face. Probably, as the nurse practitioner's expanded role gains more acceptance, her legal risks will decline—although they'll always be higher than a staff nurse's—and third-party reimbursement for nurse practitioner services will become more common.

In the last analysis, economics might determine the extent of the nurse practitioner's influence on health care. If nurse practitioners can provide efficient medical and nursing services at reduced cost to consumers, chances are this expanded role for nurses will find a secure place in our health-care system.

# 7 Working as a private-duty nurse

No doubt you've been frustrated, sometimes, when you've had to divide your attention and skills among many patients. Well, would you like a job that lets you devote all your nursing skills to the care of one patient? That's one advantage of working as a private-duty nurse.

Who's a private-duty nurse? She's any RN or LPN/LVN that a patient (or his family) hires for total nursing care. The patient pays her directly, or she

### KEY TERMS IN THIS ENTRY

**independent contractor** • A self-employed person who renders services to clients and independently determines how the work will be done.

**malpractice** • A professional person's wrongful conduct, improper discharge of professional duties, or failure to meet standards of care—any such actions that result in harm to another person.

bills a third-party insurer directly. She's an *independent contractor*, not an employee (except of her patient). This employment status is the major factor in distinguishing the private-duty nurse from the agency nurse (see Entry 10). (Of course, a hospital or other health-care institution may also hire a private-duty nurse. See the discussion of *Emory v. Shadburn*, 1933, below.)

Besides focusing all your skills on one patient, the other advantages of working as a private-duty nurse include choosing where you work, when you work, the type of patient you care for, and the fee you feel your skills are worth—although your community's prevailing fees will influence this decision.

Patients are referred to a private-duty nurse through nurse registries and referrals from other nurses and doctors familiar with the nurse's practice. Many hospitals maintain referral lists of private-duty nurses. If you work as a private-duty nurse long enough, you can expect that you'll build up a list of hospitals, other health-care institutions, nurses, doctors, and families who will call you when they need a private-duty nurse.

A private-duty nurse performs most of the tasks a hospital staff nurse performs, and she's expected to have the same degree of skill. She plans a patient's care, observes and evaluates his condition, reports signs and symptoms, carries out treatments under a doctor's direction, and keeps accurate records so that the patient's doctor has the data he needs to diagnose and prescribe. It is a private-duty nurse's obligation to perform her job within the scope of her state nurse practice act—the same as a staff nurse. And as you probably know, a private-duty nurse working in a hospital can expect the hospital to provide her with adequate *equipment* and *support services* for proper patient care.

But private-duty nursing poses unique *legal risks* and problems you ordinarily wouldn't face as a hospital staff nurse. For example, a private-duty nurse doesn't retain professional liability insurance through an employer. As an independent contractor, she's solely liable for any damages assessed as the result of a lawsuit—although a court may decide a hospital shares liability for her actions. So she (and you, if you work as a private-duty nurse) must obtain her own professional liability insurance.

Besides the additional legal risks, you must manage certain financial burdens if you work as an independent contractor. For example, you'll be responsible for making social security payments and for paying federal, state, and local taxes on schedule. And you won't be eligible for workmen's compensation benefits if you're injured on a job. The courts have repeatedly rejected private-duty nurses' claims for workmen's compensation. For example, in a Maryland case, *Edith Anderson Nursing Homes, Inc. v. Bettie Walker* (1963), a private-duty nurse was hurt caring for a nursing home patient who was in a wheelchair. The nurse attempted to collect workmen's compensation benefits from the nursing home because her injury occurred there, but her claim was denied. The nurse was an independent contractor who was paid by the patient's family, did no work for the home, and took her orders only from the patient's doctor. As an independent contractor, the court ruled, she wasn't entitled to the benefits available to the nursing home's employees. A subsequent appellate court decision upheld the denial of the nurse's claim.

## WORKING WITH A PRIVATE-DUTY NURSE

If you're working on a unit where a private-duty nurse (PDN) is working, you're responsible for seeing that the PDN receives any help she needs. However, your responsibility doesn't end there. Even though a PDN is caring for one of her patients, you're responsible for the patient as well.

Monitor the PDN's care. If you're a staff nurse and you see the PDN performing care negligently, inform your charge nurse. If you're the charge nurse, intervene immediately. If you see the PDN negligently performing emergency care when the patient's life is in danger—regardless of your staff position—you must intervene. You're protecting your patient, yourself, and your hospital. If you ignore the PDN's negligence, you and the hospital could be liable for negligence if the patient (or the patient's family) files a malpractice lawsuit.

If you're a charge nurse, remember that the PDN's contract outlines her responsibilities. Read over that contract and keep its provisions in mind when you make assignments. Never assign a PDN a job that involves responsibilities not included in her contract.

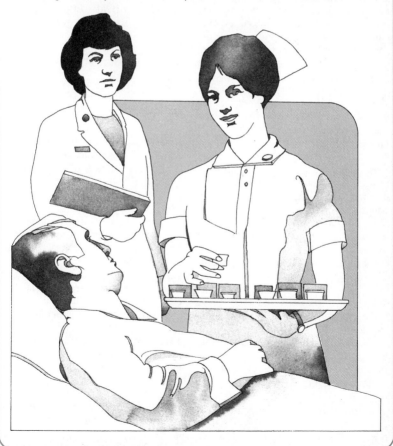

## Your legal risks working as an independent contractor

If you work as a private-duty nurse for a patient, you're legally considered an independent contractor. In this situation, your legal risks are highest when you care for a patient in his home. Why? Because you're responsible not only for giving proper patient care but also for obtaining and correctly using any equipment the patient care requires. These added responsibilities naturally increase your chances of making a mistake. And because you're self-employed, legally you're solely responsible for paying court-ordered damages if you're sued and found negligent.

Making written contracts with your patient can help reduce your legal risks as an independent contractor. A contract spells out the conditions of your employment—but remember, having a contract doesn't prevent a lawsuit, nor can it provide evidence that definitely will exonerate you if you're sued.

The case of *Emory University v. Shadburn* (1933) set the precedent for a hospital's liability for a private-duty nurse's wrongful conduct. A patient jumped out of a window after the assigned private-duty nurse—who had reason to know that his condition warranted continuous watching—left him unattended. The court ruled that the hospital was liable for this nurse's negligence because the hospital had hired and paid the nurse on a private-duty basis.

A hospital will usually insist on tight control of a private-duty nurse's practice, both to protect patients and to demonstrate "reasonable supervision" if the hospital is sued. Because of the trend to make hospitals share liability, you'll probably face liability alone only if you commit a negligent act *despite* the hospital's reasonable supervision.

Hospital controls include checking every private-duty nurse's credentials and approving her nursing qualifications. The case of *Ashley v. Nyack Hospital* (1979) established that a hospital has the right to refuse practice privileges to a nurse if the hospital doesn't approve her qualifications. Hospitals generally also establish policies to govern how private-duty nursing practice will relate to hospital nurses' practice (see *Working with a Private-Duty Nurse,* page 57). Hospitals are obligated to inform all health team members about private-duty nurses' responsibilities and rights in the hospital.

## A final word

Private-duty nursing offers you the opportunity to work in different practice settings and to give complete nursing care to individual patients. If you're a "take-charge" person who seeks new challenges, you may decide that the rewards of private-duty nursing are worth the increased legal risks.

# 8 Working in geriatric facilities

America is growing gray. U.S. census statistics show that the number of Americans over age 65 is growing. By 1990, they'll probably make up about 12% of the population; by 2000, about 13%.

As you know, this trend means that more and more patients will be cared for in geriatric facilities, including nursing homes and extended-care facilities. In fact, surveys already show that more patients are in geriatric facilities than in hospitals.

This growth in the number of patients in geriatric facilities began in 1965, when Congress passed the Medicare and Medicaid amendments to the Social Security Act. Because these amendments provided government reimbursement for geriatric care, the number of nursing homes (and their patients) began increasing dramatically.

The Medicare and Medicaid amendments also provided reimbursement for skilled nursing care in extended-care facilities. These were initially planned to deliver short-term nursing care to elderly patients who no longer needed intensive medical and nursing care in a hospital. Today, about 80% of the patients admitted to extended-care facilities do come directly from hospitals or other health-care facilities. But because many patients remain in extended-care facilities for long periods of time, the distinction between extended-care and geriatric facilities has blurred.

### Geriatric care today

You're probably aware that all geriatric facilities should provide nursing and medical care that is preventative, protective, restorative, and supportive. Unfortunately, the care provided today in many geriatric facilities falls short of these goals. (See *Helping Your Patient Select an Extended-Care Facility*, page 60.) A 1974 U.S. Department of Health, Education, and Welfare survey showed that many geriatric facilities failed to meet standards for patients' safety, nutrition, medical care, and rehabilitation. This survey also discovered frequent violations of patients' rights. The relatively small number of licensed nurses employed by geriatric facilities may be a large part of this problem. A recent Institute of Medicine study states that sickness and disability have increased among nursing home patients, but that employers' demands for nursing services haven't kept pace. Why? Because Medicare and Medicaid payments aren't sufficient to pay for the nursing staff that would be needed. So Medicare and Medicaid payments, begun by Congress to help elderly patients, have inadvertently resulted in substandard care for many of them.

Many RNs and LPNs/LVNs working in geriatric facilities are aware of this problem, and most are concerned about their legal rights and responsibilities. The three areas these nurses are most concerned about are staffing patterns, quality of care, and ensuring patients' rights.

### Understanding staffing patterns in geriatric facilities

Health-care professionals use the term *minimal licensed-personnel staffing* to describe the current staffing situation in many geriatric facilities. The following are characteristic of nursing homes:

- Only about 1 of every 20 nursing home employees is an RN.
- Only about 1 licensed health-care professional is employed for every 100 nursing home patients.
- Doctors spend only about 2 hours a month with their nursing home patients.
- Licensed nurses usually must process the paperwork while comparatively untrained aides provide most of the patient care.

In some extended-care facilities, about 6 of 10 charge nurses on the 3 p.m. to 11 p.m. shift and about 7 of 10 charge nurses on the 11 p.m. to 7 a.m. shift are LPNs/LVNs.

Health-care experts testifying before

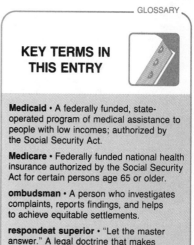

GLOSSARY

### KEY TERMS IN THIS ENTRY

**Medicaid** • A federally funded, state-operated program of medical assistance to people with low incomes; authorized by the Social Security Act.

**Medicare** • Federally funded national health insurance authorized by the Social Security Act for certain persons age 65 or older.

**ombudsman** • A person who investigates complaints, reports findings, and helps to achieve equitable settlements.

**respondeat superior** • "Let the master answer." A legal doctrine that makes an employer liable for the consequences of his employee's wrongful conduct while the employee is acting within the scope of his employment.

## HELPING YOUR PATIENT SELECT AN EXTENDED-CARE FACILITY

Your elderly or disabled patient may need the care provided at an extended-care facility. As a nurse, you can help the patient and his family choose a facility by explaining the three types of extended-care facilities available and what type of care each offers.

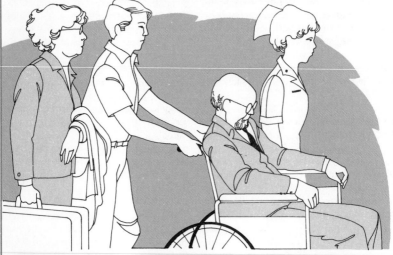

### RESIDENTIAL CARE FACILITY

Best for a patient who needs minimal medical attention, this type of facility provides meals, modest medical care, and a life-style free of most housekeeping responsibilities. Some offer recreational and social programs as well. Federal and state subsidy programs don't usually cover the cost of residential care facilities.

### INTERMEDIATE-CARE FACILITY

The best choice for a patient who can't manage independently, this type of facility provides room, board, and daily nursing care. The cost may be covered by government subsidy programs. Some offer rehabilitation programs as well as recreational programs.

### SKILLED NURSING FACILITY (SNF)

Best for a patient who needs constant medical attention, this type of facility provides 24-hour nursing care, medical care when needed, and such rehabilitation services as physical and occupational therapies. Depending on the patient's eligibility, both Medicare and Medicaid may pay the cost of the patient's care.

the Select Committee on Aging of the U.S. House of Representatives have alleged that Medicare's regulations created the staffing patterns that are causing inadequate care. For instance, federal Medicare regulations only require geriatric facilities to have one LPN/LVN on all shifts and one RN on the day shift. This means that many such facilities hire only this minimum number of licensed nurses, to qualify for federal funds. Few state Medicaid

programs provide reimbursement to geriatric facilities for additional licensed nurses.

In most geriatric facilities, RNs hold administrative positions, shouldering broad supervisory responsibility for the quality of care. LPNs/LVNs often work as charge nurses, performing most nursing procedures and supervising nurses' aides. Obviously this arrangement creates potential legal problems concerning both supervision and the scope of nursing practice.

## Legal risks of staffing problems

As you know, every nurse is legally responsible for her own actions. A supervisor is responsible for her supervisory acts and decisions. Suppose a supervisor knows—or should know—that a subordinate is inexperienced, untrained, or unable to perform a task safely. A court may find that supervisor liable in a malpractice lawsuit for delegating such a task to the subordinate. Of course, if the subordinate performs that task negligently, she'll be liable, too. And if the court finds that the supervisor and the subordinate were working within the scope of their employment, the nursing home may share liability under the doctrine of respondeat superior.

The courts judge lawsuits involving nursing malpractice by determining whether the defendant-nurse's actions met professional standards for her position. As part of this determination, the courts may review details of the staffing situation. For example, a New York court found that nurses were negligent when an unsupervised patient jumped from a balcony (*Horton v. Niagara Falls Memorial Medical Center*, 1976). The court reached this conclusion after reviewing evidence detailing the number of patients on the unit, the number of staff members, and what each staff member was doing. During this review, the court discovered that a charge nurse had permitted the only available aide to go to supper when she had the authority to prevent it, leaving the disoriented patient unsupervised.

Whether you're an RN or an LPN/LVN working in a geriatric facility, you *must* practice within the legal limits set by your state nurse practice act, meet professional standards for your position, and be familiar with state regulations for the type of facility in which you work. If you're an RN, be sure you possess the management and supervisory skills that your job requires. Keep in mind that if you're sued for mal-

practice, you'll be judged according to how a reasonably prudent nursing supervisor would act in similar circumstances. You can't defend yourself by claiming that you weren't trained to supervise.

If you're an LPN/LVN working in a geriatric facility, remember that no individual or institution can force you to practice beyond the limits of nursing care outlined in your state nurse practice act (see Entry 2). If you do exceed the legally permissible scope of nursing in your state, your state board of nursing can suspend or revoke your license. You won't be able to use your employer's expectations to excuse your actions (see Entry 5).

Under the law, an LPN/LVN who performs a nursing function legally restricted to RNs will be held to the RN

---

*"Nurses working in geriatric facilities are particularly concerned about fragmentation of the nursing process."*

---

standard if she's sued for malpractice. In *Barber v. Reinking* (1966), involving an LPN who had performed an RN function, the court stated, "In accordance with public policy of this state, one who undertakes to perform the services of a trained or graduate nurse must have the knowledge and skill possessed by the registered nurse."

## Quality of patient care

RNs and LPNs/LVNs working in geriatric facilities are concerned about the quality of patient care they're able to provide. They're particularly concerned about fragmentation of the nursing process; although an RN *remains responsible* for overall patient assessment and evaluation, an LPN/LVN decides on the daily assessments, planning, and evaluation, and a nurse's aide *implements* the assessment plan. This fragmentation of the nursing process can greatly reduce the quality of patient care. And it can also have legal consequences if nursing actions are performed improperly—or not performed at all. Here's a list of legally risky actions that occur more frequently in geriatric facilities, largely because of inadequate staffing:

- failing to make a nursing diagnosis
- observing a patient's condition carelessly
- failing to document
- writing illegibly when documenting
- failing to keep up with geriatric-nursing knowledge
- failing to use nursing consultants
- delegating improperly
- failing to insist on clear institutional policies

## HOSPICE CARE: SOME LEGAL CONSIDERATIONS

As you probably know, a hospice is a health-care facility that provides terminally ill patients with therapy and psychosocial and spiritual services until life ends. If you work in a hospice, you assume the same patient-care responsibilities as nurses in other settings. Your legal responsibilities, however, differ as follows:

• *Standing orders.* A hospital staff nurse can follow standing orders for pain medication. When working in a hospice, however, you should never rely on standing orders as authorization to administer pain medication. Always obtain specific orders signed by the patient's doctor.

• *Advice on making a will.* In a hospice, never give your patient advice concerning his will. If he asks you about it, tell him you can't help him, but suggest that he discuss it with his attorney or family.

• *Living wills.* Unlike the hospital nurse, whose duty with respect to living wills varies from state to state, the nurse who works in a hospice *must* respect the patient's living will. Don't violate it in any way, unless a court order instructs you to do so.

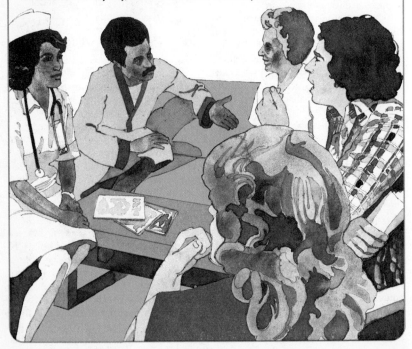

• failing to question a doctor's order
• taking a dangerous patient-care shortcut
• excluding family from patient care
• failing to call the doctor whenever nursing judgment indicates that a patient needs medical attention.

## Protecting patients' rights in geriatric facilities

In recent years, a number of states have enacted patients' rights legislation patterned after the Patient's Bill of Rights published by the American Hospital Association (see Entry 11). Twenty-eight of these states have passed laws that make reporting maltreatment of patients a legal responsibility. Some states have even established an ombudsman's office that has the authority to investigate complaints of abuse and the obligation to post complaint procedures in all geriatric facilities. So in most states, RNs and LPNs/LVNs working in geriatric facilities have a professional obligation (and in some states, a legal responsibility) to protect their patients' rights.

If you work in a geriatric facility, you should request that your institution adopt patient's rights policies that:
• require a patient's signature for any release of information
• clearly specify who has access to medical records and impose penalties for unauthorized disclosure of patient information (see Entry 14)
• restrict the use of chemical (drug) and physical restraints, which should be used only when the patient's record gives evidence that they're necessary (see Entry 29); and even then, of course, only with a doctor's order
• foster a patient's right to know about his condition, and provide for informed consent for his treatment (see Entry 12)
• help combat drug abuse and misuse by requiring that nurses administering drugs know the drugs' effects and know how to assess a patient's changing needs (see Entry 23)
• insure prompt, effective communi-

cation between doctors and nurses (see Chapter 13)
• acknowledge and respect a patient's right to refuse treatment (see Entry 13)
• encourage nurses to evaluate the quality of nursing services and to work cooperatively with patient representatives and accreditation agencies in the evaluation process.

Most health-care professionals are patient-rights advocates, but the patient-rights issue can create an adversary relationship between a nurse and a doctor or between a nurse and an institution. This situation presents a paradox for nurses: you have a professional obligation to protect your patient's constitutional rights—but doing so could cost you your job. Unfortunately, your legal protection in this situation is limited. If you're an employee working without a contract, you can be dismissed for any reason your employer wants to give. You do have legal grounds to protest your dismissal if:
• your contract clearly states you can't be fired on these grounds
• your hospital guarantees you the right to notice and a hearing prior to dismissal
• your state's laws prevent your employer from retaliating if you report violations to the appropriate agency
• you're a government employee and can claim the First Amendment right to free speech.

## A final word

In a geriatric facility, where doctors' involvement with patients is limited, RNs and LPNs/LVNs have a good opportunity to grow professionally and to affect the quality of patient care. If you're an RN, you'll need to learn not only geriatric nursing but also good management. If you're an LPN/LVN, you may have the chance to fill a charge-nurse position and to expand your nursing skills. (Depending on the limits of your nurse practice act, you may also learn how to perform nursing assessment and patient teaching.) For all nurses, along with opportunity comes responsibility—for practicing within legal limits and for continuing your education to meet professional standards for your position.

# 9 Working in alternative settings

Practicing nursing outside of traditional settings—such as hospitals, clinics, and nursing homes—isn't new. In fact, in the 19th century, *most* nurses worked outside hospitals: in doctors' offices, in patients' homes, and on battlefields. Today, many nurses are practicing in *alternative settings.* Their employers include factories, schools, community public health services, insurance companies, and claims review agencies (see *Working in Alternative Settings*). Some nurses—such as those working in schools and factories—may choose their alternative settings because they offer more independence and a challenging variety of responsibilities. Others—such as nurses in public health agencies—may want to devote themselves to public service.

GLOSSARY

## KEY TERMS IN THIS ENTRY

**liability** • Legal responsibility for *failure to act,* so causing harm to another person, or for *actions* that fail to meet standards of care, so causing harm to another person.

**malpractice** • A professional person's wrongful conduct, improper discharge of professional duties, or failure to meet standards of care—any such actions that result in harm to another person.

**workmen's compensation** • Insurance that reimburses an employer for damages he's required to pay when an employee is injured on the job.

These nurses find that along with benefits come additional responsibilities and legal risks. For instance, a nurse working alone doesn't have the daily support of senior nurses, doctors, and specialized equipment that a hospital setting offers. And of course, greater individual responsibility for patient care means greater legal risks. In this sense, a nurse working in an alternative setting is similar to a private-duty nurse (see Entry 7).

As you know, two of the most important challenges for a nurse working in *any* setting are to know her legal responsibilities and to minimize her legal risks. A nurse must be particularly careful when working in an alternative setting—she may not have anything like the legal services of a hospital's administration to help her.

## Understanding professional standards for licensure

As you probably know, your state nurse practice act defines professional qualifications for RN and LPN/LVN licensure. (See Entries 1 to 3.) But nurse practice acts generally don't describe professional standards for nurses working in various settings. If you work in an alternative setting, you must meet the same practice standards as a hospital nurse. If you violate those standards, your state board of nursing may suspend or revoke your license, just as it would if you were a hospital nurse (see Entry 4), and your patient may be able to sue you for malpractice.

Few court cases involving nurses working in alternative settings have been reported. In one such case, *Stefanik v. Nursing Education Committee* (1944), a state board of nursing recommended that the state revoke the license of a district welfare department nurse. The board found that the nurse, who saw patients without their doctors' consent and contradicted their doctors' orders, was guilty of unprofessional conduct. The nurse appealed to the court, which sustained the board's decision. In reaching its decision, the

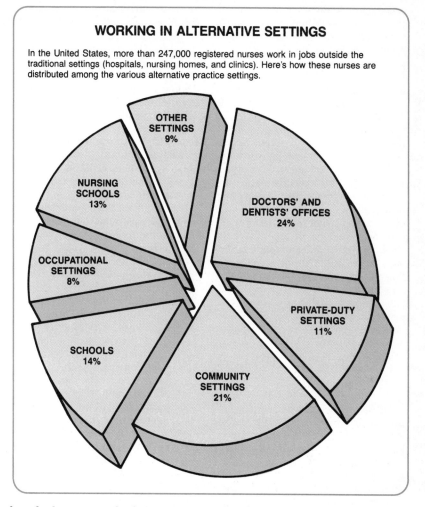

## WORKING IN ALTERNATIVE SETTINGS

In the United States, more than 247,000 registered nurses work in jobs outside the traditional settings (hospitals, nursing homes, and clinics). Here's how these nurses are distributed among the various alternative practice settings.

- OTHER SETTINGS 9%
- NURSING SCHOOLS 13%
- DOCTORS' AND DENTISTS' OFFICES 24%
- OCCUPATIONAL SETTINGS 8%
- PRIVATE-DUTY SETTINGS 11%
- SCHOOLS 14%
- COMMUNITY SETTINGS 21%

board of nursing judged this nurse's conduct by the state's standards for nursing practice. Neither the court nor the board considered that this nurse could be judged by any special standards because she worked in an alternative setting.

### Understanding your liability

A few legal differences exist between nurses working in traditional settings and in alternative settings.

Usually, if you work for a privately owned business (such as a manufacturer, an insurance company, or a small medical practice group), you may be sued by anyone who believes you're guilty of failing to meet standards of nursing care or of practicing beyond the scope of your license. In some states, however, you can't be sued by a fellow employee you've treated for a job-related injury. That's because state workmen's compensation laws, which protect the employer from excessive business costs, also protect you.

If you work for certain government agencies, you may be immune from lawsuits because of the doctrine of sovereign immunity. Depending on the state in which you're working, this immunity may be complete or partial. Check with your personnel office or agency attorney to find out if you have this legal protection.

You know that a nurse in an alternative setting must meet the same practice standards as a hospital staff nurse. A California malpractice case, *Cooper v. National Motor Bearing Co.* (1955), illustrates this point. The lawsuit concerned an occupational health nurse who failed to diagnose suspected cancer and so didn't refer the patient for further evaluation and treatment. At the trial, the court ruled that the only point of law to be considered in deciding the case was whether the nurse met the standards of nursing practice in her area. When expert testimony showed that she'd breached those standards, the court found her guilty of negligence. Her occupational setting was irrelevant to the court's decision. Similar court cases illustrating this principle include *Johnston v. Black Co.* (1939); *Barber v. Reinking* (1966; see Entry 3); and *Stahlin v. Hilton Hotels Corp.* (1973; see Entry 5).

The Canadian approach to such cases is similar to the American approach. In *Dowey v. Rothwell* (1974), a nurse who worked in a doctor's office knew that an epileptic patient was about to have a seizure, yet she failed to stay with the patient. This patient did have a seizure, fell, and fractured an arm. The court found that the nurse failed "to provide that minimum standard of care which a patient has a right to expect in an office setting." The court based its findings on testimony about the expected performance standards of experienced RNs in many settings.

## Should you buy your own professional liability insurance?

Private *medical* employers generally have coverage that includes the nurses they employ, but private *industrial* employers, especially small companies, may not. Check your employer's coverage thoroughly: if you've any doubt about whether you're fully protected, consider buying your own insurance.

You may also need your own professional liability insurance if you work for a peer review organization or a state or federal government agency, unless the law grants you complete immunity from job-related lawsuits. (For more information, see Entries 42 and 43.)

## Knowing your rights as an employee

Can you join a union if you work in an alternative setting? It depends on the setting—but usually you can. In fact, if you work as an occupational health nurse in a factory with a closed shop, you may be required to join a union. (See Entry 48.)

If you work for a state or local government, state laws may permit you to join a union but forbid your union to strike. Remember that the National Labor Relations Act exempts state and local governments, and so doesn't protect government nurses—such as community health nurses and public school nurses—in unionization disputes.

If you work in an alternative setting, can you be fired? That depends on whether or not you have a contract. If you don't have one, your employer may fire you at his discretion. Actually, your situation is the same as that of the hospital nurse—nothing but a contract clause, a union agreement, or a civil service law can legally protect you from being fired. Even if you have such protection, you may be vulnerable to discretionary firing until after an initial probationary period. Following this period, however, any of these forms of protection guarantees you the right to appeal your employer's decision.

If you work in an alternative setting, you should know what coverage your employer as well as your state, federal, or Canadian provincial government provides for on-the-job injuries. Generally, workmen's compensation will cover you. But not always.

The majority of states and Canadian provinces require that most *privately owned businesses* participate in workmen's compensation plans. If you work for such a business, you'll probably receive workmen's compensation for job-related injuries. But you should be aware that if the money you receive from this fund is inadequate, workmen's compensation laws prevent you from suing your employer for additional compensation.

If you work for *an employer with few employees or limited income* (for instance, a doctor with a small-scale practice), you may not be covered by workmen's compensation. That's because some states don't require such employers to participate in the workmen's compensation plan. If you're in this situation, you *can* sue your employer directly for any job-related injury. Most of these employers buy their own insurance to cover workers' in-

juries. If your employer doesn't have such insurance, you can buy your own insurance.

If you work for *a state or federal government agency,* you may receive compensation from the state workmen's compensation plan or by making a claim under a state or federal tort claims act, depending on the applicable laws. However, if the sovereign immunity doctrine applies, you may not be eligible for any compensation (see *Understanding the Doctrine of Sovereign Immunity*).

No matter what kind of compensation plan you have, it usually covers *any* on-the-job injury. For example, if you're a school nurse and a student kicks you, workmen's compensation will normally cover you. Typically, you also have the legal right to sue the person who caused the injury. If you win

## UNDERSTANDING THE DOCTRINE OF SOVEREIGN IMMUNITY

If you work as a government employee, you'll find that the law provides you with special legal protection. Most important is the doctrine of sovereign immunity, also called government immunity. The doctrine of sovereign immunity goes back to the days when a person couldn't sue a sovereign (or his agents) unless the sovereign consented. In the United States the courts transferred this privilege, applicable in most circumstances, to the elected government and its appointed agents—government employees. So government employees ordinarily can't be sued for their on-the-job mistakes.

In the past, this immunity has had some unfair results: a patient harmed in a private hospital could sue the hospital and its employees, but a patient harmed in a municipal or state hospital could not.

Perhaps because of this immunity, public hospitals gained a reputation for substandard practice; the public suspected that because public hospitals couldn't be sued for malpractice, their standards of care were lax.

In recent decades, most state legislatures have recognized the unfairness of this system. Many have passed laws that allow

patients to sue public hospitals and other government agencies. In some states, legislatures have created special courts—often called courts of claims—in which such lawsuits must be heard. In other states, legislatures have set dollar limits on the amount a patient can recover from a government agency if he wins his suit. Some states have done both.

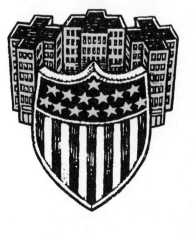

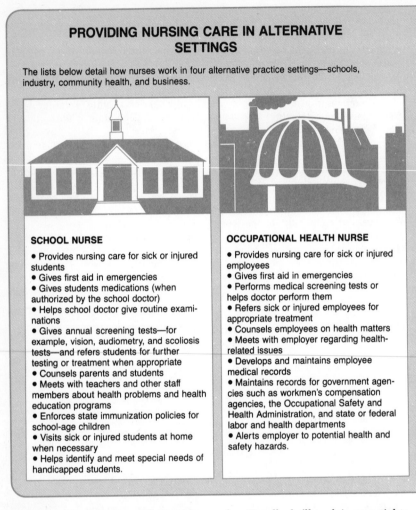

## PROVIDING NURSING CARE IN ALTERNATIVE SETTINGS

The lists below detail how nurses work in four alternative practice settings—schools, industry, community health, and business.

**SCHOOL NURSE**

• Provides nursing care for sick or injured students
• Gives first aid in emergencies
• Gives students medications (when authorized by the school doctor)
• Helps school doctor give routine examinations
• Gives annual screening tests—for example, vision, audiometry, and scoliosis tests—and refers students for further testing or treatment when appropriate
• Counsels parents and students
• Meets with teachers and other staff members about health problems and health education programs
• Enforces state immunization policies for school-age children
• Visits sick or injured students at home when necessary
• Helps identify and meet special needs of handicapped students.

**OCCUPATIONAL HEALTH NURSE**

• Provides nursing care for sick or injured employees
• Gives first aid in emergencies
• Performs medical screening tests or helps doctor perform them
• Refers sick or injured employees for appropriate treatment
• Counsels employees on health matters
• Meets with employer regarding health-related issues
• Develops and maintains employee medical records
• Maintains records for government agencies such as workmen's compensation agencies, the Occupational Safety and Health Administration, and state or federal labor and health departments
• Alerts employer to potential health and safety hazards.

your lawsuit, the court will consider any money you've already received, either from workmen's compensation or other insurance, in deciding the amount of damages you should receive. (Because these lawsuits are costly and can take years to resolve, most nurses don't sue.)

Do you know what to do if your employer violates your legal rights? If the employer's violation is an action—such as a breach of a contract or civil service regulation, sexual harassment, or racial discrimination—you should see an attorney or your union's legal coun-

selor. Usually, he'll explain your rights and the legal actions you can take according to applicable state, national, or Canadian provincial laws. Under most laws that protect employees' rights, however, you must file a complaint quickly (as dictated by state or provincial law) or risk losing your right to compensation.

### Choosing an alternative setting

Many options exist for the nurse who wants to work outside traditional practice settings (see *Providing Nursing Care In Alternative Settings*). First,

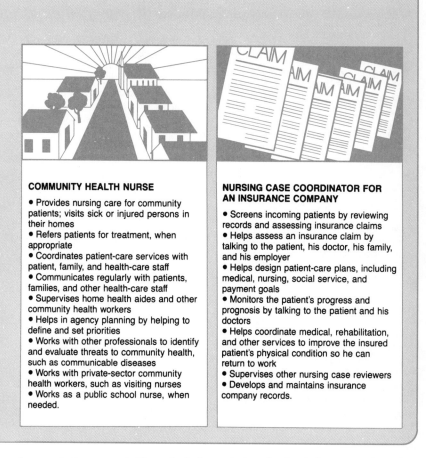

**COMMUNITY HEALTH NURSE**

- Provides nursing care for community patients; visits sick or injured persons in their homes
- Refers patients for treatment, when appropriate
- Coordinates patient-care services with patient, family, and health-care staff
- Communicates regularly with patients, families, and other health-care staff
- Supervises home health aides and other community health workers
- Helps in agency planning by helping to define and set priorities
- Works with other professionals to identify and evaluate threats to community health, such as communicable diseases
- Works with private-sector community health workers, such as visiting nurses
- Works as a public school nurse, when needed.

**NURSING CASE COORDINATOR FOR AN INSURANCE COMPANY**

- Screens incoming patients by reviewing records and assessing insurance claims
- Helps assess an insurance claim by talking to the patient, his doctor, his family, and his employer
- Helps design patient-care plans, including medical, nursing, social service, and payment goals
- Monitors the patient's progress and prognosis by talking to the patient and his doctors
- Helps coordinate medical, rehabilitation, and other services to improve the insured patient's physical condition so he can return to work
- Supervises other nursing case reviewers
- Develops and maintains insurance company records.

know what you want. Then, look for the alternative setting that can give it to you.

If you want more independent responsibility, for example, look into school nursing or occupational health nursing. You'll probably be the only health-care professional on duty. (Working in a doctor's office offers little opportunity for independent decision making.)

Or maybe your chief desire is plenty of patient contact. Then a doctor's office may be the place for you. Other settings where you'd see plenty of patients include schools, industry, and public-health agencies.

If your main interest is public service, check out public health agencies and social service departments. If you get a job with one of these organizations, you may be able to influence policy and thus improve the quality of health-care services for a large number of people.

### A final word

Of course, if you accept a nursing position in an alternative setting, you'll also be accepting the special challenges of knowing your legal responsibilities and minimizing your legal risks. But if an alternative setting appears to offer you the job satisfaction you want, these challenges shouldn't discourage you.

# 10 Working for an agency

How'd you like a job that lets you continuously choose not only where you work but also the hours and the days you work? You can get that kind of work-schedule flexibility if you work for a temporary-nursing service agency. And agencies generally pay higher salaries than hospital staff nurses receive.

Keep in mind, however, that the professional relationships and responsibilities of agency work are still evolving, and no set of uniform policies and procedures has yet been formally identified or administratively defined. For example, if an RN and an LPN/LVN are assigned to care for the same patient in his home but on different shifts, what responsibility does the RN have for the LPN's/LVN's work? Does the RN have the responsibility for supervising home health aides? Also, should communication between the RN and the patient's doctor be direct or channeled through an agency supervisor?

Large agencies, especially those with nationwide placement, may have specific policies for how RNs and LPNs/LVNs should function in situations like these. But smaller, more regional agencies may not. So when you work as an agency nurse, you may have few clear-cut guidelines. Sometimes you may have to rely heavily on your professional nursing judgment when you care for patients. *But remember: The courts will generally apply the same traditional legal principles governing staff-nurse malpractice cases to agency nurses as well.* This policy means you need to be thoroughly aware of the legal risks involved in agency nursing and how you can minimize them.

## Understanding your legal status as an agency nurse

When you work for an agency, you have an employee-employer relationship. The agency charges, for your services, a fee from which it pays your salary. It may also provide such benefits as social security and other tax deductions, workmen's compensation, sick pay, and professional liability insurance. (Traditional nursing registries, of course, also refer nurses to clients. But they refer private-duty nurses, who don't have employee-employer relationships with the registries. See Entry 7.)

As you know, a nurse is *always* liable for her own wrongful conduct. She can't escape liability if a court makes that decision. But if an agency nurse is judged to have been working within the legally permissible scope of her employment (see Entry 1), then she's still liable. The agency is held *vicariously liable* and is required to pay any damages awarded to the plaintiff. The court can use the doctrine of *respondeat superior* to interpret the nurse's legal status. This doctrine makes an employer

> *"You need to be thoroughly aware of the legal risks involved in agency nursing and how you can minimize them."*

responsible for the negligent acts of his employees—so the agency is responsible for the actions of the nurses it employs. The situation is different, however, if the court finds that the nurse was *exceeding* the scope of her employment. This makes her solely responsible for paying any damages.

As an agency employee, you may be assigned to work in a patient's home, to care for a single patient in a hospital or other health-care institution, or to temporarily supplement an institution's staff. These different practice circumstances can influence how a court decides who's liable in a lawsuit. At present, any malpractice lawsuit involving an agency nurse will probably name as defendants the nurse, the temporary-nursing service agency, and (if applicable) the hospital or other health-care institution where the alleged malpractice happened. *When you work as an agency nurse in a patient's home,* your agency-employee status is generally clear-cut. This is also true *when you care for a single patient in a hospital or other health-care institution.*

The courts have more difficulty assigning legal liability, however, in cases involving agency nurses *working as supplemental hospital or institutional staff.* In this situation, you're still an agency employee, of course, but you're also in the "special service" of another "employer"—the hospital or institution. Courts frequently apply the *borrowed-servant* doctrine to these situations, holding that the regular employer (the agency) isn't liable for injury negligently caused by the employee ("servant") while in the special service of another "employer." When a court interprets a case this way, the legal liability shifts from the agency to the hospital or institution.

To help protect yourself against a lawsuit, be sure you fully understand what's expected of you when you accept an agency job. And be prepared to have your practice scrutinized in court.

## Professional guidelines for agency nursing

As you try out the new job opportunities agencies offer, be prepared to adjust to different policies and procedures. When you work in a patient's home, for example, your *agency's* policies and procedures govern your actions. Be sure you understand them thoroughly and follow them carefully.

### KEY TERMS IN THIS ENTRY

**borrowed-servant doctrine** • A legal doctrine that courts may apply in cases when an employer "lends" his employee's services to another employer who, under this doctrine, becomes liable for the employee's wrongful conduct.

**respondeat superior** • "Let the master answer." A legal doctrine that makes an employer liable for the consequences of his employee's wrongful conduct while the employee is acting within the scope of his employment.

**workmen's compensation** • Insurance that reimburses an employer for damages he's required to pay when an employee is injured on the job.

How competently you follow them can affect such important matters as whether a claim for workmen's compensation is allowed, or whether your agency will be included as a defendant with you in a malpractice suit. Don't perform any nonnursing functions when you work in a patient's home, or arbitrarily change his nursing-regimen policies and procedures from what your agency has specified. If you do, and the patient or his family decides to sue, you may find yourself solely liable if you can't prove you acted the way a reasonable and prudent nurse would ordinarily have acted under similar circumstances. (See Entries 2 and 41.)

The American Nurses' Association has issued guidelines outlining the responsibilities of temporary-nursing agencies and agency nurses. These guidelines say that an agency has a duty to select, orient, evaluate, and assign nurses and to provide them with professional development. Agency nurses, according to these guidelines, should:
• keep their licenses current
• select reputable employers
• maintain their nursing skills

• observe the standards of professional nursing practice
• document their nursing practice
• adhere to the policies and procedures of their agencies and clients.

The last point is particularly important if an agency assigns you to work in a hospital or other health-care institution. As always, you must be sure you understand the hospital's or institution's policies and procedures for the nursing tasks you're expected to perform. Get to know the head nurse or unit supervisor, and seek clarification from her whenever you're in doubt (see Entry 18).

The hospital or institution, in turn, is obligated to supply equipment you need for patient care and to keep its premises and equipment in safe condition.

## What's the future of agency nursing?

Today's nursing shortages dictate that health-care institutions will suffer frequent imbalances in the number of nurses available to work regularly scheduled shifts. In this situation, temporary-nursing service agencies provide a valuable service by supplying skilled nurses on short notice. You should be aware, however, that use of agency-provided RNs and LPNs/LVNs as supplemental staff in hospitals, nursing homes, and extended-care facilities is a fairly new and controversial practice. Critics point out problems—for example, the morale problems that inequities in salaries between hospital and agency nurses—performing the same functions—can cause. Proponents of agency-based supplemental staffing, on the other hand, stress the cost-effectiveness of the practice and believe its flexibility helps keep nurses working and prevents nurse burnout. Proponents and critics alike urge that nursing administrations *plan* supplemental staffing programs, instead of bringing in agency nurses on a few hours' notice before a shift begins. This policy would help maintain the quality and continuity of patient care and would aid long-term planning for nursing services.

So far, no plaintiff in a lawsuit has ever charged a hospital with inadequate staffing caused by a failure to obtain available supplemental staff from an agency. But observers of the nursing profession feel that this may happen soon. Already, in the Louisiana case *McCutchon v. Mutual Insurance Co.* (1978), a court has required an insurance company to pay the agency fees of two LPNs/LVNs recruited to care for a critically ill patient whose doctor had ordered RNs (and whose insurance policy allowed payment only for RNs). The court reached its decision after reviewing evidence that neither the temporary-nursing service agency, the hospital, nor the insurance company could locate any available RNs at the time the LPNs/LVNs were assigned. Also considered was the fact that the assigned LPNs/LVNs were closely supervised by an RN at all times.

## WORKING WITH AN AGENCY NURSE: WHAT'S YOUR RESPONSIBILITY?

Suppose you're a hospital staff nurse and an agency nurse is assigned to your unit. At first, she handles herself well and seems to have no problem performing her nursing duties. But later, you see her performing a procedure in a way that may harm her patient. In this situation, you have the same responsibility—to *stop the procedure*—that you'd have when working with your regular health-team colleagues. If an agency nurse performs a procedure incorrectly but without potential harm to the patient, you should report your observation to your nursing supervisor.

What legal responsibility do you have when working with her? Actually, your responsibility when working with her isn't any different than when working with others on the health-care team. If the patient may be harmed, you have a responsibility to stop the procedure.

## A final word

Temporary-nursing service agencies represent an innovative approach to the delivery of nursing services—one response to the need for practical, efficient, and cost-effective nursing care. If you, as a nurse, continue your efforts to understand the economic, professional, and legal basis of your practice, you'll be able to evaluate such new approaches accurately. And you'll be able to decide how *you* can influence the direction of nursing—and benefit from its growth and change.

## Selected References

Brown, S.P. "Some Concerns on Certification," *AORN Journal* 31(1):51-2, January 1980.

Bullough, Bonnie, ed. *Law and the Expanding Nursing Role*, 2nd ed. East Norwalk, Conn.: Appleton-Century-Crofts, 1980.

Cazalas, Mary W. *Nursing and the Law*, 3rd ed. Rockville, Md.: Aspen Systems Corp., 1979.

Chaska, Norma, ed. *The Nursing Profession*. New York: McGraw-Hill Book Co., 1977.

Cohn, Sarah D. "Revocation of Nurses' Licenses: How Does it Happen?" *Law, Medicine and Health Care* 11(1):22-4, February 1983.

Creighton, Helen. *Law Every Nurse Should Know*, 4th ed. Philadelphia: W.B. Saunders Co., 1981.

Creighton, Helen. "Law for the Nurse Supervisor: Licensure Problems," *Supervisor Nurse* 11:68-9, January 1980.

Curtin, Leah, and Flaherty, M. Josephine. *Nursing Ethics: Theories and Pragmatics*. Bowie, Md.: Robert J. Brady Co., 1981.

Cushing, M. "When Medical Standards Apply to Nurse Practitioners," *American Journal of Nursing* 82:1274, August 1982.

Cushing, Maureen. "A Judgment on Standards: Circumstances Under Which a Patient Should Be Placed in Seclusion," *American Journal of Nursing* 81:797-98, April 1981.

Deloughery, Grace L. *History and Trends of Professional Nursing*, 8th ed. St. Louis: C.V. Mosby Co., 1977.

DeYoung, Lillian. *The Foundation of Nursing: As Conceived, Learned and Practiced in Professional Nursing*, 3rd ed. St. Louis: C.V. Mosby Co., 1976.

Fenner, Kathleen M. *Ethics and Law in Nursing*. New York: Van Nostrand Reinhold Co., 1980.

Gunn, I.B. "Certification for Specialty Practice," *AORN Journal* 31(1):48-51, January 1980.

Hemelt, M., and Mackert, M. *Dynamics of Law, Nursing and Health Care*, 2nd ed. Reston, Va.: Reston Publishing Co., 1982.

Hollowell, E.E. "Legal Liability and the LPN/LVN," *Journal of Practical Nursing* 32:30, February 1982.

Howe, Marilyn, et al. *A Plan for Implementation of the Standards of Nursing Practice*. Kansas City, Mo.: American Nurses' Association, 1977.

Kelly, L.Y. "Credentialing of Health Care Personnel," *Nursing Outlook* 25:562-9, September 1977.

Kelly, Lucie Y. *Dimensions of Professional Nursing*, 4th ed. New York: Macmillan Publishing Co., 1981.

McDowell, Doris. "How Well Do You Know Your Board of Nursing?" *Nursing and Health Care* 2:557-63, December 1981.

Markowitz, Lucille A. "How Your State Board Works for You," *NursingLife* 2:25, May/June 1982.

Murchinson, Irene, et al. *Legal Accountability in the Nursing Process*, 2nd ed. St. Louis: C.V. Mosby Co., 1982.

Notter, Lucille E., and Spalding, Kennedy. *Professional Nursing: Foundation, Perspectives and Relationships*, 9th ed. New York: J.B. Lippincott Co., 1976.

"A Plan for the Implementation of the Standards of Nursing Practice," *American Nurse* 9:5, February 1977.

Reid, D., and Deane, A.K. "Licensure: For Whose Protection?" *Dimensions in Health Service* 59:30-2, January 1982.

Schwartz, Bernard. *Administrative Law: A Casebook*. Boston: Little, Brown & Co., 1977.

Swansburg, R.C. "The Consumer's Perception of Nursing Care," *Supervisor Nurse* 12:30-3, May 1981.

# Patients' Rights

## Introduction

Today's patient is different. He's more aware, assertive, and involved in his health care than the patients you used to care for. He questions his diagnosis, seeks corroboration through a second opinion, expects assurances that the treatment chosen is appropriate, and takes action when his care doesn't meet his expectations. Sometimes this action is a lawsuit, and it may involve you.

Patients' bills of rights, endorsed by major health-care providers and consumer groups across the country, have increased the awareness and reinforced the assertiveness of today's patients.

And the courts have sometimes used these documents as standards for judging your nursing care. Chapter 2 discusses your professional obligations and potential liabilities regarding patients' rights of informed consent, privacy, and confidentiality.

### A new perspective on consent

If you've been in nursing for several years, you remember when nurses were forbidden to give a patient even the most basic information about his care or his health. Answering a patient's questions about his condition was the doctor's domain.

The consumer movement of the 1960s changed these rules in a hurry. Encouraged by patients' bills of rights, which first appeared in the late 1950s, patients began demanding to know more about their care. And, because nurses were available almost constantly, patients began demanding the information from them.

### Understanding patients' rights

How can you respond to patients' demands without exceeding the legal limits of your nursing practice?

Each entry in Chapter 2 takes an in-depth look at a different aspect of patients' rights—from a basic definition to a discussion of the complex professional and legal situations that can arise.

Entry 11, "Understanding the patient's bill of rights," explains the meaning and significance of patients' rights, and it gives you a brief history of the development of bills of rights for patients. Reading this entry will give you the guidelines you need for developing a working partnership with your patient that respects his rights.

Entry 12, "Consent requirements for treatment," discusses the development and current concept of informed consent, defines the situations that require informed consent, and explores your role as a witness when you think a patient has been improperly or inadequately informed.

Entry 13, "The patient who refuses

treatment," discusses the patient's right to refuse, how you should respond, and when you should challenge his refusal.

Entry 14, "Protecting your patient's privacy," explores the patient's right to privacy and the possible legal consequences of compromising this right by divulging confidential information.

Entry 15, "The patient who demands to read his chart," discusses the importance of understanding why a patient wants to read his chart. And it tells you how to handle his demand.

Entry 16, "The patient who leaves against medical advice," looks closely at your responsibilities and possible liabilities when a patient leaves the hospital against medical advice. You'll learn when you shouldn't restrain a patient who wants to leave. And you'll learn how to document the episode and notify appropriate hospital personnel.

Entry 17, "When a patient dies," considers the rights of a patient and his family after he dies. You'll learn about

---

> *"Nurses face issues involving patients' rights every day."*

---

the legal confusion over a definition of death as well as who's responsible for pronouncing the patient dead, signing the death certificate, and getting consent for an autopsy.

### You and patients' rights

Like all nurses, you face issues involving patients' rights every day. How you respond depends partly on your legal responsibilities set forth by your state's nurse practice act. But it also depends on your ethical responsibility to respond when questions arise about a patient's rights.

This chapter will help you apply your legal and ethical responsibilities regarding patients' rights to your everyday nursing practice.

# 11 Understanding the patient's bill of rights

A patient's bill of rights defines a person's rights while he's receiving health care. It helps protect his basic human rights at a time when he's most vulnerable.

Some consumers, civil rights activists, and attorneys feel that a patient's bill of rights is unnecessary. They claim it simply reiterates the basic rights that courts and laws recognize anyway.

In institutions that have prepared patients' bills of rights, the bills make patients aware that they have recourse to the institutions' grievance procedures.

Generally, patients' bills of rights are designed to protect such basic rights as human dignity, privacy, confidentiality, informed consent, and refusal of treatment. And they assert the patient's right to explanations about medical costs—and medical research, if he's asked to consent to experimental treatments.

Consumer-promoted bills emphasize the patient's right to decide and control his health care. These bills also include the patient's right to information about his care.

### The trend toward guaranteed rights

The concept of patient's rights is a relatively recent development in the health-care field. The first professional group to publish a statement on patients' rights, in 1959, was the National League for Nursing (NLN). In its position statement, "What People Can Expect of Modern Nursing Practice," the NLN called the patient a partner in health care whose ultimate goal is self-care.

Patients' rights received increasing public support during the 1960s as more people became aware of their rights as consumers. In a 1962 message to Congress, President John F. Kennedy further heightened this awareness when he outlined four basic consumer rights: the right to safety, the right to be informed, the right to choose, and the right to be heard.

The American Hospital Association (AHA) responded to the consumer movement in 1973 with its "Statement on a Patient's Bill of Rights." The statement—the result of a study the AHA had conducted with consumer groups—listed 12 patient rights. (See *Your Patient's Rights,* page 80.)

That same year, the Pennsylvania Insurance Department (PID) issued "Citizens Bill of Hospital Rights," the first patient's bill of rights formulated by a government agency. This bill outlined the kinds of treatment a patient should expect in a hospital. And it pointed out omissions in the AHA bill. The PID also warned that it would enforce this bill by stopping Blue Cross/Blue Shield payments to hospitals and other health-care institutions that failed to protect the rights mentioned in the bill.

Also in 1973, Minnesota became the first state to make patients' rights a law. That law requires all state health-care facilities to post Minnesota's bill of rights conspicuously and to distribute it to their patients.

Since these first milestones, other states and groups have developed their own bills of rights.

## Patients' bills of rights—legally binding or not?

As with any standard, formal or informal, written or verbal, a bill of rights has only as much authority as the group that issues it.

Bills of rights that have become laws or state regulations have the most authority because they give the patient legal recourse. If a patient believes a hospital has violated his legal rights, the patient can report the violation to the appropriate legal authority, usually the state health department. If an investigation shows that the hospital violated the patient's rights, the state will demand that the institution modify its

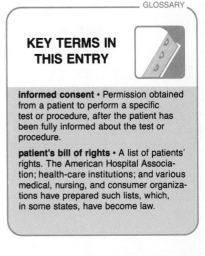

practices to conform to state law. (In Canada, the courts usually accept a professional tribunal's decisions about patients' rights violations.)

Some bills of rights protect the rights of specific types of patients. Canada has a Charter of Rights and various provinces have Human Rights Acts. And, in the United States, the Rehabilitation Act was passed by Congress in 1973. This act guarantees the physically or mentally handicapped person the right to any service available to a nonhandicapped person. This may require a health-care institution to redesign its facilities or equipment, transfer a handicapped patient to a better-equipped facility, offer home visits, hire an interpreter of sign language for a deaf patient, or supply auxiliary aids for a patient with impaired vision or manual skills.

Bills of rights issued by health-care institutions and professional associations aren't legally binding. But hospitals could jeopardize certain federal fundings, such as Medicare and Medicaid reimbursement or research funding, if they violated federal regulations or the standards of the Joint Commission on Accreditation of Hospitals, which establishes industry-wide standards.

Patients' bills of rights are also

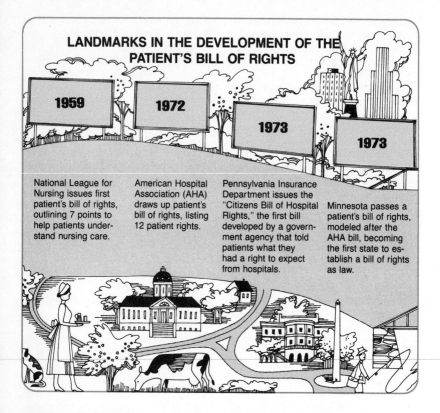

**LANDMARKS IN THE DEVELOPMENT OF THE PATIENT'S BILL OF RIGHTS**

**1959**
National League for Nursing issues first patient's bill of rights, outlining 7 points to help patients understand nursing care.

**1972**
American Hospital Association (AHA) draws up patient's bill of rights, listing 12 patient rights.

**1973**
Pennsylvania Insurance Department issues the "Citizens Bill of Hospital Rights," the first bill developed by a government agency that told patients what they had a right to expect from hospitals.

**1973**
Minnesota passes a patient's bill of rights, modeled after the AHA bill, becoming the first state to establish a bill of rights as law.

professionally binding on you. If your hospital has a bill of rights, you're required to uphold those rights.

You're also expected to uphold the bills of rights published by professional organizations such as the NLN.

### Interpreting the patient's rights

The theory is clear, but the practice is full of conflict. That's why defending a patient's rights without exceeding the bounds of nursing practice isn't easy. The case of *Tuma v. Board of Nursing* (1979), shows how the bounds of nursing practice are sometimes unclear.

In the Tuma case, a patient with myelogenous leukemia was admitted to a hospital in Idaho for chemotherapy. Although she had agreed to the chemotherapy, she was openly distressed about it. But instead of asking her doctor about alternative treatment, she

asked Jolene Tuma, RN, MSN, a nursing instructor at the College of Southern Idaho who supervised nursing students at the hospital. Ms. Tuma had asked to be assigned to the patient because of her interest in the needs of dying patients.

Ms. Tuma told the patient, in detail, about alternative treatments. She discussed laetrile therapy and various natural food and herbal remedies, comparing their side effects with those of chemotherapy. She also gave the patient the name of a therapist who practiced alternative treatments and offered to arrange an appointment with the therapist.

At no time did Ms. Tuma encourage the patient to alter her treatment plan or indicate that alternative treatments were better than the prescribed therapy or would cure her.

At the patient's request, Ms. Tuma

also discussed the alternative treatments with the patient's son and daughter-in-law. They told the patient's doctor, and, as a result, he interrupted the chemotherapy until he could discuss the situation with the patient. The next day the patient, again, agreed to undergo chemotherapy. Two weeks later, she went into a coma and died.

The patient's doctor demanded that the hospital remove Ms. Tuma from her position as clinical instructor at the College of Southern Idaho.

At the hospital's request, the board of nursing conducted an investigation and hearing. The board interpreted Ms. Tuma's behavior as unprofessional, under the Idaho Code. They agreed that she'd interfered with the doctor-patient relationship, and that this constituted unprofessional conduct. And they suspended her nursing license for 6 months.

Ms. Tuma appealed, lost, and appealed again. This time, 3 years after the incident, the Idaho State Supreme Court ruled that she couldn't be found guilty of unprofessional conduct because the Idaho Nurse Practice Act neither clearly defines unprofessional conduct nor provides guidelines for avoiding it.

This decision illustrates the nurse's evolving role in protecting patients' rights. But the decision fails to define the nurse's specific role in upholding a patient's right to information, and that leaves many troubling questions unanswered. For example, Ms. Tuma's patient asked her, not the doctor, for information about alternative therapies. The doctor testified that he wasn't knowledgeable about these therapies, so what recourse did that give his patient? If a doctor can't or won't answer such questions, does the patient have the right to get answers from a knowledgeable nurse?

Until the courts or legislatures address such questions, you won't find any easy answers. But guidelines are available.

## Sizing up your responsibilities

The best guideline you can follow to protect your patient's interests is the NLN's position statement on nursing's role in patients' rights. According to the NLN statement, you begin by viewing your patient as a partner in the health-care process. That's the underlying premise of all patients' bills of rights.

In planning your patient's care, recognize his right to participate in the decisions. Help him set realistic goals for his health care, and teach him the various approaches he can use to achieve them.

Throughout the decision-making process, keep assessing the patient's understanding of his illness. When he needs and wants more information, first determine if you or the doctor should provide it. (See Entries 12, 24, 36, and 37). Then, let the patient decide on his care plan. A care plan you formulate with your patient helps you communicate and demonstrates your respect for his wishes and rights.

Such supportive nursing practice also has the long-term benefit of opening health care to new ways of doing things. For example, nurse-midwives and other maternity nurses have acted as advocates for patients who challenge traditional childbirth practices. The results? Many hospitals have introduced birthing rooms, as an alternative to traditional delivery rooms; use less intervention and medication during delivery; and allow patients to use a birthing chair, walk at will during labor, and enjoy the company and support of a "coach"—husband, other relative, or friend—during labor and delivery.

## A final word

You aren't alone in your efforts to protect your patient's rights. Increasing interest in patients' rights has led many hospitals to employ full-time patient advocates, or ombudsmen. They mediate between the patient and the hospital when a patient is dissatisfied with the care he's receiving. Patient advo-

# YOUR PATIENT'S RIGHTS

Most hospitals design their own patient's bills of rights. The American Hospital Association's bill of rights, shown below, is one of the bills they use as a model. Two other bills, developed by The National League for Nursing and the American Civil Liberties Union, can be found in the Fact Finder section.

## A PATIENT'S BILL OF RIGHTS

**1** The patient has the right to considerate and respectful care.

**2** The patient has the right to obtain from his physician complete current information concerning his diagnosis, treatment, and prognosis in terms the patient can be reasonably expected to understand. When it is not medically advisable to give such information to the patient, the information should be made available to an appropriate person in his behalf. He has the right to know, by name, the physician responsible for coordinating his care.

**3** The patient has the right to receive from his physician information necessary to give informed consent prior to the start of any procedure and/or treatment. Except in emergencies, such information for informed consent should include but not necessarily be limited to the specific procedure and/or treatment, the medically significant risks involved, and the probable duration of incapacitation. Where medically significant alternatives for care or treatment exist, or when the patient requests information concerning medical alternatives, the patient has the right to such information. The patient also has the right to know the name of the person responsible for the procedures and/or treatment.

**4** The patient has the right to refuse treatment to the extent permitted by law and to be informed of the medical consequences of his action.

**5** The patient has the right to every consideration of his privacy concerning his own medical care program. Case discussion, consultation, examination, and treatment are confidential and should be conducted discreetly. Those not directly involved in his care must have the permission of the patient to be present.

**6** The patient has the right to expect that all communications and records pertaining to his care should be treated as confidential.

**7** The patient has the right to expect that within its capacity a hospital must make reasonable response to the request of a patient for services. The hospital must provide evaluation, service, and/or referral as indicated by the urgency of the case. When medically permissible, a patient may be transferred to another facility only after he has received complete information and explanation concerning the needs for and alternatives to such a transfer. The institution to which the patient is to be transferred must first have accepted the patient for transfer.

**8** The patient has the right to obtain information as to any relationship of his hospital to other health-care and educational institutions insofar as his care is concerned. The patient has the right to obtain information as to the existence of any professional relationships among individuals, by name, who are treating him.

**9** The patient has the right to be advised if the hospital proposes to engage in or perform human experimentation affecting his care or treatment. The patient has the right to refuse to participate in such research projects.

**10** The patient has the right to expect reasonable continuity of care. He has the right to know in advance what appointment times and physicians are available and where. The patient has the right to expect that the hospital will provide a mechanism whereby he is informed by his physician or a delegate of the physician of the patient's continuing health-care requirements following discharge.

**11** The patient has the right to examine and receive an explanation of his bill, regardless of source of payment.

**12** The patient has the right to know what hospital rules and regulations apply to his conduct as a patient.

Reprinted with permission from the American Hospital Association.

cates are your ally, helping you uphold your responsibilities to your patient. But patient advocates don't diminish those responsibilities. Whether you're an RN, LPN, or LVN, you must respect and safeguard your patient's rights.

# 12 Consent requirements for treatment

Suppose you're caring for a patient scheduled for surgery. He's talked to his doctor and signed the consent form. But the night before surgery, he doesn't seem to understand the implications of the procedure. What should you do? This question arises from a more fundamental question: What *is* informed consent?

## What is informed consent?

Informed consent has two elements: *informed* refers to information given to the patient about a proposed procedure or treatment; *consent* refers to the patient's agreement to the procedure or treatment. To be informed, a patient must receive, in terms he understands, *all* the information that would affect a reasonable person's decision to consent to or refuse a treatment or procedure. The information should include:

• a description of the treatment or procedure
• the name and qualifications of the person who'll perform the treatment or procedure
• an explanation of the potential for death or serious harm (such as brain damage, paralysis, or disfiguring scars) or for discomforting side effects during or after the treatment or procedure
• an explanation and description of alternative treatments or procedures
• an explanation of the possible effects of not having the treatment or procedure.

The patient must also be told that he has a right to refuse the treatment or procedure without having other care or support withdrawn, and that he can withdraw his consent after giving it.

## The origins of informed consent

The right of *informed* consent didn't exist at the beginning of this century. At that time, a patient had no legal right to *information* about his medical treatment. If a doctor performed surgery without the patient's consent, the patient could sue for battery. (As you know, battery means one person touching another without consent.) However, a patient could claim battery only if he'd refused consent or hadn't been asked to give it—not because he hadn't had enough information to make an appropriate decision.

Most battery lawsuits were unsuccessful, because courts usually took the doctor's word over the patient's. Two cases that patients did win were *Mohr v. Williams* (1905)—in which the patient consented to surgery on one ear, but the doctor performed it on both—and *Schloendorff v. Society of New York Hospitals* (1914)—in which the patient consented to an abdominal examination, but the doctor performed abdominal surgery.

The right to give an informed consent wasn't introduced until 1957, when the California Supreme Court introduced the theory in the case of *Salgo v. Leland Stanford, Jr. Univ. Board of Trustees* (1957). This case involved a doctor and a patient who had acute arterial insufficiency in his legs. The doctor recommended diagnostic tests, but he did *not* describe the tests or their risks. The day after the patient underwent aortography, his legs became permanently paralyzed. The court found the doctor negligent *for failing to explain the potential risks of aortography to the patient.*

This decision established the basic rule: A doctor violates "his duty to his patient and subjects himself to liability

GLOSSARY

## KEY TERMS IN THIS ENTRY

**battery** • The unauthorized touching of a person by another person, such as when a health-care professional treats a patient beyond what the patient consented to.

**consent form** • A document, prepared for a patient's signature, that discloses his proposed treatment in general terms.

**informed consent** • Permission obtained from a patient to perform a specific test or procedure, after the patient has been fully informed about the test or procedure.

**negligent nondisclosure** • The failure to completely inform a patient about his treatment.

**substantive laws** • Laws that define and regulate a person's rights.

**substitutive consent** • Permission obtained from a parent or guardian of a patient who's a minor.

**therapeutic privilege** • A legal doctrine that permits a doctor, in an emergency situation, to withhold information from the patient if he can prove that disclosing it would adversely affect the patient's health.

**tort** • A private or civil wrong outside of a contractual relationship.

if he withholds any facts that are necessary to form the basis of an intelligent consent by the patient to the proposed treatment."

Since this landmark ruling, a patient can sue for negligent nondisclosure if his doctor fails to give him enough information to make an informed decision.

But the ruling also raised a difficult question: How much information is enough? To help answer this question, the courts have developed two standards—the reasonable doctor standard and the reasonable patient standard.

Today, most state courts use the reasonable doctor standard (also called the malpractice model). Essentially, this standard is based on what another doctor would disclose to a similar patient

under similar circumstances. A famous example is *Natanson v. Kline* (1960). In this case, the doctor failed to inform the patient of the side effects of cobalt radiation therapy. The patient suffered the side effects and sued the doctor. The court ruled that the doctor had a duty to disclose information "which a reasonable medical practitioner would [disclose] under the same or similar circumstances."

In *Kinikin v. Heupel* (1981), a Minnesota court provided a variation on the reasonable doctor standard. This court ruled that a doctor must disclose as much information as any reasonable doctor would under similar circumstances who knew the *particular patient.*

The other standard courts use to decide how much information a patient should be given is the reasonable patient standard. The landmark decision using this standard occurred in *Canterbury v. Spence* (1972). In this case, a patient had a laminectomy, then fell and developed paralysis. The patient charged the doctor with failing to warn him of the inherent risks. The court ruled that the doctor had a duty to disclose as much information as he knew—or should have known—a reasonable patient would need to know to make an informed decision.

Courts may eventually develop variations of this reasonable patient standard based on the information a *particular* patient needs to make his decision. If so, the courts might weigh such personal factors as a patient's intelligence, hopes, fears, and idiosyncrasies.

## Laws that require informed consent

Recently, many state legislatures have passed laws that support the standards of informed consent set by the courts. Twelve states have substantive laws—laws that define informed consent or specify the claims and defenses that can be made in informed consent cases. (The 12 states are Alaska, Delaware,

Hawaii, Kentucky, Nebraska, New Hampshire, Oregon, Pennsylvania, Tennessee, Texas, Utah, and Vermont.)

Five other states have procedural laws on informed consent—laws that describe the tort of negligent nondisclosure and possible defenses to such a lawsuit. (These states are Florida, Maine, New York, North Carolina, and Rhode Island.) In addition, Washington State has a law that is both substantive and procedural.

Five other states (Mississippi, Arkansas, Louisiana, Georgia, and Missouri) have laws that deal with consent but not *informed* consent. And other states (including Idaho, Iowa, Nevada, and Ohio) have laws limited to the legal effect of documents, such as consent forms.

Among state laws on informed consent, Georgia's is unique. It says that a signed consent form disclosing the treatment in general terms is *conclusive* proof of a valid consent. Thus, in Georgia, a patient who signs a consent form has no legal right to claim he didn't fully understand a medical treatment or that the doctor didn't explain the information in the consent form.

In most other states, a signed consent form is *evidence* of informed consent, but it's not *conclusive proof.* Even if a patient signs a form, he may still challenge his consent's validity in court—claiming, for example, that he didn't understand the information or that he wasn't given relevant information. Most state laws don't even *require* a signed consent form. Some states accept as evidence of informed consent a doctor's handwritten progress notes, stating that he discussed the proposed procedure, its risks, benefits, and alternatives with the patient, and that the patient consented.

### When is informed consent required?

Implied consent is required before any treatment or procedure. As a nurse, you get this kind of consent by explaining the procedure before you perform it. At that point, any conscious, mentally competent adult has a right to refuse to let you perform the nursing treatment or procedure. The controversy over informed consent centers on medical and surgical treatments and procedures that are invasive, risky, experimental, or unlikely to succeed. For these, the doctor must obtain express consent for treatments and procedures (see *Key Terms in this Entry*) unless delaying necessary treatment to get consent will adversely affect the patient's health.

### Who's responsible for obtaining informed consent?

The responsibility for obtaining a patient's informed consent rests with the person who'll perform the treatment or procedure. Usually this is the attending doctor.

Ideally, each doctor would disclose the information necessary for informed consent, then have the patient sign a consent form. The doctor would also sign the form to indicate that he'd witnessed the patient's signing. In reality, however, some hospitals have a policy requiring their nurses to witness patients' signatures. If your hospital has such a policy, you need to understand

---

## THERAPEUTIC PRIVILEGE: WHEN WITHHOLDING INFORMATION IS ALLOWED

The doctrine of informed consent assumes that an informed patient can act in his own best interests. But what if information about his condition seems likely to act against his interests—if the information itself would jeopardize his health? In these situations, the courts recognize a doctor's *therapeutic privilege.* This legal concept permits the doctor to withhold information he believes would jeopardize the patient's health. This concept of therapeutic privilege may be extended to allow the doctor to provide care to the patient before obtaining his informed consent. But after the risk has passed, the doctor must inform the patient.

ADVICE

# PATIENT CONSENT: ACTING LEGALLY AND RESPONSIBLY

### Consent before or after sedation?

*We have an ongoing conflict with the anesthesiologist on our short-stay surgical unit. The problem is, some patients arrive for surgery without signed consent forms. (Their surgeons bring the forms when they come to the hospital just before surgery.)*

*Our problem is that the anesthesiologist wants us to sedate the patient before the surgeon arrives with the consent form. We contend that we can't legally sedate the patient before we see the signed consent. The anesthesiologist argues that we shouldn't clinically withhold sedation because the patient needs it to be properly prepared for general anesthesia.*

*Can we legally give the sedative after we inform the anesthesiologist there's no consent? Or should we continue to sedate the patient until the signed consent arrives?—RN, Ariz.*

Check your hospital's preoperative checklist. If it requires a signed operative consent before a patient is sedated (most hospital policies stipulate this), then the surgeon, the anesthesiologist, and *you* must abide by this policy. You must continue to refuse to sedate the patient until *you* see the signed consent.

If you don't have a preoperative checklist (or the checklist doesn't require a consent form before sedation), document the problem, and ask the administration's help. In the meantime, have the patients bring their own consents. Or, if the surgeons are concerned that the patients will forget, the surgeons can have their secretaries deliver the consents well ahead of surgery.

### Nonconsensual procedures

*For the past year, I've been working in the emergency department (ED) of a large metropolitan hospital, where we frequently treat victims of assault and battery, rape, alcohol-related incidents, and other violence. We're sometimes asked to cooperate with investigating police officers by obtaining blood specimens for legal evidence.*

*Just last month I was asked to take a blood smear from a patient, allegedly involved in a murder, whose arm was streaked with blood. I did it, but I was unsure whether my action was legal.*

*Since the man was fully conscious, should I have obtained his consent before I took the blood sample? Since the procedure was noninvasive, was his verbal or written consent necessary at all? And how about informing him of his rights before I took the specimen as legal evidence?—RN, Vt.*

An informed consent signed by the patient is always your best protection against liability. Ideally, the consent form should describe *what* the procedure is, *why* it's being done, and *how* the results will be used. If you get this straight before each procedure, there is no question of the patient having been misled.

A 1966 U.S. Supreme Court decision *(Schmerber v. California)* held that a health-care provider could obtain a blood sample against the patient's wishes *only if the patient was under arrest and the test was likely to produce evidence.* If these criteria are met, we suspect that a noninvasive procedure like taking a blood smear sample would be legally permissible. As an

your responsibilities as a witness.

## What your signature means

Your signature as a witness indicates that you saw the patient sign the consent form and that he was awake, alert, and aware of what he was signing. So, before you give a consent form to a patient to sign, check his records to be sure he hasn't recently received any

preanesthetic drugs, narcotics, barbiturates, or anesthesia. If he has, put the unsigned form back in his chart, and notify your supervisor and the attending doctor.

If the patient is alert, have him read the consent form, or read it to him, before he signs it. If the patient doesn't understand the information or wants more information, you can answer any

added precaution in the future, you should tell the arresting officer you'll get the sample after he reads the patient his legal rights.

### Overstepping my bounds?

*As an operating room nurse, I have the job of explaining preoperative procedures to patients scheduled for next-day surgery.*

*Recently, I stopped in to see a middle-aged man scheduled for a bilateral orchiectomy. I explained the preoperative procedures to him and then, almost routinely, asked if he had any questions. I couldn't believe my ears when he asked, "Exactly what is a bilateral orchiectomy?"*

*When I explained that it was removal of both testicles, the patient was clearly shaken. He said he hadn't fully realized what the surgery involved because the doctor had described it in vague terms.*

*I tried to reassure the patient, and I advised him not to sign the surgical consent form until he'd talked to his doctor again.*

*I reported the conversation to my charge nurse and my supervisor, and they advised me to call the patient's doctor at once and explain the problem to him.*

*The doctor was wild. He accused me of "practicing medicine" and said he had told the patient "all he needed to know." Then he warned me: "If you ever overstep your bounds again, I'll file a complaint against you."*

*I can't believe I was wrong. If the patient had signed the consent form and went into surgery without realizing what it entailed, couldn't he have sued the doctor and the hospital? (By the way, the patient did sign the consent form, but I understand that the doctor had a lot of talking to do first.) What's your viewpoint?*—RN, Ill.

The doctor shouldn't have accused you—he should've *thanked you,* but that's beside the point. The real issue is: *Were* you overstepping your bounds? The answer—a very defininte *no.* The patient could've looked up "orchiectomy" in a medical dictionary and found the answer to his question. But he didn't. He asked you, and you answered him truthfully.

The doctor is responsible for getting the patient's informed consent. So he took a big risk when he failed to explain the procedure adequately. If the patient had signed the form without an explanation, the consent would not have been "informed." The patient might have sued—and won.

If you encounter this problem again (and chances are you will), do just what you did before. Reassure your patient, tell him *not* to sign the consent form until he talks to the doctor again, and tell your supervisor and the doctor about your action. Next time, go one step further, and *document* everything in your nurses' notes.

Chances are the doctor won't thank you *next* time, either. But good documentation will ensure your administration's support if the doctor complains.

---

These letters were taken from the files of *Nursing* magazine.

---

questions that are within the scope of your practice. However, you *aren't* obligated to answer any of the patient's questions. Your role as a witness doesn't include the legal responsibility for disclosing all relevant information to the patient. That's the doctor's legal responsibility, and he *cannot* delegate it to you.

That doesn't mean that you have no legal responsibility to the patient regarding informed consent. If you see that a patient is confused about explanations he's received, and *you* don't provide the information he needs, you're responsible for documenting your observation in the patient's chart and making sure the patient gets the information from his doctor or another appropriate source.

## The legal risk involved in doing nothing

If you know a patient hasn't been informed and you do nothing, you, and sometimes your hospital, can be held legally responsible.

Usually, the courts won't hold the hospital responsible if the patient charges the doctor with battery for performing a procedure without the pa-

tient's consent. But the courts might hold *you* responsible if you took part in the battery or knew it was taking place and didn't try to stop it.

Similarly, the courts won't usually hold the hospital responsible if the patient charges the doctor with negligent nondisclosure for failing to provide adequate information for consent. But, again, the court might hold you re-

---

## THE RIGHT TO CONSENT: FROM BIRTH TO ADULTHOOD

As you know, a minor's rights in making independent decisions about medical treatment are more restricted than an adult's rights. However, in certain instances, a doctor or judge may decide a minor is mature—has a sufficiently developed awareness and mental capacity. In these instances, the minor, not his parents, has the right to make decisions about his medical treatment. This chart details how medical rights change from birth to adulthood.

From birth, everyone has the right to:
- confidentiality concerning medical records
- privacy during treatment
- legal protection from malpractice.

A minor—anyone under the age of 18 or 21, depending on the state where he lives—has the right to:
- consent to treatment for sexually transmitted diseases, serious communicable diseases, and drug or alcohol abuse (although the minor's parents may have to be notified).

A mature minor—a minor that a doctor or judge considers *mature*—has the right to:
- consent to, or refuse, medical experimentation and emergency care, as well as routine care
- obtain contraceptives and advice about contraception (although the minor's parents may have to be notified)
- obtain an abortion (although the minor's parents may have to be notified)
- request a second opinion if his parents have him committed to a mental health facility.

An adult—anyone who's reached majority or who's legally emancipated—has the right to:
- consent to, or refuse, medical treatment
- consent to, or refuse, medical treatment for a spouse or children in certain circumstances.

sponsible if—knowing the doctor hasn't provided adequate information to a patient—you don't perform your professional and legal duty to try to stop the procedure by informing your supervisor.

Usually though, you can meet your legal obligation for informed consent by ensuring that the consent form has been signed and witnessed and that it's attached to the patient's chart.

### Informed consent for treating the sedated patient

If you know a doctor is going to seek consent from a patient receiving a sedative, narcotic, or tranquilizer, make sure the doctor is aware of the patient's medication schedule. Then the doctor can select an appropriate time to explain the procedure or treatment and thus ensure that a valid consent has been obtained.

If the patient receives such medication before the doctor explains the procedure or treatment, the doctor should evaluate the patient's mental status. If his mental status is impaired, his consent will be invalid, and someone else will have to give consent for him.

If the patient is comatose from a long-term disease process, the doctor may ask the court to appoint a guardian for the patient. But if immediate treatment is needed, the doctor may, as a practical matter, seek consent from the nearest relative.

### Informed consent to treat incompetent adults

A patient who's been declared incompetent by a court (such a patient is called an *adjudicated incompetent*) cannot give a valid consent. In such instances, a court-appointed guardian must give consent: consent from a relative or friend may *not* be legally binding.

When a patient is incompetent but hasn't been adjudicated as such, the doctor has two alternatives. He may seek consent from the patient's next of kin—usually his spouse. (Note that de-

termining who's the next of kin is a legal question and varies from state to state.) Or the doctor or hospital may petition the court to appoint a legal guardian for the patient. The courts haven't specified which alternative a doctor should choose. When to appoint a legal guardian remains a controversial issue. Generally, doctors go to court when they don't feel comfortable with the next of kin's decision.

The decision that a patient is incompetent can be very difficult, particularly with a mentally ill patient: don't make the mistake of assuming that mental illness is the same as incompetence. Several court decisions have upheld the constitutional right of the

---

*"Generally, doctors petition the court to appoint a legal guardian when they don't feel comfortable with the next of kin's decision."*

---

alert, involuntarily confined mental patient to refuse medication and treatment even if the treatment might ameliorate the mental illness. Even a committed mental patient can be forcibly medicated *only* in an emergency when he may cause harm to himself or others.

### Obtaining informed consent to treat minors

In most situations, a minor's consent to treatment is legally invalid, so the doctor must obtain *substitutive consent* from the parents or guardians. In these instances, the doctor is legally obligated to disclose all relevant information to the parents or guardians to ensure their consent is informed.

In some situations, minors *can* give consent. For instance, some states let a minor give legal consent to treatment of a sexually transmitted disease. And most states let an emancipated minor— one who's married, a parent, or financially independent—give legal consent to treatment.

To avoid difficult judgments on whether a minor is legally emancipated, a doctor usually tries to get informed consent from both a minor and his parents (see Entry 26).

## Two exceptions to the need for informed consent

There are two situations in which the legal requirement for informed consent is waived. In one situation, the patient himself waives the requirement. In the other, the urgent nature of a medical or surgical emergency waives the requirement.

## What to do when the patient doesn't want to be informed

A patient's rights include the right *not* to be informed. If a patient exercises that right by telling his doctor that he doesn't want to know the details regarding a treatment or procedure, the doctor has two responsibilities. He must make sure that the patient understands that risks and alternatives do exist. And he must document the patient's waiver of his right to receive information.

## How to handle informed consent in emergencies

A doctor can legally treat a patient without getting his consent if the patient needs immediate treatment to save his life or to prevent loss of an organ, limb, or function, and the doctor can't get consent because the patient is unconscious and the family can't be reached. In such situations, the law assumes that if a patient could decide, he would choose to receive treatment rather than risk the consequences of no treatment.

This form of "consent" is very lim-

ited, however. It doesn't apply if the doctor knows the patient has previously said he'd refuse treatment. And it also doesn't apply if he can wait for a proper consent from the patient or his family without increasing the patient's risk. For example, a doctor may admit a minor patient with acute appendicitis, but he can't do emergency surgery without consent if he has time to obtain the parents' informed consent.

If you assist in emergency treatment without consent, make sure the doctor documents his reasons for proceeding, including the specific risks the patient would face without treatment.

What should you do if the doctor wants to provide emergency care without consent, but you feel the patient could wait? First, tell the doctor why

---

*"In an emergency, the law assumes that if a patient could decide, he would choose to receive treatment...."*

---

you feel that way. If the doctor insists on treating the patient anyway, evaluate the likely consequences of two courses of action:
- If your refusal to help would harm the patient or create an unsafe situation (a doctor caring for a patient without assistance), you should assist, even if you know you're right.
- In all other situations, you should refuse to participate, and then notify your nursing supervisor. She, in turn, should report to hospital administration.

## When does a patient's informed consent become invalid?

You should know that informed consent can become invalid if a change in a patient's medical status alters the risks and benefits of the treatment he consented to. In such situations, the doctor must explain the new risks and benefits to the consenting patient to be sure he still consents to the treatment. And the doctor must explain any new risks or benefits to a nonconsenting patient to be sure he still wants to refuse the treatment.

### A final word

Don't let the legal complexities of informed consent frighten you. You should take the time to know your state laws, but you shouldn't be overwhelmed by them. If you're in doubt, get advice from your hospital's legal services department. Above all, remember these two important guidelines: The patient has a legal right to determine the treatment he receives, and you have a professional responsibility to protect that right.

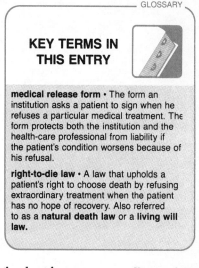

GLOSSARY

## KEY TERMS IN THIS ENTRY

**medical release form** • The form an institution asks a patient to sign when he refuses a particular medical treatment. The form protects both the institution and the health-care professional from liability if the patient's condition worsens because of his refusal.

**right-to-die law** • A law that upholds a patient's right to choose death by refusing extraordinary treatment when the patient has no hope of recovery. Also referred to as a **natural death law** or a **living will law.**

# 13 The patient who refuses treatment

You're in the business of saving lives, so you probably have a hard time accepting a patient's decision to refuse treatment. You may be very disturbed, for example, when a patient refuses treatment he can't live without—just to avoid unpleasant side effects. But as a professional, you know you must respect that decision. Laws and court rulings give almost all patients the right to refuse treatment.

When your patient refuses treatment, you must understand his right and your responsibilities. If you don't, you increase your legal risks on the job.

### Where did the right to refuse treatment come from?

Most right-to-privacy court cases have involved patients or their families who want to discontinue life-support treatment for a terminal illness. In one of the best-known cases, Karen Ann Quinlan's parents argued that unwanted treatment violated their comatose daughter's right to privacy. In 1976, the parents successfully petitioned the court to discontinue her life-support treatment.

Many right-to-religious-freedom court cases have involved Jehovah's Witnesses. Members of this sect oppose blood transfusions because a section of the Bible forbids "drinking" blood. Some sect members believe that even a life-saving transfusion given against their will deprives them of everlasting life. The courts usually respect their refusals because of the constitutionally protected right to religious freedom. In the case of *Osborne* (1972), for example, the court respected a Jehovah's Witness' right to refuse consent.

Most other religious freedom court cases involve Christian Scientists, who oppose many medical interventions, including medicines. For example, in *Winters v. Miller* (1971), a psychiatric patient claimed she involuntarily received treatment and medications at a New York state hospital. After her discharge, she sued for damages based on a violation of her religious freedom as a Christian Scientist. The trial court dismissed her complaint, but an ap-

# WHEN A PATIENT SAYS NO

As you know, a patient must give his consent before you can perform any treatment. Do you know what to do if he refuses?

If the patient refuses, start by telling him the risks involved in not having the treatment done. If the patient understands the risks but still refuses, notify your supervisor and the doctor. Record the patient's refusal in your nurses' notes.

Next, ask the patient to fill out a refusal-of-treatment release form, like the one shown below. The signed form indicates that the appropriate treatment would have been given had the patient consented. This form protects you, the patient's doctors, and your institution from liability for not providing treatment.

If the patient refuses to sign the release form, document this in your nurses' notes. For additional protection, your institution's policy may require you to get the patient's spouse or closest relative to sign another refusal-of-treatment release form. Document whether or not the spouse or relative does this.

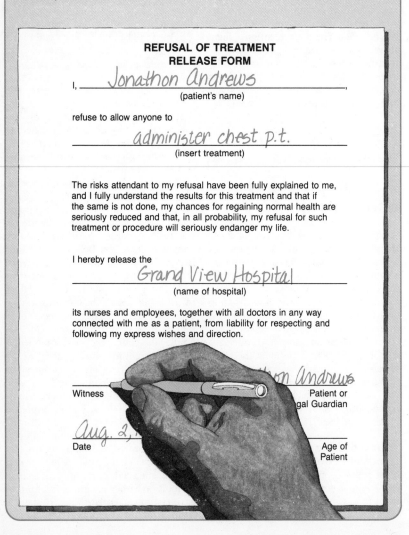

## REFUSAL OF TREATMENT RELEASE FORM

I, _Jonathon Andrews_ ,
(patient's name)

refuse to allow anyone to

_administer chest p.t._
(insert treatment)

The risks attendant to my refusal have been fully explained to me, and I fully understand the results for this treatment and that if the same is not done, my chances for regaining normal health are seriously reduced and that, in all probability, my refusal for such treatment or procedure will seriously endanger my life.

I hereby release the

_Grand View Hospital_
(name of hospital)

its nurses and employees, together with all doctors in any way connected with me as a patient, from liability for respecting and following my express wishes and direction.

_____
Witness

_____ _Andrews_
Patient or
gal Guardian

_aug. 2,_
Date

_____
Age of
Patient

peals court ordered a new trial on the grounds that the unwanted treatment might have violated her rights.

Besides court rulings, most patients' bills of rights also support the right to refuse treatment—starting with the bill of rights adopted by the American Hospital Association in 1973 (see Entry 11).

### What part do state laws play?

State laws provide another legal authority for the right to refuse treatment. Twenty-three states have informed-consent laws that require you to explain the risks of nontreatment to a patient who refuses nursing treatment. Thirteen states and the District of Columbia have right-to-die laws (also called *natural death laws* or *living will laws*). These laws recognize the patient's right to choose death by refusing extraordinary treatment when he has no hope of recovery. For example, they would support a terminally-ill patient's (or his family's) insistence that a hospital discontinue life support (see Entry 30).

Each state has established its own guidelines, so ask your employer for a summary of your state's right-to-refuse-treatment laws. In general, the same right-to-refuse-treatment laws apply in Canada and the United States.

### Reasons to challenge the right to refuse

Any mentally competent adult can legally refuse treatment if he's fully informed about his medical condition and about the likely consequences of his refusal. This leaves you two grounds for challenging a patient's right to refuse. You can claim that the patient is incompetent, or you can claim that compelling reasons exist to overrule his wishes.

The courts consider a patient incompetent when he lacks the mental ability to make a reasoned decision, such as when he's delirious.

The courts also recognize several compelling reasons to overrule a patient's refusal of treatment. Here are some of the reasons:

• Refusing treatment endangers the life of another. For example, a court may overrule a pregnant woman's objection to treatment, in order to save her unborn child's life.

• A relative wants to withhold treatment of an incompetent patient.

• A parent wants to withhold lifesaving treatment from his child. For example, a court may overrule parents' religious objections to their child's treatment when the child's life is endangered. When the child's life isn't in danger, however, the courts are more likely to

---

## AVOIDING BATTERY CHARGES

Can you be sued for battery—intentionally touching another person without authorization to do so—for simply doing what a doctor has ordered? Yes—if the patient refuses the treatment. Here's a fictional example:

Albert Proxy, age 69, is hospitalized with a gastrointestinal disorder. He's also depressed and uncooperative. His day-shift nurse, Bernice Bransted, reads on his chart that the doctor ordered an enema.

Disgruntled and surly, Mr. Proxy has other ideas. He bluntly tells the nurse: "Leave me alone. I'm not getting an enema now!"

Despite his protests, Ms. Bransted insists. She gently turns him in his bed and administers the enema.

Later, Mr. Proxy's son becomes angry when his father tells him what happened. The son confronts the nursing supervisor and warns her that he intends to pursue the matter.

Does Mr. Proxy have a case for battery against the nurse? Yes. As a conscious, coherent adult, even though depressed, Mr. Proxy has the right to refuse treatment. After he—or any other adult patient—refuses any nursing treatment, giving it will make the nurse liable for battery.

## WHEN THE COURT MAY OVERRULE THE PATIENT

Can your patient refuse life-support treatment under any circumstances? Can a relative of an unconscious adult patient force you to withhold treatment? Can parents stop you from treating their child?

Usually, the court respects a patient's right to refuse treatment if the patient is capable of making a reasoned decision. And it usually lets the parent or legal guardian of a child decide about the child's care, provided that the parent doesn't refuse lifesaving treatment. But the court will intervene in certain circumstances, even when the patient's or parent's decision rests on constitutionally protected grounds, such as religious beliefs. If you ever get caught between a patient and his family and a court, you'll be better prepared to deal with the situation if you know about previous court rulings in this area. Here are some delicate legal situations the court has ruled on:

• If an adult patient becomes physically or mentally incapacitated, a relative can't always refuse treatment for him. The court reserves the right to overrule even a spouse in the patient's behalf. For example, in *Collins v. Davis* (1964), the court overruled the wife's refusal of surgery for her unconscious husband.

• If a patient who's responsible for the care of a child refuses lifesaving treatment, the court may reverse the patient's decision. In *Application of the President and Directors of Georgetown College, Inc.* (1964), the court ordered a blood transfusion for a Jehovah's Witness who was the mother of an infant and who refused to give consent for the transfusion. In the *Melideo* case (1976), the court said that it might have ordered a lifesaving transfusion for the patient if she had had a child.

• If a patient who's pregnant refuses treatment, thereby threatening not only her health but also that of her unborn child, the court has reversed the patient's decision. In *Jefferson v. Griffin Spalding County Hospital Authority* (1981), the court awarded temporary custody of the unborn child to a state agency. The mother had a complete placenta previa but had refused to consent to a cesarean section. The court's custody award included full authority to give consent for a surgical delivery.

• If a patient is a minor, the court will allow his parents or legal guardian to consent to medical treatment, but not allow them to deny him lifesaving treatment. *In re Sampson* (1972) was such a case.

---

respect the parents' religious convictions. In the *Green* case (1972), the court upheld the parents' wish to withhold treatment from their 16-year-old child.

• The patient links his refusal of treatment with a strong indication that he wants to live, by making statements to you such as that he fears death. For example, some Jehovah's Witnesses who oppose blood transfusions say or imply that they won't prevent the transfusions if a court takes responsibility for the decision. In *Powell v. Columbian-Presbyterian Medical Center* (1965), the court authorized transfusions when a Jehovah's Witness indicated she wouldn't object to receiving blood, although she'd refused to give written consent.

• Public interest outweighs the patient's right. For example, the law re-

quires school-age children to receive polio vaccines before they can attend classes.

### What to do when a patient refuses treatment

A patient planning to refuse treatment may tell *you* first. When he tells you he's going to refuse treatment or he simply refuses to give consent, stop preparations for any treatment at once. Then immediately report your patient's decision to your supervisor. She'll notify the doctor and hospital administrator. Never delay informing your supervisor, especially if a delay could be life-threatening. Any delay you're responsible for will greatly increase your legal risks. The doctor and hospital have the responsibility to take action, such as trying to convince the patient to accept treatment or asking him to sign a re-

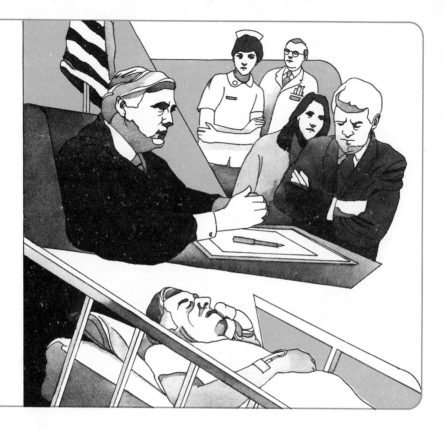

lease form. This form relieves the hospital and its health team of liability for any consequences the patient might suffer by refusing treatment. (However, the release form doesn't release the health team from its obligation to continue providing care.)

If the patient has refused life-sustaining treatment and you're asked to participate in terminating treatment, be sure you fully understand your state's right-to-die law first. (See Entries 30 and 70.) Otherwise—even with a signed release form—you could face criminal or civil charges for honoring *or* violating the request. For example, some states could prosecute you on criminal charges if you allowed a patient to die by withholding the life-support treatment he refused. In other states, a patient or his family could sue you for battery for continuing life-

support measures they refused. (A patient can sue you for battery even if you administer a treatment that helps him.)

### How can you challenge the patient's refusal?

To overrule the patient's decision, the doctor or your hospital must obtain a court order. Only then are you legally authorized to administer a treatment your patient doesn't want.

If the doctor or hospital tries to convince the court to overrule a patient's refusal on the grounds that he's incompetent, they'll need proof that he lacks the mental ability to make a reasoned decision. That proof can come from your documented observations about your patient's mental status.

The refusal itself, no matter how serious the patient's condition, isn't evidence of incompetence. In *Lane v.*

*Candura* (1978), for example, a Massachusetts diabetic patient first agreed to have her leg amputated, then changed her mind and refused the surgery. The doctors applied for a court order, arguing that by changing her mind the patient had shown incompetence. The court disagreed. It upheld the patient's right to withdraw her consent.

### How emergencies affect the right to refuse

A competent adult has the right to refuse even emergency treatment. His family can't overrule his decision, and his doctor may not give the expressly refused treatment even if the patient becomes unconscious.

Sometimes, however, *not* giving emergency treatment that the patient has refused can incur liability. For example, a patient who refuses treatment in an irrational way—with disjointed statements and gestures—could be considered incompetent. In that situation, the doctor could be held liable for not treating him.

Obviously, for your protection as well as your patient's, you need to exercise great care when dealing with a difficult patient in an emergency. Make sure the doctor waits till he has consent, if that's possible. And make sure he has a court order before you assist in giving emergency care to a competent patient who refuses treatment.

If you have no grounds for seeking a court order to overrule your patient's refusal, you have an ethical duty to defend his right to refuse treatment in the face of all opposition, even his family's. If they disagree with his decision, try to explain why he made it. But emphasize that the decision is his as long as he's competent.

You also have a responsibility to continue to inform your patient about treatment, because he may change his mind.

### A final word

Even if you disagree with a patient's refusal, you must let him know that you'll abide by his decision. To do otherwise will compromise your credibility, your patient's trust in you, and your professional integrity.

# 14 Protecting your patient's privacy

Have you ever had to obtain highly personal, even embarrassing, information from a patient to care for him properly? If so, you probably remember how uncomfortable you both felt. You may have tried to put him at ease by reassuring him that you'd keep his information confidential. But did you stop to think about the complexities of that responsibility?

How do you exercise that responsibility when your patient's spouse, other health-care professionals, the media, or public health agencies ask you to disclose confidential information? Find out by reading this entry on your responsibility to maintain your patient's privacy.

### In the eyes of the law

Privacy and confidentiality were first proposed as basic legal rights in 1890 in a *Harvard Law Review* article entitled "The Right to Privacy."

The U.S. Constitution doesn't explicitly sanction a right to privacy. But in *Griswold v. Connecticut* (1965), *Katz v. United States* (1967), *Stanley v. Georgia* (1969), and *Roe v. Wade* (1973), the U.S. Supreme Court cited several constitutional amendments that imply the right to privacy.

Essentially, the right to privacy is the right to be left alone—and to make personal choices without outside interference. In the landmark case of *Griswold v. Connecticut* (1965), for example, the U.S. Supreme Court recognized a married couple's right to privacy in contraceptive use. In *Eisenstadt v. Baird* (1972), the Supreme Court extended the privacy right to include unmarried persons. In *Carey v. Population Services International* (1977), the Supreme Court said a state law that prohibited the sale of contraceptives to anyone under age 16 was unconstitutional. The court held that the decision to bear a child is a fundamental right and that the state law could only be justified if it protected a compelling state interest.

Recently, the Department of Health and Human Services tried to modify the Court's ruling in the *Carey* case. The department published a regulation, "Parental Notification Requirements Applicable to Projects for Family Planning Services." Also known as the "squeal rule," it proposes that any federally funded clinic or health agency that gives contraceptives to a minor must inform the minor's parents or guardian. A New York federal district court has already declared that divulging such confidential information invades the minor's privacy and is unconstitutional.

The Supreme Court ruling in *Roe v. Wade* (1973) protects a woman's right to privacy in having an abortion during the first trimester. The ruling permits a woman and her doctor to decide to terminate the pregnancy free from state intrusion until the end of the first trimester. After the first trimester, a state may regulate abortion to protect the mother's health. And the state may prohibit an abortion if the fetus is judged able to live outside the womb.

The *Roe v. Wade* decision played an important role in getting abortion rights extended to minors.

In *Planned Parenthood of Central Missouri v. Danforth* (1976), the Supreme Court overruled a law that prevented first trimester abortions for minors without parental consent. Its decision hinged on the *Roe v. Wade* decision that a state could not interfere with a woman's personal choice to abort her pregnancy during the first trimester.

GLOSSARY

## KEY TERMS IN THIS ENTRY

**confidentiality** • A professional responsibility to keep all privileged information private.

**fiduciary relationship** • A legal relationship of confidentiality that exists whenever one person trusts or relies on another—such as a doctor-patient relationship.

**privilege doctrine** • A doctrine that protects the privacy of persons within a fiduciary relationship, such as a husband and wife, a doctor and patient, or a nurse and patient. During legal proceedings, a court can't force either party to reveal communication that occurred between them unless the party who'd benefit from the protection agrees to it.

In a similar case, *Belotti v. Baird II* (1979), the Court acknowledged that the privacy rights of a minor are not equal to the constitutional rights of adults. But it held that a state law requiring a minor to obtain parental consent for an abortion infringed on the minor's rights.

In some cases of abortion involving minors, parental notification may be necessary. In *H. L. v. Matheson* (1981), the Supreme Court ruled that a state may require parental notification before an abortion if the minor is immature or unemancipated. The law has been judged to be constitutional because it doesn't prohibit a minor from getting an abortion. (See Entry 73.)

## How the states support the patient's right to privacy

The right to privacy has received even more attention at the state level. Ten states—Alaska, Arizona, California, Florida, Hawaii, Illinois, Louisiana, Montana, South Carolina, and Washington—have written some type of privacy provision into their constitutions. And nearly all states have recognized the right to privacy through statutory or common law.

The state courts have been strong in protecting the patient's right to not have confidential information revealed about him. Even in court, your patient is protected by the privilege doctrine. According to this doctrine, people who have a protected relationship—such as a doctor and patient—can't be forced, even during legal proceedings, to reveal communication between them unless the person who'd benefit from the protection—usually the patient—agrees to it.

State law determines which relationships are protected by the privilege doctrine. Most states include husband-wife, lawyer-client, and doctor-patient relationships.

At present, only four states (New York, Arkansas, Oregon, and Vermont) recognize the nurse-patient relationship as protected. But some courts have said the privilege exists when a nurse is following doctor's orders. Whether the privilege applies to LPNs/LVNs as well is uncertain.

Some courts have allowed a hospital or doctor to withhold confidential information on the patient's behalf. But the hospital's motive cannot be self-protection, as it was in *People v. Doe* (1978). In this case, a nursing home was being investigated for allegedly mistreating its patients. The court ruled that the nursing home's attempt to invoke patient privilege was unjust, since the issue at hand was the patient's welfare.

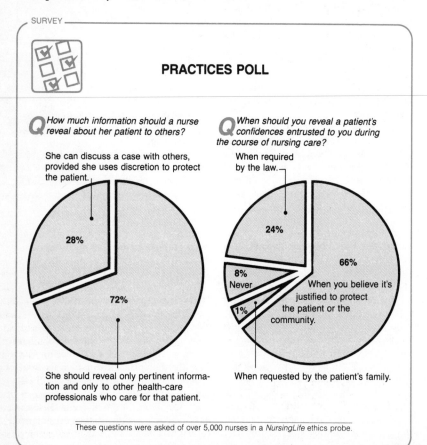

SURVEY

## PRACTICES POLL

**Q** How much information should a nurse reveal about her patient to others?

She can discuss a case with others, provided she uses discretion to protect the patient.

28%

72%

She should reveal only pertinent information and only to other health-care professionals who care for that patient.

**Q** When should you reveal a patient's confidences entrusted to you during the course of nursing care?

When required by the law.

24%

66%
When you believe it's justified to protect the patient or the community.

8% Never

1%

When requested by the patient's family.

These questions were asked of over 5,000 nurses in a *NursingLife* ethics probe.

## How far does the privilege extend?

State laws also determine the extent of the privilege in protected relationships. In some states, a patient automatically waives his right to doctor-patient privilege when he files a personal injury or workmen's compensation lawsuit.

The purpose of the privilege doctrine in patient relationships—doctor-patient, nurse-patient—is to encourage the patient to reveal confidential information that may be essential to his treatment. The doctrine guarantees that no one will reveal his confidential information without his permission. In *Hammonds v. Aetna Casualty and Surety Co.* (1965), the court reinforced that guarantee by declaring that protecting a patient's privacy is a doctor's legal duty. It further ruled that a patient could sue for damages any unauthorized person who disclosed confidential medical information about him. Similarly, a patient can sue for invasion of privacy any unauthorized personnel, such as student nurses, who observe him without his permission. The only hospital personnel who have a right to observe a patient are those involved in his diagnosis, treatment, and related care.

## Canada's view of patient privacy

Canadian common law recognizes the privilege doctrine in doctor-patient relationships, but not in nurse-patient relationships. (Cases that suggest the doctor-patient privilege include *Dembie*, 1963; *Re SAS*, 1977; and *Geransky*, 1977.) However, the Canadian Nurses Association and the provincial licensing authorities have adopted the International Council of Nurses Code of Ethics. (See *International Council of Nurses Code of Ethics*, in the appendices.) The code requires you to keep confidential any personal information you receive from a patient during the course of your nursing care. Consequently, although violation of a patient's right to privacy isn't subject to criminal prosecution in Canada, it is deemed professional misconduct. So in Canada, a nurse who violates a patient's right to privacy can lose her nursing license.

## Nurses' responsibilities in protecting patient privacy

Despite the *legal* uncertainties regarding nurses' responsibilities under the privilege doctrine, you have a professional and ethical responsibility to protect your patient's privacy, whether you're an RN or an LPN or an LVN, a Canadian or an American.

This responsibility requires more of you than sealed lips. You may have to educate your patients about their right

> *"The court has declared that protecting a patient's privacy is a doctor's legal duty."*

to privacy. Some of them may be unaware of what their right to privacy means, or that they even have such a right. In such situations, you must inform the patient of his rights and make sure his wishes are carried out. Explain that he can refuse to allow pictures to be taken of his disorder and its treatment, for example. And tell him he can choose to have information about his condition withheld from others, including family members. (For additional information about a patient's rights, see Entry 11.)

## When can you disclose confidential information?

If your patient is exercising his right to privacy in such a way that others' well-being is threatened, you may have to violate his privacy and reveal confidential information.

Under certain circumstances, you can lawfully disclose confidential in-

## KEEPING PATIENT INFORMATION CONFIDENTIAL: HOW TO HANDLE A REPORTER'S QUESTIONS

Imagine this: A reporter approaches you in the hospital and asks if a local government official is being treated for cancer. Would you know how to answer?

Usually, you'd answer a reporter's question directly and honestly. As a general rule, you can release the patient's name, age, address, and condition—as good, fair, serious, or critical—with one exception: Don't release a patient's name until you know that his family has been notified.

But what do you say when a direct, honest answer would violate your patient's right to confidentiality?

The best answer is, "Call my nursing supervisor or the hospital's public relations officer." If neither is available, answer as honestly as you can *without releasing confidential information.* Here are some sample answers to some tough questions:

**Q.** Is the sheriff being treated at your hospital for cancer?

**A.** The sheriff *is* being treated at our hospital. He's listed in fair condition. I can't release the nature of his problem because that's confidential information.

**Q.** The sheriff is a community leader. The public has a right to know if he's seriously ill. Can't you just tell me if he has cancer?

**A.** I'd like to help you, but you know that our hospital can't release confidential patient information. I'll be happy to tell the sheriff you'd like more information about him. If he gives the okay, someone will contact you.

**Q.** Mary Jones was brought to your hospital by ambulance tonight. The police say she was raped. Can you confirm that?

**A.** We never confirm whether a patient has been raped. I'm sure you can understand the harm this could cause a patient.

**Q.** Did you treat Mary Jones?

**A.** Yes. Mary Jones was treated and released.

**Q.** Did you treat a child-abuse victim today?

**A.** We can't confirm that a patient is a victim of child abuse. That's for courts to decide.

**Q.** But this child was brought by ambulance. That makes the case a public record. Can you confirm that you treated a child who was the victim of child abuse?

**A.** If you can provide the child's name, I can only confirm whether he was treated here, and I can tell you whether he's listed in good, fair, serious, or critical condition.

formation about your patient. For example, the courts allow disclosure when the welfare of a person or a group of people is at stake.

Consider the patient who's diagnosed as an epileptic and asks you not to tell his family. Depending on the circumstances, you may decide this isn't in the patient's and his family's best interest, particularly in terms of safety. In that situation, inform the patient's doctor; he may then decide to inform the family of the patient's condition to protect the patient's well-being.

You're also protected by law if you disclose confidential information about a patient that's necessary for his continued care, or if your patient consents to the disclosure. But be sure you don't exceed the specified limit of a patient's consent. Taking pictures is the largest single cause of invasion of privacy lawsuits. In *Feeney v. Young* (1920), a woman consented to the filming of her cesarean delivery for viewings by medical societies. But the doctor incorporated the film into a generally released movie entitled *Birth*. The court awarded damages to the woman under the state's privacy law.

The courts have also granted immunity to health-care professionals who, in good faith, have disclosed confidential information to prevent public harm. In *Simonsen v. Swenson* (1920), a doctor who believed his patient had

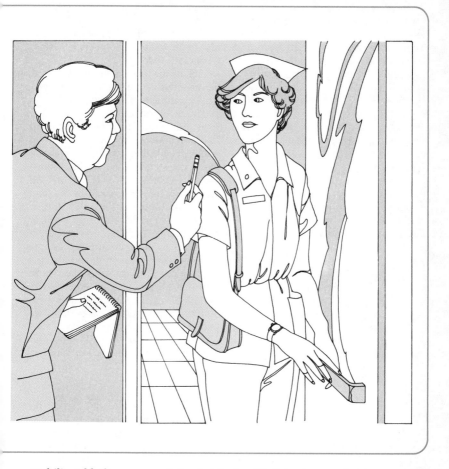

syphilis told the owner of the hotel where the patient was staying about the patient's contagious disease. The court ruled that doctors are privileged to make disclosures that will prevent the spread of disease.

A controversial California case established a doctor's right to disclose information that would protect any person whom a patient threatened to harm. In *Tarasoff v. Regents of the University of California* (1976), a woman was murdered by a mentally ill patient who had told his psychotherapist that he intended to kill her. The victim's parents sued the doctor for failing to warn their daughter. The Supreme Court found the doctor liable because

he didn't try to avert the danger posed by the patient's condition. The Court ruled similarly in *McIntosh v. Milano* (1979).

In some situations, the law requires you to disclose confidential information. For example, all 50 states and the District of Columbia have disclosure laws for child abuse cases. Except for Maine and Montana, all states also grant immunity from legal action for a good-faith report on suspected child abuse.

Courts may also order you to disclose confidential information in cases of child custody and neglect. One case involving such an order was *D. v. D.* (1969). Despite the doctor-patient privilege, the court ordered the doctor to turn the mother's medical records over to the court for a private inspection. The mother had a history of illness, and the court said the inspection would help it decide which parent should be granted custody. The courts made a similar ruling in the custody case of *In re Doe Children* (1978). The court stated that the children's welfare outweighed the parent's right to keep their medical records private.

Some laws create an exemption to the privilege doctrine in criminal cases so that the courts can have access to all essential information. In states where neither a law nor an exemption to the law exists, some courts will *find* an

exemption to the doctrine in criminal cases.

Certain government agencies can also order you to reveal confidential information. Federal agencies that can do so include the Internal Revenue Service, the Environmental Protection Agency, the Department of Labor, and the Department of Health and Human Services. State agencies that can do this include revenue, or tax, bureaus and public health departments. For example, most state public health departments require reports of all communicable diseases, births and deaths, and gunshot wounds.

The newsworthiness of an event or person can also make disclosure acceptable. In such circumstances, the public's right to know must outweigh an individual's right to privacy, as in the assassination attempt on President Ronald Reagan in 1981. Another example was the precedent-setting implantation of an artificial heart in 1982 into Seattle dentist Barney Clark. (See *Keeping Patient Information Confidential: How to Handle a Reporter's Questions,* page 98.)

Even when the public has a right to know about a confidential matter, the courts will not allow the public disclosure to undermine a person's dignity. In *Barber v. Time, Inc.* (1942), *Time* magazine was sued by a woman whose picture and name they published in an article which said the patient suffered from an illness that caused her to eat as much food as 10 people could eat. The court ruled that publishing the patient's name and picture was an unnecessary invasion of her privacy and that ethics required keeping such information confidential.

*Doe v. Roe* (1977) is a similar case: a patient sued a psychiatrist for publishing the patient's biography and thoughts verbatim. Even though the doctor didn't use the patient's name, the court said the patient was readily identifiable by the article. It found the doctor liable for violating the doctor-patient privilege.

## A final word

Other court cases that involve violations of patients' confidences include *Griffin v. Medical Society* (1939) and *Bazemore v. Savannah Hospital* (1930). As these cases and the others discussed show, you're responsible for protecting patients' privacy even when the circumstances allow some disclosure. Clearly, your patient's right to privacy is one that you must carefully uphold.

# 15 The patient who demands to read his chart

Suppose your patient says to you, "I'm paying for the tests; I have a right to know the results." Does he have the legal right to know what's in his medical records?

Yes. And because patients increasingly want explanations about what's being done to them and why, you should know what to do when your patient asks to see his medical records.

## The disclosure debate

For years, health-care experts have debated the merits of letting a patient see his medical records. Proponents argue that the information helps the patient better understand his condition and care and makes him more cooperative.

Opponents—usually doctors and hospitals—argue that the technical jargon and medical abbreviations found in medical records will confuse and perhaps frighten a patient. In addition, opponents claim that opening medical records to a patient will increase the risks of malpractice lawsuits. However, evidence to support this contention doesn't exist.

Legally, the right-to-access debate has centered on other issues. The first issue the courts had to answer involved ownership.

## Who owns a patient's medical records?

The hospital owns the hospital medical records, and the doctor owns his office records, according to court decisions. Generally, the courts have decided that a patient sees a doctor for diagnosis and treatment, not to obtain records for his personal use.

The second issue the courts had to resolve involved access. While granting ownership of medical records to doctors and hospitals, the courts have expressed their own right to get the records anytime they need them for a case review.

For this reason, any patient in any state can file a lawsuit to subpoena his medical records. But some court decisions and some states' laws have given patients the right to direct access. Nine states' laws guarantee a patient's right to his medical information. And in states without such laws, the courts have recognized a patient's right to see the information.

In *Cannell v. Medical and Surgical Clinic S.C.* (1974), the court ruled that a doctor had the duty to disclose medical information to his patient. However, the court said doctors and hospitals needn't turn over the actual files to the patient. Instead, they need only show the complete medical record—or a copy—to the patient.

The court based the patient's limited right to access on two important conclusions:

• A patient has a right to know the details about his medical treatment under common law.

• A patient has a right to the information in his records because he pays for the treatment.

Despite the laws and court decisions, hospitals don't always make access to records easy. Some hospitals discourage a patient from seeing his medical records by putting up bureaucratic barriers. For example, requiring the patient to have an attorney make the request can stifle a patient's attempt to gain access to his records.

## KEY TERMS IN THIS ENTRY

**medical record** • A written, legal record of every aspect of the patient's care.

**right-to-access laws** • Laws that grant a patient the right to see his medical records.

Other hospitals charge high copying fees in an effort to discourage patient record requests. Some states, such as Pennsylvania, have passed laws requiring reasonable copying fees.

In rare circumstances, hospitals can legally deny a patient access to his medical record information. For example, in *Gotkin v. Miller* (1975), a patient wanted access to all her medical records for the 8 years she spent in various New York mental hospitals. She wanted the information for a book she was writing about treatments for mental illness. The court said Mrs. Gotkin's records possibly contained many references to and statements by other patients. Since releasing the Gotkin records would violate the privacy of the other mental patients, the courts said the hospitals didn't have to give Mrs. Gotkin access to her records.

### What to do when your patient asks to see his records

A patient's request should, first, make you question whether you and your colleagues have done enough to communicate with him. When you get such a request, try to assess why. Your patient could simply be curious; but his request may reflect hidden fears. For example, maybe he feels that he isn't being told enough about his treatment.

Next, notify your nursing supervisor that the patient has asked to see his medical records. Also, notify the risk manager, if your facility has one. Why? To alert administrative staff—and legal counsel, if necessary—so they can pro-

tect the hospital's interests.

After your patient gets approval to see his records, stay with him while he reads them. Explain to him that state laws prohibit him from changing or erasing information on his records, even information he considers incorrect. Tell him to show you any information he considers incorrect. Offer to answer any of his questions you can; assure him that his doctor will answer questions, too. In fact, encourage the patient to write down specific questions for his doctor, and offer to contact his doctor for him.

While your patient reads, help him interpret the abbreviations and jargon used in medical charting. One patient hospitalized for hypertension was greatly relieved when her nurse explained that the "malignant hypertension" notation on her chart had nothing to do with cancer.

Observe how the patient responds while he reads. If he becomes apprehensive, puzzled, or angry, be sure he receives calm, professional explanations about his treatment. He may simply seem relieved: some patients want to read their records just to be sure you and the doctors aren't hiding any information. For example, one patient who demanded to see her medical records merely flipped through the pages. The hospital's willingness to share information about her treatment apparently satisfied her.

### Can a patient's relative see the records?

A relative can see a patient's medical records only under these conditions:
• The relative is the patient's legal guardian, and the patient is incompetent.
• The relative has the patient's approval.
• Circumstances indicate that the patient routinely involves the relative in treatment discussions and decisions.

### A final word

Don't be upset or feel defensive when

your patient asks to see his records. You'll probably find he'll gain confidence in you and in his treatment after reading his medical records. Seeing his accurate, well-kept medical records will assure him that he's receiving efficient and safe care.

# 16 The patient who leaves against medical advice

The patient's bill of rights and the laws and regulations based on it give a competent adult the right to refuse treatment for any reason without being punished or having his liberty restricted (see Entries 11 and 13).

Some states have turned these rights into law. And the courts have cited the bills of rights in their decisions.

The right to refuse treatment includes the right to leave the hospital against medical advice (AMA) any time, for any reason. Since the law prohibits you from detaining most patients and upholds their right to leave, all you can do is try to talk them out of it.

But if you think your responsibilities to your patient end if he leaves AMA, you're mistaken. You still have a legal and professional responsibility to your patient and to the hospital to manage the situation properly.

## Managing an AMA situation

Because you have more contact with your patient than any other health-care professional, you're likely to be the first person to suspect that a patient is contemplating leaving AMA.

His complaints or hostile behavior may indicate his extreme dissatisfaction with hospital routine or with the care he's receiving—valid reasons, in his mind, for getting out. By carefully observing, listening, and talking with him, you may be able to resolve the problems by giving him a new perspective on his situation that will change his mind about leaving.

If you discover that a specific problem has caused his dissatisfaction, try to resolve it. If the problem lies outside the scope of your practice, call the patient's doctor or the house doctor.

Recognize, too, that a patient may tell you he's changed his mind about leaving just to divert your attention. If you suspect this, check on him more often and ask other nurses to do the same. And stay with him when you escort him to another part of the hospital.

Suppose, however, your patient insists on leaving AMA. If your hospital has a policy on managing the patient who wants to leave, follow it exactly. It's designed to protect the hospital, your co-workers, and you from the risk of a lawsuit for malpractice (unlawful restraint, false imprisonment). If you don't have a policy, follow these steps:

• Contact the patient's family (if you or the patient hasn't already called them) to explain that the patient is getting ready to leave. If you can't reach the family, contact the person listed in the patient's records as being responsible for him (or for his body and valuables if he should die).

• Explain the hospital's AMA procedures to the patient if hospital policy delegates this responsibility to you. If it doesn't, have the house officer or other appropriate person do it.

• Give the patient the AMA form to sign (see *Documenting AMA Incidents*, page 105). His decision to leave is the same as a refusal of treatment, so make sure he's aware of the implications of his decision. Tell him the medical risks if he leaves the hospital and explain the *alternatives available at the hospital* and at other locations, such as regular visits to the hospital's outpatient clinic or admission to another facility. His signature on the AMA form is evidence of his refusal of treatment. You should witness the signature. (See Entry 20.)

• Provide routine discharge care. Even though your patient is leaving AMA,

GLOSSARY

## KEY TERMS IN THIS ENTRY

**AMA** • Against medical advice; refers to when a patient decides to leave a health-care facility when his doctor advises him to stay.

**false imprisonment** • The act of confining or restraining a person without his consent, or for no clinical or legal reason.

his rights to discharge planning and care are the same as those for a patient who's signed out with medical advice. So if the patient agrees, escort him to the door (in a wheelchair, if necessary), arrange for medical or nursing follow-up care, and offer other routine health-care measures. These procedures will protect the hospital as well as the patient.

### When your patient refuses to sign out or escapes

What if your patient refuses to sign the AMA form? In this situation, you're responsible for documenting his refusal in his medical chart. Be sure to include what you told him about signing the form, his response, and your efforts to involve his family in his decision.

What if you discover that the patient is missing from the hospital? Your first priority is to notify the hospital and nursing administrations immediately. If the patient was in police custody or if he poses a threat to anyone outside the hospital, the administration may contact the police. Subsequently, the hospital administration may ask you to notify the patient's family or friends, collect the patient's belongings, and document the escape in the patient's medical chart and incident report. (See *Documenting AMA Incidents.*)

### What's false imprisonment?

At no time should you attempt to detain a competent adult who has a right to leave. Any attempt to detain or restrain him may be interpreted as unlawful restraint or false imprisonment, for which you can be sued or prosecuted. (See Entry 28.)

Your hospital's policy should reflect your state's laws and should specifically answer such questions as: How long and for what reasons may a patient be detained? When can you use forcible restraints? Who may order the use of restraints? Who may apply the restraints? Know the policies and the court rulings they're based on.

In general, the courts disapprove of detaining a patient arbitrarily or for an unreasonably long time, which may be ruled false imprisonment. Some court cases involving false-imprisonment charges resulted when institutions threatened to hold patients or their personal belongings until bills were paid. In most cases of this type, the courts ruled against the institutions.

A hospital or nursing home can, however, delay a patient's discharge until routine paperwork is complete— if the delay is reasonable. *Bailie v. Miami Valley Hospital* (1966) was a case in which the court ruled in favor of a hospital.

A typical case in which the courts found an institution guilty of false imprisonment was *Big Town Nursing Home v. Newman* (1970).

Mr. Newman, 67, had Parkinson's disease, arthritis, heart trouble, hiatus hernia, a speech impediment, and a history of alcoholism. Four days after his nephew signed him into the nursing home, Mr. Newman decided to leave. But employees at the nursing home stopped him, locked away his suitcase and clothes, restricted his use of the phone, and restricted his right to visitors. When Mr. Newman tried to walk off the grounds, employees locked him in a wing with severely emotionally disturbed patients and patients addicted to drugs and alcohol. He made other unsuccessful escape attempts, so staff tied Mr. Newman to a chair for

## DOCUMENTING AMA INCIDENTS

An AMA (against medical advice) form differs from the paperwork you deal with every day in one very important way. It's not a medical record; it's purely a legal document that's designed to protect you, your co-workers, and your institution should any problems result from the patient's unapproved discharge or escape.

To document an AMA incident, begin by getting your institution's AMA form. The form may look like the one shown below. You'll notice the form clearly states that the patient:
• knows he's leaving against medical advice
• has been advised of and understands the risks of leaving
• knows he can come back.

Discuss this form with the patient and ask him to sign it. You should sign it, too, as a witness. The patient, of course, doesn't *have* to sign the form, so don't try to force him.

Add the AMA form to the patient's medical chart, and write a detailed description of how you first learned of the patient's plan to leave AMA, what you and the patient said to each other, and what alternatives to the patient's action were discussed.

Also, check your institution's policy concerning incident reports. If the patient leaves without anyone's knowledge, or if he refuses to sign the AMA form, you'll probably be required to file an incident report. Be sure to include the names of any other employees involved in the discovery of the patient's absence. Hospital administration or your head nurse may also want to solicit corroborating reports from other employees, such as other RNs, LPNs/LVNs, doctors, aides, orderlies, and clerical staff.

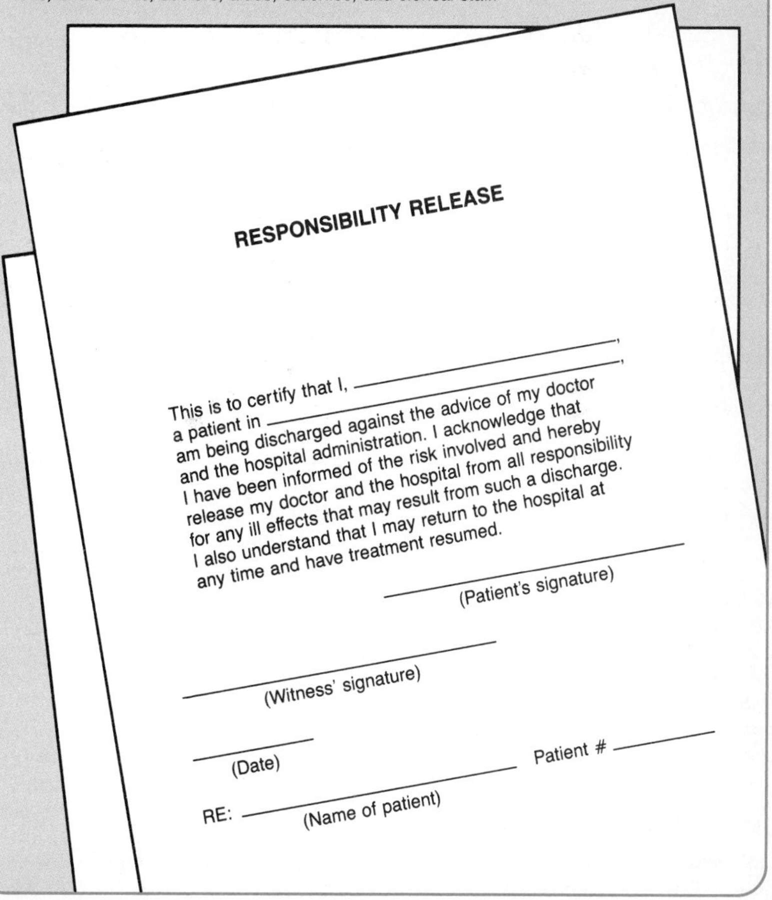

### RESPONSIBILITY RELEASE

This is to certify that I, _____,
a patient in _____
am being discharged against the advice of my doctor
and the hospital administration. I acknowledge that
I have been informed of the risk involved and hereby
release my doctor and the hospital from all responsibility
for any ill effects that may result from such a discharge.
I also understand that I may return to the hospital at
any time and have treatment resumed.

_____
(Patient's signature)

_____
(Witness' signature)

_____
(Date)                                   Patient # _____

RE: _____
(Name of patient)

long periods of time. Twenty-two days after his admission, Mr. Newman escaped. Eventually, he sued.

The court ruled in favor of Mr. Newman. Despite his physical infirmities, Mr. Newman had not legally been declared incompetent and was, therefore, legally entitled to exercise his rights.

In a few cases, because of extenuating circumstances, the courts have ruled against a patient who sued on grounds of false imprisonment. The case of *Pounders v. Trinity Court Nursing Home* (1979) is one such example.

Mrs. Pounders, 75, was a disabled widow. When her niece and nephew

---

> *"Patients who pose a threat to themselves or others cannot legally leave the hospital under any circumstances."*

---

no longer wanted her to live with them, the niece arranged for her to move to Trinity Court Nursing Home. Mrs. Pounders did not object.

During her 2 months at Trinity Court, Mrs. Pounders complained only once to a nurse's aide that she wanted to leave. Unfortunately, the aide failed to report the complaint to anyone in authority at the home.

Mrs. Pounders was finally released, through the aid of an attorney, into another niece's care. Eventually, she sued the nursing home.

But because Mrs. Pounders couldn't prove she'd been involuntarily detained, the court absolved the nursing home of the false imprisonment charges.

### A final word

The right to leave the hospital AMA isn't absolute. Certain patients who pose a threat to themselves or others cannot legally leave the hospital. In these situations, restraint, when necessary, is lawful:

• *The mental patient or prisoner.* If a patient transferred to your hospital from a prison or mental hospital threatens to escape, notify the custodial institution immediately. They're responsible for sending personnel to guard the patient or for making new arrangements for his care. Restrain the patient only if his medical condition indicates it or if the police or mental hospital authorities instruct you to do so. (See Entries 28 and 29.)

If the prisoner or mental patient escapes, you or your hospital or nursing administration should call the authorities at the custodial institution or the police and ask them to intervene.

• *The violent patient.* If you suspect that a patient with a history of violence or violent threats is planning to leave AMA, notify hospital and nursing administrators immediately. If state law allows it, your hospital administrators may decide to get police assistance to restrain the patient. (See Entry 28.)

If the violent patient has escaped, notify your nursing or hospital administration immediately. They will contact the police and mental health authorities. If the patient ever expressed an intention to harm a known person, the administration should also contact that person.

• *The patient with a communicable disease.* If your patient with a communicable disease warns you that he's going to leave AMA, notify your nursing or hospital administration. They'll alert appropriate public health authorities and the police. Your hospital may decide to restrain the patient until the authorities arrive or until a court issues a restraining order. The hospital will determine how to restrain the patient and how long to detain him, depending on his disease. Leprosy, smallpox, bubonic plague, and an untreated sexually transmitted disease present different risks of contagion to the community.

# 17 When a patient dies

When a patient dies, his rights don't end—they transfer to his estate. But in recent years, legally determining when death has occurred has become very difficult. That, in turn, makes your role difficult.

How can you be sure a patient is legally dead? Who has the right to pronounce death? What are your responsibilities after the patient dies? This entry will answer those questions.

## The changing definition of death

Determining death used to be fairly simple. When a person's circulation stopped, he was dead. But in the last 30 years or so, advances in medical technology have made death pronouncements more difficult. Because medical equipment (such as respirators, pacemakers, and intraaortic balloon pumps) can maintain respiration and circulation, some patients continue to "live" even after their brains have died.

To help doctors determine death in such cases, an ad hoc committee at Harvard Medical School published a report, in 1968, defining brain death (see *Defining Brain Death*, page 108). This report set the following criteria for death:

• a failure to respond to the most painful stimuli
• an absence of spontaneous respirations or muscle movements
• an absence of reflexes
• a flat EEG.

Other groups also issued definitions of brain death, and several court decisions have been based on brain death definitions.

In *State v. Brown* (1971), an Oregon court was among the first to recognize brain death. In this case of second degree murder, the defendant argued that he hadn't caused the victim's death by inflicting a gunshot wound to the brain. Instead, he claimed, a doctor killed the victim by removing artificial life support. But the court ruled that the defendant caused the victim's death because the gunshot wound resulted in brain death.

In 1975, several New York hospitals initiated a lawsuit to get a legal ruling on the definition of death when the patient was a potential donor of an anatomic organ (*N.Y.C. Health and Hospitals Corporation v. Sulsona*).

Expert testimony in the case showed that the common law definition of death apparently raised the failure rate of organ transplants. According to testimony, when death was defined as the cessation of circulation and respiration, the incidence of renal failure in kidney recipients was about 88%. But when death was defined by the brain death standard, the incidence of renal failure in recipients was only about 15%. (Bear in mind, however, that medical advances have improved the success rate of almost all types of transplant surgery since 1975.)

The court ruled it would recognize brain death in transplantation cases to encourage anatomic gifts, even though the state had no law defining brain death. This ruling applied to transplantation cases *only*.

In 1979, a Colorado court also accepted the criteria for brain death, in *Lovato v. Colorado*. In this case, a

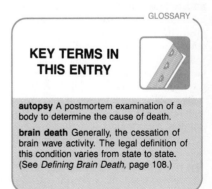

GLOSSARY

### KEY TERMS IN THIS ENTRY

**autopsy** A postmortem examination of a body to determine the cause of death.

**brain death** Generally, the cessation of brain wave activity. The legal definition of this condition varies from state to state. (See *Defining Brain Death*, page 108.)

# DEFINING BRAIN DEATH

Despite recent efforts, doctors and medical authorities have yet to agree on a definition of brain death. Several states have statutory law definitions of death.

The most familiar definition was formulated in 1968 by the Ad Hoc Committee of the Harvard Medical School to Examine the Definition of Brain Death. The committee established these criteria for establishing brain death:
• unreceptiveness and unresponsiveness even to the most painful stimuli
• absence of spontaneous respiration or muscle movement
• absence of reflexes
• a flat EEG.

The committee recommended that all the above tests be repeated after 24 hours and that hypothermia and the presence of central nervous system depressants, such as barbiturates, be ruled out.

Other groups have also defined brain death. They include the Baylor University Medical Center, the American Bar Association, and the American Medical Association. Baylor University Medical Center is considering using the following criteria to determine death in patients whose bodily functions continue with the aid of artificial support:
• The patient will show no perceptible signs of mental awareness of environment or external stimulation. He'll also be unable to maintain, without artificial support, one or more vital body functions essential to recovery and the maintenance of consciousness.
• This state will be a permanent and irreversible cerebral state, or the condition causing this state will be irreversible, precluding any reasonable expectation of patient recovery.
• The doctors determining death will employ resources of examination, observation, and such tests and consultations as may be appropriate to make this determination. The merit of consultation in this inherently grave determination is self-evident.

Representatives of the American Bar Association, American Medical Association, and the Uniform Law Commission met in 1980 to draft the Uniform Determination of Death Act to replace the Uniform Brain Death Act. The 1980 act states that "an individual who has sustained either irreversible cessation of circulatory and respiratory functions or irreversible cessation of all functions of the entire brain, including the brain stem, is dead. A determination of death must be made in accordance with accepted medical standards."

mother was charged with abusing her child. The child was comatose, with a flat EEG, with pupils fixed and dilated, and without spontaneous respirations or reflexes, or responses to painful stimuli. The mother petitioned the court to maintain the child on a respirator. But the court ruled that the child was dead because he met the criteria for brain death.

In 1980, representatives of the American Bar Association, the American Medical Association, and the Uniform Law Commission drafted the Uniform Determination of Death Act. Basically, this act defines death as *either* the irreversible cessation of the circulatory and respiratory systems *or* the irreversible cessation of all brain functions.

No state has yet adopted this act verbatim. However, many state legislatures have passed laws that describe how to determine brain death. In states without such laws—or judicial precedents—the common law definition of death (cessation of circulation and respiration) is still used. In these states, doctors are understandably reluctant to discontinue artificial life support for brain-dead patients. If you are likely to be involved with patients on life-support equipment, protect yourself by finding out how your state defines death.

In Canada, defining the moment of

death has traditionally been left to medical professionals. Human-tissue gift legislation says death is determined according to accepted medical practice.

## Who's responsible for pronouncing death?

Legally, only a doctor or a coroner can pronounce a person dead. However, in some health-care facilities, such as nursing homes, nurses pronounce death when a doctor isn't available. If you work in such a facility, you should understand, however, that pronouncing death isn't a nursing responsibility (see *Could You Be Liable for Pronouncing Death?* page 110).

The attending doctor is usually responsible for signing the death certificate, unless the death comes under the jurisdiction of a medical examiner or coroner. State laws specify when this occurs. Usually, the coroner or medical examiner has jurisdiction over deaths with violent or suspicious circumstances: suspected homicides and suicides, and deaths following accidents, abortions, surgery, or hospital stays of less than 24 hours.

The Canadian provincial laws on autopsies are similar. Any death occurring in violent or suspicious circumstances comes under the jurisdiction of a medical examiner or coroner. Depending on the province, other types of death—including a prisoner's death, a sudden death, or a death not caused by a disease—may also come under the jurisdiction of a medical examiner or coroner.

When a patient dies, you're responsible for *accurately* and *objectively* charting all his signs and any actions you take. For example, an appropriate entry in the nurses' notes would be: "Midnight. No respirations or pulses, pupils fixed and dilated. Notified Dr. York." Don't write a conclusion that borders on a medical diagnosis, such as "Patient seems dead."

You're also responsible for notifying the doctor who can be reached most

quickly. If this is the doctor on call, he should notify the patient's doctor, who should notify the family. Find out who will be notifying the family, and document it.

At the appropriate time, you should prepare the body for removal to the morgue, according to hospital procedure. When doing this, be sure you carefully identify the body. In *Lott v. State* (1962), a nurse mistagged two bodies, causing a Roman Catholic to be prepared for an Orthodox Jewish burial, and an Orthodox Jew to be prepared for a Roman Catholic burial. The court found her liable.

## Obtaining consent for an autopsy

As you know, an autopsy is a postmortem examination to determine the cause of death. If the death came under the jurisdiction of a medical examiner or coroner, the decision to perform an autopsy rests solely with him, despite the family's wishes.

In all other cases, however, the patient's family has a right to give or withhold consent. (In some states, the patient can give written consent to an autopsy before he dies.) When a doctor or other hospital representative has sought consent from a patient's family, you can help by explaining why the autopsy is needed and how autopsy arrangements are made.

## Who can give consent?

Most states have laws that specify who has the right to give consent to autopsies. Some laws simply list which relative can give consent. Others list relatives in descending order, according to their relationship to the deceased. The usual order is spouse, adult children, parents, brothers or sisters, grandparents, uncles or aunts, and cousins. The person with the right to consent may withhold consent or impose limits on the autopsy. If the autopsy exceeds these limits, the consenting relative may sue.

Of course, the relative with the right

# COULD YOU BE LIABLE FOR PRONOUNCING DEATH?

*When a patient in our nursing home dies, my nursing supervisor pronounces death if a doctor isn't available. She says the RN on duty or the supervisor can legally pronounce death if no doctor is available.*

*Can a nurse pronounce a death, or is this illegal?—RN, Ohio.*

In almost all states, including your own, a nurse *can't* legally pronounce a patient dead—only the doctor can do this. But if the doctor can't be there in person, he can pronounce death over the telephone.

You're considered qualified to determine whether a patient exhibits *evidence* of death. Based on your findings, the doctor can pronounce a patient officially dead.

As a precaution, be sure to chart the fact that the *doctor* pronounced the patient dead after you'd relayed the necessary information to him. And be sure to check whether your institution has a written policy on the matter.

By the way, telling the family about the patient's death is usually the job of the doctor or an administrator. Check your institution's policy on this matter.

One last detail: If the doctor pronounces a death on the basis of your report, but the patient is not really dead, the doctor could be liable for malpractice. You, however, would *not* be liable, because you merely reported your physical findings.

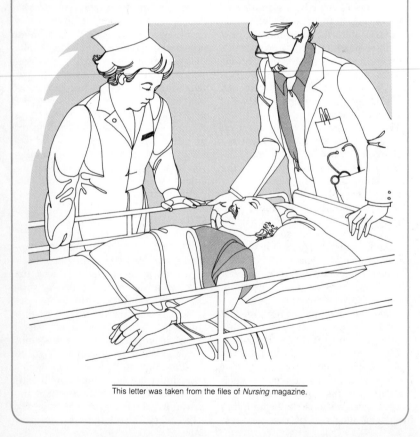

This letter was taken from the files of *Nursing* magazine.

to consent may also sue if an autopsy is performed without any consent. Usually, the grounds for such lawsuits are mental or emotional suffering.

The family also has a right to give or withhold specific consent to practice medical procedures on a corpse. In teaching hospitals, residents and medical students practice procedures, such as intubation, on corpses. But if a hospital allows this without obtaining proper consent, the family member responsible for consent may sue. In many states, the hospital may even face criminal charges for mistreating a corpse.

## Responsibility for burial
In the United States and Canada, the family member who has the right to consent to autopsy usually has the responsibility to bury the body as well. However, in one Canadian case (*Hunter v. Hunter,* 1930), the court ruled that the deceased's son, who was the executor of the will, had this responsibility—not the wife, who was the next of kin.

If no one claims the body, despite the hospital's effort to contact the person responsible, a state or county official must dispose of it. Laws in many states direct this official to deliver unclaimed bodies to an appropriate educational or scientific institution, unless the person is a veteran or has died from a contagious disease. In these situations, the state pays for burial or cremation.

In Canada, the hospital must notify an appropriate official of an unclaimed body, and the body will be delivered to a medical school.

## A final word
As state legislatures and courts continue to grapple with the definition of death, you'll find your responsibilities in a sometimes confusing period of transition. Until a single, national definition of death exists, you must know your current state or provincial laws and hospital policies defining death.

In addition, you must know what to do when a patient dies. To protect yourself legally, be sure you understand which tasks are the doctor's responsibility, and which tasks are yours.

## Selected References

Creighton, Helen. *Law Every Nurse Should Know,* 4th ed. Philadelphia: W.B. Saunders Co., 1981.

Doudera, A. Edward, and Peters, J. Douglas, eds. *Legal and Ethical Aspects of Treating Critically and Terminally Ill Patients.* Ann Arbor, Mich.: Health Administration Press, 1982.

Friloux, C. Anthony, Jr. "Death: When Does It Occur?" *Baylor Law Review* 27:10, 1975.

Harvard Medical School, Ad Hoc Committee to Examine the Definition of Brain Death. "A Definition of Irreversible Coma," *Journal of the American Medical Association* 205:337-40, August 1968.

"Informed Consent," chapter 3 in *Hospital Liability and Risk Management.* New York: Practicing Law Institute, 1981.

Pozgar, George D. *Legal Aspects of Health Care Administration.* Rockville, Md.: Aspen Systems Corp., 1979.

President's Commission for the Study of Ethical Problems in Medicine and Biomedical and Behavioral Research. *Defining Death: Medical, Legal and Ethical Issues in the Determination of Death.* Washington, D.C.: U.S. Government Printing Office, 1981.

Rocereto, LaVerne, and Maleski, Cynthia. *Legal Dimensions of Nursing Practice: A Practical Guide.* New York: Springer Publishing Co., 1982.

Rosoff, Arnold J. *Informed Consent: A Guide for Health Care Providers.* Rockville, Md.: Aspen Systems Corp., 1981.

Rozovsky, Lorne E. *Canadian Hospital Law: A Practical Guide,* 2nd ed. Canadian Hospital Association, 1979.

Warren, Samuel D., and Brandeis, Louis D. "The Right to Privacy," *Harvard Law Review* 4:193, 1890.

# 3 Your Legal Risks in Nursing Practice

## Introduction

No doubt about it—as a nurse, your chances of being named a defendant or codefendant in a malpractice lawsuit are growing.

In 1976, for example, 834 registered nurses were named in lawsuits. Just 2 years later, in 1978, that number had jumped more than 440%—to 3,775. And the number of nurses involved in work-related lawsuits continues to grow.

Why this rapid and continuing increase? Certainly one reason is today's "I'm gonna sue!" climate, which suggests that lawsuits should be used to resolve grievances against anybody and everybody, including nurses. The dynamic growth within the nursing profession, however, offers another—more substantial—reason. As nursing grows professionally, nurses are taking on expanded responsibilities that inevitably lead to increased legal accountability. What does this mean for you? It means you need to thoroughly understand your basic legal rights, responsibilities, and risks in everyday nursing practice. If you don't, you may be setting yourself up for a lawsuit. (See *Preventing the Nurse-Defendant Syndrome*, page 114.)

Entry 18, "Hospital policies and procedures—the legal implications," focuses on the ways in which hospital policies and procedures define your roles and responsibilities as a nurse and specify the procedures you must follow in giving nursing care. You know that if you give care negligently, you're vulnerable to a lawsuit. But if your negligent care takes place while you're performing a procedure that's inconsistent with your hospital's policies and procedures, a stronger case for liability can be made against you. So you need to be familiar with your hospital's policies and procedures and follow them—but not blindly, for sometimes a policy or procedure may conflict with your state or (in Canada) provincial nurse practice act. When this happens, following your hospital's rules may cause you to exceed the legal limits of your nursing practice. Entry 18 offers guidelines to giving care that meets standards according to the law *and* your employer.

Entry 19, "The liability of understaffing," deals with a major concern of many nurses today. As you know, hospitals are responsible for providing an adequate nursing staff to care for patients. Failure to do so can expose hospitals to expensive lawsuits. Most hospitals try to follow state or (in Canada) provincial staffing guidelines or those developed by self-regulating agencies, such as the Joint Commission on Accreditation of Hospitals.

Still, due to chronic nursing shortages and other causes, hospital units are often understaffed. As you know, if your unit has too few nurses or an inadequate mix of RNs, LPNs/LVNs, aides, and others on duty, your ability to provide adequate supervision and in-depth patient care decreases signif-

icantly. At the same time, your chance of making mistakes increases. And with mistakes comes the possibility of malpractice lawsuits. Entry 19 explains the liability of understaffing and suggests ways to protect yourself legally when *your* unit is understaffed.

## PREVENTING THE NURSE-DEFENDANT SYNDROME

Nurses with signs and symptoms of the *nurse-defendant syndrome* may easily end up in court. What's the nurse-defendant syndrome? Basically, it's a pattern of substandard nursing care—care that consistently fails to meet current legal standards. Nurses who exhibit this syndrome are ready targets for malpractice lawsuits.

Fortunately, you can prevent the nurse-defendant syndrome by doing the following:

● *Recognize that your first duty is to defend your patient, not his doctor.* If your judgment says your patient's condition warrants a call to his doctor, don't hesitate—in the middle of the day or in the middle of the night. If your judgment says to question a doctor's order because you can't read it, don't understand it, think it's incomplete, or think it may harm your patient, don't hesitate.

If your hospital doesn't already have a policy covering nurse-doctor communications, ask for one and keep asking till you get one. Meanwhile, for your own protection, carefully record all contacts with doctors.

● *Keep your nursing know-how up to date.* Here are some effective ways: reading nursing journals, attending clinical programs, attending inservice programs, and seeking advice from nurse specialists. If your hospital doesn't offer needed inservice programs, ask for them.

Remember, ignorance of new techniques is no excuse for substandard care. If you're ever sued for malpractice, your patient care will be judged by current nursing standards.

● *Include all parts of the nursing process in your patient care.* Taking shortcuts risks your patient's well-being and your own. If you're charged with malpractice, and the court finds out you took a dangerous patient-care shortcut, the court may hold you liable for causing harm to your patient.

● *Document every step of the nursing*

*process for every patient.* Chart your observations immediately, while facts are fresh in your mind; express yourself clearly; and always write legibly. If you're ever involved in a lawsuit, a complete patient-care record could be your best defense.

● *Audit your nursing records consistently and comprehensively, using specific criteria to evaluate the effectiveness of patient care.* Ask for a charting class—or start one yourself—to encourage staff nurses to chart patient care correctly and legibly. Use problem-oriented charting (to be sure you're documenting all parts of the nursing process) and flow sheets (to record large volumes of data). Encourage other nurses to use these documenting aids.

● *Use your nursing knowledge to make nursing diagnoses and give clinical opinions.* You have a legal duty to your patient not only to make a nursing diagnosis but also to take appropriate action to meet his nursing needs. Doing so helps protect your patient from harm and you from malpractice charges.

● *Delegate patient care wisely.* Know the legal practice limits of the people you supervise, and caution them to act only within those limits. If your delegation of skilled tasks to an unskilled person harms a patient, you can be held liable for breaching your nurse practice act.

● *Know your nursing service policies.* Review the policies at least yearly. If you think new policies are needed, ask for them. If you're ever involved in a malpractice lawsuit, good nursing service policies and your knowledge of them could be important in your defense.

● *Treat patients' families, as well as patients, with kindness and respect.* When you help relatives cope with the stress of your patient's illness and teach them the basics of home care, they'll more likely remember you with a thank-you card than with a legal summons.

While a patient is under your care, he may ask you to witness the signing of a will, consent form, or other document. Although witnessing a patient's signature may seem a simple act, it has important legal implications, as described in Entry 20, "Witnessing and signing documents." Knowing when and how to document your reasons for signing—and for refusing to sign, too—are important, especially if the incident should ever become part of a court proceeding.

Entry 21, "Special risks in special-care units," discusses the legal risks involved in working in a critical care

---

## "The more you know about specialized nursing's legal risks, the better."

---

or intensive care unit, in an emergency department, in the operating room, and in other specialized nursing settings. As you probably know, your legal responsibilities and risks in these settings differ from those of a nurse who works on a general unit. That's because the standards used in judging your care differ. For example, if you're a specialist in emergency nursing, a higher standard of care will be expected of you in the emergency department than if you're a nurse-generalist. The more you know about the legal risks that go with working in specialized nursing settings, the better—for you, your hospital, and your patients.

Entry 22, "Your legal responsibility for patients' safety," emphasizes the fact that hospitals are legally obligated to provide a safe environment for their patients. As a nurse, one of your major responsibilities is patient safety. Among other things, this means you must help make sure that facilities and equipment are in good repair and that they're used for their intended pur-

poses. If they aren't, you may not only endanger your patients but also expose yourself and your hospital to malpractice liability.

Improper drug administration is one of the most common malpractice accusations patients make against nurses. Entry 23, "Your legal risks in administering drugs," stresses the five "rights" of giving drugs: the right medicine for the right patient, in the right dose, at the right time, and by the right route. Of course, it's not really that simple: Entry 23 also describes the various drug laws affecting your practice and gives you guidelines for supervising others who give drugs to patients.

"Your legal responsibilities in patient teaching," Entry 24, describes how you, as a nurse, can be held legally accountable for teaching your patients. As you know, patient teaching has traditionally been a part of nursing care, and its importance today is greater than ever. Yet, although many state and Canadian provincial nurse practice acts include patient teaching in their definitions of nursing, few define the nurse's role in patient teaching. To find out your rights and responsibilities in this area, you must turn to the few available court decisions for guidance. Entry 24 discusses some of these and shows how you can adapt your patient teaching to avoid similar outcomes.

Entry 25, "What to do after a patient incident," discusses the legally correct ways to report patient incidents—any occurrences that are inconsistent with routine patient care or a hospital's (or other health-care institution's) routine operation.

You know that, when an incident occurs, you must immediately report and document it, stating clearly and factually what happened, who was involved, and what you did to resolve the problem. Entry 25 describes your rights and responsibilities when patient incidents occur, as well as your need to follow applicable rules and regulations when you report an incident.

Entry 26, "Caring for minors—your

legal responsibilities," discusses informed-consent issues in caring for minors. At one time, as you probably know, minors had few (if any) rights concerning their health care. Currently, however, their rights have increased—a fact you must acknowledge if you want to avoid legal complications. Entry 26 spells out how you should proceed when a minor's parents must consent to treatment for their child, and when—as happens in some situations—parental consent may not be necessary (for example, when the patient is an emancipated minor).

Are you sure of your legal responsibilities regarding child or spouse abuse? Entry 27, "The abused child or adult—your legal responsibility," can help. As a nurse, you've no doubt had to care for a child or adult who's been abused. (You may even have been the first professional to identify the abuse.) You know that when you suspect abuse, you're required by law to report the case to specified local authorities for investigation and possible action. But many questions arise from this simply stated requirement. What, for example, does the law say about documenting abuse cases? How does it apply to any specific patient? What kind of special help can you—and should you—offer? And what about your own immunity from civil or criminal liability—especially if your suspicions are found groundless? Check Entry 27 for the answers to these and other questions about this very troubling subject.

In Entry 28, "Special risks in caring for 'special' patients," you'll read about the special legal risks involved in caring for mentally ill and developmentally disabled patients. Until the 1960s, mentally ill and developmentally disabled persons had little opportunity to direct their own health care. Since then, however, their rights have increased dramatically. For example, state, provincial (Canada), and federal laws currently grant the right to consent to treatment (unless the patient has been

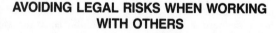

## AVOIDING LEGAL RISKS WHEN WORKING WITH OTHERS

To help you steer clear of legal dangers when working with the health-care team, here are some questions and answers that deal with the legal responsibilities you face:

**Q** *Can I be held liable for mistakes made by a student nurse under my supervision?*

**A** Yes, if you have primary responsibility for instructing the student and correcting her mistakes.

**Q** *If a student nurse performs tasks that only a licensed nurse should perform, and does so with my knowledge but without my supervision, am I guilty of breach of duty?*

**A** Yes, because as a staff nurse, you should know that a student nurse can perform nursing tasks *only* under the direct supervision of a nurse licensed to perform those tasks.

**Q** *What should I do if I see another health-team member perform a clinical procedure incorrectly?*

**A** If the incorrect procedure can harm the patient, you have a legal duty to stop the procedure—tactfully, when possible—and immediately report your action to your nursing supervisor. If the incorrect procedure doesn't threaten to harm the patient, don't stop the procedure—but report your observation to your supervisor.

**Q** *Can I face legal action if I ask a hospital volunteer to help me give patient care and she does something wrong?*

**A** Yes. Don't ask a volunteer to participate in any task she isn't trained and professionally qualified to perform.

declared incompetent by a court) and the right to refuse treatment (including medications). The laws also restrict the use of restraints, seclusion, and sterilization in caring for these patients.

Keeping yourself updated about how the law protects these patients is a challenge. Why? Because the laws are still changing. Entry 28 offers guidelines for protecting your patients' legal rights *and* protecting yourself against liability for violating those rights.

Entry 29, "When your patient is a suspected criminal," helps you manage a potentially difficult situation. You need to be aware of the legalities involved in obtaining and handling evidence. You need to protect this patient's legal rights without prejudice, no matter what his alleged crime is. Entry 29 will help you give your patient the care he's entitled to, and it will show you how to avoid creating legal difficulties for the police, the hospital, and yourself.

In Entry 30, "Your responsibility for a patient's living will," you'll read about your legal responsibility to a terminally ill patient who's drawn up such a will. Do you know how to respond when a patient or his family asks you to honor a living will's provisions and not go out of your way to prolong the patient's life? Should you fulfill such a request? And if you do, what are the legal consequences?

Although some states, such as California and New Mexico, have legally recognized the validity of living wills, others have not. But even in those states where the wills are legal, difficulties remain. Entry 30 demonstrates that the more you know about living wills, the less likely you'll be to make a mistake that could place you in a courtroom.

### Understanding the issues
As you know, whether you're an RN or an LPN/LVN, you're always legally accountable for your nursing actions. In any practice setting, your care must meet these baseline legal standards:
• Does your care fall within the scope

of your nurse practice act?
• Does your care measure up to established practice standards?
• Are you protecting your patient's rights?

Remember these points as you read the entries in this chapter. Each entry is designed not to restrict your patient-care options, because of legal issues, but to free you to give your patients the best care possible—because you understand those issues.

# 18 Hospital policies and procedures—the legal implications

Every hospital and other health-care institution has *policies*—a set of general principles by which it manages its affairs. If you work for a hospital, you're obligated to know those policies and to follow the established *procedures* that flow from them.

But never do this blindly. As a nurse, you're also obligated to maintain your professional standards, and these standards may sometimes conflict with your employer's policies and procedures. At times, you may be forced to make decisions, and take actions, that risk violating those policies and procedures. At times like these, you need help balancing your duty to your patient with your responsibility to your employer. Your best help is a well-prepared nursing department policy manual, coupled with high standards of performance. This combination is the mark of a successful nursing department—one whose first concern is to deliver high-quality patient care.

### What makes a good nursing department manual?
Although manuals will differ, most good ones will do the following:
• show how general hospital policies

GLOSSARY

## KEY TERMS IN THIS ENTRY

**malpractice** • A professional person's wrongful conduct, improper discharge of professional duties, or failure to meet standards of care—any such action that results in harm to another person.

**proximate cause** • A legal concept of cause and effect, which says a sequence of natural and continuous events produces an injury that wouldn't have otherwise occurred.

and procedures apply to the nursing department
• outline the nursing department's roles and responsibilities, both internally and in relation to other hospital departments
• identify the expected limits of nursing action and practice
• offer guidelines for handling emergency situations
• provide standing orders for nurses who work in special areas, such as the intensive care unit (ICU) or the coronary care unit (CCU)
• show the steps to be taken before—and after—arriving at nursing-care decisions. These steps can then become a well-thought-out statement of the care standards applied in the institution, and the manual itself can be used as evidence in malpractice cases. (See the discussion of *Utter v. United Health Center,* 1977, below.)

Any good nursing department manual should always be in the process of revision—especially today, when hospitals are rapidly revising and expanding their basic policies and procedures. Some of these procedure and policy changes result from efforts to streamline and standardize patient care. Others result from efforts to comply with new state, provincial (Canada), and federal regulations or to implement recommendations of the Joint Commission on Accreditation of Hospitals.

## How hospital policies can affect court decisions

Hospital policies are meant to be followed. Policies aren't laws, but courts have generally ruled against nurses who violated their employers' policies. Courts have also held hospitals liable for poorly formulated—or poorly implemented—policies.

Take, for example, the matter of reporting doctors who fail to give their patients adequate medical care. In *Darling v. Charleston Community Memorial Hospital* (1965), the court found the attending nurses negligent because they failed to monitor the condition of a patient's broken leg that, because of improper casting, became necrotic and had to be amputated.

Specifically, the court found that because the attending nurses did not bring the patient's worsening condition to the medical staff's attention, the nurses had failed to exercise proper judgment concerning the adequacy of the patient's medical care. The nurses should have informed the attending doctor of complications; then, if he'd failed to act, they should have advised the hospital authorities of the patient's unsatisfactory medical care. These measures would have helped to ensure that appropriate action was taken.

Since the *Darling* case, the generally accepted rule of law is that staff actions that deviate from established hospital policies and procedures constitute a breach of duty. But this case also showed that a hospital can be held liable for failure to have a system for monitoring the quality of care and taking action to correct any deficiencies. Because Charleston Community Hospital didn't provide enough trained nurses and adequate hospital policy guidelines, the judge allowed the jury to evaluate standards of accreditation, state licensing regulations, and hospital bylaws in determining the applicable standard of care for deciding the case.

Although the *Darling* case and others have established a nurse's duty to report certain matters to proper authorities, how this should be done hasn't been clearly spelled out. In many instances, this reporting consists of verbally notifying the attending doctor about the problem. If he doesn't act, then the nurse can report the situation to the chief of the service. Of course, all this should be documented in the nurses' notes on the patient's chart.

In *Utter v. United Health Center* (1977), the court relied on a provision in the hospital's nursing manual, which said that if the doctor in charge—after being notified—did nothing about adverse changes in a patient's condition, or acted ineffectively, the nurse was to "call this to the attention of the Department Chairman." The nurses cited in this case failed to report to the chairman and so caused a critical 24-hour delay in the patient's treatment. Because of this, the judge told the jury that it could label the nurses' failure as the proximate cause of the patient's injury. So the nurses shared the blame for the inaction of the patient's doctor because they did not go a step further and make sure the patient got the needed medical attention. (For more examples, see *Following Policy and Avoiding Legal Problems*, page 123.)

Another policy question that could arise involves exactly when to take a patient's history after he's admitted to your unit. Suppose, for example, you admit a patient who has pneumonia and, unknown to you, a history of GI bleeding. On admission, his doctor writes a stat order for aspirin for fever. Following his order, you give the aspirin right away. A half hour later, before you can take his history, the patient begins to have GI bleeding.

Who's liable in a situation like this? The doctor might be, assuming he knew the patient's history. But you might be, too, for not taking the patient's history that would have revealed the prior GI bleeding.

You know, of course, that legally you're personally and primarily responsible for everything you do while on hospital duty. But if you're sued for malpractice, the hospital will have to assume secondary responsibility in the lawsuit, provided you were practicing within the scope of your job description (see Entry 46). Whether you've acted properly is ordinarily determined, in court, by the patient's condition on admission and the hospital's nursing service policy.

The case of *O'Neill v. Montefiore Hospital* (1960) illustrates the dilemma a nurse faces when she must choose between hospital policy and her professional standards. This case involved a nurse who, following hospital policy, refused to admit a patient because he belonged to an insurance plan her hospital didn't accept. The man returned home and died. Although the trial court ruled in favor of the nurse, the New York Supreme Court (Appellate Division) reversed the decision and ruled the hospital nurse negligent for refusing to admit the patient. (For other examples, see *What Are the Limits of Your Liability?* pages 120 and 121.)

## How laws affect hospital policies

As you probably know, many hospital policies and procedures are mandated by state or (in Canada) provincial licensing laws, or by such federal regulations as the conditions for participation in Medicare. Once made law, these requirements must be embodied in hospital policy.

Many such mandatory requirements exist. In the United States, for instance, the Civil Rights Act of 1964 compels any hospital receiving federal funds to adopt policies against discrimination based on race, creed, color, national origin, handicap, or sex. (These requirements mainly refer to admitting patients, not to giving bedside care.) The Freedom of Information Act requires hospitals to give consumers and patients access to certain data previously considered privileged. And the Department of Health and Human Services' regulations require that hospi-

# WHAT ARE THE LIMITS OF YOUR LIABILITY?

As a nurse, do you know the limits of your professional responsibility—and liability? Most nurses think they do. But a large number of your colleagues who took part in a recent staff-nurse survey, which tested this knowledge, were in for a surprise.

In this survey, each question was based on an actual court case that measured nursing performance against current standards. For each case, the nurses surveyed were asked to judge whether or not the court found the defendant-nurse (or nurses) liable. The survey respondents averaged only about 11 correct answers out of 20.

Below are five questions selected from the survey. To test yourself, jot down *Yes* if you think the court considered the nurse or nurses liable. Jot down *No* if you think the court did not consider the nurse or nurses liable. Then read the court decisions and the corresponding survey results.

A boy, age 19, was hospitalized after his leg was broken in a football game. Nurses reported signs of infection to the doctor and charted them. The doctor took no action and the leg eventually had to be amputated. Were the nurses liable?

A staff nurse took a patient, on a stretcher, to the radiology department and left him with several other patients in the crowded hall. The patient was injured when his stretcher was knocked against the wall. Was the nurse liable?

A staff nurse called a medical resident when a patient complained of soreness in her jaw and difficulty opening her mouth, 3 days after she'd had a cesarean section. The resident examined the patient and ordered treatment. The staff nurse documented these events, treated the patient as ordered, and stayed in constant communication with the resident when the patient's condition worsened. She did not call the patient's doctor. The patient developed a serious postoperative complication and sued. Was the nurse liable?

An operating room (OR) nurse prepared a 17-year-old boy's left leg instead of the right one, and the surgeon operated on a normal knee. Was the OR nurse liable?

A nurse wasn't familiar with one of the medications ordered. So she talked to two available doctors about it. After they told her the dosage "wasn't out of line," she gave the medication. The patient died as a result of the medication. Was the nurse liable?

The courts found that, in all five cases, the nurses were liable. Here's a summary of each court decision, along with the corresponding survey results:

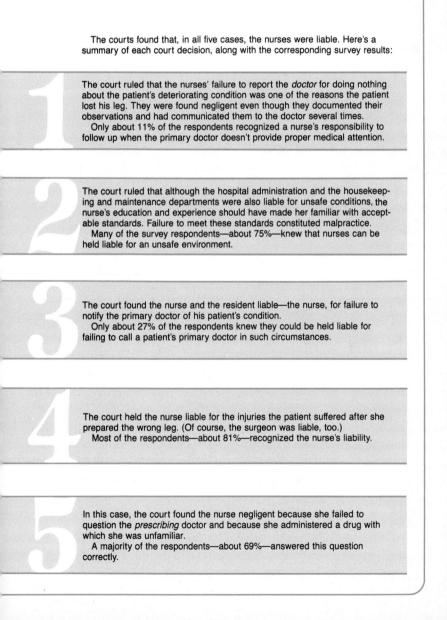

**1**

The court ruled that the nurses' failure to report the *doctor* for doing nothing about the patient's deteriorating condition was one of the reasons the patient lost his leg. They were found negligent even though they documented their observations and had communicated them to the doctor several times.

Only about 11% of the respondents recognized a nurse's responsibility to follow up when the primary doctor doesn't provide proper medical attention.

**2**

The court ruled that although the hospital administration and the housekeeping and maintenance departments were also liable for unsafe conditions, the nurse's education and experience should have made her familiar with acceptable standards. Failure to meet these standards constituted malpractice.

Many of the survey respondents—about 75%—knew that nurses can be held liable for an unsafe environment.

**3**

The court found the nurse and the resident liable—the nurse, for failure to notify the primary doctor of his patient's condition.

Only about 27% of the respondents knew they could be held liable for failing to call a patient's primary doctor in such circumstances.

**4**

The court held the nurse liable for the injuries the patient suffered after she prepared the wrong leg. (Of course, the surgeon was liable, too.)

Most of the respondents—about 81%—recognized the nurse's liability.

**5**

In this case, the court found the nurse negligent because she failed to question the *prescribing* doctor and because she administered a drug with which she was unfamiliar.

A majority of the respondents—about 69%—answered this question correctly.

tals observe strict guidelines when using patients in research studies.

In Canada, each province has its own laws governing hospitals, both public and private. According to the Ontario Public Hospitals Act, certain classes of hospitals receiving provincial aid must, with few exceptions, admit patients needing treatment.

The provincial legislatures also pass laws governing hospitalization in psychiatric facilities. Matters of criminal law, however, are in the hands of the federal parliament, so hospital policymakers look to the federal parliament for guidance on issues such as narcotics and abortions.

## U.S. and Canadian policy similarities and differences

Hospital policies in the United States and Canada generally show more similarities than differences.

One difference involves control at the federal level. Federal agencies in the United States exert more power than their Canadian counterparts do.

Under English common law, people are usually not obligated to help each other—not even in emergencies. However, where hospitals are concerned, Canadian provincial legislatures have departed from this tradition. For example, the Public Hospitals Act of Nova Scotia states that when a qualified medical practitioner makes application for a patient and the (publicly funded) hospital has room, it must admit the patient—even if he can't pay for his care. (Private hospitals, however, needn't do this.)

Similarly, in the United States, if an uninsured patient tries to get emergency treatment in a hospital but is turned away, the hospital can be found negligent if the patient's condition becomes significantly worse while he's seeking treatment elsewhere. One such case was *Hunt v. Palm Springs General Hospital* (1977). It involved a patient who died from brain damage due to prolonged seizures after one hospital refused to admit him because he hadn't paid past-due bills. He wasn't treated until another hospital admitted him, 4 hours later.

## How hospital policies affect your job as a staff nurse

Remember that top management originates policies specifically to guide workers in the hospital's daily operations. Policies stem from the hospital's philosophy and objectives and are part of the hospital's planning process. So they affect your job very directly.

If you're considering employment at a hospital, study its policies carefully. If they're well defined, they may give you an indication of how satisfied and secure you can expect to be in your job.

If you're working in a specialized nursing area, such as the ICU or CCU, give special attention to any policies that directly or indirectly apply to you. Make sure your specialty is clearly defined in keeping with your state or provincial nurse practice act—and with the standards recommended by accrediting agencies and professional medical and nursing associations.

Besides reading policies—the general principles by which a hospital is guided in its management—read the hospital's rules, too. These describe the actions that employees should or should not take in specific situations. "No smoking in the patient's room," for example, is a rule and must be enforced without exception.

If you feel reasonably comfortable with the hospital's philosophy, objectives, policies, rules, and quality of care, you'll probably feel comfortable on the job. But if the hospital's policy calls for nursing procedures that conflict with your personal nursing standards or ethics, then you'll probably do better if you look elsewhere for employment.

## What should you do when hospital policy conflicts with your state board of nursing's definition of care?

You must refuse to follow hospital pol-

# FOLLOWING POLICY AND AVOIDING LEGAL PROBLEMS

### When in doubt, stick with policy

*I'm a new nursing graduate, working the night shift on an oncology floor. Maybe because this is my first nursing job, I've read the hospital's policy manual carefully and I try to follow instructions. But not everybody does the same. Let me explain.*

*According to our hospital's written policy, only certified chemotherapy nurses may administer any chemotherapeutic drug. This regulation also stipulates that if a chemotherapy nurse isn't available, the attending doctor must administer the drug himself.*

*The policy couldn't be clearer. But on our floor, uncertified nurses do hang 5-fluorouracil (5-FU) when a chemotherapy nurse isn't available.*

*I checked with my supervisor about this practice. She took out and read her policy manual and then said "Look— everyone else hangs 5-FU. It's not a potent chemotherapeutic drug and won't cause damage if it should infiltrate. If we don't have a chemotherapy nurse available, the attending doctor isn't about to come in to hang a bottle of 5-FU at midnight."*

*She was telling me, without using the words, to hang the drug if I had to— despite what the manual said.*

*What should I do now? If I follow my supervisor's advice and I run into trouble, will my malpractice insurance protect me?*—RN, Mass.

You're in a precarious position. If a written hospital policy says one thing and a nurse does another, she's probably legally liable for any trouble that may arise. Nurses *have* been sued for administering drugs improperly. What's more, if a nurse is acting contrary to hospital policy, she's *not* acting as an agent of the hospital. Therefore, the hospital's insurance doesn't have to cover her.

If you're going to correct this situation, you'll have to document all the facts. Then take your documentation through channels to the patient's doctor, to the hospital and nursing administrators, and to the hospital's policy committee.

### Put it in writing

*I'm writing for myself and for three other RNs in a hospital outpatient clinic. We're all concerned about our role in giving immunizations at the clinic. Usually, a local doctor gives the injections. But some days, he can't get to the clinic. On those days, his receptionist sends a typewritten note, saying the doctor won't be in and giving us the hospital phone number where we can reach him in an emergency. She always signs his name and initials the signature.*

*When the doctor isn't there, he expects us to give the immunizations ourselves. So far, we've done as he wishes, and we haven't had any problems. But we're worried about our liability. Our state doesn't allow nurses to prescribe drugs, and we don't have standing orders for administering immunizations. We've talked with the doctor, and he says we don't need to worry. But we'd like another opinion. Is the receptionist's note adequate authorization? Will it protect us legally if something goes wrong?*—RN, Mich.

No. You definitely need a written protocol to handle this situation. In the current situation, you're administering prescription drugs without a doctor's order, and the receptionist's note wouldn't protect you legally if someone accused you of practicing medicine without a license.

Here's what you can do to protect yourselves and your patients: ask your state health department to send you current immunization recommendations from the Centers for Disease Control in Atlanta. (Or contact the centers yourself: Centers for Disease Control, 1600 Clifton Rd., NE, Atlanta, Ga. 30333.)

Put the information in a manual, and ask the clinic doctor to review and sign it. Revise the manual every year, and get the doctor's signature after each revision. The result: You'll have a *procedure manual,* as well as a standing order for immunizations. Clinic nurses who've prepared such manuals say they can offer excellent protection in touchy situations.

---

These letters were taken from the files of *Nursing* magazine.

icy. Why? Because your state legislature has given the board of nursing power to monitor nursing practice in the interest of public health and safety. Any willful violation of board rulings, even with your hospital's knowledge and encouragement, could result in suspension or revocation of your license (see Entry 4).

So if your hospital policy calls for nurses to remove sutures from postoperative patients, but your state board of nursing says you may not, don't do it. (In Pennsylvania, the state board of nursing sent a notice to all RN licensees stating that suture removal was not a nursing function. The notice also stated that a nurse who removed a patient's sutures would be violating the Pennsylvania Nurse Practice Act.) But *do* tell your hospital administration about the discrepancy.

### Understanding how hospital policies apply to LPNs and LVNs

LPNs and LVNs aren't RNs. They shouldn't be asked to exceed limits that law and education place on their practice. You'll find exceptions to this, of course. Both state law and national health commissions have recognized LPNs/LVNs' right to perform in an expanded role—for example, to administer drugs, if the LPN or LVN is properly trained for the task, and it's one that other nurses perform in the hospital where she works.

But you should protect yourself. Make sure the conditions for your doing this work are included in your hospital's *written* policies. And make sure the policies have been established by a committee representing the medical staff, the nursing department, and the administration, and that the written version is available to all medical and nursing staff members. If these LPN/ LVN policies *aren't* stated in writing, you'd better not administer drugs. If you're sued on this basis and can't back up your actions with written hospital policy, you could be found liable.

### How can you go about getting hospital policies changed, if you don't agree with them?

You have two ways to bring nursing policy problems to your hospital administration's attention. You can involve your health-team colleagues by discussing policy problems at committee meetings, conferences, and interdepartmental meetings. Or you can communicate directly with your hospital administration via the grievance procedure, counseling, attitude questionnaires, and formal and informal unit management committees. Both ways give you a voice in determining the policies that affect your job.

# 19 The liability of understaffing

*Understaffing*—failure to provide enough professionally trained personnel to meet a patient population's needs. If you're like most nurses, you're very familiar with understaffing and the problems it can cause.

Statistics about understaffing are sketchy, but the fact that a number of court cases have addressed this issue suggests not only that understaffing is widespread but also that understaffing results in substandard bedside care, increased mistakes and omissions, and hasty documentation—all of which increase nurses' (and their employers') liability.

For example, if during hospitalization a patient is harmed and can demonstrate that the harm resulted from the hospital's failure to provide enough qualified personnel to care for him, the hospital may be found liable in a malpractice lawsuit, *along with any nurse who cared for that patient*. Even if a nurse can demonstrate that she was too busy to perform all her assigned duties for that patient, the court may still find her liable.

## What constitutes adequate staffing?

You won't find many legal guidelines to help you answer this question. So if you want to determine whether your floor has too few nurses, you may have a problem. The few guidelines that do exist vary from state to state and are limited mainly to specialty care units (such as intensive care, coronary care, and recovery room care). Even the Joint Commission on Accreditation of Hospitals (JCAH) offers little help. The JCAH staffing standard sets no specific nurse-patient ratios. It just states generally that "nursing personnel staffing shall... be sufficient to assure prompt recognition of an untoward change in a patient's condition and to facilitate appropriate intervention by the nursing, medical, or hospital staffs."

In the absence of well-defined staffing guidelines, the courts have had no reliable standard to use in deciding cases where understaffing is alleged. So each such case has been decided on an individual basis.

The first case decided partly on the basis of this issue was *Darling v. Charleston Community Memorial Hospital* (1965). A young man broke his leg while playing football and was taken to Charleston's emergency department, where the on-call doctor set and cast his leg. The patient began to complain of pain almost immediately. Later, his toes grew swollen and dark, then cold and insensitive, and a stench pervaded his room. Nurses checked the leg only a few times a day, and they failed to report its worsening condition. When the cast was removed 3 days later, the necrotic condition of the leg was apparent. After several surgical attempts to save the leg, it had to be amputated below the knee.

After an out-of-court settlement with the doctor who'd applied the cast, the court found the hospital liable for failing to have enough trained nurses available at all times to recognize the patient's serious condition and to bring it to the attention of the medical staff.

GLOSSARY

**KEY TERMS IN THIS ENTRY**

**liability** • Legal responsibility for *failure to act*, so causing harm to another person, or for *actions* that fail to meet standards of care, so causing harm to another person.

**malpractice** • Professional wrongful conduct, improper discharge of professional duties, or a professional person's failure to meet the standards of care—any such action that results in harm to another person.

Since the *Darling* case, several similar cases have been tried (for example, *Cline v. Lund*, 1973 and *Sanchez v. Bay General Hospital*, 1981). Almost every case involved a nurse who failed to continuously monitor her patient's condition—especially his vital signs—and to report significant changes to the attending doctor. In each case, the courts have emphasized:
• the need for sufficient numbers of nurses to continuously monitor a patient's condition
• the need for nurses who are specially trained to recognize signs and symptoms that require a doctor's immediate intervention.

## Understanding the hospital's liability

Courts hold hospitals primarily liable in lawsuits where nursing understaffing is the key issue. A hospital can be found liable for patient injuries if it accepts more patients than its facilities can accommodate or its nursing staff can care for. The hospital controls the purse strings and, in the courts' view, is the only party that can resolve the problem.

Hospitals accused of failing to maintain adequate nursing staffs have offered various defenses. Some have argued they acted reasonably because their nurse:patient ratio was equal to that found in other area hospitals. This

## FLOATING: WHEN CAN YOU REFUSE?

An order to float to an unfamiliar unit can cause worry and frustration in the best of nurses—and understandably so. It may cause you worry about using skills that have grown rusty since nursing school, or frustration at being pulled away from work you enjoy.

Unfortunately, floating is necessary. Hospitals must use it to help solve their understaffing problems. And you'll have to go along with it unless:

• you have a union contract that guarantees you'll always work in your specialty
• you can prove you haven't been taught to do the assigned task.

Legally, you can't refuse to float simply because you fear that the skills you need for the assignment have diminished or because you're generally concerned about legal risks in the assigned unit. However, if your supervisor gives you a task you definitely haven't been taught to do, *tell* her that. Usually, she'll accommodate you by changing your assignment. But if she insists that you perform the task you don't know how to do, refuse the assignment. If the hospital reprimands or fires you, you can appeal the action taken against you in a court of law.

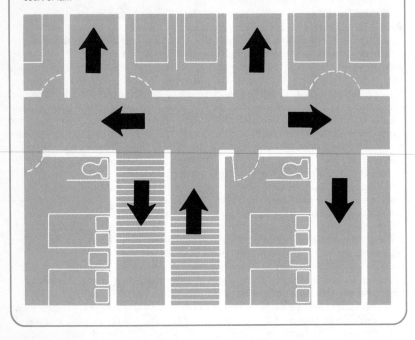

argument fails if any applicable rules and regulations contradict it.

Other hospitals have defended understaffing by arguing that no extra nurses were available. The courts have hesitated to accept this defense, however, especially when hospitals have knowingly permitted an unsafe condition to continue despite their inability to correct it. And the day may come when a hospital is charged with failing to use the nursing personnel available from temporary-nursing service agencies (see Entry 10) or nursing registries (see Entry 7) during understaffed periods.

Still other hospitals have excused understaffing by pleading lack of funds. The courts have repeatedly rejected this defense.

Of course, hospital liability for understaffing isn't automatic. Suppose a hospital finds itself understaffed on the night shift and assigns one nurse to cover two adjacent units. If a patient is injured because of the nurse's unmanageable work load, the hospital may be held liable if it could have reasonably provided adequate staff. But if it couldn't—because, for example, a nurse suddenly called in sick and no substitute could quickly be found—the hospital may escape liability. This is known as a *sudden emergency exception* when used as a defense during a trial. The emergency could not have been anticipated—in contrast to chronic understaffing.

Except for the sudden emergency exception defense, a hospital has only two alternatives for avoiding liability for understaffing: either hire sufficient personnel to staff an area adequately or else close the area (or restrict the number of beds) until adequate staff can be found.

## The charge nurse's liability

Any nurse who's put in charge of a unit, even temporarily, may find herself liable in understaffing situations, including the following:
• She knows understaffing exists but fails to notify the hospital administration about it.
• She fails to assign her staff properly and then also fails to supervise their actions continuously.
• She tries to perform a nursing task for which she lacks the necessary training and skills.

In *Horton v. Niagara Falls Memorial Center* (1976), the charge nurse, one LPN, and one nurse's aide were responsible for 19 patients on a unit. During their shift, one patient became delirious and tried to climb down from a balcony off his room. The attending doctor, when notified, ordered that someone stay with the patient at all times to keep him from going out on the balcony again.

The charge nurse, instead of calling for additional help from within the hospital or notifying the hospital administration, called the patient's wife and summoned her to the hospital to sit with him. The wife agreed to send her mother, but said her mother would

need a while to get there. During this period, the charge nurse provided no supervision of the patient, who did go out on the balcony again. He jumped and sustained injuries. In the lawsuit that followed, the court held the charge nurse liable.

In *Norton v. Argonaut Insurance Company* (1962), a temporary staff shortage led the assistant director of nurses to volunteer her nursing services on a pediatric floor. Because she had been an administrator for several years and was unfamiliar with pediatric care, she proceeded to give a newborn 3 ml of Lanoxin (digoxin) in injectable rather than elixir form. The infant died of cardiac arrest, and the court held the assistant director liable.

Assignment of liability to the charge nurse isn't automatic, however, in lawsuits where understaffing is a factor. The charge nurse isn't necessarily liable unless she knew, or should have known, that the nurse who made the mistake:
• had previously made similar mistakes
• wasn't competent to perform the task
• had acted on the charge nurse's erroneous orders.
And remember, the plaintiff-patient has to prove two things: that the charge nurse failed to follow customary practices, thereby contributing to the mistake; and that the mistake actually caused the patient's injuries.

## Coping with a sudden overload

You know it happens. You begin your shift and suddenly you find yourself assigned more patients than you feel you can reasonably care for. What can you do to protect yourself?

First of all, make every effort to protest the overload and get it reduced. Begin by asking your supervisor or director of nursing service to supply relief. If they can't or won't, notify the hospital administration. If no one there will help either, write a memorandum detailing exactly what you did and said and the answers you got. Don't walk off the job (if you do, you may be liable for abandonment), but do the best you can. After your shift is over, prepare a written report of the facts and file it with the director of nursing.

Filing a written report isn't guaranteed to absolve you from liability if a patient is injured during your shift and sues you for malpractice. You may still be found liable, especially if you could have foreseen and prevented the patient's injury. But a written report will impress a jury as a sincere attempt to protect your patients. And the report could provide you with a defense if the alleged malpractice involves something you should have done, but didn't do, because of understaffing.

If you're a Canadian nurse faced with a sudden patient overload, you may have only two choices: tolerate the situation or refuse to work under such conditions and suffer suspension from duty without pay. Consider the case of *Re Mount Sinai Hospital v. Ontario Nurses Association* (1978).

This case involved three nurses in the hospital's intensive care unit. Because they were already caring for many critically ill patients, they refused to accept still another from the emergency department. The nurses argued that admitting the new patient would endanger the patients already under their care. The hospital disagreed and suspended them for three shifts without pay.

The case was settled in favor of the hospital, on the premise that a hospital is legally obligated to provide care for patients it admits and can insist that certain instructions be carried out. If the hospital had to defer to its employees' opinions, the decision stated, it would be placed in an intolerable legal position.

---

ADVICE

## STAFFING SUGGESTIONS

*Our 85-bed hospital has no recovery room nurse. Every day, one of the RNs from the day shift is "floated" to the recovery room. We feel this is dangerous, for a couple of reasons:*

*Only one RN is assigned, no matter how many patients are there. Shouldn't the hospital maintain a certain nurse:patient ratio in the recovery room?*

*Also, the nurse assigned to the recovery room must work 8 to 10 hours without a break. Surely this isn't right.*

*Our director of nursing knows the whole situation but has made no improvements.*—RN, Tex.

The acceptable nurse:patient ratio varies with the types of surgical procedures and the patients' expected conditions. For example, in a large hospital one or two RNs may be needed for each open-heart surgery patient, but one RN could safely care for three or four patients after less-complicated procedures.

To determine daily averages in your recovery room, record the number and types of operations performed daily and the number of patients in the recovery room each hour. With these figures, you can document any times when the patient load is too great for one nurse.

Regarding the RN's working 8 to 10 hours without a break, if this happens frequently, check your state wage-and-hour division to find out whether your hospital can legally require such a schedule.

Why not ask for a meeting with the director of nursing after compiling the information suggested? Even if your figures don't indicate the need for a full-time recovery room nurse, you might be able to make other staffing arrangements, such as floating a second nurse into the recovery room during peak periods or for breaks or limiting nurses who can be floated to two or three nurses who've received appropriate inservice training.

---

This letter was taken from the files of *Nursing* magazine.

## Dealing with chronic understaffing

Chronic understaffing, if it occurs on your unit, presents you with a dilemma. On the one hand, your conscience tells you to try your best to help every patient. On the other hand, you feel compelled to protect yourself from liability in case a patient is harmed.

The best protection, as you might expect, is prevention—action taken to remedy the understaffing situation (see *Staffing Suggestions*). If you and your colleagues act responsibly and collectively to try to bring about institutional change, the law protects you in several important ways.

A case in point is *Misericordia Hospital Medical Center v. N.L.R.B.* (1980), which involved a charge nurse who was discharged from her job because her employer found her activities "disloyal."

She belonged to a group of hospital employees called the Ad Hoc Patient Care Committee. The committee was formed after the JCAH, which intended to survey the hospital, had invited interested parties—including hospital staff—to submit at a public meeting information on whether accreditation standards were being met. One complaint lodged by the nurse and her committee was insufficient coverage on many shifts—a situation the hospital had failed to remedy.

Even though the JCAH examiners approved the hospital, the nurse was fired shortly afterward. When the National Labor Relations Board (NLRB) ordered the hospital to reinstate the nurse, the hospital appealed. The appeals court upheld the NLRB order, citing a U.S. Supreme Court ruling that employees don't lose protection "when they seek to improve terms and conditions of employment or otherwise improve their lot as employees through channels outside the immediate employee-employer relationship."

This decision offers nurses considerable protection in conflicts with employers, especially those in which working conditions directly affect the care given patients.

Of course, you must be sure you follow the appropriate channels of communication. If you can't get help to remedy a dangerous understaffing situation, first go through all hospital channels, up to and including the board of trustees. Simply report what the problem is, the number of hours you've been forced to work without relief, the number of consecutive days you've been forced to work, and any other relevant facts. Then, if you still can't get help, and if your complaint involves an alleged unfair labor practice, you can contact the NLRB.

### A final word

Given the present uncertainty about future numbers of nursing graduates, and in view of hospitals' financial woes, understaffing probably will continue in many health-care institutions. Some hospitals are experimenting with ways to ensure adequate staffs, however, and others will surely follow. Ideas include letting nurses choose their own work schedules and hiring part-time nurses through agencies or on a private-duty basis. But don't look for this issue to disappear any time soon.

# 20 Witnessing and signing documents

You can't escape it. As a nurse, you'll sometimes be asked to witness the signing of documents, such as deeds, bills of sale, powers of attorney, contracts, and wills. You'll also find yourself—intentionally or otherwise—witnessing patients' (or others') oral statements that may have legal significance. Your actions at times like these are important. They can influence whether what you witnessed has the force of law, and they can also expose you to certain legal

## KEY TERMS IN THIS ENTRY

**causa mortis** • A state of mind in a person approaching death.

**common law** • Law derived from previous court decisions, not from statutes. Also called **case law.**

**respondeat superior** • "Let the master answer." A legal doctrine that makes an employer liable for the consequences of his employee's wrongful conduct while the employee is acting within the scope of his employment.

consequences. You may even have to testify, later, in court about the signing and the circumstances surrounding it.

## What signing as a witness means

When you sign as a witness, you're usually certifying only that you saw the person, known to you by a certain name, place his signature on the document. You're not certifying the primary signer's mental competence (although you should *not* sign if you believe he's incompetent), nor are you certifying the presence or absence of duress, undue influence, fraud, or error.

If you're ever called to testify about the signing, don't underestimate the importance of your testimony. A court looking into charges of fraud or undue influence used in executing a document often gives great weight to a nurse's perception. You may be asked about the patient's physical and mental condition at the time of the signing, and the court may ask you to describe his interactions with his family, his attorney, and others.

## Which laws apply to signing documents?

In the United States and Canada, as you know, nurse practice acts are the laws

that establish nurses' scope of professional and legal accountability. When you witness a document, other laws also apply. For example, all states have laws setting out the legal requirements for written and oral wills, dying declarations, and gifts *causa mortis* (in expectation of death). These laws establish the format of wills, the number of witnesses needed, who can be a witness, what makes a will valid or invalid, how to make a will inoperative, and how to contest a will.

In many states, your signature on a will certifies not only that you witnessed the will-signing but also that you heard the maker of the will declare it to be his will, and that all witnesses and the maker of the will were actually present during the signing.

By attesting to these last two facts, you help ensure the authenticity of the will and the signatures. (See *When You're Asked to Witness a Patient's Written Will.*) Your signature doesn't certify, however, that the maker of the will is competent.

The laws also cover dying declarations and gifts *causa mortis,* specifying when they're valid and when they aren't.

In the case of a living will, your state law may prohibit you from acting as a witness. (See Entry 30.)

## What's your liability?

You can be liable and in violation of the prevailing standards of care if the signature you witness is false or if you sign knowing the patient is incompetent or has given uninformed consent. You can also be held liable if you knowingly allow a minor, nonguardian, or other ineligible person to sign a document.

If you're the only person who informs a patient about a planned medical procedure and you then witness his signature, you can be liable for practicing outside your nurse practice act, for practicing medicine without a license, or both. And your hospital may be liable for negligence under the doctrine of respondeat superior. If you've given the patient false information in an attempt to deceive him, you may be guilty of fraud or misrepresentation.

### Before you sign—read!

Before you sign any document, read at least enough of it to make sure it *is* the type of document the primary signer represents it to be. Usually you won't have to read all the text, and legally this isn't necessary for your signature to be valid. But always examine the document's title and first page, and give careful attention to what's written immediately above the place for your signature. (The place for your signature, by the way, should be clearly labeled as such.)

### How to sign

When signing a document, write legibly and use your full legal name. When signing on hospital forms, add your title. On other documents the title is optional, but adding it will establish why you're in the hospital.

### When—and when not—to sign

When you're asked to sign as a witness, do so only if you believe the patient to be both mentally and physically competent. Legally, as you know, you don't need to have knowledge of exactly what's contained in the documents you witness. But professionally, as when you witness the signing of an informed consent form, you should know. You also should make sure the patient knows what procedure or treatment he's consenting to when he affixes his signature (see Entry 12).

When should you not sign? Here are some instances:

• when the patient is not legally able to give consent—for example, when he's

---

## WHEN YOU'RE ASKED TO WITNESS A PATIENT'S WRITTEN WILL

If a patient asks you to serve as a witness when he draws up his will, follow these precautions:

• Don't forget to notify the patient's doctor and your supervisor before you act as a witness.
• Don't give the patient any legal advice.
• Don't offer to assist him in phrasing the document's wording.
• Don't comment on the nature of his choices.
• Don't forget to document your actions in your nurses' notes.

a minor or a nonguardian
• when the patient is not who he says he is, or you can't be sure
• when the patient has no power of free choice; for example, when he's being blackmailed or otherwise pressured into signing by his family
• when the patient is uninformed about what he's consenting to because he's been given misleading information, doesn't understand the information given, or hasn't been told of the risks involved
• when a patient is obviously incompetent—for example, when he's suffering from advanced senility and is being

> *"When you witness an oral statement, document what the patient says as close to word-for-word as you can."*

pressured to sign a deed transferring a real estate title to someone else.

In such situations, simply explain that you choose not to act as a witness. Then record the incident in your nurses' notes, using a chronologic format. Chart the setting, the patient's mental and physical condition, the reason for the refusal, what you saw and heard, and what happened after your refusal (for instance, that someone else witnessed or someone else gave consent).

Finally, report the incident to other staff members affected by your refusal to sign—for example, your supervisor and the patient's doctor.

### Writing your nurses' notes

When you record in your notes that you've witnessed a patient's signature on any type of document, always include something about his apparent perceptions of his health and general circumstances.

When you witness a *written will*,

document that it was signed and witnessed, who signed it, who else was present, what was done with it after signing, and what the patient's condition was at the time.

When you witness *oral statements* such as dying declarations or oral wills, document what the patient says as close to word-for-word as you can. Also document the names of other witnesses, the patient's physical and mental condition at the time, and the patient's reaction to the statement afterwards. Make your notes carefully: remember, they could be used in court for probating the will, for resolving creditors' claims, or for prosecuting alleged criminals. The notes will also refresh your memory if you're called to testify in court.

Besides recording the event in your own notes, write up or type a copy of the patient's oral statement and, if possible, get him and other witnesses to sign it. Report the matter to the patient's doctor and to your supervisor, too. This will keep them informed and alert them that an item in the patient's medical record may have legal importance.

### Understanding Canadian procedures

The formalities of signing and witnessing documents differ between the United States and Canada. But because both countries' legal systems are based primarily on English common law, the U.S. and Canadian laws governing how a witness should sign legal documents are essentially the same.

# 21 Special risks in special-care units

As you know, recent decades have witnessed dramatic changes in the nurse's role. In many patient-care circumstances, nurses now perform tasks that only doctors used to perform. This is particularly true in special-care units, such as the emergency department (ED), operating room (OR), recovery room (RR), intensive care unit (ICU), and coronary care unit (CCU). Here, patient care offers exciting nursing challenges, increased nursing responsibilities—and extra risks of liability.

For example, if you're an ED nurse, you'll sometimes have to employ triage in patient selection. If you make a mistake, a seriously injured patient's treatment may be needlessly delayed. And you may be liable.

In the OR, you must confirm that the patient has given his informed consent and that his consent is documented. As you work with the operating team (work that today involves much more than worrying about missing instruments and sponges), you can't help but be aware of the legal risks involved.

If the RR is your assignment, you know you must watch your patients for signs and symptoms of adverse anesthetic effects, of postoperative cardiac and pulmonary complications, and of shock caused by hypoxia, hemorrhage, or infection. The same concerns apply if you work in an ICU or CCU. In these units, you may also have to administer sophisticated drugs or perform sophisticated procedures, such as passing a stylet through a patient's subclavian line to determine patency. In any of these special-care units, you must be able to take appropriate and effective action when a patient's survival depends on your judgment.

### Where you stand legally

If you work in a special-care unit, you must take the possibility of increased liability seriously. Remember, even though hospital policy requires that you perform certain tasks, or you perform them under doctor's orders as a doctor's *borrowed servant,* your individual liability continues. If a patient sues for malpractice, all the persons involved can be held separately and jointly liable. This suggests that you carefully evaluate the jobs you're asked

to do. If any task is beyond your training and expertise, don't attempt it. And even if you can do it, make sure you're permitted to do it according to hospital policy and your state or Canadian provincial nurse practice act. (See *Exercising Caution in Special-Care Units,* pages 136 and 137.)

### How the law views nurses' expanded roles

Many nurse practice acts recognize nurses' expanded roles (see Entries 1 and 6).

One such role involves diagnoses. In general, a nurse can't legally make a medical diagnosis or prescribe medical, therapeutic, or corrective measures, *except as authorized* by the hospital and the state where she's working. This means that if you perform a tracheotomy while working on a postoperative orthopedic floor (especially if you could have called a doctor), you may be found liable, if the patient sues, for performing a medical function. But you probably wouldn't be liable if you performed the tracheotomy in the ED during a disaster.

In Canada, several provinces, including Ontario and Quebec, have passed medical acts that permit the del-

## PROTECTING YOURSELF WHEN WORKING IN SPECIAL-CARE UNITS

If you're working in a special-care unit of a hospital—the emergency department, intensive care unit, operating room, or recovery room—your expanded responsibilities make you extra vulnerable to malpractice lawsuits. To protect yourself, take the following precautions:

● Request a clear, written definition of your role in the hospital. Your hospital should have an overall policy and an individual, written job description for you that specifies the limits of your nursing role. You'll be better protected if guidelines for advanced nursing competencies are formally established.

● Document everything you do, so there's no question later about your actions. Your notes, of course, should reflect the nursing process: document your assessment of the patient, your care plan, your actual care, and your evaluation of the plan's effectiveness.

● Make sure of your own competence. If your role expands, your skills have to grow, too. If this requires advanced courses and supervised clinical experience, make sure you get both.

● Insure yourself. Damages awarded to patients can be very high, and high legal fees may mean you can't afford even to *win* a lawsuit. If you don't have your own professional liability insurance, and your hospital doesn't help defend you against a lawsuit, you could face a startling bill even after all claims against you are proven groundless and dropped. (You might never even get to court—but you could still find yourself with a large bill for legal consultation.)

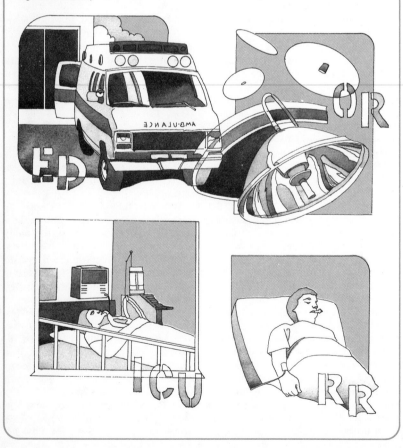

egation of specific medical functions to nurses. Some provinces require that a nurse obtain special training or certification to perform these functions. In the United States, however, current laws provide little guidance for nurses who daily face situations like these. (See *Protecting Yourself When Working in Special-Care Units*.)

Suppose, for example, you're working in an ICU, where you must often act on standing orders and without a doctor's supervision. How can you be sure that when you perform quasi-

> *"A nurse working in a special-care unit is subject to the same general rule of law as her staff-nurse colleagues."*

medical functions, even with standing orders, that you're not violating your nurse practice act?

You can't be sure, of course, because nurse practice acts don't provide specific guidelines. Treating patients on the basis of standing orders is a matter of judgment. In such situations, be sure you're qualified to recognize the problem; then follow established medical protocol.

## How nursing standards apply

In general, a nurse working in a special-care unit is subject to the same general rule of law as her staff-nurse colleagues: she must meet the standard of care that a reasonably well qualified and prudent nurse would meet in the same or similar circumstances.

However, in deciding whether a specialty nurse has acted reasonably, if she's the defendant in a malpractice lawsuit, the court won't consider what the average LPN/LVN or RN would have done. Instead, the court will seek to determine the standard of care that an

LPN/LVN or RN *specifically trained to work in the special-care unit* would have met. Thus, the law imposes a higher standard of conduct on persons with knowledge, skill, or training superior to that of other persons in the profession.

*Hunt v. Palm Springs General Hospital* (1977) illustrates how the courts evaluate the reasonable-person standard in light of prevailing practices.

The patient, Mr. Hunt, was rushed to the ED with convulsions. Once he was examined, his doctor concluded that Mr. Hunt, a known drug addict, was experiencing convulsions because he'd gone without drugs for several days. Although the doctor advised the hospital administration that the patient's condition wasn't critical, he nevertheless requested hospitalization.

The hospital refused to admit Mr. Hunt because of a history of unpaid bills. During the next 4 hours, while Mr. Hunt sat in the ED waiting area, the doctor tried to find hospitalization for him elsewhere in the city. Eventually, Mr. Hunt was admitted to a neighboring hospital. He lived for 26 hours before dying from brain damage caused by prolonged seizures.

During the lawsuit that followed, the court examined the practice of ED nurses elsewhere and found that the Palm Springs Hospital nurses had acted unreasonably. Their duty was to monitor Mr. Hunt's condition periodically while he awaited transfer to another hospital. If this duty had been carried out, the court concluded, the nurses would have noted his elevated temperature—a clear indication that he needed immediate hospitalization.

Similarly, in *Cline v. Lund* (1973), the patient, Ms. Cline, was sent to a CC step-down unit after problems developed following a hysterectomy on July 10. Except for one bout with nausea, she appeared to be making satisfactory progress. At about 2:30 p.m. on July 11, a nurse dangled Ms. Cline's legs from the side of her bed. The nurse charted that the patient tolerated the

# EXERCISING CAUTION IN SPECIAL-CARE UNITS

### Risky practice in the emergency department

*I enjoy working in the emergency department (ED) of a small community hospital near my home, but I don't enjoy one of the practices there. Our nurses routinely take doctors' telephone orders for narcotic injections.*

*What am I making a fuss about? Well, what usually happens is that when a patient comes in complaining of a headache, a staff doctor is consulted by phone, and he orders a narcotic. The patient receives his injection, then leaves without ever seeing a doctor. Supposedly, the doctor will come by the next day to sign the verbal order he gave. But many doctors here "forget" this step.*

*Several months ago, one of the ED doctors reported this practice to the hospital administration and said he felt it was ill-advised and illegal. The administration responded with a letter to all staff doctors indicating that the ED would continue to honor telephone orders as a service to staff doctors. (We were also told doctors would sign their telephone orders the next day.)*

*Maybe I'm bucking the system, but I'm not satisfied. I've discussed our policy and practice with ED nurses at other hospitals and with several staff doctors here who also work in other EDs. Everyone tells me the same thing: other hospitals consider our practice illegal.*

*I'd like to refuse to give narcotic injections under these circumstances, but I need some backup.*—RN, Tenn.

This practice is illegal. It violates the federal government's conditions for nurses' participation in medical care. And it runs counter to numerous court decisions supporting the requirement that a doctor examine every patient who comes to the ED before the patient receives treatment.

Document the telephone orders as they occur (with facts only; leave your opinions aside), and then send a memo with the facts, and the reasons for your concern, through proper channels. If you're attempting to change your hospital's policy, why not join forces with the ED doctor who's already protested the unsafe practice?

### Guarding the postoperative patient

*I've just started to work in the recovery room (RR) of our local hospital, but I'm already up in arms about an unsafe practice I see going on.*

*When a postoperative patient is ready to return to the medical/surgical unit, one of our nurses places the stretcher near the RR door to wait for an orderly. No nurse accompanies the patient back to the unit—just an orderly who isn't even trained in cardiopulmonary resuscitation.*

*But that's not all that's bothering me. If all the orderlies are busy, the patient may wait as much as half an hour at the RR door. During this time, no one's checking his vital signs. If one of these patients should run into trouble before he reached the medical/surgical unit, who'd be responsible?*

*Our charge nurse claims the hospital would be responsible. I checked the hospital's policy book, and it's vague about transport and about the RR nurse's role in discharging a patient.*

*Of course I'm worried about these patients. But I'm also worried about my responsibility as an RR nurse. I'd like to know: is transporting a patient without a nurse being present standard policy in most hospitals?*—RN, Vt.

---

dangling well. By 3:30 p.m., Ms. Cline was unresponsive, her blood pressure was rising, and she was vomiting.

At 9:00 p.m., when Ms. Cline's blood pressure reached 142/90, the attending nurse notified her supervisor, who at 9:40 p.m. notified the attending doctor.

He came to the hospital, examined the patient, and—suspecting an internal hemorrhage—ordered blood work and vital signs taken every 30 minutes. At 11:45 p.m., the patient's blood pressure was 160/90. Her arms and legs were stiff, her fists clenched.

diac arrest at 12:45 a.m., and died at 4:45 a.m.

In the ensuing lawsuit, the court found the nurse liable, stating that her care had fallen below that of a reasonably prudent nurse in the same or similar circumstances. "Nurses," the court decision said, "should notify the doctor of any significant change or unresponsiveness."

## How Canadian nursing standards apply

As you're probably aware, a Canadian nurse's performance is also measured against the appropriate standard of care.

For example, in *Laidlaw v. Lions Gate Hospital* (1969), the court held that both the RR nurse who left for a coffee break and the supervisor who permitted her to leave should have anticipated an influx of patients from the OR.

When the nurse left on her break, only two patients and the supervisor nurse were in the RR. In a short time, however, three more patients arrived— including the plaintiff, Mrs. Laidlaw. Because only one nurse was on duty to care for five patients, Mrs. Laidlaw did not receive appropriate care and suffered extensive, permanent brain damage as a result of anesthesia-related hypoxia.

When the resulting lawsuit came to trial, another nursing supervisor testified that usually two nurses were present in the RR and that nurses were not permitted to take breaks after new patients arrived. Other testimony revealed that RR nurses should know the OR schedule and so should anticipate when new patients will arrive.

The court found the nurse who left, and her supervisor, negligent in leaving only one nurse on duty in the RR.

## Staying within nursing practice limits

You know that when you work in special-care units, you mustn't presume that your increased training and

---

At no time should an RR patient be left unattended. The responsibility for that patient remains with the RR staff until that patient has been turned over to the staff of the medical/surgical unit and an appropriate report has been given.

The hospital *is* liable; but so is the RR staff, because they *know* about the dangerous practice of leaving the patient unattended but have neither documented nor remedied it.

Ideally, an RN should accompany all patients leaving the RR. In hospitals where this is routine practice, the RR nurses love it. They feel secure about the patients and about their own responsibilities.

If a nurse can't go with *every* patient, *at least* a nurse should accompany a high-risk patient—say, one with chest tubes. An orderly could accompany a patient less likely to develop difficulties.

For every departing RR patient, an RR nurse should call the medical/surgical floor, tell the staff the patient is on his way, and inform them of his progress and condition.

To remedy the situation in your hospital, try to get a detailed policy in writing. Begin by finding out how the transfer of postoperative patients is handled in other hospitals in your area. Then document the risks of your hospital's current practice. Bring all this information to the attention of your immediate supervisor. If she doesn't take action, keep going up the chain of command.

In calling attention to this risky nursing practice, you may get some flak. Just tell yourself you're not *making* trouble— you're *preventing* it. If you need professional support, consult the Association of Operating Room Nurses (AORN), 10170 E. Mississippi Ave., Denver, Colorado 80231.

---

These letters were taken from the files of *Nursing* magazine.

---

Instead of summoning the doctor again, the attending nurse once more notified her supervisor. At 12:15 a.m. on July 12, when Ms. Cline's blood pressure had reached 230/130, the doctor was called. The patient stopped breathing at 12:40 a.m., suffered a car-

broadened authority permit you to exceed nursing's legal limits. This is especially important in an area such as diagnosis, where you can easily cross the legal boundary separating nursing from medicine.

One place this sometimes happens is in the ED, where an on-call doctor may refuse to see a patient himself, instead ordering care based on a nurse's observations of the patient. Similar situations may occur in the RR, ICU, and CCU, where split-second patient-care decisions are sometimes made on the basis of nurses' phone calls to attending doctors.

If you find yourself in this situation, remember that all state and Canadian provincial nurse practice acts prohibit you from medically diagnosing a patient's condition. You can tell the doctor about signs and symptoms you've observed—but you may not make the decision about what care should be given. If you do, you'll be practicing medicine without a license. And you'll be held at least partly liable for any harm to the patient that results.

Consider the case of *Methodist Hospital v. Ball* (1961). Young Mr. Ball was brought to the ED with injuries sustained in an automobile accident. Because of a sudden influx of critically ill patients, the ED staff was unable to care for him immediately. While lying on a stretcher in the hospital hallway, Mr. Ball became boisterous and demanded care. Apparently the attending nurse decided he was drunk. Instead of being treated, Mr. Ball was put into restraints and transported by ambulance to another local hospital. There, 15 minutes after arriving, he died from internal bleeding.

An autopsy revealed no evidence of alcohol in Mr. Ball's system. The court that heard the resulting lawsuit found the attending nurse and medical resident negligent because they failed to diagnose Mr. Ball's condition properly, to give supportive treatment, and to alert personnel at the second hospital about Mr. Ball's critical condition.

## A final word

If and when you practice in a special-care unit, be sure you know—and follow—hospital policies and procedures. Know your own limitations, too—never perform a procedure you feel unsure about. Remember, admitting to inexperience is never improper. But performing a procedure that may exceed your capabilities could be, especially if it results in a patient's serious injury or death.

If you're an LPN or LVN working in a special-care unit, the same precautionary watchword applies. As you help RNs care for acutely ill patients and carry out doctors' orders, remember that you assume a significant legal risk when you perform a task that an RN ordinarily performs. If you injure the patient in the process and he sues you for malpractice, your care will be measured against what a reasonably competent RN would do in the same or similar circumstances.

# 22 Your legal responsibility for patients' safety

As a hospital nurse, one of your most important responsibilities is patients' physical safety. To prevent falls, for example, you have to make sure bed side rails are up for debilitated, elderly, confused, or medicated patients. You also have to help weak patients walk, use proper transfer methods when moving patients, and sometimes use restraining devices to immobilize patients.

In the interest of patient safety, you also have to keep an eye on your hospital's facilities and equipment. If you spot loose or improperly functioning side rails, water or some other substance on the unit floor, or an improperly functioning respirator, you have a duty to report the problem and call for repairs or housekeeping assistance. Failure to do so may not only endanger patients but also make you—and the hospital—liable if patients are injured.

## What are patient-safety standards of care?

In any malpractice lawsuit against a nurse, she's judged on how well she performed her duty as measured against the appropriate standards of care. This means that if you're ever sued for malpractice, the court, in reaching its judgment, will analyze whether you gave the plaintiff-patient care equal to that of a reasonably well qualified and prudent nurse in the same or similar circumstances. (To learn how courts establish appropriate standards, see Entry 2.)

Where patient safety is involved, your duty includes anticipating foreseeable risks. For example, if you're aware that the floor in a patient's room is dangerously slippery, your duty is to report the condition to the appropriate hospital department. If you don't, and a patient falls and is injured, you could be held liable for breaching your duty to protect that patient.

In fact, you might be held liable even if you *didn't* know the floor was slippery. Using accepted standards of care as a measure, a court might reason that part of your duty as a reasonable and prudent nurse was to check the floor of your unit regularly and report any patient hazard immediately.

Of course, the standards of care that you meet will vary with your job or the training you've had. A staff nurse's actions, for example, will be measured against staff-nurse standards, and a gerontologic nurse's actions will be measured against standards that gerontologic nurses must meet.

## Special safety concerns

You're always on guard, of course, to prevent *patient falls*. (See *Preventing Patient Falls*, page 140.) You know that almost anything can cause a patient to fall, particularly if he's elderly or re-

ceiving medication. Elderly patients are in many instances confused, disoriented, and weak. Medications can cause (or increase) confusion and lessen a patient's ability to react in situations when he might fall. Here are some important ways you can protect your patient from falls:
• Make sure his bed's side rails are kept up, when indicated.
• Orient him to where he is and what time it is, especially if he's elderly.
• Monitor him regularly—continually, if his condition makes this necessary.
• Provide adequate lighting and a clean, clutter-free environment.
• Make sure that someone helps and supports him whenever he gets out of bed, and that he wears proper shoes when walking.
• Make sure adequate staff are avail-

# PREVENTING PATIENT FALLS

When one of your patients falls down, you worry not only about his condition but also about liability—your own and your hospital's. You should know that patient falls are among the most common hospital accidents. Of course, you can't prevent all falls. But you can help minimize your patients' risks by using this handy fall-prevention checklist. When a patient is assigned to your unit, fill out this checklist and keep it with the patient's chart. Then any nurse caring for the patient can use the list to take the appropriate safety precautions.

PATIENT'S NAME: _____ AGE: _____
DIAGNOSIS: _____
NURSING UNIT & STATION: _____

|  | YES | NO | COMMENTS |
|---|---|---|---|
| • Are restraints needed? | ☐ | ☐ | _____ |
| • Are side rails up? | ☐ | ☐ | _____ |
| • Is the bed in low position? | ☐ | ☐ | _____ |
| • Are the bed wheels locked? Wheelchair brakes on? | ☐ ☐ | ☐ ☐ | _____ |
| • Is the call light within the patient's reach? | ☐ | ☐ | _____ |
| • Does the patient understand how to use the call light? | ☐ | ☐ | _____ |
| • Is the night-light on? | ☐ | ☐ | _____ |
| • Does the room have any physical hazards (e.g., is the floor slippery because of damp mopping)? | ☐ | ☐ | _____ |
| • What type of footwear does the patient have on? |  |  | _____ |
| • Are the patient's water, tissues, and urinal within his reach? | ☐ | ☐ | _____ |
| • If the patient is a surgical patient, how many hours or days postoperative is he? |  |  | _____ |
| • Does the patient have any previously identified physical or mental limitations? | ☐ | ☐ | _____ |
| • Is the patient aware of his activity limitations? | ☐ | ☐ | _____ |
| • Is the patient showing any physical or mental limitations now? | ☐ | ☐ | _____ |
| • Has the patient received any analgesics, hypnotics, sedatives, or relaxants? If yes, what are they? | ☐ | ☐ | _____ |
| • Is he receiving other medications that may cause him to fall? If yes, what are they? | ☐ | ☐ | _____ |

able to transfer him, if necessary.

Elderly patients and patients taking medications need special nursing care when doctors' orders require them to be "up in chair for 15 minutes x 3 daily" or "up in chair for meals." If you can't supervise such a patient while he's sitting up, at least make sure another member of the health-care team does so.

*Restraining devices,* often prescribed to ensure a patient's safety, unfortunately can also endanger it. So when a doctor prescribes a Posey belt or other restraining device for a patient, keep in mind that such devices don't remove your responsibility for the patient's safety. In fact, they increase it. For example, when a patient wears a Posey belt, you have to make sure he doesn't undo it or inadvertently readjust it; if he does, it could choke or otherwise injure him. You also have to make sure the belt is fitted properly; if it's too tight, it could restrict the patient's breathing or irritate his skin.

You may have to decide when the belt is no longer necessary. Failure to do this could result in an accusation of false imprisonment against you.

Be sure to document carefully any use of a restraining device. Note why the patient needed it, when you first applied it, how you supervised its use, and when and why you stopped using it. As long as you can demonstrate that the restraint is lawful—that is, clinically necessary—you're protected from false-imprisonment accusations. (See *When Can You Legally Restrain a Patient?,* page 143.)

*Preventing suicides* is another very important aspect of patient safety for every nurse. Not all self-destructive, suicidal patients are cared for by psychiatric nurses.

If a suicidal patient is in your care, your first obligation is to provide close supervision. He may require one-on-one, 24-hour-a-day supervision until the immediate threat of self-harm is over. Take from him all potentially dangerous objects, such as belts, bed linens, glassware, and eating utensils. And make sure he swallows pills when you give them; otherwise, he may retain them in his mouth and save them for use—and abuse—later.

Check his hospital environment carefully for possible dangers. If he can easily open or break his room windows, or if escape from your unit would be easy, you may have to transfer him to a safer, more secure place—if necessary, to a seclusion room.

Remember, whether you work on a psychiatric unit or a medical unit, you'll be held responsible for the decisions you make about a suicidal patient's care. If you're sued because he's been harmed while in your care, and the case is brought to court, you'll be judged on the basis of:
• whether you knew (or should have known) that the patient was likely to harm himself
• whether, knowing he was likely to harm himself, you exercised reasonable care in helping him avoid injury or death.

*Ensuring the safety of equipment,* making sure that the equipment used for patient care is free from defects, is an important duty. (See Entry 22.) You also need to exercise reasonable care in selecting equipment for a specific procedure and patient, and then help maintain the equipment. Here again, your patient care must reflect what the reasonably well qualified and prudent nurse would do in the same or similar circumstances. This means that if you know a specific piece of equipment isn't functioning properly, you must take steps to correct the defects, and document the steps you took. If you don't, and a patient is injured because of the defective equipment, you may be sued for malpractice.

Selecting proper equipment and maintaining it also means making sure it's not contaminated. When cleaning equipment, always follow hospital procedures strictly, and document your actions carefully. This will decrease the possibility that you could be held liable for using contaminated equipment.

Similarly, be sure *you* don't cause contamination or cross-infection of patients. In *Helman v. Sacred Heart Hospital* (1963), staff nurses were held responsible for causing the plaintiff-patient's *Staphyloccus* infection. According to the court decision, the nurses were negligent because after caring for the plaintiff's roommate (who originally had the infection), they did not wash their hands before caring for the plaintiff.

You can also be held liable for improper use of equipment that's functioning properly. This liability occurs in many instances with equipment that can cause burns—for example, diathermy machines, electrosurgical equipment, and hot water bottles. When you use such equipment, carry out the procedure or therapy carefully, observe the patient continually until the procedure or therapy is completed, and ask the patient frequently (if he's awake during the procedure or therapy) whether he's comfortable or having any pain.

## Understanding the hospital's responsibility

Patient safety, of course, isn't only your responsibility. Your hospital is responsible, too. This institutional responsibility for patient safety rests on the two most frequently used doctrines of malpractice liability.

The first doctrine, *corporate liability*, holds the hospital liable for its own wrongful conduct—for any breach of its duties as mandated by statutory law, common law, and applicable rules and regulations. The hospital's duty to keep patients safe includes the duty to provide, inspect, repair, and maintain reasonably adequate equipment for diagnosis and treatment. The hospital also has a duty to keep the physical plant reasonably safe. Thus, if a patient is injured because the hospital alone breached one of its duties, the hospital is responsible for the injury.

In recent years, the courts have expanded the concept of an institution's liability for breaching its duties. In a landmark case, *Darling v. Charleston Community Memorial Hospital* (1965), the Illinois Supreme Court expanded the concept of hospital corporate liability to include the hospital's responsibility to supervise the quality of patient care given to its patients. (For a discussion of this case, see Entry 19.)

The second doctrine of institutional malpractice liability is *respondeat superior* (see Entry 42). Under this doctrine, the liability for an employee's wrongful conduct is transferred to the institution. This means that both the employee and the institution can be found liable for a breach of duty to the patient—including the duty of ensuring his safety.

## How court cases have helped establish liability for patients' safety

You may be wondering which breaches of the duty to protect patients will result in liability for a hospital alone, and which will result in a nurse's sharing the liability. The answers depend on the facts involved. If, for example, a court can determine that the duty to monitor patient-care equipment and to repair any discovered defects rests with the hospital and the nurse, then both could be held liable for a breach of that duty. In *May v. Broun* (1972), the plaintiff-patient sued the hospital, the circulating nurse, and the doctor for burns she sustained when an electric cautery machine's electrode burned her during a hemorrhoidectomy.

Although the machine had been used successfully earlier in the day, when the doctor began to use it on the plaintiff, he noticed that its heat was not sufficient to cauterize blood vessels. So, he asked the circulating nurse to check the machine. She did, and after that it apparently worked properly. Nevertheless, the plaintiff was burned where the electrode had touched her body. She later sued the hospital, the circulating nurse, and the doctor.

Because the hospital and the nurse settled with the plaintiff out of court, the doctor was the only one to stand trial. The court held the doctor not liable for the patient's injuries because the hospital had the duty to monitor the equipment and to provide trained personnel to operate it. This meant that the hospital had to bear responsibility for the defective equipment and any wrongful conduct by the nurse. In this case, the hospital and the nurse were liable for the plaintiff's injury.

In *Story v. McCurtain Memorial Management, Inc.* (1981), the outcome was different. This case involved the delivery of one twin by the mother herself when she was left unattended in a shower room. The patient continuously called for help, but her calls went un-answered and the baby the mother delivered herself died.

The mother sued both the hospital and the nurse on duty at the time. The court found the nurse not liable, but it held the hospital liable (under the doctrine of corporate liability) for failing to provide safeguards in the shower room and adequate supervision on the unit. Here, then, the hospital alone was liable for breaching its duty to protect patients from harm.

### A final word

As a nurse, you have an important duty to ensure your patients' safety. Remember, all your actions directed toward patient safety must be in line with your hospital's policies and procedures, so be sure you know what these are. If no

---

ADVICE

## WHEN CAN YOU LEGALLY RESTRAIN A PATIENT?

*Recently, we had a confused elderly patient who kept wandering off the unit. We kept a "sitter" with him for several days, but that taxed our staff. Finally, our nurse said we couldn't spare anyone to sit with him anymore and told me to put restraints on him.*

*I told her I was afraid I'd get in trouble if I restrained a patient without his doctor's orders. She told me I was insubordinate and did it herself.*

*I still think I was right. Is a nurse ever justified in restraining a patient without his doctor's orders?*—RN, Calif.

Yes. In fact most hospitals expect nurses to restrain a patient if that's necessary to protect him from injury. In one court case, a patient's family accused nurses of negligence because they *didn't* restrain a patient. The family won.

Read your hospital's policy on restraints immediately, so you'll know what's expected of you next time. You were right to *question* an order you weren't sure was proper. But you weren't right to refuse it without checking further.

Despite your hospital's policy, you may still have questions about a restraint order—and rightly so. With or without a doctor's order, restraints are legal only if they're necessary to protect the patient or others from harm. You can be charged with false imprisonment or battery if you use restraints on a competent patient simply because he refuses to follow orders.

Were restraints called for in the situation you mentioned? The patient's safety clearly required some method of restraining his wandering, so no one's likely to challenge the need for restraint. If you had adequate staff to provide a sitter, that would have been the best form of restraint—because it was the least restraining. If you couldn't spare a staff member, applying a soft restraint would probably have been the safest course to take. With proper documentation explaining the need to protect the patient, the use of restraints in this situation probably wouldn't have exposed you to liability. (Presumably you contacted the doctor as soon as possible and obtained an order to continue the restraint.)

---

This letter was taken from the files of *NursingLife* magazine.

policies exist, or if they're outdated or poorly drafted, bring this to your supervisor's or head nurse's attention. Consider volunteering to help write or rewrite the policies. By getting involved in efforts to improve patients' safety, you may decrease your potential liability and, at the same time, improve the quality of patient care.

# 23 Your legal risks in administering drugs

Administering drugs to patients continues to be one of the most important—and, legally, one of the most risky—tasks you perform as a nurse.

For many years, U.S. and Canadian nurses were only permitted to give drugs orally or rectally. If a patient needed to receive a drug by injection, the prescribing doctor injected it himself.

Gradually, however, the nurse's role expanded. Today you give subcutaneous and intramuscular injections, induce anesthesia, and use I.V.s. In some states you may even prescribe drugs, with certain limitations.

In general, the law has kept pace with nurses' expanding role in administering drugs. You must meet high practice standards and adhere to the long-standing *five rights formula*:

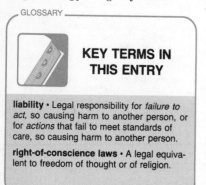

GLOSSARY

## KEY TERMS IN THIS ENTRY

**liability** • Legal responsibility for *failure to act*, so causing harm to another person, or for *actions* that fail to meet standards of care, so causing harm to another person.

**right-of-conscience laws** • A legal equivalent to freedom of thought or of religion.

- the right drug
- to the right patient
- at the right time
- in the right dosage
- by the right route.

And you'd be wise to add a sixth right to this checklist:

- by the right technique.

## How are drugs legally defined?

Legally, as you probably know, a *drug* is any substance listed in an official state, Canadian provincial, or national formulary. It may also be any substance (other than food) "intended to affect the structure or any function of the body . . . (or) for use in the diagnosis, cure, mitigation, treatment, or prevention of disease" (N.Y. Educ. Law).

A *prescription drug* is any drug restricted from regular commercial purchase and sale. Why? Because a state, provincial, or national government has determined that it is, or might be, unsafe unless used under a qualified medical practitioner's supervision.

## Understanding drug laws

Two federal laws mainly govern the use of drugs in the United States: the Comprehensive Drug Abuse Prevention and Control Act (incorporating the Controlled Substances Act), which regulates those drugs thought to be most subject to abuse; and the Food, Drug, and Cosmetic Act, which restricts interstate shipment of drugs not approved for human use and outlines the process by which drugs are tested and approved.

On the state and (in Canada) provincial level, the main laws affecting the distribution of drugs are the pharmacy practice acts. These laws give pharmacists (and sometimes doctors, in Canada) the *sole legal authority* to prepare, compound, preserve, and dispense drugs. *Dispense* refers to taking a drug from the pharmacy supply and giving or selling it to another person. This contrasts with *administering* drugs—actually getting the drug into the patient. As you know, your nurse

## HOW COMMON ARE DRUG ERRORS?

Did you know that one out of every six drug administrations in hospitals is given in error? Some studies have tried to calculate how many patients are actually harmed by such errors. These studies reveal that injuries from drug errors are all too common.

In four independent studies published between 1972 and 1978, researchers reported that 9% to 30% of all malpractice claims arose from drug-related injuries.

A 1981 study of the hospital-induced illnesses and injuries of 815 hospitalized patients showed that drugs were the major cause. Nearly 20% of these patients developed serious disabilities from drug-related complications.

Another study, published in 1979, analyzed the types of drug-related incidents reported in a Michigan hospital. This study uncovered seven kinds of errors, detailed below, and pinpointed how frequently they occurred.

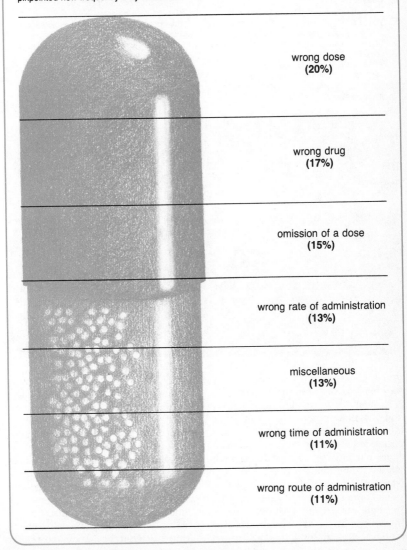

wrong dose
**(20%)**

wrong drug
**(17%)**

omission of a dose
**(15%)**

wrong rate of administration
**(13%)**

miscellaneous
**(13%)**

wrong time of administration
**(11%)**

wrong route of administration
**(11%)**

## TAKING DRUG ORDERS AND CARRYING THEM OUT: HOW TO PROTECT YOURSELF

When a doctor writes a drug order for his patient and signs it—or when another health-care professional writes an order and the doctor countersigns it—the courts usually will not question the legality of the order. But if a doctor gives you an oral drug order—either in person or by telephone—protect yourself legally, as follows:
• Write down the order *exactly* as he gives it.
• Repeat the order back to him so that you're sure you heard the doctor correctly.

Once you've given the drug to the patient, make sure you document all necessary information:
• Record *in ink* the type of drug, the dosage, the time you administered it, and any other information your institution's policy requires.

• Sign or initial your notes.

If your institution keeps drug orders in a special file, make sure that you transfer the doctor's drug order, which you wrote on the patient's chart, to that file.

If a doctor orally gives a drug order during an emergency, your first duty is to carry it out at once. When the emergency is over, document what you did.

Here's what can happen if you don't document drug orders:
• You could face disciplinary measures for failing to document.
• You could damage your defense or your hospital's in any malpractice lawsuit.
• Other nurses, not knowing what drugs have been given, may administer other drugs that could have harmful interactions.

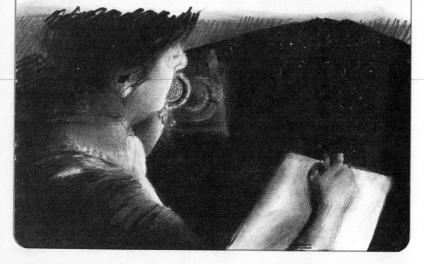

practice act is the law that most directly affects how you administer drugs.

In general, most nursing, medical, and pharmacy practice acts first define the tasks that belong uniquely to the profession being regulated, and then state that anyone who performs such tasks without being a licensed or registered member of the defined profession is breaking the law. (See Entry 1.) In some states and Canadian provinces, certain tasks overlap. For example, both nurses and doctors can

provide bedside care for the sick and, in Canada, both doctors and pharmacists can prepare medicines.

In many states, if a nurse prescribes a drug, she's practicing medicine without a license; if she goes into the pharmacy or drug supply cabinet, measures out doses of a drug, and puts the powder into capsules, she's practicing pharmacy without a license. For either action, she can be prosecuted or lose her license (or both), even if no one is harmed by what she does. In most states and Canadian provinces, to practice a licensed profession without a license is, at the very least, a misdemeanor.

In *Stefanik v. Nursing Education Committee* (1944), a Rhode Island nurse lost her nursing license in part because she'd been practicing medicine illegally: she'd changed a doctor's drug order for a patient because she didn't agree with what had been prescribed. No one claimed she had harmed the patient. But to change a prescription is the same as writing a new prescription, and Rhode Island's nurse practice act didn't—and still doesn't—consider that to be part of nursing practice.

The federal Food, Drug, and Cosmetic Act and the federal and state drug-abuse laws are less important to nursing practice than the state nursing, medical, and pharmacy practice acts. Why? Because most nurses don't test drugs, prescribe them, compound them, or dispense them. But you should know what the federal and state drug-abuse laws do. They seek to categorize drugs by how dangerous they are (forbidding the use of some, limiting the use of others), and they provide for rehabilitating drug-abuse victims.

*Randal v. California State Board of Pharmacy* (1966) involved a state's nursing, medical, and pharmacy practice acts as well as its drug-control laws. In that case, a pharmacist lost his license to practice partly because he'd taken telephone orders for controlled substances (amphetamines) from a nurse. The law in his state clearly treats telephone orders as prescriptions and, as such, requires that they be taken only from a doctor.

## How nurses get involved in drug-related lawsuits

Unfortunately, lawsuits involving nurses' drug errors are common.

In *Derrick v. Portland Eye, Ear, Nose & Throat Hospital* (1922), an Oregon nurse gave a young boy a pupil-contracting drug when the doctor had ordered a pupil-dilating drug. As a result, the boy lost his sight in one eye, and the nurse and the hospital were found negligent.

As you're probably aware, a diagnostic drug can also prompt a lawsuit. In a 1967 case in Tennessee, *Gault v. Poor Sisters of St. Francis Seraph of Perpetual Adoration*, a nurse was supposed to give a patient a saltwater gastric lavage in preparation for a gastric cytology test. Instead, she gave the patient dilute sodium hydroxide, causing severe internal injuries. The hospital lost the verdict and also an appeal.

Getting the dose right is also important. In a Louisiana case, *Norton v. Argonaut Insurance Co.* (1962), a nurse inadvertently gave a 3-month-old infant a digitalis overdose that resulted in the infant's death. At the malpractice trial that followed, the nurse was found liable, along with the hospital and the attending doctor.

Similarly, in *Dessauer v. Memorial General Hospital*, a 1981 New Mexico case, an emergency department doctor ordered 50 mg of lidocaine for a patient. But the nurse, who normally worked in the hospital's obstetrics ward, gave the patient 800 mg. The patient died, the family sued, and the hospital was found liable.

In *Moore v. Guthrie Hospital*, a 1968 West Virginia case, a nurse made a mistake in the administration route, giving the patient two drugs intravenously rather than intramuscularly. The patient suffered a seizure, sued, and won.

All the court decisions in these cases were based on, and in turn help to define, the standard of care you must apply when administering drugs to patients. In some of these court cases, if the nurse had known more about the proper dose, administration route, or procedure connected with giving the drug, she might not have made the mistake that resulted in the lawsuit. But even when a nurse can demonstrate her competence, one point still stands: The courts will not permit carelessness that harms the patient. (See *How Common*

## ADMINISTERING CONTROLLED DRUGS: PRECAUTIONS TO TAKE

As you know, in the United States and Canada, government agencies regulate certain drugs that have a high potential for abuse. In the United States, the Food and Drug Administration divides these controlled substances into five groups, Schedules I to V. In Canada, the Health Protection Branch groups all controlled drugs into one group, Schedule G. The chart below lists the drugs in each category.

You'll never administer Schedule I drugs; they have the highest potential for abuse and aren't accepted for any medical use. But you may administer Schedule II to V drugs, or Schedule G drugs in Canada.

Remember that all these drugs are potentially habit-forming and addictive. Before administering them, take these precautions:
- Check your hospital's policy for special procedures.
- Sign out, on the narcotics form, any drugs you remove from the narcotics cabinet.
- Follow the proper disposal procedures if any part of the drug remains after use.
- Never leave any drugs lying on the counter.
- Relock the narcotics cabinet after you've removed the drugs you need.

| SCHEDULE | EXAMPLES |
|---|---|
| **In the United States:** | |
| I | heroin, lysergic acid diethylamide (LSD), marijuana derivatives, mescaline, peyote, and psilocybin |
| II | amobarbital, amphetamine, cocaine, codeine, hydromorphone, meperidine, methadone, methamphetamine, methaqualone, methylphenidate, morphine, opium, oxycodone, oxymorphone, pentobarbital, phenmetrazine, and secobarbital |
| III | barbituric acid derivatives (except those listed in another schedule), benzphetamine, chlorphentermine, glutethimide, mazindol, methyprylon, paregoric, and phendimetrazin |
| IV | barbital, benzodiazepine derivatives, chloral hydrate, diethylpropion, ethchlorvynol, ethinamate, fenfluramine, meprobamate, methohexital, phenobarbital, paraldehyde, and phentermine |
| V | diphenoxylate compound and expectorants with codeine |
| **In Canada:** | |
| G | all salts and derivatives of the following: amphetamine, barbituric acid, benzphetamine, butorphanol, chlorphentermine, diethylpropion, methamphetamine, methaqualone, methylphenidate, pentazocine, phendimetrazine, phenmetrazine, and phentermine |

*Are Drug Errors?*, page 145.)

## Your liability for dispensing drugs

In rare instances, adequate patient care may require that you give a certain drug that isn't available on the floor. Normally, of course, you'd call the hospital pharmacist and ask that the drug be sent. But what can you do if you're working on the night or weekend shift and no pharmacist is available?

In this situation, a nurse can't escape liability if she dispenses the drug herself and a lawsuit results. Some hospitals and nursing homes have written policies that permit the charge nurse under special circumstances to go into the pharmacy and dispense an emergency dose of a drug. But whether the institution has a written policy or not, a nurse who dispenses drugs is doing so unlawfully—unless her state's pharmacy practice act specifically authorizes her to do so. If she makes an error in dispensing the drug and the patient later sues, the fact that she was practicing as an unlicensed pharmacist can be used as evidence against her.

You can, of course, choose to disregard the laws that govern your practice if you think your patient's well-being requires it. But clearly you do so at your own risk. And even if you don't harm your patient, you can still be prosecuted and you can still lose your license. In extraordinary circumstances —when ethics and the law conflict, and you have to weigh concern for your patient's life or health against concern for your license—you must make up your own mind about what action you're going to take.

### Your role in drug experimentation

At times, you may participate in administering experimental drugs to patients or administering established drugs in new ways or at experimental dosage levels. Your legal duties in these situations are the same as when you normally administer drugs. But if you have any questions, you'll get your answers from the experimental protocol, not your usual sources (books, product labels, or package inserts). You'll also need to make sure no drug is given to a patient who hasn't consented (in writing, if it's a federally funded experiment) to taking part in the experiment.

### Your responsibility for knowing about drugs

Once you have your nursing license, you're expected—by law—to know

## WHEN YOUR PATIENT IS ABUSING DRUGS

If you suspect your patient is abusing drugs, you have a duty to do something about it. If such a patient harms himself or anyone else, and a lawsuit results, the court may hold you liable for his actions. However, your legal responsibilities vary, depending on how much you know about the patient's drug or alcohol abuse.

For instance, suppose you know for certain that a patient is abusing drugs—if you're an emergency department nurse, you may find drugs in a patient's clothes or handbag while looking for identification. Your hospital's policy may obligate you to confiscate the drugs and take steps to see that the patient doesn't acquire more.

What if a patient's erratic or threatening behavior makes you *suspect* he's abusing drugs, but you have no evidence? Your hospital's policy may require that you conduct a drug search. The legal question here is whether your search is justified. As a rule of thumb, if you strongly believe the patient poses a threat to himself or others, and you can document your reasons for searching his possessions, you're probably safe legally.

Before you conduct a search, review your hospital's guidelines on the matter. Then follow those guidelines carefully. Most hospital guidelines will first direct you to contact your supervisor and explain why you have legitimate cause for a search. If she gives you her approval, next ask a security guard to help you. Besides protecting you, he'll serve as a witness if you do find drugs. When you're ready, confront the patient, tell him you intend to conduct a search, and tell him why.

Depending on your hospital's guidelines, you can search a patient's belongings as well as his room. If you find illegal drugs during your search, confiscate them. Remember, possession of illegal drugs is a felony. Depending on your hospital's guidelines, you may be obligated to report the patient to the police.

If you find alcoholic beverages, take them from the patient and explain that you'll return them when he leaves the hospital.

After you've completed your search, tell the patient's doctor about it and record your findings in your nursing notes and in an incident report. Your written records will be an important part of your defense (and your hospital's) if the patient decides to sue.

about any drug you administer. This means you're expected to know a drug's safe dosage limits, toxicity, side effects, potential adverse reactions, and indications and contraindications for use. If you're an LPN or LVN, you assume the same legal responsibility as an RN once you've taken a pharmaceutical course or have some other authorization to administer drugs.

Increasingly, judges and juries expect nurses to know what the appropriate observation intervals are for a patient receiving any type of medication. And they expect you to know this even if the doctor doesn't know, or if he doesn't write an order stating how often to check on the newly medicated patient. A case that was decided on this basis is *Brown v. State*, a 1977 New York case. After a patient was given 200 mg of Thorazine, the nurses on duty left him largely unobserved for several hours. When someone finally checked on the patient, he was dead. The hospital and the nurses lost the resulting lawsuit.

In *LaMade v. Wilson* (1975), a nurse applied Ophthaine to the eye of an ophthalmology-unit patient. The anesthetic stopped his eye from hurting, but it also stopped it from healing. As a result, the hospital and attending nurses were sued.

When the case was appealed, the appellate court presumed that a reasonably experienced nurse specialist would know a great deal about the drugs she was ordered to give—including contraindications. The burden was on the nurse and on the hospital to prove that the appropriate standard of care was lower. (See Entry 40.) The appellate court decided that the lower court should have heard evidence to determine whether the nurse knew, or should have known, that Ophthaine might be contraindicated in post-trauma and postoperative situations. If she did know or should have known and she hadn't at least questioned the order, the court implied, she and the hospital would be liable.

## When you're not sure—ask!

If you have a question about a drug order, follow your hospital's policies. Usually they'll tell you to try each of the following actions until you receive a satisfactory answer:
● Look up the answer in a standard drug reference.
● Ask your charge nurse.
● Ask the hospital pharmacist.
● Ask your nursing supervisor or the prescribing doctor.
● Ask the chief nursing administrator, if she hasn't already become involved.
● Ask the prescribing doctor's supervisor (service chief).
● Get in touch with the hospital administration and explain your problem.

## When you must refuse to administer a drug

All nurses have the legal right not to administer drugs they think will harm patients.

You may choose to exercise this right in a variety of situations:
● when you think the dosage prescribed is too high
● when you think the drug is contraindicated because of possible dangerous interactions with other drugs, or with nondrugs such as alcohol
● because you think the patient's physical condition contraindicates using the drug.

In limited circumstances, you may also legally refuse to administer a drug on grounds of conscience. Some states and Canadian provinces have enacted *right-of-conscience laws*. These laws excuse medical personnel from the requirement to participate in any abortion or sterilization procedure. Under such laws, you may, for example, refuse to give any drug you believe is intended to induce abortion.

When you refuse to carry out a drug order, be sure you do the following:
● Notify your immediate supervisor so she can make alternative arrangements (assigning a new nurse, clarifying the order).

# GIVING INJECTIONS: A STICKY LEGAL QUESTION

*I'm a nurse in a small-town general practitioner's office. When the doctor is out of town, he expects me to give injections—for instance, penicillin— to his regular patients who are complaining of sore throats or colds. He also expects me to give vitamin and allergy shots to those patients who receive them regularly.*

*The last time the doctor left town, he even asked me to give flu and pneumococcus injections to patients after I'd examined them—but then have each patient sign a statement saying he wouldn't hold me responsible for any side effects.*

*I've never felt comfortable giving these injections, and I've told the doctor this. But he just shrugs off my remarks.*

*What can and can't I do while the doctor is gone? Will a statement signed by the patient really protect me? The doctor says "Yes," but I disagree."*—RN, Del.

You're right—release statements can't absolve you of professional responsibility for your actions.

Aside from the issue of responsibility, what would you do if a patient *did* have an unexpected reaction to an injection? Is there another doctor on call to handle these emergencies?

And what if a patient does sign a statement releasing you from responsibility? Who'll accept responsibility? Your boss?

You may administer certain injections during the doctor's absence—but only under specific conditions. Give injections only if the doctor left standing orders for those patients who need vitamin or allergy shots for preexisting conditions; and even then, only if another doctor is available to handle any emergencies.

Don't ever administer injections for *new* conditions. For example, don't give penicillin shots to patients complaining of sore throats or colds. If you do, you're diagnosing patients and prescribing medicine without the required licenses.

Discuss this problem with your boss immediately—and don't let him shrug off your concern. Protect yourself now. If an emergency ever does occur, you'll need all the protection you can get.

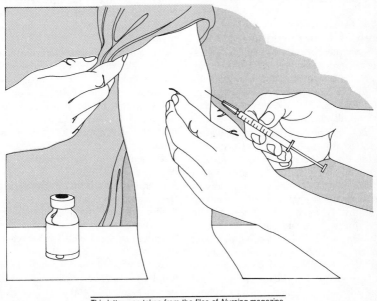

This letter was taken from the files of *Nursing* magazine.

• Notify the prescribing doctor if your supervisor hasn't done this already.
• If your employer requires it, document that the drug wasn't given, and explain why.

### Protecting yourself from liability

If you make an error in giving a drug, or if your patient reacts negatively to a properly administered drug, protect yourself by documenting the incident thoroughly. (See *Taking Drug Orders and Carrying Them Out: How to Protect Yourself*, page 146.)

Some of the documentation belongs in the patient's chart. In addition to normal drug-charting information, include information on the patient's reaction and any medical or nursing interventions taken to minimize harm to the patient.

Other documentation should be confined to the incident report. Here, identify what happened, the names and functions of all personnel involved, and what actions were taken to protect the patient after the error was discovered. (See Entry 25.)

### The LPN's/LVN's role in administering drugs

A few states' and Canadian provinces' nurse practice acts don't permit LPNs/ LVNs to administer drugs to patients at all, even under supervision. If you're an LPN or LVN working under such a law, don't administer any drugs—ever.

Most nurse practice acts, however, now permit LPNs and LVNs to give drugs under the supervision of an RN, a doctor, or a dentist, assuming that the LPN or LVN has the appropriate educational background or on-the-job training. What constitutes appropriate training or educational background? No clear-cut definitions exist, but most courts probably would be satisfied if an LPN or LVN could prove that her supervising RN or doctor had watched her administer drugs and had judged her competent.

Of course, if you're a newly graduated LPN or LVN, don't expect to administer drugs your first few days on the job—unless you've completed the qualifying courses.

### A final word

Both U.S. and Canadian laws restrict the nurse's role in regard to drugs. And within that narrow role, the laws impose exceptionally high standards. The standards probably won't be lowered— but the role may expand.

No matter what the future holds, the legal watchword for nurses where drugs are concerned is still "Take care."

# 24 Your legal responsibilities in patient teaching

Anytime you give a patient information about his care or treatment, you're involved in patient teaching—a professional nursing responsibility *and* a potential source of liability. This entry explains your legal risks in patient teaching and how you can minimize them.

You teach patients both formally and informally. You teach *formally* when, for example, you prepare instructions on stoma care for a colostomy patient. Before giving the patient this detailed information, you follow a typical patient-teaching process that includes these steps:
• assessing what the patient wants or needs to know
• identifying goals that you and the patient want to reach
• choosing teaching strategies that will help reach the goals
• evaluating how well you've reached the goals.

You teach *informally* when, for example, you answer your postoperative patient's question about the fact that he has a 100° temperature. When you explain to him that a low-grade temperature is common for a day or two after surgery, you're reassuring him and teaching him that this sign isn't unusual.

For best results, patient teaching should include the family and others involved in the patient's care. The family that understands the reason for a patient's treatment will support him as he acquires new information and skills.

## Nurses' role in giving health-care information

You know, of course, that people have traditionally turned to nurses as important sources of health-care information in and out of the hospital. Informally, friends often ask nurses about such concerns as caring for a child with a fever, why grandmother has been prescribed certain drugs, and what immunizations are needed for traveling overseas. (See Entry 32.) Community health nurses, in particular, teach families how to maintain good health. And, of course, hospital nurses give patients information about their care, such as when a nurse tells a patient what to expect when he undergoes a diagnostic test.

The trend toward nurses doing patient teaching has accelerated in recent years, largely because patients are spending less time in hospitals. Now that patients are being discharged earlier, they need more understanding of their illness and how to manage it at home. And so do their families.

## How the law defines nurses' patient-teaching responsibilities

Most nurse practice acts in the United States and Canada contain wording about promoting patient health and preventing disease or injury. But they don't specify a nurse's responsibility for patient teaching. Nurses can find this information in the practice standards developed by professional organizations, in nursing job descriptions, and in statements about nursing practice from national commissions.

The nursing practice standards pub-

## KEY TERMS IN THIS ENTRY

**common law** • Law derived from previous court decisions, not from statutes. Also called **case law.**

**patient's bill of rights** • A list of patients' rights. The American Hospital Association; health-care institutions; and various medical, nursing, and consumer organizations have prepared such lists, which, in some states, have become law.

**statutory law** • A law passed by a federal or state legislature.

lished in 1973 by the American Nurses' Association (ANA) provide a good example (see Entry 2). Standard IV states, "The plan of nursing care includes priorities and the prescribed nursing approaches or measures to achieve the goals derived from the nursing diagnoses." To help nurses understand this standard, the ANA suggests making sure that "teaching-learning principles are incorporated into the plan of care and objectives for learning stated in behavioral terms."

The standard clearly recognizes the dynamic nature of the teaching-learning process: that it is a means to an end, and that its effectiveness is measured by an objective goal. The standard merges the patient-teaching process into the expected outcome.

## Understanding the patient's right to be taught

Both statutory law and common law support the patient's right to have information about his condition and treatment. In fact, when a patient is admitted to a hospital, he may be handed a patient bill of rights that clearly indicates his right to such information (see Entry 11). The doctrine of informed consent further supports the patient's right to know (see Entry 12).

Despite RNs' deep involvement in patient teaching (RNs, not LPNs/LVNs, are primarily responsible for patient teaching), the courts have rarely addressed nurses' liability in this area of patient care. Why? Perhaps because, in the past, patients have usually sued doctors rather than nurses. But some legal experts believe that nurses will increasingly become the target of such lawsuits, in part because of their increasing patient-teaching responsibilities.

One case that did address the question of a nurse's liability for patient teaching was *Kyslinger v. United States* (1975). In that case, a veterans' hospital sent a hemodialysis patient home with an artificial kidney. He eventually died (apparently while on the machine), and his wife sued the federal government—because a veterans' hospital was involved—alleging that the hospital and its staff had failed to teach neither her nor her late husband how to properly use and maintain a home hemodialysis unit.

After examining the evidence, the court ruled against the patient's wife, as follows:

"During those 10 months that plaintiff's decedent underwent biweekly hemodialysis treatment on the unit (at the VA Hospital), both plaintiff and decedent were instructed as to the operation, maintenance, and supervision of said treatment. The Court can find no basis to conclude that there was any course of conduct on the part of the defendant or any of its personnel which would support the finding of any liability or any evidence which would lead the Court to conclude that the plaintiff or plaintiff's decedent were not properly informed on the use of the hemodialysis unit."

According to present law, a court faced with a question involving a nurse's responsibility for patient teaching will probably examine the question under the general category of a patient's right to know (*Gerety v. Demers*, 1978, and *Canterbury v. Spence*, 1972).

Health care requires the patient's participation and cooperation, so this right to know becomes an inherent part of successful treatment. When the right to know becomes critical to the patient's health (as in the home-hemodialysis situation described above), a court is likely to view patient teaching as a health-care provider's legal duty. This is similar to the way courts view the act of supplying information as essential to obtaining a patient's informed consent.

---

*"A team approach to patient teaching ensures teaching continuity— and a better educated patient."*

---

Suppose you're sued for malpractice, and your alleged wrongful act involves patient teaching. The court will consider whether patient teaching was your legal duty to the patient—the standard of care you should have met—and whether you met or breached it. If the evidence indicates you did breach your duty to the patient and so caused him harm, you could be found liable.

### What's the LPN's/LVN's role in patient teaching?

Unlike RNs, LPNs and LVNs aren't taught the fundamentals of patient teaching as part of their school curriculum—nor is patient teaching included in their scope of practice. RNs are primarily responsible for patient teaching and may delegate to LPNs/LVNs only the responsibility to reinforce what has already been taught. For example, if an RN is preparing a patient for a barium enema, she could ask an LPN or LVN to tell the patient about the X-ray room and what to expect there. (The LPN/LVN should know what to tell the patient, because LPNs/LVNs are trained in the technical aspects of patient care.) The RN could add to the information as necessary.

## What if a patient refuses your teaching?

Suppose you begin teaching a patient about the medications he's taking, only to hear him say, "Oh, just tell my wife; she gives me all my pills." When something like this happens, be sure to document the incident. Include the patient's exact words; then describe what you taught his wife, and how.

## When should you teach patients?

What you teach a patient while he's in the hospital can help him adjust to the medical regimen or altered life-style he may have to follow after returning home—and benefit more from it, too. Be prepared to arrange for a community health nurse to continue the teaching program you've begun.

Patient teaching also helps patients being admitted to other health-care agencies. For example, when an elderly patient is transferred into a nursing home, he needs information about the home's rules and regulations, its recreational opportunities, and the paramedical support systems available. If a social service worker doesn't provide such information, an RN can.

RNs can also teach children who are being moved to foster or adoptive homes. And if you're a nurse involved in community education programs, you can help families adjust to healthier life-styles by teaching them about good nutrition, regular exercise, and the use of health resources.

Patients taught about their health care are more cooperative because they recognize the reasons for their treatments, medications, and restrictions. They also adapt more readily to changes resulting from medical regimens or new health routines. All this helps reduce patients' stress and the tensions that stem from dependence on health-care personnel.

Patient teaching also helps reduce the likelihood of medical emergencies. For example, diabetic patients who've been taught to assess their urine for ketones generally require fewer admissions to emergency departments for treatment of ketoacidosis. And when community health nurses teach the mothers of young children ways to prevent accidents at home, those children also require fewer emergency department visits.

Last, but not least, patient teaching saves patients money. For example, the mother who's taught to manage her child's colostomy or orthopedic prosthesis will need fewer costly doctor's visits. And the patient who's taught to manage his permanent central venous catheter (for nutrition or chemotherapy) will spend less time in the hospital.

## Avoiding conflicts about patient teaching

Doctors, nurses, and other health-team members sometimes disagree about how patient teaching should be done and who should do it. To avoid conflict, always consult doctors and other health-team members (if appropriate) when you're preparing routine patient-teaching protocols. A team approach to patient teaching not only decreases conflicts but also ensures continuity in teaching—and a better educated patient.

You can also avoid conflicts by listening to the instructions that doctors, respiratory therapists, dietitians, and others give the patient. Then, you'll know exactly what's already been said to him, and you can structure your teaching accordingly.

Candor and diplomacy, of course, also help reduce conflict. Everyone profits when health-team members share their patient-teaching approaches and work together to achieve patient-teaching goals.

## A final word

As a nurse, you provide the most constant care to patients and can best evaluate how well they understand what they're taught. Your responsibility for patient teaching is steadily increasing. And it will continue to increase as people become more aware of their rights and grow more knowledgeable about health and illness.

# 25 What to do after a patient incident

Many times, despite the best training and intentions, "incidents" occur in the hospital. As you know, these incidents are events that are inconsistent with the hospital's ordinary routine. In most hospitals (and other health-care institutions), *any* injury to a patient requires an incident report. Besides patient injuries, patient complaints, medication errors, and injuries to employees and visitors require incident reports.

An incident report serves two main purposes:
• to inform hospital administration of the incident so it can consider changes that will help prevent future similar incidents (risk management)
• to alert the administration and the hospital's insurance company to the possibility of liability claims and the need for further investigation (claims management). Even when the incident isn't investigated, the report helps identify witnesses if a lawsuit is started months or even years later.

## The benefits of incident reports
A patient who's injured in a reported incident benefits from prompt response to his new medical needs. Future patients also benefit if action is taken to prevent a recurrence of the incident. And the hospital and the nurse benefit in two ways: by identifying and eliminating problems, and by gathering and preserving information that may

be vitally important in a lawsuit.

Of course, an incident report is useful only if it's filed promptly, thoroughly, and appropriately (see *Completing an Incident Report,* page 158).

## Understanding your legal duty
Whether you're an RN, an LPN, or an LVN, a staff nurse or a nurse manager, your legal duty is to report any incident of which you have first-hand knowledge. Failure to report an incident not only can lead to your being fired, it can also expose you to personal liability for malpractice—especially if the breach of your duty to report the incident causes injury to a patient.

Only a person with first-hand knowledge of an incident should report it. And only the person making the report should sign it. *Each person with first-hand knowledge should fill out and sign a separate report.* Never sign a report describing circumstances or events you haven't personally witnessed.

## What—and what not—to include in an incident report
An incident report should include only the following:
• the identities of the patient and any witnesses
• information about what happened, and what were the consequences to the patient (supply enough information so the hospital administration can decide whether the matter needs further investigation)
• any other relevant facts.

Statements like these should never be included in an incident report:
• mention of events not seen by the reporter (such as something another employee said happened)
• opinions (such as the reporter's opinion of the patient's prognosis)
• conclusions or assumptions (such as what caused the incident)
• suggestions of who was responsible for causing the incident
• suggestions to prevent the incident

from happening again.

Including this type of information in an incident report could seriously hinder the defense in any lawsuit arising from the incident.

Remember, the incident report serves only to notify the administration that an incident has occurred. In effect, it says, "Administration: please note that this incident happened, and please decide whether you want to investigate it further." Such items as detailed statements from witnesses and descriptions of remedial action are normally part of an investigative follow-up, so don't include them in the incident report itself.

Be especially careful that the hospital's reporting system does not lead to improper incident reporting. For example, some hospitals require nursing supervisors to correlate reports from witnesses and then to file a single report. And some incident report forms

---

*"Failure to report an incident can lead to your being fired and to your being personally liable for malpractice."*

---

invite inappropriate conclusions and assumptions by asking, "How can this incident be prevented in the future?"

Avoid these potential pitfalls by following the guidelines given above. If your hospital's reporting system or forms contain such potential pitfalls, alert the administration to them.

### How an incident report compares with the patient's medical record

As you're probably aware, an incident report doesn't become part of the patient's medical record. In fact, the record shouldn't even mention that an incident report has been filed. The record should include *only* clinical ob-

> GLOSSARY
>
> ## KEY TERMS IN THIS ENTRY
>
> **discovery** • A pretrial procedure that allows the plaintiff's and defendant's attorneys to examine relevant materials and interrogate all parties to the case.
>
> **liability** • Legal responsibility for *failure to act*, so causing harm to another person, or for *actions* that fail to meet standards of care, so causing harm to another person.
>
> **malpractice** • A professional person's wrongful conduct, improper discharge of professional duties, or failure to meet the standards of care—any such actions that result in harm to another person.
>
> **qualified privilege** • A conditional right or immunity granted to the defendant because of the circumstances of a legal case.

servations relating to the incident. (Again, avoid value judgments.)

By the way, entering your observations in the nurses' notes section of the patient's record doesn't take the place of completing an incident report. Nor does completing an incident report take the place of proper documentation in the patient's chart.

### What happens to an incident report?

An incident report, once it's filed, may be reviewed by the nursing supervisor, the doctor called to examine the patient, appropriate department heads and administrators, the hospital attorney, and the hospital's insurance company. (See *What Happens to an Incident Report?* pages 160 and 161.) The report may be filed under the involved patient's name or by the type of injury, depending on the hospital's policy and the insurance company's regulations. Reports are rarely placed in the reporting nurse's employment file.

A currently controversial question concerns whether a patient's attorney may "discover" (request and receive a copy of) an incident report and intro-

## COMPLETING AN INCIDENT REPORT

When an incident involves one of your patients, you know you must document it by filling out an incident report form. Report forms vary from institution to institution, but all incident reports generally require the same information. The report form shown here is a typical example.

---

USE ADDRESSOGRAPH
IF PATIENT

**INCIDENT REPORT**

Mary J. Smith
68 Oakwood Circle
Haddenville, Pa. 19008

| **PERSON INVOLVED** | *Smith* | *Mary* | *J.* |
|---|---|---|---|
| | Last Name | First Name | Middle Initial |
| | ☐ Male  ☑ Female | Age: *63* | |

| **EMPLOYEE:** | Department | | Job Title |
|---|---|---|---|
| **VISITOR:** | Home Address | | Home Telephone |
| **OTHER:** | Home Address | | Home Telephone |
| **PATIENT:** | Room Number *439* | State Cause of Hospitalization *Diabetes Mellitus* | |

| Exact Location of Incident | Date of Incident | Time of Incident |
|---|---|---|
| *Bathroom in 439* | *9/1/83* | *9:30 a.m.* |

Describe exactly what happened (Facts, no opinions):

*Patient found sitting on floor in bathroom. Patient states she slipped on floor when getting out of the shower and hit left arm on door. Patient complaining of pain in left shoulder. No abrasions, lacerations or swelling evident. Pt escorted back to bed. BP 124/80, P.84. MD notified*

Name, Address and Telephone Number of Witness(es)
*none*

| Date of Report *9/1/83* | Signature of Person Preparing Report *Sally Jones, R.N.* |
|---|---|
| Was Person seen by a Physician  ☑ Yes  ☐ No | Time seen *9:45 am* | Where *Patient's room* |
| Date of receipt *9/1/83* | Signature of Department Head/Supervisor Receiving Report *Sarah Miller, RN* |

duce it into evidence in a malpractice lawsuit. The law on this issue varies from state to state. To avoid discovery, the hospital may send copies of the incident report to its attorney, or the hospital attorney may write a letter stating that the report is being made for his use and benefit only.

Actually, concern about incident-report discovery should be minimal if an incident report contains only properly reportable material. After all, the information in a properly completed incident report is readily available to the patient's attorney through many other sources. Only when an incident report contains second-hand information, opinions, conclusions, accusations, or suggestions for preventing such incidents in the future does discovery of the incident report become an important issue for attorneys and the courts.

### What to do when your error causes a reportable incident

If an incident results from an error you made, you have the duty to file an incident report immediately. Making a mistake is serious and may invite corrective action by your hospital, but attempting to cover it up is worse—and so are the potential consequences.

For one thing, the likelihood that an incident report will be used against you is slight. A hospital wants its nurses to report incidents and to keep proper records. They may not do this consistently if they're always reprimanded for even small errors. Most hospitals, in fact, will reprimand a nurse severely for *not* filing an incident report if irreversible injury is done to the patient.

Of course, if an incident results from your act of gross negligence or irresponsibility or is one of a series of incidents in which you've been involved, then the hospital may take action against you. And that possibility increases if the patient sustains irreversible injury because of your error.

If a fellow employee's error causes a reportable incident, your safest course

is to factually and objectively report what you observed. Remember, the truth isn't libel. By properly fulfilling your duty to your patient and your hospital, you'll also minimize any potential liability if the employee files a lawsuit against you.

Here's another point to remember: Most states have laws granting "qualified privilege" to those who have a duty to discuss or evaluate their co-workers, employees, or fellow citizens. This privilege means that no liability for libel exists unless the person giving the information knows it's false or has acted with a reckless disregard for the truth.

### Understanding risk-management strategy

How can you minimize the chances that a patient will sue after an incident? And how can you protect yourself and your hospital in case he does? The best way is to follow the "three Rs" of risk-

---

*"Making a mistake is serious—but covering it up is worse."*

---

management strategy: rapport, record, and report.

*Maintain rapport with the patient.* Answer his questions honestly. Don't offer any explanation if you weren't personally involved in the incident; instead, refer the patient to someone who can supply answers. If you try to answer his questions without direct knowledge of the incident, inconsistencies could arise and the patient could interpret these as a cover-up.

Don't offer any explanation if doing so might make you visibly nervous. Ask your supervisor, hospital patient-relations specialist, or an administrator for advice on how to answer the patient. If you still feel uncomfortable, have one of them talk to the patient,

## WHAT HAPPENS TO AN INCIDENT REPORT?

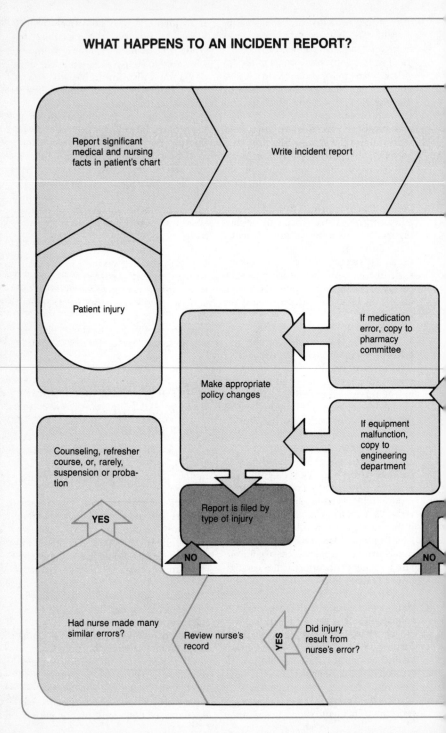

Report significant medical and nursing facts in patient's chart

Write incident report

Patient injury

If medication error, copy to pharmacy committee

Make appropriate policy changes

If equipment malfunction, copy to engineering department

Counseling, refresher course, or, rarely, suspension or probation

YES

Report is filed by type of injury

NO

NO

Had nurse made many similar errors?

Review nurse's record

YES

Did injury result from nurse's error?

Do you know what happens to an incident report after it's filed? This chart gives you a comprehensive overview of incident-report routing.

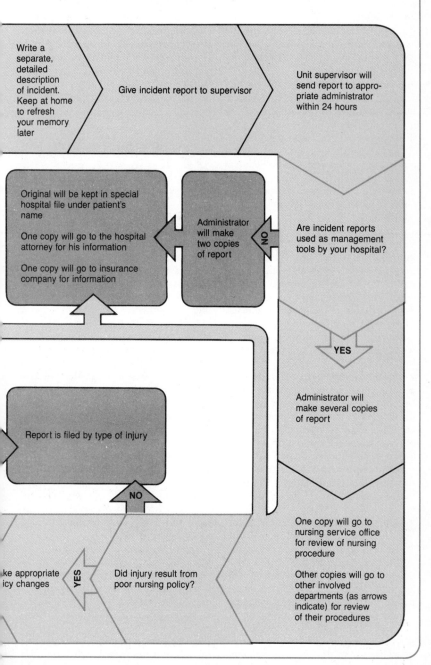

Write a separate, detailed description of incident. Keep at home to refresh your memory later

Give incident report to supervisor

Unit supervisor will send report to appropriate administrator within 24 hours

Original will be kept in special hospital file under patient's name

One copy will go to the hospital attorney for his information

One copy will go to insurance company for information

Administrator will make two copies of report

NO

Are incident reports used as management tools by your hospital?

YES

Administrator will make several copies of report

Report is filed by type of injury

NO

One copy will go to nursing service office for review of nursing procedure

Other copies will go to other involved departments (as arrows indicate) for review of their procedures

ke appropriate icy changes

YES

Did injury result from poor nursing policy?

but still try to maintain rapport.

Don't blame anyone for the incident. If you feel someone was at fault, tell your charge nurse or supervisor—not the patient.

If an incident necessarily changes the way you care for the patient, tell the patient about it and clearly explain the reasons for the change.

*Record the incident in the medical records.* Remember, truthfulness is the best protection against lawsuits. If you try to cover up or play down an incident, you could end up in far more serious trouble than if you'd reported it objectively. Never write in the medical record that an incident report has been completed. An incident report is *not* clinical information, but an administrative tool.

*Report every incident.* Some nurses think incident reports are more trouble than they're worth and, furthermore, that they're a dangerous admission of guilt. That's false. Here's why incident reports are important:

• Incident reports jog our memories. Much time may pass between an incident and when it comes to court. So we simply can't trust our memories—but we can trust an incident report.

• Incident reports help administrators act quickly to change the policy or procedure that seems to be responsible for the incident. An administrator can also act quickly to talk with families and offer assistance, explanation, or other appropriate support. Sometimes helpful communication with an injured patient and his family can be the balm that soothes a family's anger and prevents a lawsuit.

• Incident reports provide the information hospitals need to decide whether restitution should be made. When a patient is injured instead of helped during his hospital stay, the hospital sometimes decides it has a moral obligation to compensate the patient. In fact, this moral obligation is another reason (besides protection against having to pay damages awarded in a lawsuit) why hospitals

carry professional liability insurance.

## A final word

Incident reporting will become increasingly important as health-care consumers become more aware of their rights. Remember, a long period may elapse between an incident and subsequent court proceedings. Documentation may be the only objective proof of what happened.

# 26 Caring for minors—your legal responsibilities

That patient you're caring for, the one who's a minor—do you know his rights as a patient? And what your legal obligations to him are? For answers to these and other questions, keep reading.

A *minor* is any person under the age of majority, which is usually 18 or 21, depending on state or Canadian provincial law. When you care for a minor, you should keep in mind the way minors' legal rights are structured. What legal rights a minor has depend largely on his age. He may also have special legal status.

## Understanding a minor's rights

A minor's rights fall into three categories:

• *Personal rights that belong to everyone from birth.* Examples include the right to privacy and the right to protection against crimes.

• *Rights that can be exercised as a minor matures.* These fall into two groups. The first includes the right to drive a car, to work at a paying job, and to have sexual relations—as long as *both* partners are of legal age. These rights are granted at certain ages, according to state laws, whether or not the minor is mature enough to exercise the right intelligently.

The second group includes rights granted by the courts rather than by statutory law, which are given to any minor who shows the mental and emotional ability to handle them. (See the discussion of the nonemancipated but mature minor, below.)

• *Rights that belong to adults and can be exercised only by adults and so-called emancipated minors.* Examples include many financial and contractual rights, such as the right to consent to medical treatment. (See the discussion on obtaining consent from a minor, below, and *The Right to Consent: From Birth to Adulthood,* page 86.)

The law provides special rights for minors that they may exercise only *after* reaching the age of majority. For example, because a minor cannot sue in court, most states give minors a grace period after they reach the age of majority to bring any lawsuit relating to the time when they were of minor age. This includes suing persons their parents could have sued earlier on the minors' behalf but chose not to. Because this can include a lawsuit for medical malpractice, most hospitals keep the records of pediatric patients longer than the legally required period, which can be fairly short.

## Emancipation basics

Under the laws of most states and Canadian provinces, a person can become emancipated from the legal restrictions of being a minor in the following ways:

• marrying (in which case emancipation continues after separation, widowhood, or divorce)

• becoming a parent (even if not married)

• becoming pregnant (or believing she's pregnant)

• joining the armed forces

• living away from home and earning an independent living, managing his own finances, and in general assuming an adult role.

Under most circumstances, you

GLOSSARY

## KEY TERMS IN THIS ENTRY

**age of majority** • Either 18 or 21 years, depending on the state or Canadian provincial laws.

**emancipated minor** • A minor who's legally considered an adult, free from parental care, and completely responsible for his own affairs.

**guardian ad litem** • A person appointed by the court to look after a minor's legal interest during certain kinds of litigation.

**statutory law** • A law passed by federal or state legislature.

should treat an emancipated minor the same as if he were an adult.

## Mature minor

A mature minor is a nonemancipated minor in his middle to late teens who shows clear signs of intellectual and emotional maturity. A mature minor may be able to exercise certain adult rights, depending on laws in his state.

Note that even an emancipated minor may not exercise some rights. If he's 18 and the drinking age in his state is 21, he still can't legally buy a drink. Some states set a minimum age for making a will (usually the age of majority). In those states, even if the minor is married or has a child, any will he draws up won't be valid.

The laws of most states provide that some contracts made by minors are valid but voidable. In theory, this protects the minor from recklessness. Many hospitals won't allow a minor to sign a contract to pay his hospital bills unless a parent or guardian at least guarantees his contract. This legal arrangement, of course, should not influence anything you do as a nurse.

## Guardians ad litem

When a court decision is needed for a minor, the court may appoint a guardian ad litem even if the minor already has a guardian. The court may even do this if one or both parents are still living and interested in the minor's welfare. In this situation, the court assumes that the interests of the minor's parents or legal guardians probably don't coincide with the minor's welfare.

## Obtaining consent

By far the most common problem with minors is obtaining proper consent for their medical care. Although the doctor bears the legal responsibility for this, you'll often be involved in the process. Here are 11 different situations you may face in helping to obtain a minor's consent:

*Under normal circumstances.* If the minor isn't emancipated, his mother, father, or legal guardian has the right to refuse or consent to treatment for him. Whenever possible, consent should be obtained from both parents, or both guardians when joint guardians have custody of the minor.

If the parents are divorced or separated, the usual policy is to obtain consent from the parent who has custody. If the custodial parent is unavailable, the other parent may be asked to make the decision.

If the minor's parents are incompetent or dead, and he has no legal guardian, the court will usually appoint a legal guardian for him. The guardian can consent or refuse, just as if he were a parent.

*When parents or joint guardians disagree.* Problems can arise when parents (whether married, divorced, or separated) or joint guardians disagree about consenting to treatment for a minor. The hospital's only recourse may be to go to court, where a judge either makes the decision himself or assigns responsibility to one parent or guardian. You may find yourself caught in a situation where a minor's parents or guardians can't agree on consenting to his treatment. When this happens, tell the hospital administrators immedi-

ately so they can talk to the parents or guardians and, if necessary, alert the hospital's attorney.

*When the minor is emancipated.* An emancipated minor can refuse or consent to treatment himself. But if he's unable to do so (for example, because he's unconscious following an accident), you have to try to find someone who can give consent for him. Possibilities, in descending order of preference, include his spouse, parents or guardians, and nearest living relative. You may waive this requirement for consent only in an emergency situation, when your failure to treat a minor immediately could result in further injury or in death.

*When your patient is a nonemancipated but mature minor.* In Canada, nonemancipated mature minors can consent to medical treatment themselves. For example, in *Booth v. Toronto General Hospital* (1910), the court ruled that a minor who was working for his living but residing at his parents' home could give his own consent to surgery.

In the United States, nonemancipated but mature minors' rights are not so broad. In some cases, however, even young minors' wishes have been taken into account—for example, in *Hart v. Brown* (1972), an organ-transplant case involving minor twins. And in a series of rulings on abortion and contraception, discussed below, the U.S. Supreme Court has ruled that mature minors have certain rights of consent and privacy.

*When a minor needs emergency care.* The legal rule here is the same as for adults: If necessary, treat first and get consent later. Some courts have held that any mature minor, emancipated or not, may give a valid and binding consent to emergency treatment. For example, in *Younts v. St. Francis Hospital and School of Nursing* (1970), a nonemancipated but mature 17-year-old was held able to consent to surgical repair of a severed fingertip.

*When a minor asks for an abortion.*

Under common law, all pregnant minors have the right to consent to abortion. In most states, however, this common-law right has been modified or eliminated by statutory law or court decision. But recent U.S. Supreme Court rulings, including *Planned Parenthood of Central Missouri v. Danforth* (1976), *Bellotti v. Baird I* (1976), and *Bellotti v. Baird II* (1979), make clear that state laws can't stop a mature or otherwise emancipated minor from seeking and getting a legal abortion—although a judge may have to certify that the minor is mature enough to make the decision. Also, the law in some states may require notification of the parents of a minor who's seeking an abortion (*H.L. v. Matheson*, 1981).

For the rules your state requires you to follow, check with your hospital's attorney. (See Entry 73.)

*When a minor asks for contraceptives.* In *Carey v. Population Services International* (1977), the U.S. Supreme Court ruled unconstitutional various state laws that are more stringent about providing contraceptives (to minors or adults) than the laws about abortions. This means that laws about giving minors contraceptives (or advice about contraceptives) will be equally or less restrictive than the laws about obtaining abortions. Again, check with your hospital's attorney if you have questions.

*When a minor needs treatment for sexually transmitted or other communicable diseases.* Most states and Canadian provinces have laws that permit minors to consent to treatment for serious communicable diseases (including sexually transmitted diseases) without parental approval.

If you must deal with a minor who's refusing diagnosis or treatment for a communicable disease, check your state's laws. Most states permit public health authorities to deal with a nonconsenting minor as an adult, including when he must be quarantined.

*When a minor needs treatment for drug abuse.* State and federal laws generally permit minors to consent to take part in drug-abuse treatment and rehabilitation programs just as though they were adults. Like adults, minor patients in drug treatment programs are entitled to have their records kept confidential.

*When religious beliefs conflict with a minor's treatment.* If your patient or his parents or guardians are Jehovah's Witnesses or Christian Scientists, you may have special problems getting consent to treatment.

Although competent adults or emancipated minors may refuse treatment for religious reasons, unemancipated minors may not. In most states where the question has come before the courts, judges have ruled that parents and guardians can't stop a hospital from treating their child solely on religious grounds, if a reasonable chance exists that the treatment will help the patient.

Note, however, that in this situation a court will have to appoint a guardian ad litem for the sick minor. This may take some time, so to avoid delaying the minor's treatment unnecessarily, notify your hospital administration as quickly as possible.

*When a minor seeks or receives mental health care.* Minors, like adults, may be treated at private and state-run mental health facilities. When the minor and his parents agree to seek such treatment for the minor, the facility will follow its normal medical guidelines and procedures in deciding whether to admit him.

The U.S. Supreme Court, in *Parham v. J.R.* (1979) and in *Secretary of Public Welfare v. Institutionalized Juveniles* (1979), held that nonconsenting minors can be admitted to state-run mental health facilities at the request of either or both parents. Such minors, however, always have the right to have a psychiatrist or other trained fact-finder review the request at or before admission, and at least once thereafter. The fact-finder may be the facility's regular admissions officer.

In many states, however, the rules controlling admission of minors to state inpatient mental facilities are more rigorous. The rules may call for a full-scale hearing, with attorneys present, within a set time after admission (if not concurrent with admission). For example, in *Melville v. Sabbatino* (1973), a minor challenged the validity of his admission to a state mental-health facility. The court ruled that the minor was entitled to a hearing. (The outcome of the hearing wasn't reported.)

As yet, no restrictions of legal rights exist for out-patient or clinic treatment of minors. And, of course, a minor's admission to any private mental-health facility concerns only the facility and a competent adult relative (or the minor's spouse, if he's married).

### A final word
As you can see, caring for minors generally presents no special legal problems for the staff nurse. In most respects, problems in obtaining consent for nonemancipated minors' treatment are exactly the same as those in getting consent for incompetent adults.

The laws and regulations governing care of minors probably won't change much in the near future. One exception: The area of contraception—specifically, whether parents must be told when their nonemancipated minor daughter is seeking contraceptives.

Whether or not the laws concerning minors' medical treatment change, remember that you're responsible for knowing them.

# 27 The abused child or adult—your legal responsibility

As you're surely aware, nurses have long had to care for abused patients. Often these are children—victims of parents, relatives, or so-called friends. But just as often they are adults.

You know that abuse takes many forms. Sometimes abuse is physical battering, such as when a son regularly beats his aging father. At other times, abuse involves verbal, sexual, or emotional attack, or neglect.

Why abuse occurs is uncertain. It may be a product of stressful situations or sudden crises. But nonabusers also face stress and crisis—so this explanation leaves much to be desired.

## What kinds of people become abusers?
People who abuse others come from all socioeconomic levels and all ethnic groups. No specific psychiatric diagnosis encompasses the abuser's personality and behavior. However, many abusers have a history of being abused themselves when young, or of having witnessed abuse of parents or siblings. (These childhood experiences are often profound and can influence a person's behavior throughout his adult life.) Abusive persons often lack self-esteem and the security of being loved—qualities that help support nonabusers during stressful periods.

In times of crisis, abusers resort to the behavior they learned as children. They abuse just as they were abused—all in an attempt to restore their own feelings of self-control and to foster self-esteem. After all, if abuse was an acceptable behavior for their parents, why can't it be the same for them now?

Abusers are often unable to tolerate personal failure or disapproval from spouses, children, or friends. When an abuser's self-esteem is low, he expects rejection and often will act in ways that cause others to reject him. In turn, this allows the abuser to verbally or emotionally abuse those same people. Abusers commonly have unrealistic expectations of the people they abuse. These expectations show themselves in different ways, but the result is the same: When a person can't or won't live up to an abuser's expectations, he feels compelled to control, mortify, reject, and, if necessary, physically injure that person.

Sometimes low self-esteem will prompt an abuser to choose a partner much like himself. Each will then feed into the other's forms of abuse. If the couple has children, they often become targets of their parents' abusive behavior. And what the children witness, and suffer, begins another cycle of abused child to child abuser.

### Who are the abuser's victims?

How much do you know about the types of people most likely to be abused? As a nurse, you need to familiarize yourself with the attributes that frequently characterize abuse victims.

Children, of course, are commonly abused, especially children between the ages of 4 months and 3 years. (See *Caring for the Abused Child*, page 169.) Some children are particularly vulnerable to abuse. Among them are children with behavior problems as well as those who are malformed, developmentally disabled, born prematurely, or born to unmarried parents. From the abusive parent's perspective, such a child represents an unplanned disruption or a stress-producing crisis. If the child has mental or physical defects, the parent may see this as reaffirming his own inadequacy and weakness. And if the child's defects are severe, the parent may be unable to admit that the child is his: he may pour on abuse to destroy this "alien being."

Parents may also view children as extensions of persons they hate. Sometimes this results from similarities in physical appearance or similarities in behavior. If a child resembles a spouse who deserted the family, he may be blamed for the spouse's failures and abused accordingly.

Of course, adults abuse other adults as well as children. Spouses and elderly parents or relatives are the most common victims.

One important characteristic of an abused spouse is lack of self-esteem.

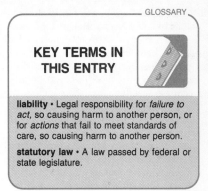

Often an abused spouse's parents abused each other, or one parent abused the other. Having witnessed these attacks as a child, the present-day abused spouse accepts that she, or sometimes he, will be abused. By behaving passively toward their partners, such spouses make it easy for the partners to abuse them repeatedly without fear of retaliation.

Like children, adults can become abuse victims if they're viewed as too dependent, too sickly, or too much like a hated person. Ill or elderly persons who make financial, emotional, or personal demands will often end up injured when the stress they create becomes intolerable for their abusers.

Among abusers of adults, men who abuse women seem to predominate. But sometimes the reverse is true. Abused men, married or not, often show the same low self-esteem and passivity as abused women. Sometimes an abused man is the less aggressive and more subservient member of the relationship, and accepts a certain level of abuse in the hope that it won't get worse. At other times, he may be so ashamed by his inability to provide adequately that he invites abuse to give himself a feeling of atonement.

### How the law relates to abusers and their victims

Until 1875, no U.S. laws specifically protected abuse victims—unless they were animals! In 1874, grossly battered

"Mary Ellen," age 9, was found chained to her bed in a New York City tenement. Etta Wheeler, a church worker, tried to find help for Mary Ellen, but she quickly discovered that New York had no laws to protect children. Her only recourse was the American Society for the Prevention of Cruelty to Animals, which agreed to intervene on Mary Ellen's behalf.

A year after Mary Ellen's case reached the courts, New York State adopted the country's first child-protection legislation. This gave child-protection agencies a legal base, and it proved a breakthrough for other disadvantaged groups as well.

Since then, child abuse has gained increasing attention from the public, from legislators—and from concerned health-care professionals. In 1946, for example, radiologists reported that subdural hematomas and abnormal X-ray findings in the long bones were commonly associated with early childhood traumatic injuries. In 1961, an American Academy of Pediatrics symposium on child abuse introduced the term *battered child*.

The first statutory laws calling for mandatory reporting of child abuse resulted from a 1963 report by the Children's Bureau of the (then) U.S. Department of Health, Education, and Welfare. Most states, using the model in the report, developed protective legislation by the early 1970s. Unfortunately, the diversity of these laws makes uniform interpretation impossible.

To help remedy this, the Early Childhood Project Education Commission published a nationwide model law in 1973. During the same year, Congress passed the Child Abuse Prevention and Treatment Act. This act required states to meet certain uniform standards in order to be eligible for federal assistance in setting up programs to iden-

## ORGANIZATIONS THAT HELP THE ABUSED AND THE ABUSER

Here's one simple but important way you can help the abuse victim and his abuser. Encourage them to call the organizations listed below for support and counseling.

| | |
|---|---|
| Child Abuse Prevention Effort | (215) 831-8877 |
| National Clearinghouse on Marital Rape | (415) 548-1770 |
| National Coalition Against Sexual Assault | (612) 296-7084 |
| National Committee for Prevention of Child Abuse | (312) 663-3520 |
| Parents Anonymous | (800) 421-0353 in California: (800) 352-0386 |
| Parents United | (408) 279-1957 |

tify, prevent, and treat the problems caused by child abuse. The act also established a national center on child abuse and neglect.

Currently, two common features characterize most state child abuse legislation:
• empowering of a social welfare or law enforcement bureau to receive and investigate reports of actual or suspected abuse
• granting of legal immunity from liability, for defamation or invasion of privacy, to any person reporting an incident of actual or suspected abuse.

Laws protecting abused spouses are still being written. Although many domestic-relations laws exist, more are needed for the specific protection of victims of domestic violence.

## Understanding your legal duty to report abuse

As a nurse, you play a crucial role in recognizing and reporting incidents of suspected abuse. While caring for patients, you can readily note evidence of apparent abuse. When you do, you must pass the information along to the appropriate authorities (see Entry 14).

If you've ever hesitated to file an abuse report because you fear repercussions, remember that the Child Abuse Prevention and Treatment Act protects you against liability. If your report is bona fide (that is, if you file it in good faith), the law will protect you from any suit filed by an alleged abuser. (Caution: This protection may not be available in Maine and Montana.)

To have a bona fide belief that abuse has occurred, you must carefully assess not only the abused child's or adult's injuries but also the relationship between him and the possible abuser. Make your report as complete and accurate as possible. At the same time, be careful not to let your personal feelings affect either the way you make out a report or whether you should file the report at all.

Abuse cases often raise many difficult emotional issues. Remember, however, that not filing a report may have more serious consequences than filing one that contains an error. Better to risk error than to risk breaching the child-abuse reporting laws—and perpetuating the abuse.

Besides your duty to report abuse, you also have a duty to teach the public about abuse. The Child Abuse Prevention and Treatment Act encourages health-care institutions to develop programs to identify, report, and ultimately prevent abuse. You can help reduce the incidence of abuse by teaching people about its signs and symptoms, diagnosis, and treatment.

## How to recognize signs and symptoms of abuse

You can learn to become adept at recognizing both the events that trigger abuse and the signs and symptoms that mark the abused and the abuser. Early in your relationship with an abused patient, you'll need to be adept in order to spot the behavioral and interactional clues that can signal an abusive situation. Why? Because many of the clues are subtle, or not easily distinguished from nonabusers' behavior.

For example, abused people tend to be passive and fearful. An abused child often fails to protest if his parent is asked to leave the examining area. An abused adult, on the other hand, often wants his abuser to stay with him.

Here's another clue: Abused persons often react to hospital procedures by crying helplessly and incessantly. And they tend to be wary of physical contacts, including physical examinations.

The abuser may also give important clues. Sometimes he'll appear overly agitated when dealing with hospital personnel; for example, he'll get impatient if they don't carry out procedures instantly. At other times, he may exhibit just the opposite behavior: a total lack of interest in the patient's problems.

When you take an abused victim's history, he may be vague about how he was injured and tell different stories to

# CARING FOR THE ABUSED CHILD

You're on duty in the emergency department when Mrs. Collins comes in with her son Jeff, age 5. She tells you, "My son was in an accident while riding in a friend's car. I didn't think Jeff was injured, but later on his knee swelled up. I decided I'd better have a doctor look at it."

You look closely at Jeff for head and neck injuries. You don't see any, but you do notice some bruises on his left arm and on his legs that look several weeks old. You question Mrs. Collins about the accident, but she offers few details. Then, when you question Mrs. Collins about Jeff's injuries, she gets very defensive. Although his injuries look painful, Jeff sits quietly while you examine him.

Considering the evidence, you suspect Jeff has been abused.

If you were faced with such a situation, would you know what to do? Here are some guidelines:

• Tell the doctor that you suspect child abuse and ask him to order a total-body X-ray. If he resists your request, talk directly with the radiologist; he can do it on his own authority. Don't hesitate to take this action into your own hands. Also, inform your supervisor of the situation.
• If you suspect the child has been forced to ingest drugs or alcohol, get an order for toxicology studies of the child's blood and urine.
• If the child is severely bruised, get an order for a blood coagulation profile.

• If X-rays or other studies suggest the child has been abused, talk with the doctor about confronting the parents. Ask how you might help him do this.
• If a parent admits to abusing the child and appears to want help, supply the address and telephone number of a local group, such as the Child Abuse Prevention Effort, and encourage the parent to call.
• Whether or not the parent admits to abusing the child, report all suspected abuse to the state-designated agency empowered to investigate the situation.

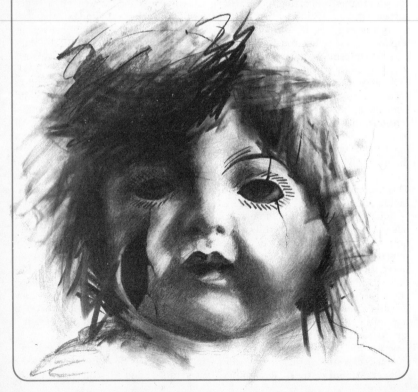

## CONSENT TO PHOTOGRAPH THE ABUSED CHILD

Imagine you work in the emergency department (ED) of a hospital. One day a social worker brings in a girl, age 11, a suspected victim of child abuse. The social worker asks you to photograph the girl's injuries to document them.

Can you legally take photographs of the patient?

No, but you can arrange for it. In most states, either an agency caseworker or the local police can photograph child-abuse injuries without parental consent. In states that don't specifically grant the right to photograph, the examining doctor has the responsibility to authorize photographs, because the duty to report implies a responsibility to preserve any evidence. If the parents are present and object to photographs, the doctor should contact law-enforcement officials to secure a court order.

All 50 states now have laws requiring that doctors and social workers (among other professionals) report suspected child abuse in children under age 16 or 18, depending on the state. These laws also offer professional care givers some immunity from liability, as long as they act in good faith.

Some states have designated reporting agencies. These agencies have 24-hour-a-day coverage and will send a caseworker to investigate, night or day. Find out the appropriate agency you should contact when you suspect child abuse, and post the number near the ED telephone.

Child abuse reporting laws are far from standardized, so ED personnel should request a specific procedure from the hospital administration. Obviously, the administration should design a procedure that meets all state reporting laws.

---

different people. When you ask directly about specific injuries, he may answer evasively or not at all. Sometimes he'll minimize or try to hide his injuries.

When examining an abused victim, look for characteristic signs of abuse. Often you'll find old bruises, scars, or deformities the patient can't (or won't) explain. X-ray examinations may show the presence of many old fractures.

Always document your findings objectively; try to keep your emotions out of your charting. One way to do this is to use the SOAP technique (see Entry 35), which calls for these steps:
• In the subjective (S) part of the note, record information in the patient's own words.
• In the objective (O) part, record your personal observations.
• Under assessment (A), record your evaluations and conclusions.
• Under plan (P), list sources of hospital and community support available to the patient following discharge.

### Offering support services
Many support services have become available for both abusers and their victims. For example, if a female victim is afraid to return to the scene of her abuse, she may find temporary housing in an established shelter. If no shelter is available, she may be able to stay with a friend or family member.

Social workers or community liaison workers may also be able to offer suggestions for shelter. Another possibility is a church, synagogue, or mosque, which may have members willing to take the patient in. If no shelter can be found, the patient may have to stay at the hospital to guarantee safety.

Alert the patient to state, county, or city agencies that can help protect him. The most obvious is the police department, which should be called to collect evidence if the patient wants to press charges against the abuser. If the patient is a child, the law may require filing a report with a government family-service agency.

As a nurse concerned about abuse, you need to evaluate the abuser's ability to handle stress. He'll probably pose a continued threat to others until he gets help in understanding his behavior and how to change it. When you question

him (or his family), try to get answers to questions like these:
• Has he recently lost his job or other means of support?
• Does he have problems with alcohol or drugs?
• Is his wife pregnant with a child he doesn't want? (This is often a triggering factor in wife abuse.)
• Does he have unusual problems?

For abusive fathers or mothers, a local chapter of Parents Anonymous (PA) may be helpful. (see *Organizations that Help the Abused and the Abuser*, page 168). PA, a self-help group made up of former abusers, attempts to help abusing parents by teaching them how to redirect their anger and deal with it.

Besides helping short-circuit abusive behavior, a self-help group like PA takes abusing parents out of their isolation and gives them someone understanding to talk to. It also provides help in a crisis, when members may be able to prevent an abusive incident.

Telephone hot lines to crisis intervention services also give abusers someone to talk with in times of stress and crisis, and may help prevent abuse. Commonly staffed by volunteers, telephone hot lines provide a link between those who seek help and those willing and trained to provide counseling and reassurance.

These and other kinds of help are also available through family service agencies and hospitals. Be sure you know what resources are available, nationally and in your area. Then when an abuser or his victim needs your help, you can respond quickly and authoritatively.

**A final word**
As you know, protecting patients' rights is a primary nursing responsibility (see Chapter 2). Abuse violates those rights. To protect your patients, be alert to recognize signs and symptoms of abuse. Accept your responsibility for reporting possible incidents of abuse. Learn about community resources that can

help abusers and their victims. And remember, *both* need your help.

---

# 28 Special risks in caring for "special" patients

When your hospitalized patient is mentally ill or developmentally disabled, take care. Despite his often dependent condition, he has most of the same rights as your other patients. And if you violate these rights, even unwittingly, you could face serious legal complications.

Part of today's concern for the rights of the mentally ill and developmentally disabled stems from attempts to correct past abuses. Under the United States Constitution, a person's rights can't be limited or denied merely because of his status. Many health-care professionals still don't realize that the courts have generally interpreted the Constitution to mean that mentally ill and developmentally disabled persons have a right to fair and humane treatment, including during hospitalization. Under most circumstances, such a patient can't be kept in a hospital against his will, for example. Nor can he be denied the right to refuse treatment or to receive information so he can give informed consent to proposed surgery.

State governments have tried to assure the rights of this special population by enacting legislation specifically addressing the problems of the mentally ill and developmentally disabled. This legislation describes and authorizes specific services and provides the necessary funding. The federal government also provides for the mentally ill and developmentally disabled. The Rehabilitation Act of 1973, for example, earmarked funds specifically for rehabilitative programs. For instance, it provides cash assistance for persons who, because of their disabilities, aren't able to provide adequately for themselves or their families. The act also outlines 14 patient's rights to ensure high standards of health care. Facilities that participate in Medicare must comply with these 14 rights and make sure that the patient, his guardian, next of kin, or sponsoring agency knows about them, too.

Canada makes similar provisions for mentally ill and developmentally disabled persons. As in the United States, Canadian legislation seeks to prevent maltreatment and to fund programs that help these persons to function successfully in society.

### Understanding issues of legal responsibility

When a mentally ill or developmentally disabled child is admitted to a hospital, legal responsibility for him must be established immediately.

If the patient is accompanied by a parent, usually the parent will be legally responsible.

If the child has been institutionalized prior to entering the hospital, the institution may have responsibility.

---

*"Restricting a 'special' patient's liberty is almost never legally permissible."*

---

However, this is true only if the parents have waived responsibility and the institution has written evidence to prove it.

If the courts have found the parents unfit or unable to care for the child, a legal guardian will have been appointed. This person has the legal right to assume responsibility for the child.

When no guardian has been appointed for the child, the state may act as a guardian under the doctrine of *parens patriae*. This is true of mentally

GLOSSARY

## KEY TERMS IN THIS ENTRY

**doctrine of parens patriae** • A doctrine that appoints the state as legal guardian of a child or incompetent adult when an individual hasn't been appointed as guardian.

**Medicare** • Federally funded national health insurance authorized by the Social Security Act for certain persons age 65 or older.

**writ of habeas corpus** • A constitutional right to a court hearing that any person has when imprisoned or detained for allegedly breaking the law.

ill or developmentally disabled adults, as well, who must have guardians.

Whenever your mentally ill or developmentally disabled patient is an adult, check his chart to see if he requires a legal guardian and to establish who it is. It may be a parent. Or if the patient is married, it may be the patient's spouse.

Sometimes an adult patient and his guardian will seriously disagree about the patient's care. When this happens, get clarification by going through proper hospital channels.

As a nurse, you have no right to control the life of a mentally ill or developmentally disabled patient. Restricting his liberty for any reason is almost never legally permissible, except when he may otherwise harm himself or others. You must analyze each situation carefully to determine at what point the patient needs help in managing his affairs.

### Obtaining informed consent

When consent is required from a patient who's mentally ill or developmentally disabled, three questions should immediately come to mind:
• Is consent for treatment or a special procedure obtained the same way it is from any other patient?

• Does the patient fully understand the procedure that he's to undergo, including risks?

• Does the patient have the authority to give his own consent, or must someone else give it?

The answers to these questions, of course, will vary with each patient. Clearly, if the patient is of unsound mind and can't understand the nature, purpose, and risks of the proposed treatment, he can't legally consent. In such a case, consent must be obtained from the patient's legal guardian.

If the legal guardian is unavailable, a court authorized to handle such matters may allow treatment.

As you know, a doctor must always explain the nature, purpose, and risks of the treatment to the person giving consent, whether it's the patient or someone else. This explanation allows the person to make an informed decision that will be in the patient's best interest. Failure to obtain a truly informed consent can result in legal action against the doctor, the nurse (if she knew the patient's consent wasn't informed), and the hospital or other health-care institution.

Sometimes a doctor or nurse may doubt a patient's capacity to consent, even though he hasn't been judged incompetent. This often happens during an illness that causes temporary incompetence. In such a situation, the nearest relative's consent must be obtained or, if none can be found, the court must authorize treatment.

In the New York case of *Collins v. Davis* (1964), a hospital administrator sought a court order to permit surgery on an irrational adult whose life was considered to be in danger. The patient's wife had previously refused to give consent, allegedly for reasons she felt served the patient's best interest. The court, after considering the entire situation—especially the patient's prognosis if surgery wasn't performed—agreed that the hospital and the doctor had only two choices: either let the patient die, or perform the operation against his wife's wishes. The court overruled the wife's refusal, holding that the patient had sought medical attention and that treatment normally given to a patient with a similar condition should be provided.

You can best protect the mentally ill or developmentally disabled patient's legal rights to informed consent by making sure a doctor has provided him or his guardian with complete, accurate information.

Of course, you know you should never help with procedures on a patient whose informed consent hasn't been obtained. If you do, you can be held liable along with the doctor and hospital (see Entry 12). In fact, if your patient is a minor, you could face double liability: his parents could sue you now, and he could sue you when he comes of age.

Adolescents who protest their hospitalization may obtain a court review and be represented by appointed legal counsel (see Entry 26).

## Understanding forced hospitalization and use of restraints

Mentally ill or developmentally disabled persons may be involuntarily kept in hospitals if they're at risk of taking their own lives, or if they pose a threat to other persons' property or lives. However, mental illness alone is not a sufficient legal basis for detaining a patient. The U.S. Supreme Court, in *O'Connor v. Donaldson* (1975), held that a state cannot constitutionally confine a patient, without treatment or without the rehabilitation necessary to reintegrate him into society, "who is capable of surviving safely in freedom by himself or with the help of willing and responsible family members or friends."

Similar restrictions apply to physical restraint of patients. Most states require a doctor to write the restraint order and place it in the patient's medical record before restraints can be applied.

## CARING FOR A PATIENT IN RESTRAINTS OR SECLUSION

Before you can keep a patient in restraints or in seclusion, you must get an order from the patient's doctor authorizing it. New York State law, typical of most states, says this order must include:

- the results of the doctor's physical examination of the patient
- a description of the patient's behavior that makes restraints or seclusion necessary
- a description of the type of restraint or seclusion you should use

- the period during which the restraint should be used
- an order indicating how frequently you should take the patient's vital signs and check on his overall safety and comfort.

In an emergency situation, if a patient becomes violent, you may need to restrain him immediately without a doctor's order to prevent him from harming himself or others. In this situation, apply the restraints, then notify the doctor to examine the patient and write the restraint order.

When you're caring for a patient in restraints or seclusion, the law says you must:

- monitor the patient's vital signs according to the doctor's order. If you can't do this because the patient is violent, explain why in your nurses' notes. Observe his level of consciousness, verbal content, activity, color, appearance, hydration, perspiration, and skin temperature, and record your findings.
- check on the patient as the doctor has ordered, paying close attention to his comfort, safety, and personal needs, including proper placement of restraints

and circulation in hands and feet, if appropriate.
- release the patient in restraints every 2 hours, if he's awake. Be sure to take proper precautions. If his actions no longer threaten others or himself, tell this to the doctor immediately. He may discontinue his order.
- feed the patient in restraints in an upright position to minimize his risk of choking.

---

Restraint (or seclusion) may be used only to prevent a patient from seriously injuring himself or others—and only when all other physical and psychological therapies would likely fail to prevent such injuries. Whenever possible, use minimal restraint—only that amount necessary to protect the patient and safeguard the staff and others. Restraint should never be used for punishment, for the convenience of staff, or as a substitute for treatment programs. Use of restraints is usually limited to a specific period of time (see *Caring for a Patient in Restraints or Seclusion*). Except in emergencies, you may normally apply restraints only after a doctor has examined the patient and

written an order to restrain him. In an emergency situation—such as a violent outburst with actual or potential harm to persons or property—any person may apply restraints to the patient. But obtain an order for the restraint as soon as possible, and document the incident carefully.

As a nurse, you may be held liable in a lawsuit if you can't verify that—in your judgment—a patient needed to be restrained, and that he was restrained only as long as necessary. If you restrain or seclude a patient simply for shouting obscenities, for example, you risk a lawsuit for false imprisonment.

When applying restraints, take care to avoid undue force; otherwise, you may invite a lawsuit for battery. Even threatening to use force may be sufficient cause for legal action.

When a doctor isn't available in an emergency, you're responsible to see that restraints and seclusion are used only to the extent necessary to prevent injury. Until the doctor authorizes the use of restraints, you must provide one-

---

*"Restraint is a form of imprisonment, so it should only be used as a last resort."*

---

to-one patient supervision. Make sure, too, that the staff uses only legally permissible forms of restraint.

Restraint is a form of imprisonment, so it should only be used as a last resort. Before restraining a patient, consider alternatives, such as constant observation or walking with the patient.

Tranquilizing drugs may be another possibility. However, use them sparingly, with caution, and of course only with a doctor's order. The patient's right to the least restrictive treatment or to an open-door policy that allows patients to move about "freely" means little if accompanied by indiscriminate drug use as a substitute for restraints.

### Protecting these patients' right to privacy

The law has tried to protect all citizens from unwarranted intrusion into their private lives. Unfortunately, mentally ill and developmentally disabled patients' right to privacy is easily violated. A good definition of privacy, first presented at the International Commission of Justice in 1970, reads: "Privacy is the ability to lead one's life without anyone: A) interfering with family or home life; B) interfering with physical or mental integrity or moral and intellectual freedom; C) attacking honor

and reputation; D) placing one in a false light; E) censoring or restricting communication and correspondence, written or oral; F) disclosing irrelevant or embarrassing information; and G) disclosing information given or received in circumstances of professional confidence."

Keep this definition in mind as you work with these patients, and do all you can to protect their rights. Despite their handicaps, these patients should never be treated as second-class citizens.

### These patients' right to writ of habeas corpus

Institutionalization may, at times, breach a patient's rights, giving him cause to petition for a writ of habeas corpus. This writ seeks to ensure the timely release of any person who claims that he's being detained illegally and deprived of his liberty.

### Understanding right-to-treatment issues

In *Wyatt v. Stickney* (1972), the court upheld the legal right of a mentally ill person hospitalized in a public institution to receive adequate psychiatric treatment. This decision suggests that when a patient is involuntarily committed because he needs treatment, his rights are violated if such treatment isn't given. Furthermore, if the underlying reason for a patient's commitment is danger to himself or others, treatment must be provided to make him less dangerous.

To qualify as adequate, treatment must be given as follows:
- by adequate staff
- in the least restrictive setting
- in privacy
- in a facility that ensures the patient a comfortable bed, adequate diet, and recreational facilities
- with the patient's informed consent, prior to unusual treatment
- with payment for work done in the institution, outside of program activities

• according to an individual treatment plan.

You must ensure that any mentally ill or developmentally disabled patient knows what treatment he needs and how he will get it. To help him, you must know what his major problems are and what he can do for himself— or what others must do for him—to help him get ready for discharge. You should also involve him in formulating his treatment plan, unless you have a documented reason why he can't or won't be involved.

### Sexual-rights issues

Many questions regarding the care of mentally ill and developmentally disabled patients have so far eluded definitive answers. Some have to do with sexual matters. For example, should developmentally disabled persons be given sex education? Should they be allowed to reproduce, practice contraception, undergo voluntary sterilization? Although the general inclination is to let guardians make these decisions, the issue of the individual's right to make his own decisions will not go away. If good care can be given to both the developmentally disabled and their offspring, who's to say that they should be denied the opportunity to enjoy the same satisfactions others do?

Many U.S. Supreme Court decisions have upheld the following rights of mentally ill or developmentally disabled patients:

• to marry
• to have children
• to employ contraception, abortion, or sterilization, if desired
• to follow a life-style of their own choosing.

These rights were upheld in such cases as *Sengstack v. Sengstack* (1958), *Wyatt v. Stickney* (1972), *O'Connor v. Donaldson* (1975), and *N.Y. State Association for Retarded Children, Inc. v. Carey* (1977).

Involuntary sterilization of mentally disabled patients isn't employed as often today as in previous years, although

its constitutionality was upheld in *Buck v. Bell* (1927). In its ruling, the court held that the state has the right to sterilize a developmentally disabled or insane person provided that:

• the sterilization is not prescribed as punishment
• the policy is applied equally to all persons
• the unborn child's interest is sufficient to warrant the sterilization.

The courts apply this ruling only when absolutely necessary. When it is applied, the patient's legal guardian must consent to the procedure, and usually a separate, independent presterilization review of the case is ordered. (In New York State, an independent medical review board must review and approve every planned involuntary sterilization before it can be performed.) If the patient refuses to submit to surgery, the matter may go to court, which may call for use of a less permanent birth-control method.

### What's involved in patient participation in research?

Another troublesome area involves using mentally ill and developmentally disabled persons as subjects for medical or other research—especially if risks are involved. Guidelines for consent to experimentation and drastic, questionable, or extreme forms of treatment are complicated and raise many unresolved questions. The so-called Willowbrook decision (*N.Y. State Association for Retarded Children, Inc. v. Carey*, 1977), however, decreed that both voluntary and involuntary residents of an institution have the constitutional right to be protected from harm. The proper authority (often a research-proposal review board) should allow the patient to participate in the research only if it's relevant to his needs and the needs of others like him. For example, a depressed patient shouldn't be asked to participate in research involving anxiety and schizophrenia.

## Should you give these patients special consideration?

Because of their limitations, mentally ill or developmentally disabled patients often make "ordinary" requests that require special consideration.

For example, a patient may demand to smoke a cigarette *now*. Probably his doctor hasn't written an order for the request. If the patient should smoke only under supervision because of the danger of fire, you may decide to stay with him while he does so. But if you have a duty to be elsewhere, you should refuse his request, explaining why and telling him when he'll be able to smoke. Or, if you know a refusal will agitate and anger him, you can ask another nurse to supervise the patient while he smokes.

But maybe you feel the patient's demand is really a challenge to your authority. If so, you may decide to refuse the request, explaining the need to follow the hospital's social and safety policies.

If the patient's behavior is part of a pattern that includes, for example, refusing to shower, refusing to go to bed by a certain time, and demanding to make an immediate phone call, then you need to refer the situation to the treatment team for a well-thought-out decision—one that serves the best interests of both patient and hospital. Once it's made, reinforce the decision with the patient, and ask all the health-team members to enforce it consistently.

## A final word

When you care for patients who are mentally incapacitated or developmentally disabled, you must remember this: *They do not have any less legal protection than the rest of society has.* In fact, often the law covers these patients' rights in extra detail, to ensure that they receive the proper care and treatment that they're due. As a nurse, your responsibility is to provide that care and treatment skillfully, safely, and humanely.

# 29 When your patient is a suspected criminal

Suppose you're asked to care for an injured suspect who's accompanied by police. Because the police need evidence, they ask you to give them not only the patient's belongings but also a sample of his blood. Should you comply?

If he's under arrest, you can legally handle his belongings and take the blood sample for evidence (with a doctor's order, of course). If he *isn't* under arrest, be careful. Make sure a valid search warrant is in effect before you proceed. If you don't, the patient may be able to sue you for invasion of privacy as well as assault and battery. Here's another consideration: If you assemble the requested evidence without a search warrant, the evidence may be inadmissible in court.

Also involved here is the suspect's right to be considered innocent until proven guilty. Despite his police guard, you have no business judging him. His guilt or innocence will be for the courts to decide.

## Some constitutional rights

The Fourth Amendment to the U.S. Constitution provides that "the right of the people to be secure in their persons, houses, papers and effects, against unreasonable searches and seizures shall not be violated, and no warrants shall issue, but upon probable cause." Ironically, this means that every individual, even a suspected criminal, has a right to privacy, including a right to be free from intrusions that are made without search warrants. So the Fourth Amendment doesn't absolutely prohibit all searches and seizures, only unreasonable ones.

Even after conviction, an individual doesn't forfeit all constitutional rights. Among those retained is the Eighth Amendment's proscription against cruel and unusual punishment. This implies that prison officials and health-care workers must not deliberately ignore a prisoner's medical needs.

Probably the *exclusionary rule* is the most common rule affecting nurses in relation to suspected criminals and their victims. This rule stems from the Fourth Amendment's prohibition of unreasonable searches and seizures. In the landmark case of *Mapp v. Ohio* (1961), the U.S. Supreme Court held that evidence obtained through an unreasonable or unlawful search cannot be used against the person whose rights the search violated.

A search without a warrant isn't reasonable unless an arrest is involved. A law enforcement official may conduct a search without a warrant if it's incidental to an arrest and if it doesn't extend beyond the accused person's body or an immediate area where he could reach for a weapon. Generally, *a search may not precede an arrest* unless probable cause has been established. So if evidence obtained during a pre-arrest search is used to *provide* probable cause for the arrest, the courts will consider that an unreasonable search. Of course, if an accused person consents to a search, any evidence found would be considered admissible in court.

Evidence in plain view can be confiscated. As a nurse, if you find a gun, knife, drug, or other item that the suspect could use to harm himself or others, you have a right to remove it. You should, however, notify the hospital administration immediately and maintain control over the evidence until you can give it to an administrator or a law enforcement official.

In *Burdreau v. McDowell* (1921), the court said that Fourth Amendment protections applied only to governmental (such as police) action and not to searches conducted by private persons. Although several courts have criticized this rule, it has been repeatedly upheld.

In *State v. Perea* (1981), a nurse took a suspect's shirt for safekeeping, then

## KEY TERMS IN THIS ENTRY

**assault** • An attempt or threat by a person to physically injure another person.

**battery** • The unauthorized touching of a person by another person, such as when a health-care professional treats a patient beyond what the patient consented to.

**privileged communication** • A conversation in which the speaker intends the information he's giving to remain private between himself and the listener.

turned it over to the police even though they hadn't requested it. The court allowed the shirt to be admitted as evidence. The reason: Since no governmental intrusion was involved, the suspect's Fourth Amendment right wasn't violated.

The case of *United States v. Winbush* (1970) produced a similar result. Here the court ruled that evidence found during a routine search of an unconscious patient's pockets was admissible because the purpose of the search was to obtain necessary identification and medical information.

*Commonwealth v. Storella* (1978) involved a bullet that a doctor removed during a medically necessary operation. After the operation, the doctor turned the bullet over to the police. The court allowed the bullet to be admitted as evidence because the doctor was acting according to good medical practice, and not as a state agent, in removing the bullet.

This doesn't mean, of course, that doctors (and nurses) have a right to become private police forces. Generally, searches that occur as part of medical care don't violate a suspect's rights. But searches made for the sole purpose of gathering evidence—especially if done at police request—very well may. Several courts have said that a suspect subjected to an illegal private search has a right to seek remedy against the unlawful searcher in a civil lawsuit. One such case was *Stone v. Commonwealth* (1967).

The major difference between U.S. and Canadian law regarding searches is that, in Canada, evidence obtained during an illegal search is still admissible in court. However, a police officer properly should have a search warrant before searching a suspected criminal, to protect his rights.

### Refusal to consent

Opinions differ as to whether a blood test, such as a blood alcohol test, is admissible in court if the person refused consent for the test. In *Schmerber v. California* (1966), the U.S. Supreme Court said that a blood extraction obtained without a warrant, incident to a lawful arrest, is not an unconstitutional search and seizure and is admissible evidence. Many courts have held this to mean that a blood sample must be drawn *after* the arrest to be admissible, and must be drawn in a medically reasonable manner.

So when a suspect is pinned to the floor by two police officers while a doctor draws a blood sample (as in *People v. Kraft*, 1970), or when a suspect's broken arm is twisted while a policeman sits on him to force consent to a blood test (as in *State v. Riggins*, 1977), the courts have ruled the test results inadmissible. The courts have also ruled as inadmissible—and as violating due process rights—evidence gained by forcibly administering an emetic to remove a suspect's stomach contents (*Rochin v. California*, 1952).

Courts have admitted blood tests as evidence when the tests weren't drawn at police request but for medically necessary purposes, such as blood typing (*Commonwealth v. Gordon*, 1968). Some courts have also allowed blood work to be admitted as evidence when it was drawn for nontherapeutic reasons and voluntarily turned over to police (*Turner v. State*, 1975). Be careful, though. As with unlawful private searches, a doctor or nurse who does blood work without the patient's consent may be liable for committing battery, even if the patient is a suspected criminal and the blood work is *medically* necessary.

Many states have enacted so-called implied-consent laws as part of their motor vehicle laws. This means that by applying for a driver's license, a person implies his consent to submit to a blood alcohol test if he's arrested for drunken driving. Many of these laws state specifically that if an individual refuses to submit to the chemical test, it may not

> *"A nurse who does blood work without the patient's consent may be liable for committing battery."*

be given, *but* the driver then forfeits his license. Check to see whether such laws exist in your state, because a blood alcohol sample is inadmissible in court if it's been drawn without a suspect's consent.

### Documenting your procedures

Needless to say, be careful and precise in documenting all your procedures when you care for a suspected criminal. Note any blood work done, and list all treatments and the patient's response to them.

If you turn anything over to the police or administration, record what it was and the name of the person you gave it to. Record a suspect's statements, too, but distinguish between those that are privileged and those that aren't. If a suspect says, "I wasted four cops tonight," that's not a privileged communication. But if he says, "I think I was shot in the leg by a cop," that relates directly to his medical care and is privileged.

## Caring for evidence

Before any evidence can be admissible in court, the court must have some guarantee of where, and how, it was gathered. Someone must account for evidence from the moment you collect it until it appears in court. You can't leave it lying around, unattended, where it might be tampered with.

If you discover evidence, mark it in some way. Before doing so, however, check with a police officer or a forensic expert, so you don't destroy valuable information.

When a suspect dies, most states provide that the coroner can claim the body. Police are free to gather any evidence that will not mutilate the body. A dead body has no constitutional rights, so no rights are violated by a search. (See Entry 17.)

## Working in prison

If you work in a prison hospital or infirmary, remember the Eighth Amendment's prohibition against cruel and unusual punishments.

The U.S. Supreme Court, in *Estelle v. Gamble* (1976), stated that the Eighth Amendment prohibits more than physically barbarous punishment. The amendment embodies "broad and idealistic concepts of dignity, civilized standards, humanity, and decency against which we must evaluate penal measures."

The state has an obligation to provide medical care for those it imprisons. The Court concluded that: "deliberate indifference to serious medical needs of prisoners constitutes the unnecessary and wanton infliction of pain proscribed by the Eighth Amendment. This is true whether the indifference is manifested by prison doctors in response to a prisoner's needs or by prison personnel in intentionally denying or delaying access to medical care or intentionally interfering with the treatment once prescribed."

In *Ramos v. Lamm* (1980), the court outlined several ways in which prison officials show deliberate indifference to prisoners' medical needs:

• preventing an inmate from receiving recommended treatment
• denying access to medical personnel capable of evaluating the need for treatment
• allowing repeated acts of negligence that disclose a pattern of conduct by prison health staff
• allowing such severe deficiencies in staffing, facilities, equipment, or procedures to exist so that inmates are effectively denied access to adequate medical care.

Working daily with prisoners is difficult and demanding, both professionally and emotionally. Along with exhibiting a host of other unpleasant behaviors, prisoners can be abusive, manipulative, and angry. In spite of this, health-care professionals can't forget their ethical and legal duty to provide quality care.

Several courts have stated that individuals have a constitutional right to privacy based on a high regard for human dignity and self-determination. This means a competent adult may refuse medical care, even lifesaving treatments. For instance, in *Lane v. Candura* (1978), an appellate court upheld the right of a competent adult to refuse a leg amputation that would have saved her life.

A suspected criminal may refuse unwarranted bodily invasions. However, an arrested suspect or convicted criminal does not have the same right to refuse lifesaving measures. In *Commissioner of Correction v. Myers* (1979), a prisoner with renal failure refused hemodialysis unless he was moved to a minimum security prison. The court disagreed, saying that although the defendant's imprisonment did not divest him of his right to privacy or his interest in maintaining his bodily integrity, it did impose limitations on those constitutional rights.

As a practical matter, inform your hospital administration anytime a patient refuses lifesaving treatments. In the case of a suspect or prisoner, notify law enforcement authorities as well.

### A final word
Caring for a suspected criminal presents some special problems that deserve close attention. Whenever you're in this situation, be sure to check your hospital's policy on caring for suspected criminals (if one exists), and follow its guidelines carefully.

# 30 Your responsibility for a patient's living will

When a legally competent person draws up a living will, he declares the steps he wants or doesn't want taken when he's terminally ill. The will doesn't apply to initial treatment decisions; it applies only to decisions that will be made after a terminally ill patient is comatose and has no reasonable possibility of recovery. Generally, a living will authorizes the attending doctor to withhold or discontinue lifesaving procedures.

The will is called *living* because its provisions take effect before death. By clearly stating his wishes regarding terminal-illness procedures, the patient also helps relieve any guilt his family and the health-care team might otherwise feel for having done too little (or too much) to keep him alive (see Entry 71).

Living wills stem from action by the public, not by the medical community. Persons active in promoting living wills are often part of a "right to die" or "quality of life" movement.

State legislatures have recognized the movement's importance. In every state, a living will is considered a legal—but not necessarily legally binding—statement of the patient's wishes (see Entry 11). California, in 1976, was the first state to adopt a living-will law (also called a natural death law). Currently, only 14 states and the District of Columbia have laws specifically governing living wills. These laws help guarantee that the patient's wishes will be carried out.

### Understanding the health team's responsibility
In three of the states with living-will laws, and in the District of Columbia, the laws make living wills binding on doctors and impose penalties for noncompliance. Five of the states impose no penalties for noncompliance, and six make the wills advisory only. (See *Living-Will Laws,* pages 186 to 189.)

### What living-will laws do
Generally, living-will laws address questions such as these:
- Who may execute a living will?
- When does a living will apply?
- Who's immune from liability for following a living will's directives?
- What documentation is required?
- How long is a living will valid?
- When and how should a living will be executed? (In California, for example, a living will is binding only if executed after a terminal illness diagnosis has been made.)
- How can a living will be rescinded?

In the 36 states without living-will laws, a doctor may choose to follow or not to follow the will's provisions.

Even if the doctor must obey the living will, or would like to, he faces real difficulties in determining when it should apply. The typical wording in living wills isn't much help. What, for example, is a "reasonable expectation of recovery?" And what is a "heroic" or "extraordinary" measure? These ambiguities and the difficulty in clarifying them (particularly before the situation actually arises) are among the reasons why legislatures have been reluctant to make living wills binding.

If doctors, nurses, and other health-care providers follow the wishes expressed in a living will authorized by law, they're generally immune from civil and criminal liability. In states without living-will laws, immunity is not assured. Because of the complexities involved, no matter which state you work in, you'll do well to check your hospital's policy-and-procedures manual and get advice from your hospital's legal department, when a living will appears in a patient's record.

In Canada, not one province has enacted legislation covering living wills. Nor are any likely to do so, because the Canadian Law Reform Commission has rejected the living-will approach. So the status of living wills in Canada is uncertain. However, the commission has proposed changes in Canadian laws that would help recognize statements in a living will as accurately representing the patient's wishes, if he is unable to speak for himself.

## May children make living wills?

Although minors can't make valid testamentary wills, and adults can't make such wills for them, living wills are another matter. In Arkansas and New Mexico, adults are authorized to make living wills for their minor children.

Of course, parents don't normally plan for their child to die, so most are unlikely to make a living will before a child's terminal illness is diagnosed. Even then, a living will is usually legally unnecessary. If the parents and the child agree that no extraordinary means should be used to prolong life, or if the child is too young to understand, the parents have the legal right to act for the child. They can require that the health-care team not use extraordinary means to prolong his life. (See Entry 26.) The same principle also applies in reverse: if the child wants to die but the parents want him treated, the parents' wishes prevail.

If a terminally ill adolescent doesn't want extraordinary treatment but his parents do, and the adolescent has written a living will, a doctor or hospital may use the will to petition a court in his behalf. Even though the will itself is legally invalid because it was written by a minor, its very existence may prompt the court to consult the ado-

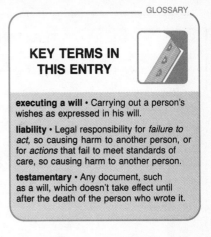

lescent and, in its ruling, grant the patient his wishes.

## When a mentally incompetent person wants to make a living will

Of the 14 states (and the District of Columbia) that have living-will laws, only Arkansas authorizes a competent adult to make a living will on behalf of an adult who's not mentally competent. The remaining states allow only competent adults to prepare such wills for themselves. But even in these states, a living will may influence a court to grant the wishes of an adult whose mental capacity is in question.

## What if a living will is from another state or country?

U.S. law applies to foreign citizens treated in the United States. This means a foreign citizen may execute a living will while in the United States, and it must be honored if executed in a state with a legally binding living-will law. A state without a living-will law may honor it, but it isn't required to.

What if a patient produces a living will executed in a foreign country? This situation is the equivalent of executing a living will in a state that doesn't have a living-will law. The patient's doctor may honor it, but the law doesn't require that he do so.

You may be wondering, what about

# THE LIVING WILL

If your patient has filled out a living will, it may resemble the one here. The wording of your patient's will may differ, however, according to his wishes. So read his will carefully.

Death is as much a reality as birth, growth, maturity and old age—it is the one certainty of life. If the time comes when I can no longer take part in decisions for my own future, let this statement stand as an expression of my wishes and directions, while I am still of sound mind.

If at such a time the situation should arise in which there is no reasonable expectation of my recovery from extreme physical or mental disability, I direct that I be allowed to die and not be kept alive by medications, artificial means or "heroic measures." I do, however, ask that medication be mercifully administered to me to alleviate suffering even though this may shorten my remaining life.

This statement is made after careful consideration and is in accordance with my strong convictions and beliefs. I want the wishes and directions here expressed carried out to the extent permitted by law. Insofar as they are not legally enforceable, I hope that those to whom this Will is addressed will regard themselves as morally bound by these provisions.

Signed _____

Date _____

Witness _____

Witness _____

Copies of this request have been given to _____

_____

_____

_____

Reprinted with permission from Concern for Dying, 250 West 57th Street, New York, N.Y. 10107.

a patient who executes a living will in one state and later finds himself terminally ill in another? If both states have living-will laws, the second state will honor the patient's living will. A state without a living-will law may, but need not, honor a living will that was executed in another state.

The same general legal principle applies to U.S. citizens in Canada or in another foreign country. A foreign country's law applies to all persons, whether citizens of that country or not, and determines the extent to which a living will will be honored.

### What invalidates a living will?

A living will needn't be honored if it's been revoked, if it's out of date, if the patient asks that it be disregarded, or if the patient asks for treatment that disagrees with statements in his living will.

In the states with living-will laws, all but Arkansas provide procedures for revocation. The procedures include deliberate destruction of the document, written revocation, and the patient's statement that he intends to revoke it.

In the states that have living-will laws, the period of time before it becomes invalidated varies. If the patient's family and attending medical personnel find that the patient made the living will many years ago and his life circumstances have changed substantially since then, they may have legal justification for disregarding the will. For this reason, publishers of living-will forms suggest reviewing the will yearly, revising it if necessary, and re-dating and re-signing it.

Remember, if a patient tells his doctor to proceed with treatment that contradicts the living will, the patient's action effectively revokes the will.

### Can the family's wishes prevail?

In a state with a living-will law, the patient's family can't contradict it unless they can prove the will is invalid. Some of these states provide penalties for concealing a patient's living will or

for falsely reporting that it's been revoked.

In a state that doesn't have a living-will law, the health team or a court will consider both a patient's living will and his family's wishes before deciding on treatment or nontreatment.

### Drafting a living will

Like all legal documents, a living will must be written, signed, and witnessed. States with living-will laws specify the execution requirements; in states without laws, the patient may use a standardized form or have his attorney design one. (See *The Living Will*.) (Anyone can obtain forms from Concern for Dying or The Society for the Right to Die, two groups that currently share offices at 250 W. 57th St., New York, N.Y., 10107.) Although it's not required, a patient may want to file copies of his living will in his medical record, with his doctor, and with family members who would be with him in the event of a terminal illness.

As a nurse, you may be asked to help a patient write a living will or to witness one. You may help him write it, or refer him to someone else for help. If he asks you to witness the will, check to see if your state has laws that restrict you from doing this by referring to *Living-Will Laws,* pages 186 to 189. If it doesn't, ask your nursing supervisor for the procedure you should follow. Document the patient's actions in your nurses' notes, describing factually the circumstances under which the will was drawn up and signed.

### Oral living wills

Patients most often make oral statements expressing their wishes about further medical treatment as follows:

*Before terminal illness.* When a patient has made his treatment wishes known to his family and doctor in advance, they will usually respect his wishes even if he later becomes comatose or otherwise incompetent. But if the doctor and the family disagree about what is best for the terminally

# LIVING-WILL LAWS

Currently, 13 states and the District of Columbia have living-will laws. This chart shows you the details of each state's law.

| STATE | TESTATOR REQUIREMENTS | WITNESS REQUIREMENTS | LENGTH OF EFFECTIVENESS |
|---|---|---|---|
| Alabama | Adult of sound mind | Two witnesses, excluding relatives, heirs, persons who are financially responsible for patient | Effective until revoked |
| Arkansas | Adult of sound mind; proxy permitted for minor or incompetent person | Two witnesses; will must be notarized | Effective until revoked |
| California | Adult of sound mind | Two witnesses, excluding relatives, heirs, patient's doctor and employees where patient is hospitalized | 5 years |
| Delaware | Adult of sound mind | Two witnesses, excluding relatives, heirs, employees where patient is hospitalized, and persons who are financially responsible for patient | 10 years |
| District of Columbia | Age 18 or older and of sound mind | Two witnesses, excluding spouse, heirs, relatives, patient's doctor, employees where patient is hospitalized, and persons who are financially responsible for patient | Effective until revoked |
| Idaho | Terminally ill adult | Two witnesses, excluding relatives, heirs, patient's doctor and employees where patient is hospitalized | 5 years |
| Kansas | Adult of sound mind | Two witnesses, excluding relatives, heirs, patient's doctor and employees where patient is hospitalized | Effective until revoked |

| LEGAL STATUS | IMMUNITY FROM LEGAL ACTION FOR OBEYING WILL | PENALTY FOR NOT OBEYING WILL | PENALTY FOR DESTRUCTION, FORGERY, CONCEALMENT, OR FALSE REPORTING |
|---|---|---|---|
| Not binding | Doctor, licensed health-care professional, medical care facility or employee | No penalty; doctor "shall permit" transfer to another doctor | Destroying will or forging revocation is a misdemeanor; forging will or concealing revocation is a felony |
| Not specified | Any person and health facility | No penalty | No penalty |
| Not binding unless executed 14 days after diagnosis of terminal illness | Doctor, licensed health professional acting under doctor's direction, and health facility | Charged with unprofessional conduct unless doctor transfers patient | Destroying will is a misdemeanor; forging or concealing revocation, causing death, is homicide |
| Not clear | Doctors, nurses | No penalty | Forcing patient to sign is a misdemeanor; any action that falsely implies patient wanted to prolong his life is a felony |
| Binding | Doctor, licensed health-care professional, health facility, or employee | Unprofessional conduct if he fails to transfer patient to doctor who will comply | Destroying will or forging revocation brings a fine and a jail term; forging will or concealing revocation, causing death, is homicide |
| Not specified | Doctor, and health facility | No penalty | No penalty |
| Binding | Doctor, licensed health professional, health facility, and employee | Charged with unprofessional conduct unless doctor transfers patient | Destroying will or forging revocation is a misdemeanor; forging will or concealing revocation is a felony |

*(continued)*

## LIVING-WILL LAWS *(continued)*

| STATE | TESTATOR REQUIREMENTS | WITNESS REQUIREMENTS | LENGTH OF EFFECTIVENESS |
|---|---|---|---|
| **Nevada** | Adult of sound mind | Two witnesses, excluding relatives, heirs, patient's doctor and employees where patient is hospitalized | Effective until revoked |
| **New Mexico** | Adult of sound mind; proxy permitted for minor or incompetent person | Same number of witnesses as for regular will; court must certify a minor's living will | Effective until revoked |
| **North Carolina** | Competent person; no age provision specified | Two witnesses, excluding relatives, heirs, patient's doctor and employees where patient is hospitalized; will must be notarized | Effective until revoked |
| **Oregon** | Adult of sound mind | Two witnesses, excluding relatives, heirs, patient's doctor and employees where patient is hospitalized | 5 years |
| **Texas** | Adult of sound mind | Two witnesses, excluding relatives, heirs, patient's doctor and employees where patient is hospitalized | Effective until revoked |
| **Vermont** | Adult age 18 or older | Two witnesses, excluding spouse, heirs, creditors, patient's doctor, and other medical personnel under his supervision | Effective until revoked |
| **Virginia** | Competent adult | Two witnesses; oral declaration requires doctor and two witnesses | Effective until revoked |
| **Washington** | Adult of sound mind | Two witnesses, excluding relatives, heirs, patient's doctor and employees where patient is hospitalized | Effective until revoked |

| LEGAL STATUS | IMMUNITY FROM LEGAL ACTION FOR OBEYING WILL | PENALTY FOR NOT OBEYING WILL | PENALTY FOR DESTRUCTION, FORGERY, CONCEALMENT, OR FALSE REPORTING |
|---|---|---|---|
| Not binding | Doctor, person acting under doctor's direction, and health facility | No penalty | Destroying will is a misdemeanor; forging will or concealing revocation, causing death, is murder |
| Binding | Doctors, employees of health facility, and health facility | No penalty | Destroying will, concealing revocation, or forgery is a felony |
| Not binding | Licensed health professional and health facility | No penalty | No penalty |
| Not binding | Doctor, licensed health professional acting under doctor's direction, and health facility | No penalty, but doctor who disagrees with will must make a reasonable effort to transfer patient to another medical facility | Prohibited, but no penalties |
| Binding when executed after diagnosis | Doctor, licensed health professional acting under doctor's direction, and health facility | Charged with unprofessional conduct unless doctor transfers patient | Destroying will is a misdemeanor; forging will or concealing revocation, causing death, is criminal homicide |
| Not binding | Doctor, nurse, health professional, and health facility | No penalty; doctor must inform patient and/or assist in selecting another doctor | No penalty |
| Not binding | Doctor, person acting under doctor's direction, and health facility | No penalty | Destroying, concealing, or falsely reporting revocation is a felony |
| Not binding | Doctor, licensed health professional acting under doctor's direction, and health facility | No penalty, but doctor who disagrees with will must make a reasonable effort to transfer patient | Destroying will is a misdemeanor; concealing revocation or forging will, causing death, is first-degree murder |

ill, incompetent patient, they may have to settle the dispute in court.

*During terminal illness.* Every competent adult has the right to refuse medical treatment for himself, including the use of extraordinary means (see Entry 13). If a terminally ill patient tells a doctor or nurse to discontinue extraordinary efforts, his wishes are binding.

If a patient tells you his wishes about dying, first write what he says in your nurses' notes, using his exact words as much as possible. Next, describe the context of the discussion—for example, was the patient in pain, or had he just been informed of a terminal illness? Be sure you also tell the patient's doctor

> ## "A patient's specifically stated oral will is not legally enforceable."

about the discussion. Remember, *specifically stated oral wills are not legally enforceable,* although a patient's stated refusal of treatment *is* binding. Oral wills *should* be respected, however, as guidelines to how the patient feels about his treatment.

## When you find a living will in a patient's chart

What do you do when a patient is admitted to your care and you discover a properly executed living will attached to his chart?

First, notify your supervisor and the patient's doctor. To protect yourself, document the existence of the living will and the fact that you notified the patient's doctor about it. Include in your documentation the date the will was signed and the names of the people who signed it.

Check your nursing policy manual, too, to see what it says about living wills. If you can't find anything there, try your hospital's policy-and-procedures manual. The hospital's le-

gal department should be able to advise you as well, particularly about applicable state laws.

(Note: If you don't find a stated policy about living wills in either your nursing manual or your hospital's manual, consider organizing a committee to write a policy. Be sure to include representatives from the departments of nursing, medicine, risk management, legal affairs, and from hospital administration, on the committee. If your hospital has an ethics committee or an intensive-care committee, you may also invite their participation.)

Next, inform the patient's doctor about the will. Ask your nursing supervisor to inform the hospital administration and the legal affairs department. Make sure (with the patient's permission) that the family knows about the will; if they don't, show them a copy.

If the patient is able to talk, discuss the will with him, especially if it contains terms that need further definition. As always, objectively document your actions and findings in the patient's record.

Beyond these actions, your responsibilities for a patient's living will will be determined by the circumstances involved—including the family's and doctor's responses to the will. If you feel strongly about the patient's right to have his wishes followed, try to talk further with those involved to come up with a unified plan of care.

## A final word

If implementing a living will conflicts with your personal ethics or beliefs, you may wish to discuss the matter with a clinical nurse specialist, your nursing supervisor, a nursing administrator, the hospital chaplain, or a hospital administrator. Then, after talking over your feelings with one of them, if you're still unable to accept the idea, you can ask for reassignment to another patient. Chances are your request will be honored and no disciplinary action will be taken against you.

# Selected References

"Abused and Neglected Children in America: A Study of Alternative Policies," *Harvard Educational Review* 143:559, November 1973.

Annas, George J. *The Rights of Doctors, Nurses and Allied Health Professionals.* New York: Avon Books, 1981.

Annas, George J. "When Patients are Prisoners They Lose Their Right to Refuse Life-Maintaining Treatments," *Nursing Law Ethics* 1:3, February 1980.

Beauchamp, Tom L., and Childress, James F. *Principles of Biomedical Ethics.* New York: Oxford University Press, 1979.

Brown, G.C. "Medication Errors: A Case Study," *Hospitals* 53:61, October 1979.

Cazalas, Mary W. *Nursing and the Law,* 3rd ed. Rockville, Md.: Aspen Systems Corp., 1979.

Cohen, Ronald J. *Malpractice: A Guide for Mental Health Professionals.* New York: Free Press, 1979.

Creighton, Helen. *Law Every Nurse Should Know,* 4th ed. Philadelphia: W.B. Saunders Co., 1981.

Davis, R.W., and Hooker, J.E. "If the Patient is a Suspected Criminal," *American Journal of Nursing* 79:1250-52, July 1979.

Driscoll, Dorothy L., et al. *The Nursing Process in Later Maturity.* Englewood Cliffs, N.J.: Prentice-Hall, 1980.

Ennis, Bruce J., and Emery, Richard D. *The Rights of Mental Patients.* New York: Avon Books, 1972.

Grane, Nancy B. "How to Reduce Your Risk of a Lawsuit," *NursingLife* 3(1):17-20, January/February 1983.

Grosser, L.R. "All Nurses Can Be Involved in Teaching Patient and Family," *AORN Journal* 33:217-18, February 1981.

Hemelt, M., and Mackert, M. *Dynamics of Law, Nursing and Health Care,* 2nd ed. Reston, Va.: Reston Publishing Co., 1982.

Hershey, N., and Lawrence, R. "The Influence of Charting Upon Liability Determinations," *Journal of Nursing Administration* 6:35-7, March/April 1976.

Jervis, G. "The Mental Deficiencies," in *American Handbook of Psychiatry,* vol 2, 2nd ed. Edited by Arieti, Silvano, et al. New York: Basic Books, 1974.

Leiba, P.A. "Management of Violent Patients," *Nursing Times* 2(76):101-4, October 1980.

Lofstedt, Carol R. *Mereness Essentials of Psychiatric Nursing: Learning and Activity Guide.* St. Louis: C.V. Mosby Co., 1982.

Mikolaj, P.J. "Hospital Association Determines Nature of Closed Claims in State," *Hospitals* 52:53, February 1978.

Mills, D.H., et al. *Report on the Medical Insurance Feasibility Study.* San Francisco: Sutter Publications, 1977.

"A Patient's Bill of Rights... American Hospital Association," *Journal of Nursing Care* 14:17, March 1981.

Porter, Sharon. "Working with a Killer," *Nursing81* 11(1):136, January 1981.

"Principles of Hospital Liability," in *Hospital Law Manual: Administrator's and Attorney's Set.* Rockville, Md.: Aspen Systems Corp., 1981.

Robertson, John A., and American Civil Liberties Union. *Rights of the Critically Ill.* Cambridge, Mass.: Ballinger Publishing Co., 1983.

Robinson, Lisa. *Psychiatric Nursing as a Human Experience.* Philadelphia: W.B. Saunders Co., 1977.

Rubin, B. "Psychiatry and the Law," in *American Handbook of Psychiatry,* vol 6, 2nd ed. Edited by Arieti, Silvano, et al. New York: Basic Books, 1974.

Southwick, Arthur F. *The Law of Hospital and Health Care Administration.* Ann Arbor, Mich.: Health Administration Press, 1978.

Warren, David G. *Problems in Hospital Law,* 3rd ed. Rockville, Md.: Aspen Systems Corp., 1978.

Wiemerslage, D. "Professional Negligence," *Critical Care Update* 9(11):21-22, November 1982.

# 4

# Your Legal Risks While Off Duty

## Introduction

When you're on duty, you have ways to check on the legal limits of your practice and the legal risks you may face. That's because you have plenty of guidelines, including professional policies and rules, statutory law, and common law.

But what about when you're off duty? Very few professional or legal guidelines exist. So the legal limits of your off-duty actions aren't clear-cut. Fortunately, though, your risk of liability is low; relatively few lawsuits are brought against nurses for off-duty actions.

### Understanding legal issues

Of course, you do run some legal risks. So you should understand the legal issues surrounding nursing actions off duty. This chapter covers those issues in four key areas:

● Entry 31, "Good Samaritan acts," details what the law says your responsibilities are in most off-duty emergencies.
● Entry 32, "When you're asked for health-care advice," highlights common concerns almost all nurses have about giving health-care advice to neighbors and friends.
● Entry 33, "Donating nursing services," outlines your responsibilities and liabilities when you volunteer your nursing skills without compensation.

● Entry 34, "Disasters," discusses your legal responsibilities and liabilities in the aftermath of a man-made or natural catastrophe (such as a fire or flood).

Each entry also distinguishes between what the law requires and what it allows. You'll learn when your nurse practice act applies and when it doesn't apply to your off-duty actions. You'll also find a common theme running through the four entries: the general silence of the law, except for Good Samaritan acts, on the subject of off-duty nursing.

As you read these entries, you'll notice that relatively few legal cases are discussed. That's simply because relatively few exist.

### A final word

If only a few legal cases exist and the chances of being named in a lawsuit are fairly slim, why have a chapter on your legal risks? Well, for one thing, the few court cases that do exist make important legal distinctions. And most states do have *some* laws that cover some of the care you provide while off duty. So whether you provide care regularly when off duty or just give advice to your next-door neighbor occasionally, this chapter will tell you what you need to know to stay on sound legal footing.

# 31 Good Samaritan acts

If you come upon an automobile accident in which a motorist is injured, what should you do? As a nurse, your conscience and compassion prompt you to offer your assistance in any healthcare emergency. But you know how vulnerable nurses are to malpractice lawsuits. So while you're naturally inclined to help, you can't help thinking, "Could I get in legal trouble in this situation?"

Because you may experience this ambivalence, you need to know about Good Samaritan acts. Why? These acts address your responsibility and risk whenever you're in a position to use your nursing skills at an accident scene. This entry will explain the extent and limits of protection that Good Samaritan acts offer you.

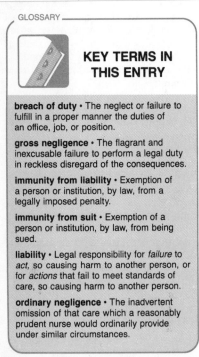

GLOSSARY

### KEY TERMS IN THIS ENTRY

**breach of duty** • The neglect or failure to fulfill in a proper manner the duties of an office, job, or position.

**gross negligence** • The flagrant and inexcusable failure to perform a legal duty in reckless disregard of the consequences.

**immunity from liability** • Exemption of a person or institution, by law, from a legally imposed penalty.

**immunity from suit** • Exemption of a person or institution, by law, from being sued.

**liability** • Legal responsibility for *failure to act*, so causing harm to another person, or for *actions* that fail to meet standards of care, so causing harm to another person.

**ordinary negligence** • The inadvertent omission of that care which a reasonably prudent nurse would ordinarily provide under similar circumstances.

## Do you have a legal duty to rescue?

Let's return to that fictional automobile accident scene. You quickly realize that you have three options:

• You can help the accident victim at the scene.

• You can pass the scene, stop at the nearest phone, and call for an ambulance, Emergency Medical Service (EMS), or other authorized rescue service.

• You can pass the scene and *make no attempt to call for help*.

In almost every state, you have the legal right to choose any of these options. Why does the law give you so much leeway? In the countries that inherited British common law, including the United States and Canada, nurses have no duty to rescue anyone. The only people with a legal duty to rescue are those who perform rescues as part of their jobs, such as firemen, EMS workers, and a few other groups, such as people who operate public transportation.

As a nurse, therefore, your decision whether or not to help is strictly voluntary and personal. But if you do decide to help the accident victim, do any laws protect you? The answer is yes. In fact, two kinds of law give you protection: common (or court-made) law and statutory (or legislature-made) law—in this situation, the Good Samaritan acts.

## How does common law protect you?

Common law is the cumulative result of many court decisions over the years. According to common law, to win a malpractice lawsuit against you a patient must prove that you owed him a duty; that you breached that duty in some way; that he was harmed; and that your breach of duty caused the harm.

Let's apply these legal rules to the auto accident situation:

Duty: As long as you pass the scene—whether or not you stop down the road to call for help—you don't owe the victim any legal duty. He's not your patient, and he can't make any legal claim on your professional services. (Remember, ethical claims aren't at issue here.) But just by stopping your car at the scene, you *do* incur a legal duty. Once you do that, you can't leave the victim until he's being cared for by another health-care professional with at least as much training as you have or until the police order you from the scene. Why? Because when you stop your car, you give the appearance to other potential rescuers that you'll take care of the victim. At that point, you establish a nurse-patient relationship. That means you owe him the normal duty you owe any patient—treatment that meets the standard of care of a reasonably prudent nurse in a similar situation.

Breach of duty: Let's assume that you've established the nurse-patient relationship because you've stopped to help. If you use the same good judgment you show on the job, you're not likely to breach your duty just because you're dealing with an off-the-job problem in a less-than-ideal situation. But what if you do breach your duty?

Harm: If you perform an act below standard, the court will ask this key question: How has your act worsened the victim's condition? If what you did hasn't made the victim measurably worse, the court is likely to find that the harm committed doesn't warrant damages. In other words, your act must cause measurable harm for the court to consider you negligent.

Cause: The victim must prove the probability is better than 50% that your error caused his injuries. The courts historically have set the 50% figure as the standard. Since the typical victim has already suffered injuries from the accident, he may have a hard time proving that your error caused or worsened his injuries.

Why have the courts made it so difficult for the victim to prove you negligent at an accident scene? Because,

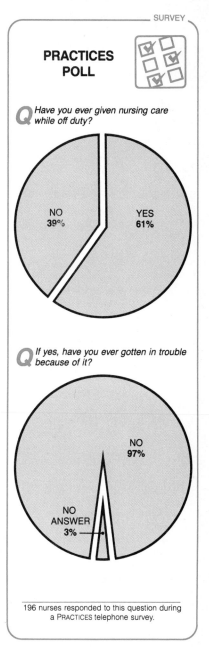

SURVEY

**PRACTICES POLL**

*Q Have you ever given nursing care while off duty?*

NO 39%

YES 61%

*Q If yes, have you ever gotten in trouble because of it?*

NO 97%

NO ANSWER 3%

196 nurses responded to this question during a PRACTICES telephone survey.

through the years, the courts have tried to balance victims' rights to justice against society's need to encourage trained professionals to use their talents in emergencies.

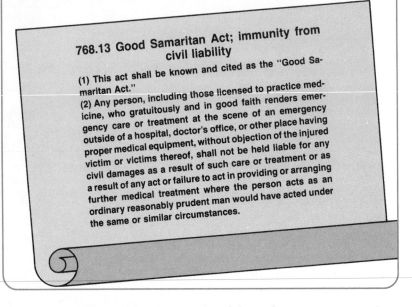

## SAMPLE GOOD SAMARITAN ACT

Almost every state and Canadian province has its own Good Samaritan act. All of the acts, however, are basically like the one reprinted in part here, from the state of Florida.

### 768.13 Good Samaritan Act; immunity from civil liability

(1) This act shall be known and cited as the "Good Samaritan Act."

(2) Any person, including those licensed to practice medicine, who gratuitously and in good faith renders emergency care or treatment at the scene of an emergency outside of a hospital, doctor's office, or other place having proper medical equipment, without objection of the injured victim or victims thereof, shall not be held liable for any civil damages as a result of such care or treatment or as a result of any act or failure to act in providing or arranging further medical treatment where the person acts as an ordinary reasonably prudent man would have acted under the same or similar circumstances.

But many health-care professionals feel that common law doesn't sufficiently reduce the likelihood that they'll be sued. For example, common law doesn't prevent a victim from pursuing a lengthy court battle against you—a battle that could cost you considerably in time, effort, and legal fees, even if you ultimately win. As a result, these health-care professionals have lobbied for a second, stronger protection, and almost all states have obliged by enacting Good Samaritan acts.

### How Good Samaritan acts work

Good Samaritan acts encourage you to volunteer your services at an accident or an emergency scene. How? By limiting your liability for any service you render. In effect, Good Samaritan acts offer you immunity from lawsuits when you help an accident victim as long as you don't intentionally or recklessly cause the patient injury. But keep in mind that no law can protect you if you commit an act that *seriously* violates the applicable standard of care.

Most Good Samaritan acts apply only to uncompensated rescue acts. If you charge or accept money for the service you render, the law usually says that you forfeit the special protections.

Also, Good Samaritan acts vary greatly from state to state. For example, some states limit the protection to nurses trained in cardiopulmonary resuscitation. One state—Wisconsin—has no Good Samaritan act. Some acts specifically include nurses, and others—such as those in Florida and British Columbia—protect any person who offers help to a victim. In some states the Good Samaritan act includes only "practitioners of the healing arts," a phrase the court has usually limited to doctors and dentists. (To learn about the Good Samaritan act that applies to you, see *Good Samaritan Acts by State and by Province*, pages 198 to 203.)

## How Good Samaritan acts are used

Regardless of the kind of Good Samaritan act your state has—if it has one at all—you should know that victims rarely sue Good Samaritans. And nurses have never had to invoke a Good Samaritan act as a defense. In effect, the common law so far has served as a deterrent.

Who, then, uses Good Samaritan acts? Ironically, auto accident victims sometimes try to claim that the acts create a duty for a nurse or doctor to respond to an accident scene. The courts have rejected this argument.

In some states, doctors being sued for malpractice have tried to use the Good Samaritan act as a defense. These doctors claim that the act protects them from liability in emergency situations, even for services they provided in a hospital. Doctors have tried this argument in California, with mixed results. But the argument won't work for nurses in California, because the Good Samaritan act that applies to nurses gives them liability protection only during emergencies "outside both the place and course" of their employment.

## Further limitations of Good Samaritan acts

Most Good Samaritan acts protect you only if your error is "ordinary" negligence. The acts won't protect you if you're grossly negligent. What's the distinction? That's decided by the jury, who'll determine the degree of negligence. The court will always measure your error against the standard of care, which can vary from locality to locality. For example, what might be considered ordinary negligence in a rural Georgia nursing case might be considered gross negligence in Boston.

---

INQUIRY

## QUESTIONS NURSES ASK ABOUT THE GOOD SAMARITAN ACTS

**Q** Am I covered by the Good Samaritan act if I respond to an emergency outside the hospital while I'm on duty?
**A** That depends on two things: the wording of the act in your state, and court decisions, if any, that interpret that act.

**Q** If I'm from out of state but I decide to help in an emergency, would that state's Good Samaritan act apply to me?
**A** If that state's act says it applies to "any person," you're covered. If the act specifically states that it applies only to "nurses," you're not; "nurse" in a law or act usually means an RN, LPN, or LVN licensed in that state.

**Q** Does the Good Samaritan act apply if I accept money from the person I've helped?
**A** The act usually doesn't apply in such a situation because, by accepting money, you've established a professional relationship with the person you've helped.

**Q** When does my responsibility end toward the person I've helped?
**A** Statutory law doesn't address this subject, but the courts have. Generally, common, or court-made, law says your responsibility ends:
• when the emergency ends—that is, when you're absolutely certain that the victim is no longer in danger.
• when an authorized rescue or other medical service takes over for you.
• when the victim dies.

**Q** If a doctor and I respond to the same emergency, does the Good Samaritan act provide us with the same coverage?
**A** Not necessarily. In some states, the Good Samaritan act for nurses is completely different from the Good Samaritan act for doctors. Contact your state's board of nursing to find out what's true for your state.

# GOOD SAMARITAN ACTS BY STATE AND BY PROVINCE

Here's a handy chart you can use to familiarize yourself with your state's or province's Good Samaritan act. You should, however, check with your board of nursing to make sure your state or province hasn't passed any amendments since 1982 that would affect how this law pertains to your practice.

| | ALABAMA | ALASKA | ARIZONA | ARKANSAS | CALIFORNIA | COLORADO | CONNECTICUT | DELAWARE | DIST. COLUMBIA |
|---|---|---|---|---|---|---|---|---|---|
| Date of act or last amendment | 1981 | 1976 | 1978 | 1979 | 1963 | 1975 | 1978 | 1974 | 1977 |
| Covers "any person" | | ● | ● | ● | | ● | | ● | ● |
| Covers in-state nurses only | | | | | ● | | | ● | |
| Includes out-of-state nurses in coverage | ● | | ● | | | ● | ● | ● | ● |
| Requires acts in good faith | ● | | ● | ● | ● | ● | | ● | ● |
| Covers only gratuitous services | ● | ● | ● | ● | | ● | ● | ● | ● |
| Covers aid at scene of emergency, accident, disaster | ● | ● | ● | ● | ● | ● | ● | ● | ● |
| Covers only roadside accidents | | | | | | | | | |
| Covers emergencies outside place of employment, course of employment | | | | | ● | | ● | | |
| Covers emergencies outside of hospital, doctor's office, or other places having medical equipment | | | | | | | | | ● |
| Protects against failure to provide or arrange for further medical treatment | ● | ● | ● | | | | | ● | |
| Covers transportation from the scene of the emergency to a destination for further medical treatment | | | | | | | | | |
| Specifically mentions that acts of gross negligence or willful or wanton misconduct are not covered | | ● | ● | ● | ● | | ● | ● | ● |

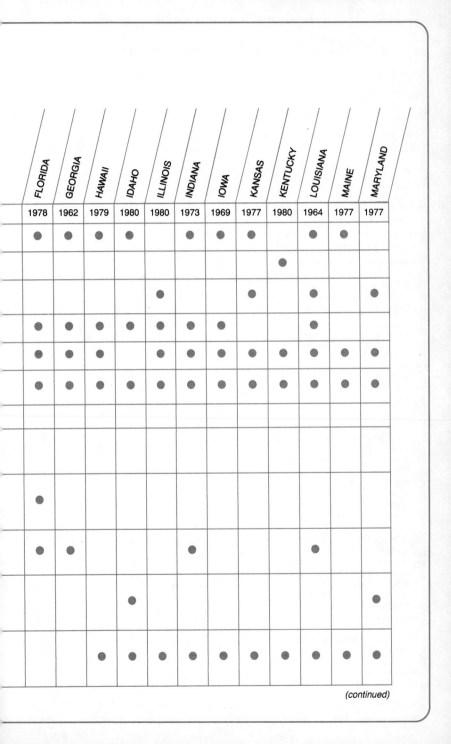

| FLORIDA | GEORGIA | HAWAII | IDAHO | ILLINOIS | INDIANA | IOWA | KANSAS | KENTUCKY | LOUISIANA | MAINE | MARYLAND |
|---|---|---|---|---|---|---|---|---|---|---|---|
| 1978 | 1962 | 1979 | 1980 | 1980 | 1973 | 1969 | 1977 | 1980 | 1964 | 1977 | 1977 |
| ● | ● | ● | ● |  | ● | ● | ● |  | ● | ● |  |
|  |  |  |  |  |  |  |  | ● |  |  |  |
|  |  |  |  | ● |  |  | ● |  | ● |  | ● |
| ● | ● | ● | ● | ● | ● | ● |  |  | ● |  |  |
| ● | ● | ● |  | ● | ● | ● | ● | ● | ● | ● | ● |
| ● | ● | ● | ● | ● | ● | ● | ● | ● | ● | ● | ● |
|  |  |  |  |  |  |  |  |  |  |  |  |
|  |  |  |  |  |  |  |  |  |  |  |  |
| ● |  |  |  |  |  |  |  |  |  |  |  |
| ● | ● |  |  |  | ● |  |  |  | ● |  |  |
|  |  |  | ● |  |  |  |  |  |  |  | ● |
|  |  | ● | ● | ● | ● | ● | ● | ● | ● | ● | ● |

*(continued)*

## GOOD SAMARITAN ACTS BY STATE AND BY PROVINCE (continued)

| | MASSACHUSETTS | MICHIGAN | MINNESOTA | MISSISSIPPI | MISSOURI | MONTANA | NEBRASKA | NEVADA | NEW HAMPSHIRE | |
|---|---|---|---|---|---|---|---|---|---|---|
| Date of act or last amendment | 1969 | 1978 | 1978 | 1979 | 1979 | 1970 | 1971 | 1975 | 1977 | |
| Covers "any person" | | | • | | • | • | • | • | • | |
| Covers in-state nurses only | | | | | | | | | • | |
| Includes out-of-state nurses in coverage | • | • | | • | • | | | • | • | |
| Requires acts in good faith | • | | • | • | • | • | | • | • | |
| Covers only gratuitous services | • | | | | • | • | • | • | | |
| Covers aid at scene of emergency, accident, disaster | • | • | • | • | • | • | • | • | • | |
| Covers only roadside accidents | | | | | | | | | | |
| Covers emergencies outside place of employment, course of employment | | | | | | | | | • | |
| Covers emergencies outside of hospital, doctor's office, or other places having medical equipment | | | • | | | | | | | |
| Protects against failure to provide or arrange for further medical treatment | • | | | | | | • | • | • | |
| Covers transportation from the scene of the emergency to a destination for further medical treatment | | | • | • | | | | | | |
| Specifically mentions that acts of gross negligence or willful or wanton misconduct are not covered | | • | | • | • | • | • | • | | |

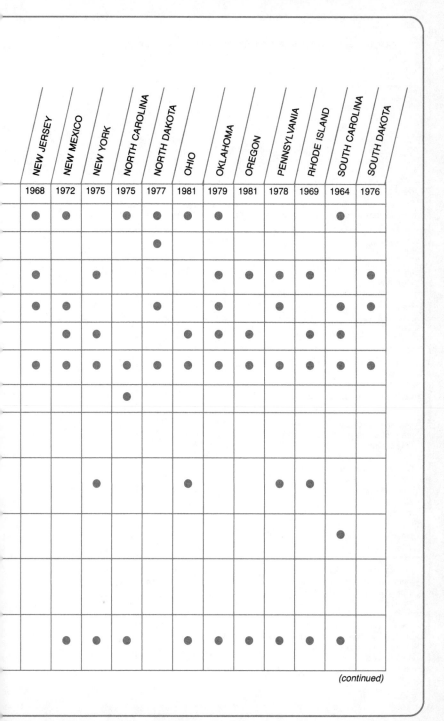

| | NEW JERSEY | NEW MEXICO | NEW YORK | NORTH CAROLINA | NORTH DAKOTA | OHIO | OKLAHOMA | OREGON | PENNSYLVANIA | RHODE ISLAND | SOUTH CAROLINA | SOUTH DAKOTA |
|---|---|---|---|---|---|---|---|---|---|---|---|---|
| | 1968 | 1972 | 1975 | 1975 | 1977 | 1981 | 1979 | 1981 | 1978 | 1969 | 1964 | 1976 |
| | ● | ● | | ● | ● | ● | ● | | | | ● | |
| | | | | | ● | | | | | | | |
| | ● | | ● | | | | ● | ● | ● | ● | | ● |
| | ● | ● | | | ● | | ● | | ● | | ● | ● |
| | | ● | ● | | | ● | ● | ● | | ● | ● | |
| | ● | ● | ● | ● | ● | ● | ● | ● | ● | ● | ● | ● |
| | | | | ● | | | | | | | | |
| | | | | | | | | | | | | |
| | | | ● | | | ● | | | ● | ● | | |
| | | | | | | | | | | | ● | |
| | | | | | | | | | | | | |
| | | ● | ● | ● | | ● | ● | ● | ● | ● | ● | |

*(continued)*

## GOOD SAMARITAN ACTS BY STATE AND BY PROVINCE *(continued)*

| | TENNESSEE | TEXAS | UTAH | VERMONT | VIRGINIA | WASHINGTON | WEST VIRGINIA | WISCONSIN | WYOMING | |
|---|---|---|---|---|---|---|---|---|---|---|
| Date of act or last amendment | 1976 | 1977 | 1979 | 1968 | 1980 | 1975 | 1967 | | 1977 | |
| Covers "any person" | ● | ● | | ● | ● | ● | ● | | ● | |
| Covers in-state nurses only | | | ● | | | | | | | |
| Includes out-ot-state nurses in coverage | | | | | | | | | | |
| Requires acts in good faith | ● | | ● | | ● | ● | ● | | ● | |
| Covers only gratuitous services | ● | ● | | ● | ● | ● | ● | | ● | |
| Covers aid at scene of emergency, accident, disaster | ● | ● | ● | ● | ● | ● | ● | NO GOOD SAMARITAN ACT | ● | |
| Covers only roadside accidents | | | | | | | | | | |
| Covers emergencies outside place of employment, course of employment | | ● | | | | | | | | |
| Covers emergencies outside of hospital, doctor's office, or other places having medical equipment | | | | | | | | | | |
| Protects against failure to provide or arrange for further medical treatment | ● | | | | | | | | | |
| Covers transportation from the scene of the emergency to a destination for further medical treatment | | | | | | ● | ● | | | |
| Specifically mentions that acts of gross negligence or willful or wanton misconduct are not covered | ● | ● | | ● | | ● | | | ● | |

| | ALBERTA | BRIT. COLUMBIA | MANITOBA | NEW BRUNSWICK | NEWFOUNDLAND | NOVA SCOTIA | ONTARIO | PRINCE EDWARD IS. | QUEBEC | NW TERRITORIES | SASKATCHEWAN | YUKON TERR. |
|---|---|---|---|---|---|---|---|---|---|---|---|---|
| | 1970 | 1979 | | | 1971 | 1969 | | | | | 1978 | 1976 |
| | ● | ● | | | ● | * | | | | | ● | ● |
| | ● | | | | | | | | | | | |
| | | | NO GOOD SAMARITAN ACT | NO GOOD SAMARITAN ACT | | | NO GOOD SAMARITAN ACT | NO GOOD SAMARITAN ACT | NO GOOD SAMARITAN ACT | NO GOOD SAMARITAN ACT | | |
| | | ● | | | ● | ● | | | | | | |
| | ● | ● | | | ● | ● | | | | | ● | ● |
| | | ● | | | | | | | | | | |
| | ● | | | | ● | ● | | | | | ● | |
| | ● | ● | | | | ● | | | | | ● | ● |

* Doctors only

## BEING A GOOD SAMARITAN: SOME DO's AND DON'Ts

When you stop at an accident scene to offer your assistance, you must still observe professional standards of nursing care, even in such an unsuitable setting. To reduce your malpractice risk, follow these guidelines:

 **DO's**

- Care for the victim in the vehicle if you can do so safely.
- Move him if he's in danger and if conditions at the scene permit.
- Keep the victim's airway patent.
- Stop his bleeding.
- Keep him warm.
- Determine his level of consciousness.
- Determine the possibility of fractures.
- Ask him where he feels pain.

 **DON'Ts**

- Don't move the victim needlessly.
- Don't try to straighten his arms and legs.
- Don't carry him or force him to walk.
- Don't speculate about who's the guilty party in the accident.
- Don't allow unskilled personnel to attend or treat the victim.
- Don't leave the scene until *skilled* personnel arrive to assume care of the victim.
- Don't give the injured person's personal property to anyone except the police or family members.

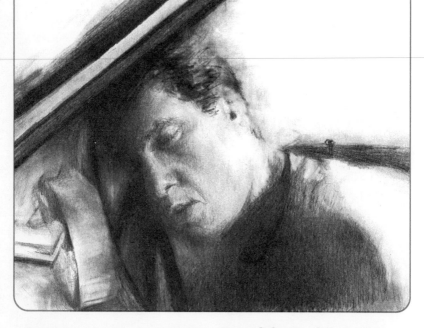

Besides your locality, the court will also take into consideration your training and experience to measure whether you've breached the standard of care. This means that RNs—even as Good Samaritans—are held to a higher standard than LPNs/LVNs.

### Beyond the Good Samaritan principle: Vermont

Vermont has taken the Good Samaritan principle a step further—as have most European countries—by *requiring* potential rescuers to help a victim. Vermont's law defines *rescuer* as any person who knows that another is exposed to grave physical harm. The law requires anyone—whether or not he's a Vermont resident—who can help a victim to do so, provided he won't then be putting himself in danger or interfering with important duties he owes to others.

Failure to comply with the law carries a fine of up to $100. The law hasn't been tested for nurses or doctors yet. How it would be applied in a roadside accident situation is uncertain. For example, if you pass an accident on the way to your dentist, the law requires you to stop and try to help. But what if you're on your way to work? Would your nursing job be considered an important duty owed to others? Answers to these questions will eventually come from the courts. Until then, you'd be wise to help the victim—acting, of course, as prudently as possible.

### A final word

A discussion of the legal aspects of being a Good Samaritan may ignore the likelihood that you feel an ethical and moral obligation to help someone in need. Because you have the skills to help save lives, you may naturally feel a duty to use those skills in any emergency—inside or outside the hospital. That attitude is certainly commendable. But when you provide rescue service, you should also be able to feel secure that you aren't legally jeopardizing your career. Good Samaritan acts, as well as common law, provide you with that security.

With the law on your side, when confronted with an emergency, let your conscience guide you. For example, suppose you're out having dinner and a patron at another table begins to choke. You don't just sit and watch him choke to death. You know how to perform the abdominal thrust maneuver, so without hesitation you take action. Other emergencies won't be so clearcut, so the decision to intervene or not to intervene won't be as easy. But, remember, the decision rests with you.

You have the final say as to whether or not you should become a Good Samaritan.

---

# 32 When you're asked for health-care advice

As a health-care professional, you're likely to find your family and friends depending on you, perhaps more than you'd prefer, for free advice. Because giving such help is an activity for which you can be sued (even though such a lawsuit is extremely unlikely), you should protect yourself. Here are several ways:
• Make sure that your advice reflects accepted professional and community nursing standards.
• Don't charge or accept money for it.
• Make sure that your professional liability insurance covers such off-the-job nursing activities.

Of course, you can also decide not to give free advice at all—the law does not require you to—but this is a difficult attitude to maintain if you want continued cordial relationships with family and friends!

### Free advice and your NPA

Giving free advice is unusual in one way: although doing it improperly can

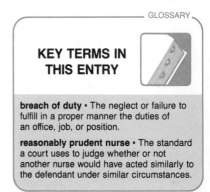

GLOSSARY

**KEY TERMS IN THIS ENTRY**

**breach of duty** • The neglect or failure to fulfill in a proper manner the duties of an office, job, or position.

**reasonably prudent nurse** • The standard a court uses to judge whether or not another nurse would have acted similarly to the defendant under similar circumstances.

be malpractice, doing it at all is not usually considered "practice." This is because the nurse practice acts (NPAs) in many states and Canadian provinces exempt services performed without pay (see Entry 33). (Of course, once you accept pay for any nursing service, even if the service is as simple as giving advice, you come under the control of the state board of nursing and your NPA.) Remember, giving health-care advice—whether you're paid for it or not—can be a problem if the advice you give is inappropriately medical. You could be liable for practicing medicine without a license.

### Free advice and the courts

In free-advice situations, the same legal rules apply as in other situations where malpractice may be alleged: the person who would sue you for harm caused by your giving the wrong advice has to prove that you owed him or her a specific duty, that you breached that duty, that he was harmed, and that the harm was a result of that breach. For a duty to exist, you must have established a nurse-patient relationship with the person asking for your advice. This rarely occurs in everyday short-lived conversations with other people. Suppose, for example, that someone at a cocktail party finds out that you're a nurse and bombards you with questions about his health. If you decide to answer, you have a duty to answer as correctly as any reasonably prudent nurse would, but you have no duty to follow up after the party is over, no duty to monitor the outcome of your advice. The person who's asking your advice hasn't established, or indicated that he intends to establish, an ongoing nurse-patient relationship with you.

The situation may be different if you decide to give advice to a neighbor. For example: The young mother next door asks you about her child's fretfulness, and you answer honestly that it doesn't appear serious enough, to you, for the mother to call the doctor. Suppose that a day later, you see the mother and child together outdoors, and the child looks particularly listless. If you go over and discover that the child is feverish,

---

## MINIMIZING YOUR LEGAL RISKS WHEN GIVING ADVICE: SOME DO's AND DON'Ts

Do you know you're assuming legal risks when you give health-care advice to your friends? In the courts' view, even a casual conversation can sometimes establish a nurse-patient relationship, making you liable for the consequences of your advice. To help minimize these risks, keep these do's and don'ts in mind:

 **DO's**

 **DON'Ts**

- Find out if your professional liability insurance (or your employer's) provides you with off-the-job coverage.
- Know whether your state's nurse practice act discusses giving advice to friends.
- Only give advice within the confines of your nurse practice act, education, and experience.
- Make sure the advice you give is up-to-date. Remember, you'll be judged on current nursing standards if your advice results in a lawsuit.

- Don't speculate about your friends' illnesses or ailments.
- Don't suggest that friends change or ignore their doctors' orders.
- Don't give any advice about medical care.
- Don't offer any advice that, if wrong, could result in serious or permanent injury.

## QUESTIONS NURSES ASK ABOUT GIVING ADVICE

**Q** *A friend and I have babies the same age. My friend isn't a nurse, and I know she relies on my judgment a lot. How can I answer her when she asks things like, "Would you take your baby with a rash like that to the doctor?"*

**A** *If you wish to advise your friend to see a doctor, you can do so without risk because no harm can result from your advice. If your advice is "Don't see a doctor," and harm does result, you may be liable. It's your decision whether to take that responsibility. Conservative advice, in this situation, is legally safer, especially when you have any doubts.*

**Q** *I seem to be the neighborhood earpiercer. Of course, with children I require a parent's permission, and I warn everyone about the risks of infection and how to reduce them. Still, I'm worried: If someone got an infection and sued me, would I be considered negligent?*

**A** *Some states have legislation or regulations governing ear piercing, so check with your state licensing board. If your state doesn't have regulations on ear piercing, your warnings about possible infection protect you only if infection results from piercing you've done according to accepted standards. The warning doesn't protect you if the infection results from your negligence.*

**Q** *One of my neighbors comes to see me whenever one of her family members is in the hospital. She's a good friend and I'm glad to help, but I'm nervous about her habit of asking me to explain everything the doctor tells her. For example, she might say, "The doctor says my husband might have adhesions from a previous operation. What does that mean? Is that common?" And so on. Can I protect myself by saying, "I can only tell you what I know from my own experience..."?*

**A** *You'd be better off saying, "I can only tell you what those terms usually mean but not what they mean in your husband's case." However, the best service you can render is to encourage your neighbor to ask the doctor to explain anything she doesn't understand.*

or shows other signs and symptoms of illness, then legally and professionally your responsibility is to tell the mother to take him to a doctor as soon as possible. This is true no matter what your original advice was. You must respond to the mother's probable reliance on you for further advice, even though you may not originally have intended to form a nurse-patient relationship with her and her child. If you realize that she *is* relying on you for further advice, you have an obligation—a legal and professional duty—to keep your advice current as the situation changes. Or you may opt to take formal steps to break off the relationship, such as telling the mother to look elsewhere for help.

The same principles, of course, apply in your regular work: the help and advice you give your patient Monday morning may have to be changed by Tuesday afternoon, and if a patient's questions reveal that his problem may be beyond the scope of nursing practice, you have a clear duty to call in the doctor.

### Your professional obligations

Whenever you establish a professional relationship with a questioner—and become responsible for giving him accurate nursing advice—you must give an answer as good as any reasonably prudent nurse would give under similar circumstances. To do this, apply the same standards that you're expected to apply in your regular work. If you know the answer, you're legally free to give it. But do this only if you're certain your answer is correct and giving it is appropriately within your scope

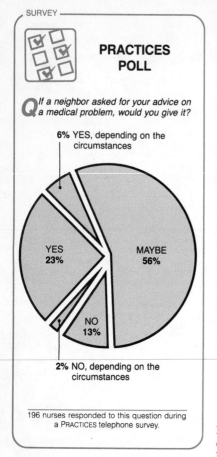

## PRACTICES POLL

**Q** *If a neighbor asked for your advice on a medical problem, would you give it?*

6% YES, depending on the circumstances

YES 23%

MAYBE 56%

NO 13%

2% NO, depending on the circumstances

196 nurses responded to this question during a PRACTICES telephone survey.

at work, and one of my patients asked the same question, what would I tell him? Try to imagine that an inquiring family member or friend is a complete stranger. Then give your best professionally considered answer.

### A final word
You alone can decide if you have a professional or ethical responsibility to give health-care advice in situations outside of your paid employment. On the one hand, you have expertise that the person requesting your advice doesn't have, and your professional advice may be helpful. On the other hand, the person requesting the advice probably hasn't stopped to consider your legal position. Decisions about whether to give nursing advice will be easier for you if you plan how you'll handle such requests *before* a neighbor knocks at your door.

## 33 Donating nursing services

Many health-care professionals, including nurses, occasionally or regularly donate their health-care services to community organizations or activities. This is unpaid work, donated in the interest of supporting the community.

Of course, as a nurse, you may find yourself "volunteering" your services for pay, such as when you provide nursing services in addition to—and outside of—your regular paid job. Here, you're volunteering your personal time while being paid for your nursing services. (To understand your legal risks in this situation, see Entries 7 and 10.) But most often, when you volunteer your nursing services, you'll be donating nursing care, and no pay will be involved.

You might donate your nursing services to family members, friends, or

of nursing practice. To protect yourself, you might say something like, "I think your problem sounds like arthritis, but it could be something more serious, and I'm not sure. You should ask a doctor."

Obviously, you're always legally protected if you refer the questioner to his doctor. However, the law doesn't require that you make that suggestion if you're honestly convinced it isn't necessary, and a reasonably prudent nurse wouldn't make it either.

Be on your guard against the temptation to say, "Don't worry," to be reassuring when family members or friends ask for advice. Reassurance is appropriate only if you're sure that nothing serious is wrong. The standard the law requires you to apply is this: If I were

such community organizations and activities as these:
- a community-run ambulance service
- a bloodmobile or hypertension outreach program
- a PTA that asks you to give a slide-lecture on children's health and development.

As a licensed nurse, whether RN or LPN/LVN, your responsibilities toward patients don't change when you donate

---

> *"When you donate your services, your responsibilities toward patients don't change, but your legal status is less well defined."*

---

your services, but your legal status is less well defined than when you're paid. Why? Because most states' nurse practice acts (NPAs) specify only the legal limits of *paid* nursing practice. (This also means that a nonlicensed or nonregistered person may provide nursing care for no pay without being subject to NPA regulations or discipline.)

### How the courts view donated nursing services
Being exempt from your state's NPA, if you donate nursing services, *doesn't* mean you'll be exempt from being sued. In such a situation, the court can use the provisions of your state NPA—together with expert-witness testimony and applicable standards of nursing care—to determine if you acted as a prudent nurse would have under similar patient-care circumstances. If the court finds that your care doesn't conform to the requirements of your state's NPA, you may be found liable for malpractice.

Even if no lawsuit results from your donated nursing services, you may be subject to discipline by your state board of nursing if the board finds your do-

nated services to be below the accepted standard of care. In such a situation, the board may suspend or even revoke your license.

If you travel to a state in which you're not licensed to practice, you're not prohibited from donating your nursing services as long as that state's NPA covers only paid nursing care. But if you're sued, the court will probably evaluate your actions—and their consequences—against whatever standard of nursing care would apply in that situation.

Remember, too, that the Good Samaritan act (see Entry 31) won't cover you in day-to-day situations in which you donate your nursing services. These acts are applicable only to emergency situations. And not all states extend coverage to nurses in their Good Samaritan acts.

### The best protection
The best way to protect yourself legally when you donate your nursing services, as you've probably realized by now, is simply to function in this situation according to the same standards of care, and scope of nursing practice, you'd follow in your regular paid job. For example, be sure that you obtain a doctor's order (or a standing order), as you would in your regular practice, before giving any treatment or medication that

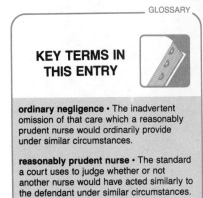

GLOSSARY

**KEY TERMS IN THIS ENTRY**

**ordinary negligence** • The inadvertent omission of that care which a reasonably prudent nurse would ordinarily provide under similar circumstances.

**reasonably prudent nurse** • The standard a court uses to judge whether or not another nurse would have acted similarly to the defendant under similar circumstances.

## WORKING WITH VOLUNTEERS

Suppose a volunteer is assigned to your unit in the hospital or nursing home where you work. Do you know what you can and can't ask her to do?

In general, you'll find the answer in the policies and rules of your institution, not in the laws of your state. In most hospitals, nonnurse volunteers perform many useful tasks, and the hospitals have guidelines that say what volunteers can and can't do. If you need help with one of your patients, and if the work involved is within your institution's guidelines, ask the volunteer if she's been trained in the task. If she hasn't, you should wait for a regular staff member to help you. In one case, *Marcus v. Frankford Hospital* (1971), in which the regular nurses on the floor forgot to obey this common-sense rule, the volunteer—untrained in the task she was given and emotionally unable to cope with it—fainted, fell, and injured herself. The hospital was held liable.

In general, the more training the volunteer has, the more the law allows you to rely on her. Still, regardless of her degree of training, you must respect a few common-sense limitations on asking for her help. If the volunteer is working as a private-duty nurse for a patient who needs round-the-clock care, you cannot call her away to help you with other duties. And if the volunteer is elderly or frail, you cannot have her help you with tasks that involve heavy lifting, such as moving an obese patient.

If you demand help from a volunteer that she cannot give, for whatever reason, she has a right to refuse. Even if she doesn't refuse, and your request leads to harm—either to her or to a patient—you may be liable. Remember that the volunteer will probably not be covered by your institution's insurance policy, and she may not have her own coverage. So the injured patient may turn against *you* as the most likely source for recovering damages.

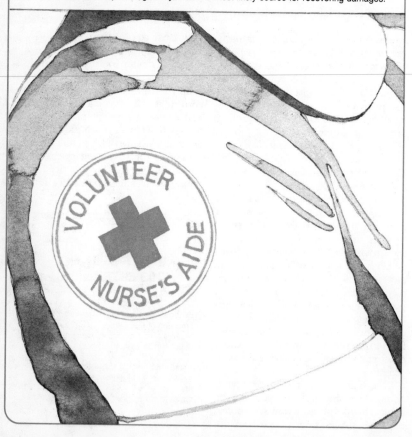

## KNOW THE LAW BEFORE YOU VOLUNTEER

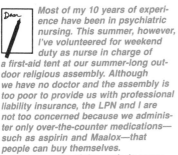

*Most of my 10 years of experience have been in psychiatric nursing. This summer, however, I've volunteered for weekend duty as nurse in charge of a first-aid tent at our summer-long outdoor religious assembly. Although we have no doctor and the assembly is too poor to provide us with professional liability insurance, the LPN and I are not too concerned because we administer only over-the-counter medications— such as aspirin and Maalox—that people can buy themselves.*

*Other aspects of the work do worry me, though. Suppose someone falls and I think it's just a simple sprain. Should I also recommend an X-ray just to be on the safe side?*

*As I said, I'm only a volunteer and not getting paid for my work.—RN, Ill.*

You're right when you say the medications you're administering could be purchased by any of the patients themselves. But there's a grave difference here. You are not a clerk in a pharmacy where the *customer* assumes the risk of taking medications from the hands of a lay person.

The law has designated you a *nurse*. As such, you'll be held to the standards of care established for a nurse. This means you're expected to know the indications, contraindications, dosages, adverse reactions, and possible drug interactions of

*anything* you administer.

Furthermore, even if you were completely confident in your knowledge of these medications, you might still be subject to disciplinary action for breaching the nurse practice act because you administered these medications without any orders from a doctor.

Do two things immediately: Get standing orders from a doctor, and get professional liability insurance to cover your volunteer work. Once you do that, we recommend that you set up some system of recording everything you do in the first-aid tent. Such records, even if not legally necessary, are good practice and good sense. And, of course, before handing out any medication, make appropriate medical inquiries of the patient (concerning possible contraindications, drug interactions, and so on) according to the accepted standard of nursing care.

Too many nurses think volunteer work is always covered by the Good Samaritan act. But not all states cover nurses or lay volunteers in their acts. Further, even if your state's act does cover you, such volunteer work as you describe would not ordinarily qualify as a true emergency.

Before you ever donate your nursing skills, make sure that you're performing within the guidelines of your state nurse practice act and that you're properly covered by insurance.

This letter was taken from the files of *Nursing* magazine.

requires it. And you'd be wise to document your care as carefully as you always do (see Chapter 5). Retain your nurses' notes so you have a permanent record of your actions should a question ever arise.

Before agreeing to donate your services to any organization, check your professional liability insurance coverage, and its limitations, from every angle. Does your personal policy cover you? Does the organization have coverage that includes you? Is the coverage adequate to cover reasonable damages and legal fees that you could be required to pay? Be sure to check whether your coverage specifically includes the type of volunteer nursing you're considering (see Entry 41).

### A final word

Should you donate your nursing services? It's your decision. Nothing in the law compels you to work without compensation. Base your decision on your sense of duty to your community, your enjoyment of the work (if that applies), the adequacy of patient-care conditions, and the extent of your professional liability insurance coverage.

# 34 Disasters

A tornado hits your community. A hurricane strikes. Heavy spring rains cause destructive flooding. A train derails, sending clouds of toxic vapor into the air in a heavily populated area. A fully loaded plane, landing in a fog, goes off the end of the runway. Any of these disastrous events can stretch local medical and nursing resources to the breaking point. As a nurse, do you know your special responsibilities, and your legal rights, in situations like these?

## Contract duties
When you give nursing care during a disaster, professional, ethical, and legal concerns figure heavily in every decision you make. In general, with the exception of declared emergencies, a nurse's responsibilities in a disaster don't differ legally from her everyday responsibilities. As a nurse, you may have specific duties to perform in specific kinds of disasters, and you may be legally bound to perform those duties, but this is likely to be based on your employment contract and not on laws or precedent-setting legal cases. If you work in a city hospital, for example, your employment contract may contain a provision that your administration can call you in to work whenever a government official declares a state of emergency. If you refuse to come in, you can be disciplined, suspended, or fired. And this rule applies even if the work you're being asked to do isn't normally part of your job description.

If you're already on the job when a disaster occurs, the same contractual provisions may be invoked to keep you from going home at the end of your shift. And the same penalties apply if you refuse to cooperate.

Similarly, if you're an unpaid volunteer for a community emergency service, such as the Red Cross or an emergency medical service, you may be expected to report for duty in any local disaster as long as your reporting doesn't conflict with your regular employment. If you refuse, the emergency service is entitled to drop you from its roster; if you're a paid part-time worker for such an emergency service, the service is entitled to fire you. These duties exist even if your work arrangements aren't written, but are merely part of an oral agreement.

By refusing to appear when people are expecting you to help in a disaster, you could make a bad situation even worse. Why? Because your agreement to be available may have led the emergency service or hospital to stop looking for, or not to hire, someone who would have been able and willing to do the job.

## Contract defenses
Because reporting for work in an emergency, including a disaster, is usually a contract matter, specific "contract defenses" apply if you're disciplined for failing to fulfill your duties. The defense of impossibility is one such contract defense. If reporting-in is impossible for you, and you can prove it—even if you're contractually required to do so and would be paid for the work—you can't be disciplined or prosecuted. For example, if a blizzard absolutely prohibits travel from your home to the hospital, or disastrous flooding causes the governor to place a ban on all travel in your area, what your contract says doesn't matter much. If you can't come, you can't. And if you're disciplined, you have a legal defense. But watch for exceptions to travel bans—for example, a ban may be announced for all but "required" personnel (you) or "persons with medical or nursing training." In these situations, obviously you'd have to report for duty.

## What the law says
No law prevents you from voluntarily donating your services, and specific statutory or common laws may protect

you if you do (see Entry 31). If you want to volunteer your help in a disaster, do it, whether or not anyone in authority has asked you.

Suppose you're working in a hospital that doesn't have a policy mandating that health-care personnel report to work when a disaster occurs. You can still volunteer to stay for extra shifts or to perform services outside your normal scope of employment. The hospital will almost certainly accept your offer—or it may ask you before you have a chance to volunteer. This is especially likely if emergency conditions prevent other staff nurses from reporting to work. But you can't necessarily expect your pay to reflect the extra work; most institutions will try to pay for the overtime, but some may not. If you're curious, find out what your institution's policy is *before* such an emergency occurs. The policy may depend on union rules or, if you work in a city or state hospital, on city ordinances or state regulations.

Your location doesn't legally restrict your ability to volunteer when a disaster happens. Your nurse practice act (NPA) doesn't even stop you. For instance, suppose you're licensed in California and while you're on vacation in Oregon, a disaster occurs. You can give your nursing services during the disaster without concern that you're breaching California's *or* Oregon's NPA. This is because most states' NPAs have a special exemption for care given in emergencies that usually includes disasters. In an unlikely instance, suppose you volunteer your nursing services in a state that doesn't have a special exemption *and* you're charged with malpractice. You could theoretically be sued for practicing nursing without a license. This, however, has never happened to a nurse.

### Taking on special duties
In a disaster, you may find yourself performing duties that you don't normally perform. If you're an LPN or LVN, you may be asked to perform duties that

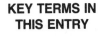 

## KEY TERMS IN THIS ENTRY

**civil defense laws** • That body of statutory law that is invoked when the jurisdiction is under attack, as in a state of war.

**contract duties** • Duties defined in your employment contract.

**declared emergency** • The situation when a government official formally identifies a state of emergency.

**defense of impossibility** • A legal defense that says a violation of a contract was literally impossible to avoid.

**disaster** • A sudden event that creates a number of victims with extensive injuries.

**state of emergency** • A widespread need for immediate action to counter a threat to the community.

ordinarily would be restricted to RNs, and aides may be asked to do work you usually do. If you're an RN, you may find yourself doing tasks normally reserved for medical residents. And either you *or* a resident may be asked to do work an aide would normally do. Provided you have the knowledge and skill to meet minimum safety requirements, you're permitted to give such substitute care in disasters based on the same exemption in NPAs that lets an out-of-state nurse volunteer her services in a disaster. This exemption may be construed as letting you expand the scope of your practice in a disaster. Even if it can't be construed this way, usually other statutory or common laws exist that permit the regulatory authorities to decide that the public welfare comes first—ahead of strict enforcement of the letter of the law.

What if you don't want to volunteer? If your hospital policy or contract doesn't require it, or in the rare instance when you don't have a contract, you generally have the right to refuse. Although most NPAs provide special exemptions to allow emergency care in

## MINIMIZING YOUR LEGAL RISKS DURING A DISASTER

As you know, volunteering your services during a disaster is not without legal risks. But you can minimize those risks if you follow these suggestions:

### BE PREPARED

Don't wait for an emergency to happen before you ask your charge nurse what you'll likely be required to do. Also, keep any equipment you're likely to need available and in good condition. (If you're being asked to go to your hospital for the duration of the emergency, carry a change of clothing and toiletries, if you wish, with you.)

### DO NOT WORK YOURSELF BEYOND YOUR POINT OF EFFECTIVENESS

If you're so tired that you're unable to make the correct decisions, no one will profit from your care. Explain your fatigue to the person in charge and ask for a rest break.

### FOLLOW INSTRUCTIONS

In any serious emergency, people in positions of public authority—such as medical personnel, public health agency staff, or governor's office staff—will probably be giving orders. Even if these people are not normally your superiors, to be truly helpful you should obey their orders as much as possible—and offer advice only when you think necessary.

### TAKE EVERY PRECAUTION TO AVOID COMMITTING MALPRACTICE

If you're helping during a disaster, you're not likely to be sued, and even if you are sued, you're not likely to lose; but being careful in the first place is always the best policy.

disasters, they don't *require* you to perform such care, any more than they require you to perform *any* care. They only *permit* such care. Similarly, Good Samaritan acts give you some legal immunity for giving emergency care, but they don't require you to provide that care—except in Vermont (see Entry 31).

Civil defense laws, also known as disaster relief laws, do not apply in most states to nurses who aren't already involved in civil defense work—although in a declared national emergency, nurses (like anyone else) can be drafted. Or martial law may be imposed, which makes all citizens subject to public authority. Many civil defense laws authorize state or federal governing bodies to enforce special regulations dealing with the duties of

medical and nursing personnel in a declared emergency. Some states already have such plans in final form, ready for use in a sufficiently serious disaster.

## Don't forget practical considerations

Your professional responsibility in particular disaster circumstances must be determined in part by assessing your actual ability to help. For example, do you have the particular skills needed to help? Caring for the disaster victims may require knowledge of a specialty such as toxicology (as in the example of the train wreck that releases toxic gases). Or the skill required may be as simple and nonprofessional as rowing a boat in a flood.

Can you get to the disaster site, or to the place where care is going to be provided? If a plane has crashed, for example, and a hundred or more badly injured passengers are being ferried by ambulance to emergency departments throughout the city, your ability to get to your hospital or *another hospital* quickly may figure in your decision whether or not to volunteer. What if the disaster is a riot taking place during a total blackout in your city, and the mayor has said, "Don't come to work unless you're within walking distance"? If you try to drive into the city from your suburban home, you'll only complicate driving conditions—and you probably won't get to your hospital in time to be of much help.

You should also consider whether volunteering in the disaster will keep you from earning your regular salary. Find out, too, whether your professional liability insurance covers off-the-job activities.

**A final word**

Two basic questions govern your response, as a nurse, when a disaster occurs. The questions are the ethical (and sometimes contractual) *"Should I help?"* and the practical *"Can I help?"* When disaster strikes, you should be ready with your answers.

## Selected References

Bullough, ed. *The Law and the Expanding Nursing Role*, 2nd ed. East Norwalk, Conn.: Appleton-Century-Crofts, 1980.

Cazalas, Mary W. *Nursing and the Law*, 3rd ed. Rockville, Md.: Aspen Systems Corp., 1979.

Fenner, Kathleen M. *Ethics and Law in Nursing*. New York: Van Nostrand Reinhold Co., 1980.

Fromer, Margot J. *Ethical Issues in Health Care*. St. Louis: C.V. Mosby Co., 1981.

Murchinson, Irene, et al. *Legal Accountability in the Nursing Process*, 2nd ed. St. Louis: C.V. Mosby Co., 1982.

Pozgar, George D. *Legal Aspects of Health Care Administration*. Rockville, Md.: Aspen Systems Corp., 1979.

Veninga, Robert L. *The Human Side of Health Administration: A Guide for Hospital, Public Health and Nursing Administrators*. Englewood Cliffs, N.J.: Prentice-Hall, 1982.

# **Documentation**

## Introduction

You may consider medical records a 20th century phenomenon. But documentation of patient information dates back to 25,000 B.C.—when Stone Age man recorded, in cave painting, his attempts to care for the sick.

Hippocrates, the famous Greek doctor of the 5th century B.C., was probably the first person to record individual patient problems.

And, in the centuries since then, medical records—like medical and nursing practice—have become increasingly more scientific and complex. They've also become more necessary—as a link between specialists.

### The key role good documentation can play

With increasing specialization in nursing and other health-care professions, now many practitioners care for every patient. A typical patient on your unit, for example, probably has several nurses besides you—and also several doctors, pharmacists, nutritionists, and therapists. With all of you observing, evaluating, and caring for the patient, careful documentation and communication are vital. And that's the key role the patient's medical record plays.

The medical record is the chief means by which you and other health-care practitioners plan, coordinate, and guarantee the continuity of each patient's care.

If you all document carefully, the medical record can help you:
● plan continuous, quality care for your patient
● coordinate the care each of you contributes
● communicate constantly to keep each other up-to-date on your patient's condition and treatment
● furnish data for continuing education and research.

### The legal significance of the medical record

Each patient's medical record is also legal proof of the quality of care you provided. And the weight it carries in the courtroom can't be exaggerated.

In fact, documentation of care has become synonymous with care itself: fail to document, and the courts are likely to assume that you also failed to provide care. That's what happened to the nurse in *Collins v. Westlake Community Hospital* (1974).

The Collins boy was hospitalized with a fractured leg, which was put in a cast and placed in traction. The evening nurse recorded the condition of the boy's toes several times during her shift. The night nurse, however, didn't record the condition of his toes until 6 a.m., when she noted that they were

## TIPS ON DOCUMENTATION:
## HOW TO PROTECT YOURSELF LEGALLY

If you've ever read a malpractice case transcript, you realize how much the jury relies on documentation.

If you're ever involved in a case, how you documented, what you documented, and what you didn't document will heavily influence the outcome. Here are some tips on how to document so that your records don't tip the scales of justice against you:

• Use the appropriate form, and document in ink.

• Record the patient's name and identification number on every page of his chart.

• Record the complete date and time of each entry.

• Be specific. Avoid general terms and vague expressions.

• Use standard abbreviations only.

• Use a medical term only if you're sure of its meaning.

• Document symptoms by using the patient's own words.

• Document any nursing action you take in response to a patient's problem. For example: "8 p.m.—medicated for incision pain." Be sure to include the medication route and site.

• Document the patient's response to medications and other treatment.

• Document safeguards you use to protect the patient. For example: "raised side rails" or "applied safety belts."

• Document any incident in two places: in your progress report and in an incident report.

• Document each observation. Failure to document observations will produce gaps in the patient's records. And these gaps will suggest that you neglected the patient.

• Document procedures after you perform them, never in advance.

• Write on every line. Don't insert notes between lines or leave empty spaces for someone else to insert a note.

• Sign every entry.

• Chart an omission as a new entry. Never backdate or add to previously written entries.

• Draw a thin line through an error. Never erase one.

• Document your own care, only. Never document for someone else.

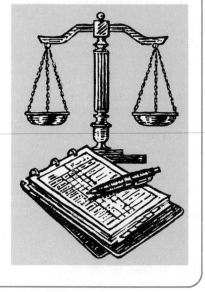

dusky and cold and that his doctor had been contacted.

Part of the boy's leg had to be amputated, and his family sued the hospital. They claimed the amputation was necessary because the night nurse had negligently failed to observe the condition of his toes during the night.

She testified that she *had* observed them and they'd been normal. Other nurses testified that only abnormal findings needed to be documented. But the blank chart spoke louder than the experts' words: the jury inferred that

no documentation meant no observation, and they found the nurse liable for malpractice.

### Why you need to know how to document properly

The standards of care for documenting require that you record your observations accurately, completely, and in a timely manner, and that you include normal as well as abnormal findings. The *Collins* case clearly shows how failure to meet the legal standards for documenting could lead to serious legal

# HOW TO AVOID SUBJECTIVE CHARTING

Do you know the most common error nurses make when they chart? It's writing value judgments and opinions—subjective, rather than factual (objective) information. This type of information is inappropriate because it tells you how the nurse feels about the patient's condition, not about the patient's condition itself. Here are some subjective entries, with their *objective* alternatives:

| SUBJECTIVE CHARTING | OBJECTIVE CHARTING |
|---|---|
| She is drinking *well*. | Drank 1500 ml liquids between 7 a.m. and noon. |
| She reported *good* relief from Demerol. | Pain in R hip decreasing, now described as "like a dull toothache." |
| Dorsalis pedis pulse *present*. *Good* pedal pulses. | Peripheral pulses in legs 2+/4+ bilaterally. |
| Moves legs and feet *well*. | Leg strength 5+/5+ bilaterally all major muscle groups. Sensation intact to light touch, pin; denies numbness or tingling. Skin warm and dry. No edema. |
| Voiding *qs*. | Voided 350 ml clear yellow urine in bedpan. |
| Patient is *nervous*. | Patient repeatedly asking about length of hospitalization, expected discomfort, and time off from work. |
| Breath sounds *normal*. | Breath sounds clear to auscultation all lobes. Chest expansion symmetrical—no cough. Nail beds pink. |
| Bowel sounds *normal*. | Bowel sounds present all quadrants—abdomen flat. NPO since 12:01 a.m. |
| Ate *well*. | Ate all of soft diet. |

consequences for you. This chapter helps you avoid such consequences by giving you an overview of your legal and professional responsibilities regarding documentation.

Entry 35, "The legal importance of documentation," discusses different methods of documentation and how documentation can protect you in court.

Entry 36, "Pitfalls of documentation," reviews the most common errors nurses make in documenting patient care and tells you how to avoid them.

Entry 37, "The altered medical record," tells you how to correct an error on a patient's medical chart. And it discusses the serious legal consequences of altering previously recorded information.

Finally, Entry 38, "Computerized record keeping: The legal aspects," takes a look at the advantages of computerized documentation. It also discusses an important problem yet to be resolved: how to ensure patient confidentiality in a computerized information system.

### A final word

As patient care becomes more complex, accurate documentation is likely to become an even greater legal and professional responsibility. Make sure you know how to document properly, so that your patients' medical records provide proof of your professionalism.

# 35 The legal importance of documentation

Good patient care is your best defense against being sued for malpractice. But if you *are* sued, clear and accurate documentation of the nursing care you provided will be your best defense in the courtroom. That's why you need to know the legal functions and impli-

cations of documentation.

What is documentation? It's the preparing or assembling of records to authenticate the care you gave your patient, as well as your reasons for giving that care. In general, you should

---

*"The days when doctors were the only ones thought qualified to provide and document patient care are gone forever."*

---

document these kinds of information for each patient:
• therapeutic measures you and other health-care providers carry out
• doctor-prescribed measures you carry out
• the patient's health-related behavior, including body action, verbal communication (always use direct quotes and describe the emotional tone), and physiologic reactions
• the patient's specific responses to therapy and care.

### How documenting became your responsibility

Doctors have been documenting their care since Hippocrates started recording his clinical observations in the 5th century B.C. For the next 2,000 years or so, doctors were thought to be the only health-care providers qualified to provide—and document—patient care. As you know, those days are gone forever.

Today, the responsibility for a major share of each patient's care rests squarely in your hands. And with that responsibility goes the responsibility for documenting accurately.

### What is the medical record?

Each patient's medical record is really a collection of records, including:
• patient's admission sheet and history
• patient's medication record

## USING FLOW SHEETS IN DOCUMENTING

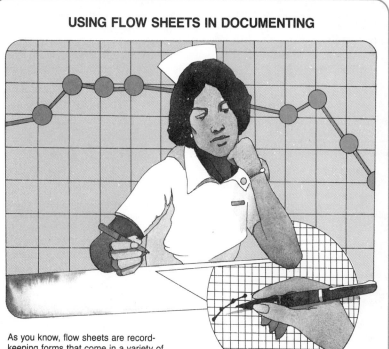

As you know, flow sheets are record-keeping forms that come in a variety of styles—blank-ruled paper, multicolumned paper, graph paper—to suit particular documenting purposes. They're perfect for recording information about routine tasks you perform throughout the day, such as giving medication or monitoring your patient's vital signs or fluid balance. Why? For four reasons. A flow sheet:

• displays a specific aspect of your patient's condition, such as his temperature, at a glance. You don't have to search through pages of notes to determine his temperature pattern over the last 48 hours.

• saves you time. You can write down the vital signs or medication given without having to write a full descriptive entry every time. You can use your nursing notes to describe how the patient is responding to treatment.

• documents that you're giving the patient the continuous care he needs. In this way, a flow sheet legally protects you and the hospital from charges of negligent care.

• provides a legal form for nonlicensed personnel to chart their care and observations. Because nonlicensed personnel can't chart in the nurses' notes, information about patient care they give may be lost. Have them enter their care and initial each entry on a flow sheet. Then, if you have a question about the status of your patient's skin, you can check the flow sheet to identify the nursing assistant who administered that day's bed bath.

Despite their usefulness, flow sheets can create a legal tangle if you don't avoid two common mistakes.

The first mistake many nurses make is to treat flow sheets casually. For instance, some nurses will routinely check off whatever the previous shift checked off on the flow sheet, regardless of the actual care given, and then carefully chart the actual care in the nurses' notes. Obviously, as part of the legal medical record, the flow sheet must accurately reflect the care given.

A second common mistake is to depend too heavily on the flow sheet. Flow sheets can help you document, quickly and accurately, what care was given and who gave it. But don't neglect to record the *patient's response to care* in your nurses' notes. Like any other chart form, retain it as part of the permanent chart so that you have a progressive picture of the patient's status and a record of your care.

## KEY TERMS IN THIS ENTRY

**block charting** • A method of charting in which you detail, in paragraph form, procedures you carried out during a block of time.

**documentation** • The preparing or assembling of written records.

**medical record** • A written, legal record of every aspect of the patient's care.

**problem-oriented medical record** • A record-keeping system in which you provide information about the patient from the standpoint of what's bothering him.

**SOAP** • An acronym for the format used in problem-oriented record keeping; it represents: Subjective data, Objective data, Assessment data, and Plans.

**source-oriented records** • A record-keeping system in which each professional group within the health-care team keeps separate information on the patient.

**time charting** • A method of charting in which you detail at regular time intervals—for example, every ½ hour—the procedures you carried out at that particular time.

• doctor's order sheet and progress notes
• nursing care plan (cardex)
• nurses' notes
• laboratory test results
• X-ray reports
• flow sheets, checklists, and graphic sheets
• discharge summary
• home-care instruction sheet.

This collection of separate records grew out of a system of record keeping called *source-oriented records*. As the name implies, in this system, each *source* of information keeps a separate record. This type of record keeping was almost universal until the 1960s, with doctors charting the progress notes and nurses charting the nurses' notes. The obvious drawback of this system is that you have to consult several sources to get an accurate picture of your patient's condition. Failing to consult all the separate records could have disastrous clinical consequences for the patient, and serious legal consequences for the patient's doctors and nurses. The case of *Villetto v. Weilbaecher* (1979) is an example. In this case, the nurses noticed that the patient had developed several blisters after surgery for a fractured kneecap. They recorded their observation in the nurses' notes and reported it to the doctor.

The patient later sued the doctor for failing to treat the blisters. The doctor couldn't defend himself successfully because *his* record, the progress notes, didn't mention the blisters until 6 days after the nurses charted them.

To avoid this kind of communication gap, many hospitals have switched to *problem-oriented records*. In this system of record keeping, all members of the health-care team, and even the patient, combine their information in a special format that goes by the acronym SOAP. Each note combines Subjective data (how the patient feels), Objective data (what you find), Assessment data, and Plans. For example, you might note: Problem: *Pain on ambulation.*

S "My side hurts when I walk"

O Favoring left side, appendectomy done on 8/15/83

A Stitches and local inflammation causing pain

P Assist when walking.

This type of record keeping provides a comprehensive picture of how well the patient is coping with his problem and responding to therapy.

## Block charting and time charting

With both systems, you can use either block charting or time charting. When using *block charting*, you note—in paragraph form—the procedures you carried out during a block of time; for example, between 11 p.m. and 7 a.m., or between 3 p.m. and 11 p.m. Block charting encourages you to note the important patient care information as briefly as possible. But it may *discour-*

# WHEN IN DOUBT, CHART EVERYTHING

Have you ever wondered what information you should chart besides your nursing care interventions and patient observations? To be on the safe side, chart as much factual information as you can about your patient's care. This includes:

• incidents
• omitted treatments
• safety precautions
• attempts to reach the doctor.

Omitting any of this information may invite misunderstanding and jeopardize the quality of your patient's care. For example, consider this fictional situation:
The doctor's order read, "Out of bed for 20 minutes, three times daily as tolerated." Mr. Cauthen's nurse, Phyllis McKay, helped Mr. Cauthen out of bed after explaining to him that the doctor wanted him to get out of bed and exercise. But as soon as she helped him stand up, he dropped to his knees. Mr. Cauthen was apparently unhurt but *certainly* angry. He complained bitterly that he fell because she made him get out of bed.

Phyllis got him back in bed, checked to be sure his vital signs were normal, and got him to stop complaining long enough for him to agree that he wasn't hurt. Then, feeling that some things are better unsaid, Phyllis went off to care for another patient without charting the incident, notifying the doctor, or completing an incident report.

Two hours later, nurse Alice Perkins read Mr. Cauthen's chart and assumed he hadn't been out of bed for his exercise. She got about as far as Phyllis did. As soon as Mr. Cauthen tried to stand, he collapsed. And this time, he fractured his hip.

Later, Mr. Cauthen complained to his doctor about his *two* falls. The doctor immediately notified Phyllis' supervisor about the uncharted incident. And Phyllis ended up on probation—all for a "minor" charting omission. Had Mr. Cauthen decided to sue the hospital, Phyllis could also have been charged with malpractice.

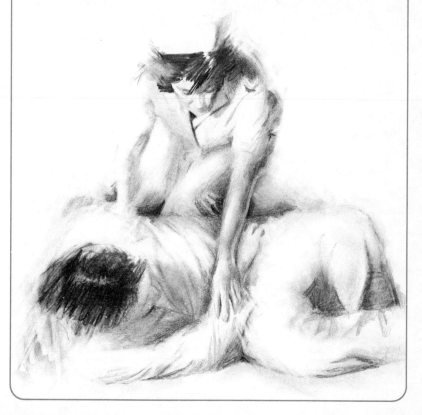

*age* you from including all the significant information. In *Engle v. Clarke* (1961), for example, a nurse recorded that she'd administered medication to a patient, but she'd failed to record the time at which the medication took effect.

Because of the danger of omitting important information, block charting isn't as popular as time charting. In *time charting*, you record the hour-by-hour care you give the patient: your observations, what you did, and when you did it.

## The basis of good documentation

The rules governing documentation come from four sources:
- federal regulations
- state and provincial (Canada) laws
- professional standards
- hospital policies.

Many federal regulations, such as those regarding Medicare and Medicaid, stipulate the form and content of the medical record. Although these regulations don't have the authority of law, most hospitals conform to the reg-

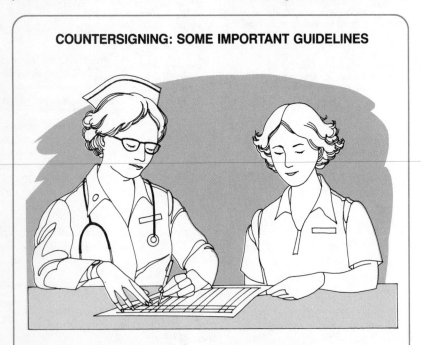

### COUNTERSIGNING: SOME IMPORTANT GUIDELINES

As an RN, have you ever worried about the legality of countersigning notes made by LPNs, LVNs, or aides when you haven't supervised their actions?

To ease your worries, find out what your hospital's policy says. Does the hospital interpret countersigning to mean that the LPN/LVN or aide performed her nursing actions *in your presence*? If so, don't countersign unless she did.

If your hospital accepts the fact that you don't always have the time to witness your co-workers' actions, then your

countersignature implies that:
- the notes describe care that the LPN/LVN or aide had the authority and competence to perform.
- you have verified that all required patient-care procedures were performed.

What should you do if another nurse asks you to document her care or sign her notes? In a word, "Don't." Unless your hospital policy authorizes—or requires—you to witness someone else's notes, your signature will make you responsible for anything you put in the notes.

## WRITING A DISCHARGE SUMMARY

The discharge summary is the final document in each patient's records. Follow your hospital's policy in deciding what format to use and what information to include in the summary. You'll probably need to list significant highlights of your patient's condition, his treatment, and his status at discharge. You may also need to include a home-care instruction sheet, the name of the person accompanying the patient, the patient's discharge address, and his mode of transportation (car, ambulance, taxi).

To make sure you perform this final responsibility well, follow these guidelines:
• Before writing your summary, review the patient's problem list, care plan, flow sheets, and progress notes to develop an overall picture of his hospitalization.
• Make a mental list of the highlights of the patient's hospitalization, including any exceptional details or unusual findings.
• Outline all patient teaching, including what you told him about his diagnosis, diet, medications, activity, special care, follow-up, and referrals. (Also write down this information on a patient instruction sheet in language he can understand so he'll have a record of what you discussed.)

After you write the summary, reread it to be sure it does the following:
• summarizes your patient's care
• provides useful information for further teaching and evaluation, and for readmission
• documents that the patient has the information he needs to care for himself or

to get further help
• shows that you've met documentation requirements of the Joint Commission on Accreditation of Hospitals for patient teaching
• helps safeguard you and your employer against malpractice charges.

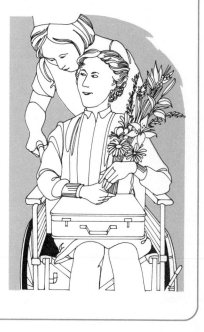

ulations to assure their eligibility for federal funds.

State and provincial laws vary, but all states and provinces require hospitals to keep records documenting a patient's care. In some states, you'll find more specific guidelines in the nurse practice act; and in Canada, in the public hospital acts. On the whole, however, the states leave the specific requirements to professional organizations.

Two professional organizations have set more stringent standards for documentation than what's required by state law.

The American Nurses' Association

(ANA) has included standards for documentation in its *Standards of Nursing Practice.* According to these ANA standards, documentation must be "systematic and continuous..., accessible, communicated, recorded," and readily available to all members of the health-care team.

The Joint Commission on Accreditation of Hospitals' standards require documentation of all phases of the nursing process for each hospitalized patient from admission through discharge.

In all likelihood, your hospital has integrated the regulations, laws, and standards into its own policy manual.

Your best assurance that you're following the law is to follow the policy manual. It will tell you who's responsible for keeping each part of a patient's chart and which charting techniques should be used.

ADVICE

## CHARTING CONSISTENTLY:
## THE BEST LEGAL PROTECTION

**Keeping charts current**
*Under our hospital's charting policy, a nurse may simply sign her name if she has nothing significant to write on a patient's chart. Hospital policy doesn't state how much time may pass before a note must be written, and I've seen charts with no nurses' notes for as many as 5 days. Don't we need a better policy?—RN, Ariz.*

If nothing significant happens to a patient for 5 days, he either doesn't need hospitalization or isn't getting proper care. In that length of time, a patient must be either responding or not responding to treatment—and that alone should be noted.

Anyone reviewing the chart—a new doctor, a hospital utilization committee, a member of an accreditation committee, or a prosecutor investigating malpractice charges—would certainly want to know what happened during those 5 days. And, obviously, a chart with only signatures wouldn't protect you or the hospital from a patient's malpractice claim.

You and the other nurses should start protecting yourselves by charting each patient's condition at least once each shift.

You should also ask for a committee of nurses, hospital lawyers, and administrators to design a new charting policy that will meet legal and accreditation requirements for your kind of institution.

**Charting exact times**
*On the 30-bed pediatric unit where I'm the medication nurse, I've always charted routine medication as given when ordered. For instance, if a doctor orders acetaminophen (Tylenol) three times a day, I write on the medication sheet: Tylenol, t.i.d., 8 a.m.—12 noon—6 p.m. Then, after I give the medication, I put my initials next to the appropriate time. Of course, with 30 patients to care for, I'm sometimes 15 to 30 minutes late with a medication.*

*My nursing supervisor says I should chart the exact times. I do this for stat and p.r.n. medications, but is it really necessary to be so specific with routinely prescribed drugs?—RN, Ill.*

Yes. A patient's chart is a legal document, so you must accurately record everything you do for a patient. This means if a drug is ordered for 8 a.m., but you don't give it until 8:30 a.m., you have to write "8:30" on the patient's medication sheet. You should also record the exact time on the medication cardex.

The most important reason for such accurate charting is to make sure a patient's medication maintains the desired therapeutic level—no drug highs or lows. If you give Mr. Smith's 8 a.m. dosage at 8:15 a.m., write "8:15." Then, be sure he gets his next dosage at 12:15 p.m., not 12 noon, especially if the drug is an antihypertensive or antibiotic, whose effectiveness depends on steady blood levels.

Charting exact times will also protect you if you're ever questioned by a doctor or attorney. As it is, you'd have a hard time explaining how you gave 30 patients their 8 a.m. medication at the same time.

**Secondhand charting**
*I'm an LPN in a hospital where aides and orderlies aren't allowed to chart the routine patient care they give. Sometimes, I'm sent to a busy unit to help with their charting.*

*I'm always uneasy about charting for a patient I've never seen, and I'm especially uneasy when the information is obviously inadequate. For some patients, the only information the aide gives me to chart for the whole 8-hour shift is an ambulation order.*

*This can't be safe for the patients, and I'm afraid it isn't safe for me. Suppose I don't chart that a patient hasn't voided or has had bloody stools. Could omitting such information make me liable for malpractice, even though I wasn't aware of it?*

*I've tried to cover myself by signing*

---

These letters were taken from the files of *Nursing* and *NursingLife* magazines.

## A good policy to follow

Hospital policy isn't law, of course, but the law tends to support the policy when documentation questions enter the courtroom. The following case, *Stack v. Wapner* (1976), illustrates this point.

Mrs. Stack was admitted to the hospital to give birth to her fourth child. At 2:45 a.m., according to her chart, intravenous oxytocin was started to induce labor by causing uterine contractions. Accepted medical practice requires constant monitoring of a patient receiving oxytocin. Otherwise, the drug may cause excessive uterine contractions, which may endanger the fetus or rupture the woman's uterus. But Mrs. Stack's labor-room charts didn't document any check on her condition until 5:15 a.m.

After the baby was born, the mother developed heavy uterine bleeding. Unable to stop the bleeding, the doctor performed a total hysterectomy. Later, the patient sued, claiming that inappropriate administration and monitoring of the oxytocin caused the complications that made a hysterectomy necessary.

Both attending doctors testified that they had monitored the administration of the drug. But they had no defense against the evidence that hospital policy required them to document all information on a patient's chart that justified a diagnosis and treatment—and all information relevant to the results. The patient was awarded damages.

## A final word

The advice "Write it down" can't be overemphasized. (See *When in Doubt, Chart Everything,* page 224.) If you've evaluated a patient, given a treatment, checked vital signs, or performed any other task that's essential to your patient's welfare, write it down in the medical record.

You may think documenting is something you do *after* you do your professional job. But—as this review of laws, standards, policies, and court judgments demonstrates—documenting *is* your professional job.

---

both names to the chart: "E. Lyons, NA/ S. Bradley, LPN." Is there anything else I can do to protect the patients and myself?—LPN, Fla.

You're right to be concerned, because your failure to report a change in a patient's condition could be considered malpractice for two reasons: first, because you failed to fulfill your legal responsibility to the patient, and second, because you failed to meet the acceptable standard of care. If a patient suffered harm because you failed to chart something, both you and your hospital could be considered liable.

Request a new hospital policy requiring nurses with personal knowledge of the patient to chart. Such a request is in the patients' best interests, as well as your own.

In the meantime, you're on the right track when you sign both your name and the aide's name to each chart. One other suggestion: Always add a statement that you haven't personally observed the patient and can't certify the truth of what you've written since your information is secondhand.

### Charting the facts

*Some nurses on our unit have been writing on the patients' charts, "Primary nursing care could not be given because nurse: patient ratio was 1:20."*

*To me, charting that primary nursing care wasn't done implies that no nursing care was given. The other nurses point out that they chart the care that's given. They just want the record to show that they're giving what care they can despite an unsafe nurse:patient ratio.*

*Does such negative "nursing" information belong on the patients' charts?—* RN, Utah

Staffing information does *not* belong on a patient's chart. A note, "primary care not given," could be used against the nurse who writes it as evidence in a malpractice suit. The nurses should avoid general statements and chart *exactly* what care they could and did give.

# 36 Pitfalls of documentation

The information you document about a patient gives other nurses the knowledge to continue that patient's care where you left off. If you leave something out or make a mistake in the chart, they may give inadequate care. If the patient is injured and sues, your charting omission or error will assume major importance.

## Legal importance of good charting

In court, your nurses' notes can be used as evidence of the quality of nursing care that you provide. If a patient is injured, the completeness, consistency, and even legibility of your notes may determine the outcome of the lawsuit. If you find that hard to believe, read these three cases. In each, the nurses' own charts provided evidence against them.

Oza Mae Rogers died of brain damage 7 days after she was admitted to the hospital for injuries suffered in an accident. In the lawsuit that followed, *Rogers v. Kasdan* (1981), the Supreme Court of Kentucky ruled against the

doctor and the hospital. The court based its ruling on the patient's medical record: the emergency room records were incomplete, the fluid input/output record was incorrectly tallied, different records contained discrepancies, and several records were illegible and contained incomplete notations.

Patricia Maslonka hemorrhaged and died 3 hours after giving birth to her fourth child. In the lawsuit that resulted, *Maslonka v. Hermann* (1980), the patient's medical record was again the determining factor in the court's decision. According to the court's interpretation of the record, two nurses and four doctors had been negligent. The nurses had poorly monitored the patient's vital signs and had failed to communicate the patient's condition.

Finally, *St. Paul Fire and Marine Insurance Co. v. Prothro* (1979) involved a lawsuit brought by a patient named Prothro. After a total hip replacement, Mr. Prothro was injured while being lowered into a Hubbard bath by an orderly. The metal basket holding him collapsed, struck his hip, and reopened his wound. The orderly stopped the bleeding and took Mr. Prothro to his room, where a staff nurse reclosed the wound with surgical tape. But no one documented the incident.

Several days later, the wound became infected. Subsequently, the doctor had to remove the hip prosthesis, leaving Mr. Prothro with a permanent limp. Mr. Prothro sued the hospital.

The court ruled in his favor and said the determining factor was the absence of crucial information on Mr. Prothro's medical chart, which would have helped the doctor and other health-care professionals provide more appropriate care.

## Nine common pitfalls of documentation

As the court cases indicate, charting errors and omissions can undermine the credibility of your nursing care in court. To protect yourself from unfore-

GLOSSARY

### KEY TERMS IN THIS ENTRY

**countersignature** · The signature you must obtain from another health professional to verify information, or your signature that verifies another health-care provider's information.

**documentation** · The preparing or assembling of written records.

**nurses' notes** · A means of documenting the nursing care you provide and the patient's response to that care.

## DOCUMENTING NARCOTIC COUNTS CORRECTLY

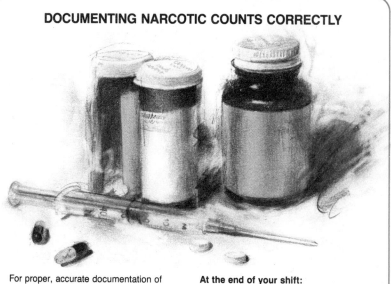

For proper, accurate documentation of narcotics, use the special narcotics records—the control sheet and check sheet—provided by your hospital pharmacy, and follow this procedure:

**Before you give a narcotic:**
• Verify the count in the narcotics drawer.
• Sign the narcotic control sheet to indicate you removed the drug.
• Get another nurse to sign the control sheet if you waste or discard all or part of a dose.

**At the end of your shift:**
• Record the amount of each narcotic on the narcotic check sheet while the nurse beginning her shift counts the narcotics out loud.
• Sign the narcotic check sheet *only* if the count is correct. Have the other nurse countersign.
• Identify and correct any discrepancies before any nurse leaves the unit.

seen legal and professional consequences, try to chart clearly, accurately, and completely, no matter how tired or busy you are. And, especially when you're tired or busy, remind yourself to watch out for these nine common charting errors:

• *Omissions.* Include all the facts other nurses need to assess your patient's needs. In a lawsuit, the court may assume that you failed to perform any task you didn't record and may suspect that you omitted information with the intention to cover up incriminating evidence.

• *Personal opinions.* Record what you saw, heard, and did. If your patient says he's mad, record it. If you think he's mad because he's quiet, record

only that he's quiet. Otherwise, your personal opinions might influence other nurses' attitudes toward your patient, which could adversely affect the care they provide.

• *Generalizations.* Be specific. Don't use meaningless phrases like, "Had a good day." Instead, describe *why* your patient's day was good. For example: "Patient ate 100% of regular diet; did not complain of pain."

• *Late charting.* Record patient information promptly. The longer you wait, the more likely you are to forget important facts. When you're unable to chart immediately because of patient needs, jot down key information on a note pad to help you recall important information later.

## USING ABBREVIATIONS

Abbreviations are a safe way to save time when you document *if* you use abbreviations whose meanings are unmistakably clear.

The abbreviations listed below *aren't* clear. Study this list, and avoid using any of the abbreviations it contains.

| ABBREVIATION | INTENDED MEANING |
|---|---|
| **Apothecary symbols** | dram |
| | minim |
| | *Aminophylline 3T tid*<br>*Tr opium 10 My* |
| **AU** | *auris uterque*<br>(each ear) |
| | *Colymycin gtts iii a u tid* |
| **Drug names**<br>MTX<br>CPZ<br>HCl<br>DIG<br>MVI<br>HCTZ<br>ARA-A | <br>methotrexate<br>Compazine (prochlorperazine)<br>hydrochloric acid<br><br>digoxin<br>multivitamins *without* fat-soluble vitamins<br>hydrochlorothiazide<br>vidarabine |
| **µg** | microgram |
| | *Vit B₁₂ 1 µg IM Now* |
| **o.d.** | once daily |
| | *KCl 15 mEq OD* |
| **OJ** | orange juice |
| | *Lugol's sol'n*<br>*gtts x in OJ* |

| MISINTERPRETATION | CORRECTION |
| --- | --- |
| Frequently misinterpreted or not understood. | Use the metric system. |
| Frequently misinterpreted as OU (*oculus uterque*— each eye). | Write it out. |
| Frequently misinterpreted as:<br>Mustargen (mechlorethamine HCl)<br>chlorpromazine<br>potassium chloride (The "H" is misinterpreted as "K.")<br>digitoxin<br>multivitamins *with* fat-soluble vitamins<br>hydrocortisone (HCT)<br>cytarabine (ARA-C) | Use the complete spelling for drug names. |
| When handwritten, frequently misinterpreted as "mg." | Use mcg. |
| Frequently misinterpreted as "right eye" (OD—*oculus dexter*). | Don't abbreviate "daily." Write it out. |
| Frequently misinterpreted as "OD" (*oculus dexter*— right eye) or "OS" (*oculus sinister*—left eye). Medications that were meant to be diluted in orange juice and given orally have been given in a patient's right or left eye. | Write it out. |

*(continued)*

## USING ABBREVIATIONS *(continued)*

| ABBREVIATION | INTENDED MEANING |
|---|---|
| $\dot{T}$/D  _T/D_ | once daily <br><br> _Diabinese 250mg T/d_ |
| per os | orally <br><br> _Lugol's sol'n gtts X per os_ |
| q.d. | every day <br><br> _Digoxin 0.25g q.d._ |
| qn | nightly or at bedtime <br><br> _Librium 10 mg qh_ |
| q.o.d. | every other day <br><br> _digoxin 0.25 mg q.i.d._ |
| sub q | subcutaneous <br><br> _Heparin 5000 units sub q 2 hrs before surgery_ |
| U or u | unit <br><br> _NPH 6U Now SC_ <br> _NPH 44 Now SC_ |

| MISINTERPRETATION | CORRECTION |
|---|---|
| Misinterpreted as "t.i.d." | Write it out. |
| The "os" is frequently misinterpreted as "left eye." | Use "P.O." or "by mouth" or "orally." |
| The period after the "q" has sometimes been misinterpreted as "i," and the drug has been given q.i.d. rather than daily. | Write it out. |
| Misinterpreted as "every hour" when poorly written. | Use "hs" or "nightly." |
| Misinterpreted as "daily" or "q.i.d." if the "o" is poorly written. | Use "q other day" or "every other day." |
| The "q" has been misinterpreted as "every." In the example, a prophylactic heparin dose meant to be given 2 hours before surgery was given *every* 2 hours before surgery. | Use "subcut." or write out "subcutaneous." |
| Misinterpreted as a zero or a four (4), causing a tenfold or greater overdose. | Write it out. |

## SIGNING YOUR NURSING NOTES

To discourage nurses from adding information to your nursing notes, draw a line through any blank spaces and sign your name on the far right side of the column.

> P: WILL CONTINUE PLAN
> AND REQUEST DIABETIC
> NURSE SPECIALIST
> TO ASSESS PATIENTS'
> KNOWLEDGE OF
> DIABETES MELLITUS
> 3RD OR 4TH POSTOP
> DAY — J. Price R.N.

If you don't have enough room to sign your name after the last word of your entry, draw a line from the last word to the end of the line. Then, drop down to the next line, draw a line from the left margin almost to the right margin, and sign your name on the far right side.

> AND HYPERGLYCEMIA
> A: EXCELLENT KNOW-
> LEDGE OF DISEASE
> AND MANAGEMENT.
> P: SEE NO NEED
> FOR ADDITIONAL
> FOLLOW-UP: —
> — S. Smith R.N.

If you have a lot of information to record and you anticipate running out of room on a page, leave room on the right side of the page for your signature. Sign the page, then continue your notes on the next page, and then sign that page as usual.

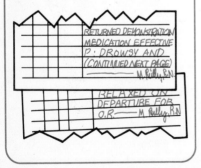

> RETURNED DEMONSTRATION
> MEDICATION EFFECTIVE
> P: DROWSY AND
> (CONTINUED NEXT PAGE)
> M. Reilly, R.N.

> RELAXED ON
> DEPARTURE FOR
> O.R. — M. Reilly, R.N.

• *Improper abbreviations.* Use commonly accepted abbreviations only, and use them correctly. Ask your supervisor to post a list of acceptable abbreviations where you do your charting, so you don't have to rely on your memory. The wrong abbreviation may endanger your patient's health. For example, suppose you write "O.D." after a medication order instead of "o.d." The significance: O.D. means right eye; o.d. means once daily. The nurse who carries out the order could irreversibly damage the patient's eye. (See *Using Abbreviations,* pages 230 to 233.)

• *Illegibility.* Write clearly and neatly. If others can't read your writing, print. If a court is unable to decipher your notes, it may doubt your credibility.

• *Incorrect spelling.* Be precise. Misspellings lead to confusion. Use a dictionary when you're unsure of spelling or usage. Use common words and expressions to make sure you convey your meaning.

• *Improperly correcting charting errors.* Draw a line through any error, label it *charting error,* and initial it. Never erase or scratch out an error. (For a complete discussion on correcting errors, see Entry 37.)

• *Improperly signing your notes.* Sign all your notes with your first initial, full last name, and title. Put your signature on the right side of the page as proof that you entered all the information between the previous nurse's signature and yours. If another nurse on your unit has the same first initial, last name, and title, include a middle initial in your legal signature.

If the last entry is unsigned, immediately contact the nurse who made the entry and have her sign it. If you can't reach her, make a notation to distinguish your entry from hers. (For a complete discussion on how to handle this situation, see Entry 37 and *Signing Your Nursing Notes.*)

### Common pitfalls in noting doctors' orders

The courts look at all aspects of docu-

## CHARTING ON PROGRESS NOTES?

*My hospital recently changed its charting system: everyone now charts on the progress notes. We've already had some problems with the new system.*

*For one thing, many doctors leave blank lines between their notes and a nurse's note. Isn't this dangerous?*

*Second, some nurses don't chart anything if the doctor has already written a note adequately covering the patient's condition and care. Is this good nursing practice?*—RN, Ore.

First things first. Leaving blank lines between entries on a patient's chart is inviting legal trouble. If someone inserted an entry out of chronological order or padded the notes, an attorney could zero in on these as suspicious entries when the notes are used as evidence in court. Therefore, ask your hospital administrator to establish a protocol that clearly states that *no one* can leave blank lines.

Your second problem is just as serious. A nurse isn't relieved of her responsibilities in charting when a doctor writes a note, even if his note describes the patient's condition and care. The nurse must still document her *own* observations, interactions with the patient, and nursing care provided. In court, the rule of thumb is—documentation means *done,* and no documentation means *not done.*

---

This letter was taken from the files of *Nursing* magazine.

mentation during a malpractice trial, so be prepared to defend your handling of medical orders, too.

When you take a doctor's order off a patient's medical chart, don't forget to make a check mark in ink on each line of the order. Draw lines through any

---

> *"Draw a line through any blank spaces to prevent later additions."*

---

space between the last written order and the doctor's signature to prevent a later addition to the order. Below the doctor's signature, sign your name, the date, and the time.

Take verbal and telephone orders only in an emergency when the doctor can't immediately attend to the patient. If time and circumstances allow, have another nurse read the order back to the doctor. Record the order on the doctor's order sheet as soon as possible. Note the date, then record the order verbatim. On the following line, write *v.o.* for verbal order or *t.o.* for telephone order. Then write the doctor's name and the name of the nurse who read the order back to the doctor. Sign your name and write the time. Draw lines through any spaces between the order and your verification of the order.

Be sure the doctor countersigns the order within the time specified by hospital policy. Without the countersignature, you can be held liable for practicing medicine without a license.

### Avoiding pitfalls in keeping narcotic records

The legal consequences of improper charting also apply to narcotics records. Be sure you're familiar with local and state regulations as well as hospital policy when you dispense narcotics. These regulations may be more stringent than Title II of the Comprehensive Drug Abuse Prevention and Control Act

of 1970, also known as the Controlled Substances Act. As you know, this act holds you accountable for storing all narcotics and barbiturates on your unit and for keeping a record of each distributed dose. (See *Documenting Narcotic Counts Correctly*, page 229.)

### A final word

Because you're human, you'll inevitably make errors in documenting patient care. But as a professional you have to strive to minimize the errors that all too frequently turn up on a patient's medical record. Being alert to commonly made errors and identifying ways to avoid them are the first steps you can take toward improving the quality of your patient charting.

# 37 The altered medical record

Suppose you're charting Mrs. Smith's vital signs at 10:00 a.m., and you discover you didn't chart them at 8:00 a.m. Or suppose you finish charting your assessment of Mrs. Stanton, and then notice that you've written it on Mr. Williams' chart. Would you know how to correct these errors properly? If you do it improperly—and the chart ends up in court—your motives as well as your nursing care may come into question.

If the court uncovers alterations during the course of a trial, it may discount the medical record's value. That's what happened to the nurse involved in a Canadian case, *Joseph Brant Memorial Hospital v. Koziol* (1978). The nurse failed to chart her observations for 7 hours on a postoperative patient who died during that period. Later, the patient's family sued the hospital, charging the nurse with malpractice. The nurse insisted that she *had* observed the patient, and, on the instruction of the assistant director of nursing, added the nursing observations to the patient's medical record. The court wasn't convinced. Suspicious of the altered record, it ruled that the nurse's failure to chart her observations at the proper time supported the claim that she'd made no such observations.

In *Thor v. Boska* (1974), the court considered a rewritten copy of a patient's record to be as suspicious as an altered record. The lawsuit was brought by a woman who had seen her doctor several times because of a lump on her breast. Each time, the doctor examined her and made a record of her visit. After 2 years, the woman sought a second opinion and learned she had breast cancer. She sued the first doctor. Instead of producing his records in court, he brought *copies*. He said he'd copied the originals, so they'd be legible. But the court inferred that he was withholding incriminating evidence from the jury.

### State laws regulate alterations

Some state laws specify penalties for tampering with medical records. Improperly adding or changing information in a chart can bring charges of fraudulent concealment or obstruction of justice. Under the California Penal Code, for example, altering a record with fraudulent intent is a misdemeanor.

### How to correct your charting errors

Clearly, correcting mistakes is a serious business. But—just as clearly—mistakes occur that *need* to be corrected. Here's how to do it properly, legally, and without charges of attempted cover-up.

To avoid legal problems, use these techniques for *changing* information on a chart. First, draw one line through any incorrect information, *without obscuring it*. Write the date and time, and sign your name. Then, depending on the type of error, do the following:

● If you've used the *wrong chart*—recording your assessment of Mrs. Stanton on Mr. Williams' chart, for

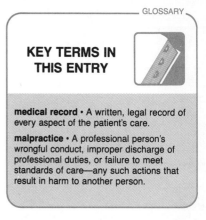

## KEY TERMS IN THIS ENTRY

**medical record** • A written, legal record of every aspect of the patient's care.

**malpractice** • A professional person's wrongful conduct, improper discharge of professional duties, or failure to meet standards of care—any such actions that result in harm to another person.

example—write "wrong chart" to explain why you've drawn a line through the entry.

● If you've written the *wrong information*, add the correct information. If the incorrect and the correct information are legible, you won't have to write the reason for your change.

● If you've *misspelled* a word, spell it correctly. If you discover the misspelling immediately, you can correct it without adding the date and time and your initials.

If, however, you've *omitted* information, chart it when you remember it. If you discover at 10 a.m., for example, that you forgot to chart Mrs. Smith's 8 a.m. vital signs, add them after your 10 o'clock entry. Simply write "10 a.m.," then "vital signs for 8/17/83, 8 a.m.." After you record the vital signs, mark the addition "late entry." Always use this method; *never* try to squeeze additional information into the original entry.

If you go home, then realize you've made an error or omitted information, decide whether anyone will need the correct information before your next shift. Call anyone who will need it. When you return to work, make the appropriate change on the chart.

If the nurse on the previous shift has omitted information, call her at home and tell her. If the information isn't needed before she returns, ask her to correct the record when she does re-

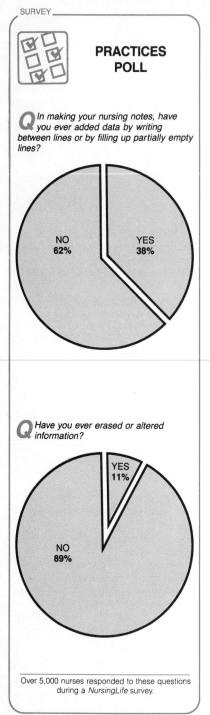

## PRACTICES POLL

**Q** *In making your nursing notes, have you ever added data by writing between lines or by filling up partially empty lines?*

NO 62%

YES 38%

**Q** *Have you ever erased or altered information?*

YES 11%

NO 89%

Over 5,000 nurses responded to these questions during a *NursingLife* survey.

turn. If it is needed before then, chart it yourself. Then write, "Charted by [your name] for [her name]." Be sure she countersigns the chart when she returns.

If she's left blank spaces, draw lines through them so no one can insert any information.

If she's made an error, tell her so she—not you—can correct it.

If she's forgotten to sign her name, begin your entry with the date, time, and the statement, "My notations begin at [specify the time]." Then, sign your name to separate your notes from hers.

### When should you leave charting errors alone?

Suppose you find out a patient is going to sue you or the hospital. You read the medical record to refresh your memory, and you find a charting error. What then? Never make corrections in a situation like that. The plaintiff's attorney may have received a copy of the records before filing the lawsuit. If you change the record after that, the court may interpret it as a cover-up, and you might be charged with tampering.

Leave the record as it is, but make your own record of what the changes should be. Then, you'll have the correct version straight in your mind, and if you're questioned about the error, you'll have something to refer to.

What if someone asks—or pressures—you to change a record before a case goes to court? The request may seem harmless. For example, someone might note a small disagreement between the progress notes and the nurses' notes over the exact time of an event or the exact size of a wound. No matter how harmless the change seems, you must refuse. For one thing, the court expects and accepts some differences between your records and the doctor's. But more importantly, changing your record would seriously weaken its credibility—and yours. If the pressure continues, report the situation to your supervisor or, if she's doing the pressuring, to *her* supervisor.

## COMPOUNDING THE ERROR

*The legal office at my hospital insists that we simply line out, then cover, any errors on a patient's chart with white, gummed labels. The long list of errors includes stamping the chart with the wrong patient's plate, making mistakes on the temperature, pulse, and respiration graph, writing notes on the wrong patient's chart, and so on.*

*I've refused to cover up mistakes because it contradicts everything I've learned in nursing. I still think what I was taught is right: Draw a single line through the error, initial it, and write in the correction. I'm always warning my colleagues about the legal problems they could face if they "gum up" mistakes, and I've complained to my supervisor about the cover-up procedure. But I feel like I'm beating my head against a wall.*

*Although the legal staff can't prove that the labeling practice is legal, they say I have to prove it's illegal before the situation can be changed. Please help—I don't want to leave this job.*

*By the way, this is a military hospital. Does that change the situation?—RN, Calif.*

Your hospital's charting strategy is a mess. Gumming over the faulty entries will cripple any legal defense for the hospital or its personnel in a court action. In fact, the charts with labels may not even be legally admissible. Your best plan is to mark an error as soon as you discover it, then refer the reader to the recorded correction.

By the way, the rules are different in a military setting. A military hospital, because of the doctrine of sovereign immunity, can't be sued without its consent. You'd be wise to visit the hospital's legal office again. Get more information about your liability and the hospital's under the Federal Torts Claims Act.

Making an effort to change your hospital's poor charting practices now may save you and your hospital from trouble later.

This letter was taken from the files of *Nursing* magazine.

## A final word

Don't compound your error by correcting a charting error improperly. When you correct it, make sure both the incorrect and the correct information are readable and that the reason for the change is obvious. Such clean corrections keep the patient's record accurate and keep you legally protected.

# 38 Computerized record keeping: The legal aspects

Like most nurses, you've probably lamented the paperwork involved in keeping your patient's medical records complete. Now modern technology is offering a method to make your record-keeping duties easier: the computerized medical record. Like the manual record system, the computerized medical record provides a documented account of your patient's illness, diagnostic tests, treatments, and medical history. But unlike the manual system, the computerized record stores all your patient's medical data in a single, easily accessible source.

Computerized record keeping also creates problems—problems that mean new burdens for you. As computers become more common in patient record keeping, you'll need to understand how these burdens affect your practice legally.

## Computers enter clinical nursing

Most hospitals and other health-care facilities have been using computers for

GLOSSARY

## KEY TERMS IN THIS ENTRY

**computerized record system** • A system that stores medical records in the memory bank of a computer.

**signature code** • A code of letters and/or numbers that you enter into the computer to identify yourself.

payrolls and patient billings since the 1960s. A few computers have also made inroads in nursing care—mostly in specialized patient-care departments, such as the intensive care unit and the cardiac care unit. But experts believe the biggest effect computers will have on nursing is in patient charting.

### The components of a computerized system

Computerized systems are expensive, and computerized record programs must be extraordinarily large to include the variables needed to chart accurately. For example, your observations of a patient's skin might include variables such as scaly, clammy, cold, dry, inflamed, and purpuric. A computer program must be large enough to offer all these choices.

A few hospitals in the United States and Canada are already using computerized record-keeping systems. Typically, a system consists of a large, centralized computer, to store information, and a much smaller terminal in each work area. These terminals—linked to the main computer by electric cable—look like small television screens with typewriter keyboards.

To use the system, a nurse "signs in" by typing on the keyboard her signature code, a series of numbers and letters that gives a person access to a patient's record. The computer recognizes by her signature code that she has authorized access to the information stored in its memory. When she types her patient's code number, the computer displays the patient's records on the screen. By typing another key, she can order a printed copy of all or part of the patient's record.

### Computers can save you time

The computerized medical record can save you the time you now spend filing, searching for, and retrieving information about your patient. It will even save you the time of calling the laboratory to track down test results that never made it up to the unit. The technicians who record these results will

*"By far, the most pressing legal question about the computerized medical record is its threat to your patient's privacy."*

have "called up" the patient's record on their terminal and added the information directly.

Besides saving you time, computers offer you other important advantages. For one thing, computers reduce the risk of misinterpretation by improving legibility—no more problems with a doctor's indecipherable handwriting when you're reading his typed orders on a screen.

Computers also reduce misinterpretation by fostering standardized formats for your assessment reports, flow charts, and care plans. And by time-stamping each entry, computers decrease the chance of scheduling mistakes.

### Legal concerns with computerized records

Computerized medical records are such a new development that their legal implications are still being debated. The Joint Commission on the Accreditation of Hospitals has informally recognized them as legitimate substitutes for manual records. But some state laws require health facilities with computerized records to retain the written records as well.

Until uniform rules are adopted, the computerized record will invite questions that could raise legal risks for you.

## The computer's threat to privacy

By far, the most pressing legal question about the computerized medical record is its threat to your patient's privacy. (See Entry 14.)

With traditional records, you can limit access to information simply by keeping it on the unit. An unauthorized person wouldn't get very far into the charts before you challenged him. But with a computerized system, your patients' records can be called up at any of the terminals. Despite the use of sig-

nature codes, many more people have easier access to the computerized record than they do to manual records. That means a much greater chance exists for exposure of your patient's highly personal, private medical information.

Various laws protect the privacy of a patient's medical records. The Federal Privacy Act of 1974 protects confidential medical information of patients in Veterans' Administration hospitals, and some of the state practice acts impose an ethical duty to guard patients' privacy. However, no one can guarantee that unauthorized persons won't gain access to computerized records.

In 1977, a patient in New York charged that a computerized record system was an invasion of his privacy. In *Whalen v. Roe,* he challenged the constitutionality of a state law that required a patient buying certain drug prescriptions to list his name, address,

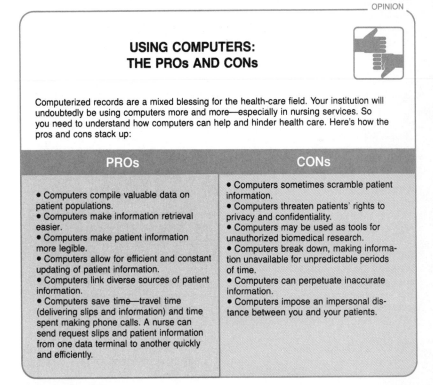

## USING COMPUTERS: THE PROs AND CONs

Computerized records are a mixed blessing for the health-care field. Your institution will undoubtedly be using computers more and more—especially in nursing services. So you need to understand how computers can help and hinder health care. Here's how the pros and cons stack up:

| PROs | CONs |
|---|---|
| • Computers compile valuable data on patient populations.<br>• Computers make information retrieval easier.<br>• Computers make patient information more legible.<br>• Computers allow for efficient and constant updating of patient information.<br>• Computers link diverse sources of patient information.<br>• Computers save time—travel time (delivering slips and information) and time spent making phone calls. A nurse can send request slips and patient information from one data terminal to another quickly and efficiently. | • Computers sometimes scramble patient information.<br>• Computers threaten patients' rights to privacy and confidentiality.<br>• Computers may be used as tools for unauthorized biomedical research.<br>• Computers break down, making information unavailable for unpredictable periods of time.<br>• Computers can perpetuate inaccurate information.<br>• Computers impose an impersonal distance between you and your patients. |

age, the drug, dosage, and prescribing doctor's name. The state then fed all the information into a computer.

The U.S. Supreme Court upheld the law, but it acknowledged the threat to privacy implicit in a centralized data system. Said Justice William Brennan: "The central storage and easy accessibility of computerized data vastly increase the potential for abuse of that information...."

Computers also threaten the doctor-patient relationship (see Entry 86). Doctors fear that patients will be less truthful in providing medical histories and details about illnesses. Why? Because patients worry that computers will be used to improperly divulge their medical information.

## Safeguarding privacy in computerized records
Health-care professionals and computer programmers have devised some safeguards to protect patients' privacy. The main safeguard is the signature code. By developing a series of access codes, programmers can limit access to the records. For example, your code would allow you to see a patient's entire record, but a technician's code would allow her to see only part of the record.

## The computer's other disadvantages
Another disadvantage of a computerized medical record system is the need for a backup system. Like all electronic devices, computers occasionally break down, making information unavailable for indeterminate periods. This is why a backup system is required to ensure completeness and continuity in charting.

Computers also sometimes scramble patient information because of mechanical or human error. When this happens, and you discover the mistake, you can't tell how many other health-team members have copies of the record containing the mistake.

Finally, some critics simply think computers are just another piece of equipment that distances you from your patient, making your practice less personal.

## How verification helps ensure accuracy
Verification is one way of reducing the chance for error in the computerized record. With verification, you check the accuracy of a doctor's order. It serves the same purpose for the computerized record that signing off a doctor's order serves for the manual record. In a computerized record system, the unit secretary enters a doctor's order into the computer. The order is held in a "suspense file" until a nurse reviews the entry and checks to be sure the unit secretary interpreted and entered the order correctly. After the nurse verifies the order, it's added to the active record file.

## Knowing how to minimize your legal risks
When you work with the computerized medical record, your liabilities are the same as when you're working with the manual system: you're liable for any patient injuries associated with your charting errors.

Here's how to minimize your legal risks:
• Always double-check all patient information you enter.
• Never tell anyone your signature code.
• Tell your supervisor if you suspect someone is using your code.
• Indicate that the doctor's order is written, verbal (in person), or verbal (by telephone) when you enter it.
• Know your institution's rules and regulations affecting patient privacy.

## A final word
As a provider of care, you should be ready to learn to use technology that promises to improve patient care. Many experts are convinced that computer technology will do that by freeing you to spend more time meeting your patient's needs.

# Selected References

American Hospital Association. *Patient's Bill of Rights.* Chicago: American Hospital Association, 1973.

American Nurses' Association. *Standards of Practice.* Kansas City, Mo.: American Nurses' Association, 1973.

Annas, George J., et al. *The Rights of Doctors, Nurses, and Allied Health Professionals.* Cambridge, Mass.: Ballinger Publishing Co., 1981.

Bennett, H.M. "The Legal Liabilities of Critical Care," *Critical Care Nurse* 2:22, January/February 1982.

Bernzweig, Eli. *The Nurse's Liability for Malpractice: A Programmed Course,* 3rd ed. New York: McGraw-Hill Book Co., 1981.

Blake, M.B. "Computerized Medical Records," *Legal Aspects of Medical Practice* 10:3, 1982.

Broccolo, Bernadette Muller. "The Importance of Proper Medical Record Entries," *Topics in Health Record Management, Legal Issues, Part 2* 2(1):67-74, September 1981.

Cazalas, Mary W. *Nursing and the Law,* 3rd ed. Rockville, Md.: Aspen Systems Corp., 1979.

Cleary, Edward W. *McCormick's Handbook of the Law of Evidence,* 2nd ed. St. Paul: West Publishing Co., 1972.

Creighton, Helen. *Law Every Nurse Should Know,* 4th ed. Philadelphia: W.B. Saunders Co., 1981.

Du Gas, Beverly W. *Introduction to Patient Care,* 3rd ed. Philadelphia: W.B. Saunders Co., 1977.

Fiesta, Janine. *The Law and Liability: A Guide for Nurses.* New York: John Wiley & Sons, 1982.

Gluck, J. "The Computerized Medical Record System: Meeting the Challenge for Nursing," *Journal of Nursing Administration* 9:17-24, December 1979.

Hemelt, M., and Mackert, M. *Dynamics of Law, Nursing and Health Care,* 2nd ed. Reston, Va.: Reston Publishing Co., 1982.

Huffman, Edna K. *Medical Record Management.* Berwyn, Ill.: Physicians' Record Co., 1981.

Joint Commission on Accreditation of Hospitals. *Accreditation Manual for Hospitals: 1983 Ed.* Chicago: Joint Commission on Accreditation of Hospitals, 1982.

Kerr, A.H. "Nursing Notes: 'That's Where the Goodies Are!'" *Nursing75* 5:34-41, February 1975.

Regan, William A., ed. "Charting Deficiencies and R.N. Liability," *Regan Report on Nursing Law* 21(8), January 1981.

Regan, William A., ed. "Charting: 'The Truth, The Whole Truth...'," *Regan Report on Nursing Law* 23(1), June 1982.

Regan, William A., ed. "Nurses and Medical Records: Legalities," *Regan Report on Nursing Law* 21(12), May 1981.

Regan, William A., ed. "Postop Infection: Poor Nursing Records," *Regan Report on Nursing Law* 21(6), November 1980.

Rocereto, LaVerne, and Maleski, Cynthia. *The Legal Dimensions of Nursing Practice: A Practical Guide.* New York: Springer Publishing Co., 1982.

Springer, Eric W. "The Medical Record in Today's World," *Topics in Health Record Management, Legal Issues, Part 1* 1(4), June 1981.

Watson, B.L. "Disclosure of Computerized Health Care Information: Provider Privacy Rights Under Supply Side Competition," *American Journal of Law and Medicine* 7:265, 1981.

Weed, Lawrence. "Medical Records That Guide and Teach," *New England Journal of Medicine* 278:593-600, March 1968.

Willig, S. *Nurse's Guide to the Law.* New York: McGraw-Hill Book Co., 1970.

# Malpractice: Understand It, Avoid It

## Introduction

Since the 1970s, the number of malpractice lawsuits filed against nurses has risen dramatically. The major reason seems to be that patients are increasingly aware of their right to receive quality health care—and increasingly willing to fight for it. When a patient feels his right has been violated, or that the care he's received falls below acceptable standards, he's likely to seek compensation through the courts.

You can protect yourself from malpractice lawsuits and help head off the upward trend of malpractice litigation in several ways. The most obvious way, of course, is to give your patients the best possible nursing care, according to the highest professional standards. This is your main strength and protection. Happily, it coincides with your constant main concern—the health and welfare of your patients. But you also need a sound knowledge of patients' rights, and you must do your best to uphold them. And your own rights— what about them? You need to know what they are and how to safeguard them.

### Understanding malpractice— the concept and the laws

Our legal system's view of malpractice evolved from negligence law and the premise, basic to all law, that everyone is responsible for the consequences of his own acts. Over the years, malpractice law developed special doctrines, or theories, to apply to cases involving subordinate-superior relationships. The law books call one such doctrine the doctrine of respondeat superior (let the master answer). In Canada, it's called the theory of vicarious liability. Simply put, this doctrine or theory holds that when a subordinate acting according to his superior's direction (servant to master, employee to employer) is found to have been negligent, he shouldn't have to bear the brunt of damages that may result from faithfully doing as directed. To the extent that a nurse was merely the hospital's functionary, she could claim protection under this theory. This doctrine is discussed many times in PRACTICES.

A derivative of respondeat superior is the borrowed-servant doctrine, which is still applied in malpractice lawsuits, but not as often as it used to be. It could apply in a situation in which you, a hospital employee, commit a negligent act while under the direction or control of someone other than your hospital supervisor, such as a doctor in the operating room. Because the doctor is an independent contractor and you're responsible to him during surgery, you're considered his borrowed servant at the time. If you're charged

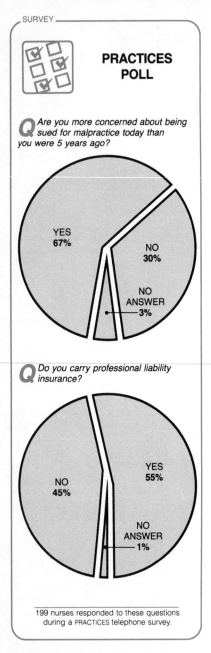

SURVEY

**PRACTICES POLL**

**Q** *Are you more concerned about being sued for malpractice today than you were 5 years ago?*

YES
67%

NO
30%

NO
ANSWER
3%

**Q** *Do you carry professional liability insurance?*

NO
45%

YES
55%

NO
ANSWER
1%

199 nurses responded to these questions during a PRACTICES telephone survey.

your patients' welfare, you've stepped out of the doctor's shadow into a personal-liability limelight of your own. Paradoxically, the increased risk you've incurred has come about because patient care is far better than it used to be—thanks to your efforts. Because you've been willing to do more, the educated consumer has come to expect more. And he looks to the courts for relief when he thinks he's gotten less than your best.

Where you and the law are concerned, you need to know how to avoid being named as a defendant in a malpractice lawsuit—how to walk that tightrope between what you perceive as your patient's needs and what your position as a nurse lets you provide. You want informed opinion about what the law says is—and isn't—appropriate nursing care. Obviously, training, background, and experience all play a part. For instance, what the law expects from an RN is sometimes different from what it expects from an LPN or LVN. You also need to know what legal and professional limits your hospital and state board of nursing put on your practice, what rules accrediting agencies have set for your professional conduct, and what guidelines apply when your hospital says one thing and your professional organizations say another.

That's where this chapter can help. It contains the latest information on:
● malpractice
● the rule of res ipsa loquitur
● professional liability insurance—the quality and quantity you need
● statutes of limitations
● what to do if you're sued for malpractice
● how you should act if you're testifying as a defendant or an expert witness.

## Malpractice
When a patient claims in court that you were negligent or committed some other form of malpractice, he must prove specific factors. In a negligence case, for example, he has to show that:

with malpractice, his liability is vicarious, meaning that even though the doctor didn't direct you negligently, he's responsible because he was in control.

By taking on more responsibility for

- you owed him a duty based on a standard of care.
- you breached that duty.
- he was harmed.
- your breach of duty is closely and causally connected to that harm.

If he convinces a judge or jury that these allegations are true, you may have to dig deeply into your own pocket to pay damages and even a penalty.

Obviously, malpractice is more than just a little carelessness. Entry 39, "Malpractice pitfalls," explores the causes of malpractice and suggests ways to avoid it.

### Res ipsa loquitur

Suppose a patient is injured while in your unit's care, but he has no way of knowing (or proving) how the injury occurred or who's directly responsible. This can happen, for example, when a patient's injured while unconscious (during surgery, or in a coma). If such

---

*"Because you've been willing to do more, the educated consumer has come to expect more."*

---

a patient brings a lawsuit against the hospital and health team, the court may apply the rule of res ipsa loquitur. If it does, *he* won't have to prove they were negligent; *they* will have to prove they weren't. Entry 40, "Understanding the res ipsa loquitur rule," spells out the three key elements that make the rule apply, gives you hints on how best to prepare for a case where it may apply, and tells why—in several real cases—courts applied the rule.

### The importance of professional liability insurance

The professional risks you take every day can make you the target of a malpractice lawsuit. And the awards to an injured claimant can be astronomical. So the sensible way to protect yourself is with professional liability insurance. In both the United States and Canada, policies come in many shapes and sizes (types and amounts of coverage) to meet a diversity of needs. By reviewing what you do as a nurse, how you do it, and where you do it, you can get a policy tailor-made to *your* needs. Entry 41, "How good is your professional liability insurance?", tells you how to be a smart insurance shopper.

### You and your employer's professional liability insurance

Once you have a handle on the jargon of professional liability insurance, you can thoroughly scrutinize the coverage your employer provides. Does the policy give you adequate coverage? Does it cover you at all? Does it protect your employer more than it does you? Entry 42, "Does your employer's insurance protect you?", gives you guidelines to find out how (and if) your employer's professional liability insurance measures up.

### Statutes of limitations

How long is too long? In both the United States and Canada, the courts can turn a deaf ear if an injured person waits too long to file suit. Because assembling evidence for a case becomes more and more difficult as time passes, states adopted statutes limiting the length of time when a person may sue for malpractice. But in some circumstances, courts may set aside statutes of limitations. This means that you could be sued for malpractice many years after the plaintiff-patient left your care. Entry 43, "Understanding statutes of limitations," probes the issues and summarizes them for you.

### When you're named in a malpractice lawsuit

Probably no one gets a better education in how the law works than a nurse-defendant in a malpractice lawsuit. When the court gears up to hear op-

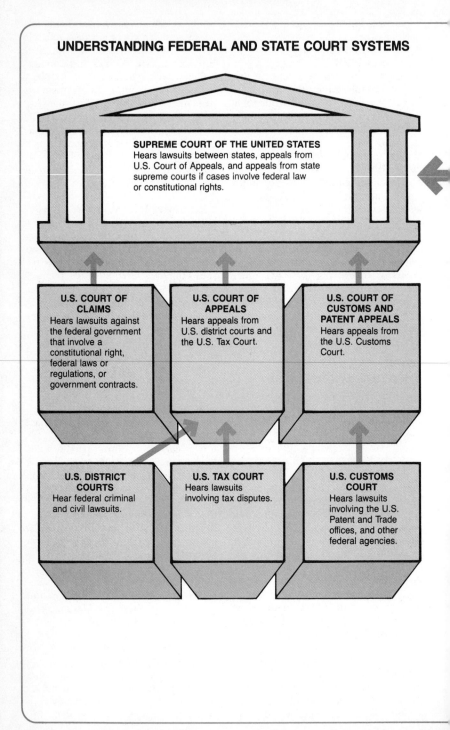

## UNDERSTANDING FEDERAL AND STATE COURT SYSTEMS

**SUPREME COURT OF THE UNITED STATES**
Hears lawsuits between states, appeals from U.S. Court of Appeals, and appeals from state supreme courts if cases involve federal law or constitutional rights.

**U.S. COURT OF CLAIMS**
Hears lawsuits against the federal government that involve a constitutional right, federal laws or regulations, or government contracts.

**U.S. COURT OF APPEALS**
Hears appeals from U.S. district courts and the U.S. Tax Court.

**U.S. COURT OF CUSTOMS AND PATENT APPEALS**
Hears appeals from the U.S. Customs Court.

**U.S. DISTRICT COURTS**
Hear federal criminal and civil lawsuits.

**U.S. TAX COURT**
Hears lawsuits involving tax disputes.

**U.S. CUSTOMS COURT**
Hears lawsuits involving the U.S. Patent and Trade offices, and other federal agencies.

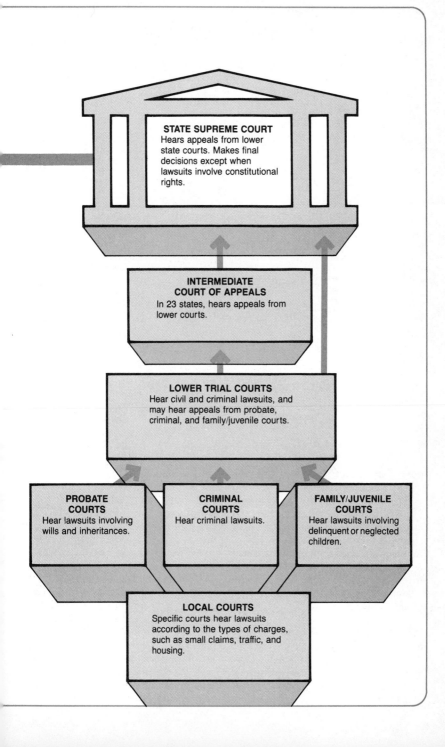

STATE SUPREME COURT
Hears appeals from lower state courts. Makes final decisions except when lawsuits involve constitutional rights.

INTERMEDIATE COURT OF APPEALS
In 23 states, hears appeals from lower courts.

LOWER TRIAL COURTS
Hear civil and criminal lawsuits, and may hear appeals from probate, criminal, and family/juvenile courts.

PROBATE COURTS
Hear lawsuits involving wills and inheritances.

CRIMINAL COURTS
Hear criminal lawsuits.

FAMILY/JUVENILE COURTS
Hear lawsuits involving delinquent or neglected children.

LOCAL COURTS
Specific courts hear lawsuits according to the types of charges, such as small claims, traffic, and housing.

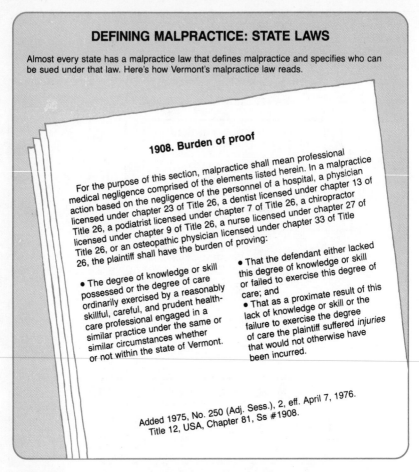

## DEFINING MALPRACTICE: STATE LAWS

Almost every state has a malpractice law that defines malpractice and specifies who can be sued under that law. Here's how Vermont's malpractice law reads.

### 1908. Burden of proof

For the purpose of this section, malpractice shall mean professional medical negligence comprised of the elements listed herein. In a malpractice action based on the negligence of the personnel of a hospital, a physician licensed under chapter 23 of Title 26, a dentist licensed under chapter 13 of Title 26, a podiatrist licensed under chapter 7 of Title 26, a chiropractor licensed under chapter 9 of Title 26, a nurse licensed under chapter 27 of Title 26, or an osteopathic physician licensed under chapter 33 of Title 26, the plaintiff shall have the burden of proving:

- The degree of knowledge or skill possessed or the degree of care ordinarily exercised by a reasonably skillful, careful, and prudent health-care professional engaged in a similar practice under the same or similar circumstances whether or not within the state of Vermont.

- That the defendant either lacked this degree of knowledge or skill or failed to exercise this degree of care; and
- That as a proximate result of this lack of knowledge or skill or the failure to exercise the degree of care the plaintiff suffered *injuries* that would not otherwise have been incurred.

Added 1975, No. 250 (Adj. Sess.), 2, eff. April 7, 1976.
Title 12, USA, Chapter 81, Ss #1908.

posing arguments, you've got to know what's going on and how to act and what to say—as well as what *not* to say.

Your attitude in the courtroom can be critical to your defense. So can your choice of an attorney: he defines your role as a defendant every bit as much as you do. Read Entry 44, "What to do if you're sued," for some no-nonsense guidelines to getting through a malpractice lawsuit.

### When you're called to testify in a malpractice lawsuit

As a defendant in a malpractice lawsuit, be prepared to present your side of the story clearly and logically. As an expert witness, be prepared to give a clear statement of your professional opinion on the proper standards of care. Entry 45, "Techniques for testifying in a malpractice lawsuit," shows you how to appear to advantage in either role.

You won't find a more compelling reason to read this chapter than *State of New Jersey v. Winter* (1982). In this criminal negligence case, a nurse was charged with administering blood of an incompatible type to a patient undergoing surgery. When she discovered her error, she attempted to cover up her negligence instead of correct her error. In the prosecution that resulted, the jury found her actions "reckless and wanton negligence... Show[ing] an utter disregard for the safety of others under circumstances likely to cause death." The jury found the nurse guilty of simple manslaughter, and the court sentenced her to 5 years in prison.

# 39 Malpractice pitfalls

As you know, nursing has changed. No one expects you to blindly follow doctors' orders anymore. Today, you're a professional in your own right. And you make your own professional decisions. Of course, you're always legally responsible for those decisions. But this needn't worry you if you consistently practice nursing according to the laws and professional standards of care that govern your practice.

Sounds pretty simple, doesn't it? But you know it isn't. You know that nursing is a much more complicated job than it used to be. Making moment-to-moment decisions about patient care is harder than ever. Under such conditions, your chances of making mistakes have increased—along with your chances of being sued for malpractice.

Can you guess why negligence is by far the largest category of nursing malpractice charges? Because negligence is *unintentional.* Nurses found liable for negligence didn't set out deliberately to commit negligent acts. They were trying to do their best for their patients, just like you. So why did they end up in court? Here's a good bet: Most of them ran afoul of malpractice pitfalls.

What are malpractice pitfalls? They're liability-producing behaviors that nurses can avoid by using caution, common sense, and heightened awareness of how the law affects nurses. Some common malpractice pitfalls are described below. (See *Understanding Tort Claims,* page 254.) Avoid them, and your chances of avoiding malpractice charges will improve.

## Discussion and documentation
Avoid being rude or disrespectful to patients or their families. Always remain calm when a patient or his family becomes difficult. Trial attorneys have a saying: "If you don't want to be sued, don't be rude."

Don't offer your opinion when a patient asks you what you think is the matter with him. If you do, you could be accused of making a medical diagnosis—practicing medicine without a license. Don't discuss possible treatments for the patient's condition, or possible choices of doctors, either.

Be careful not to discuss a patient's care or personal business with anyone except when doing so is consistent with

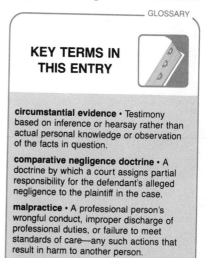

GLOSSARY

## KEY TERMS IN THIS ENTRY

**circumstantial evidence** • Testimony based on inference or hearsay rather than actual personal knowledge or observation of the facts in question.

**comparative negligence doctrine** • A doctrine by which a court assigns partial responsibility for the defendant's alleged negligence to the plaintiff in the case.

**malpractice** • A professional person's wrongful conduct, improper discharge of professional duties, or failure to meet standards of care—any such actions that result in harm to another person.

**negligence** • Failure to act as an ordinary prudent person; conduct contrary to that of a reasonable person under similar circumstances.

**res ipsa loquitur** • "The thing speaks for itself." A legal doctrine that applies when the defendant was solely and exclusively in control at the time the plaintiff's injury occurred, so that the injury would *not* have occurred if the defendant had exercised due care. When a court applies this doctrine to a case, the defendant bears the burden of proving that he wasn't negligent.

# NEGLIGENCE: WHO'S RESPONSIBLE?

Here's a test. Read these three cases. Decide for yourself who's negligent—the nurse or the doctor. Then check our answers to see how well you did.

## NEGLECTING TO SEARCH

In *Piehl v. Dallas General Hospital* (1977), Willi Piehl entered the hospital with stomach ulcers and almost left with a 14-square-inch laparotomy sponge packed around his colon. An X-ray revealed the sponge, which had to be removed through a second operation. Later, Piehl sued the doctor and the hospital—as the employer of the surgeons, the scrub nurse, and the circulating nurse assigned to his case.

Why hadn't the surgeon seen the sponge and removed it? "We take all the sponges we can see or feel," the surgeon testified. "After a pyloroplasty, we don't like to dig around and spread the infection around. If the sponge count is correct, we have no reason to believe a sponge is inside the abdominal cavity or in the wound."

Laparotomy sponges come in packages of five, witnesses at the trial testified. And the smaller 4" x 4" sponges come in packages of 10. Before surgery, the nurses count the sponges when they prepare the operating room. During surgery, the nurses routinely lay the used sponges out and count them, together with the unused sponges, in units of 5 for the laparotomy sponges and in units of 10 for the 4" x 4" sponges. They do this twice—before and after the patient's abdomen is closed.

Piehl's nurses said the count checked out and they noted this in the medical record. Still, a sponge showed up on Piehl's X-ray.

**Who was responsible?**

**ANSWER**
The court concluded that apparently the nurses had miscounted the sponges, but it found the surgeon and his employer, the hospital, guilty. Its reasoning? "Even a summary poking around for all the sponges, in the exercise of ordinary care, would have resulted in the discovery of something the size of a laparotomy sponge. And no emergency made time a critical factor."

## NO-SHOW DOCTOR

In *Taylor v. Baptist Medical Center, Inc.* (1981), Robin Taylor was 26 weeks pregnant when she told her obstetrician that labor pains had started. He told her to go to the hospital. The time was 3 a.m.

At the hospital, two experienced obstetric nurses attended Mrs. Taylor. They called the obstetrician several times during the next 8 hours, and each time he said he'd be right over. At 11:30 a.m., Mrs. Taylor gave birth to a stillborn premature infant—10 minutes before the obstetrician arrived.

Mrs. Taylor sued the hospital for failing to provide another doctor or a competent medical attendant, and she sued her obstetrician for failing to care for her during labor and delivery.

**Were both the hospital and doctor negligent?**

**ANSWER**
The court found the hospital innocent. The nurses had fulfilled their duty by keeping the obstetrician informed, the court said, and they had no reason to doubt his assurance that he'd "be right over." Furthermore, the two nurses who'd attended Mrs. Taylor were well qualified and provided Mrs. Taylor with skillful and diligent care.

But the court found the doctor liable. His failure to attend his patient constituted a breach of contract, and Mrs. Taylor had a right to recover damages.

proper nursing care (see Entry 14).

Document every verbal order thoroughly, and obtain a corresponding signed order from the doctor as soon as possible. (See Entries 18 and 23.)

Never sign your name as a witness without fully understanding what you're signing *and* the legal significance of your signature (see Entry 20).

Don't ever correct or revise a patient's medical record—particularly after he's filed a lawsuit. (See Entries 36 and 37.) The case of *Carr v. St. Paul Fire and Marine Insurance Company* (1974) illustrates the liability a hospital may have when nurses or other employees alter or destroy patient records. The patient in this case was a man who came to the hospital emergency department (ED) suffering severe pain. One of the nurses on duty refused to call a doctor for the patient, so he returned home—and died a short time later. The nurses who'd been on duty in the ED that night testified they'd taken the patient's vital signs—but this couldn't be proved or disproved, because the patient's records had been destroyed. In instructing the jury, the judge indicated that they could find the hospital negligent.

## Doctors' orders

Never treat any patient without orders from his doctor (except in an emergency, of course). And don't dispense any medication. Only doctors and pharmacists may legally perform these functions. (See Entries 5 and 23.) Don't carry out any order from a doctor, *particularly a medication order*, if you have any doubt about its accuracy or appropriateness. Don't carry out *any* order you don't fully understand (see *Protecting Yourself: Always Question These Orders*, page 255).

In *Norton v. Argonaut Insurance Company* (1962), a hospital's assistant director of nursing services temporarily covered a pediatric unit when the charge nurse's help was needed in an emergency. She did question a seemingly high dosage of injectable digoxin

---

## FAILURE TO REPORT

The case of *Kolakowski v. Voris* (1979) involved Edward Kolakowski, who'd undergone a diskectomy. Several hours later, he told his nurses that he couldn't bend his left leg and that his right side was weak and numb. They noted the complaints. And noted them again 1 hour later, 2 hours later, and 4 hours later. One of the nurses called the neurosurgeon but couldn't locate him.

Kolakowski's neurosurgeon saw him the next day and attributed his poor movement and sensation to spinal cord edema. Two days later, a myelogram showed spinal cord compression, and Kolakowski was taken back to the operating room, where the surgeon removed extruded bits of disk and performed a laminectomy. The operation left Kolakowski a quadriplegic.

Kolakowski sued the doctor and the hospital. Hospital attorneys pointed out that Kolakowski's doctor didn't act immediately, even after a day's delay, so the nurses and their employer—the hospital—were not negligent despite the nurses' delay in contacting the doctor. The attorneys asked the courts to drop the lawsuit against the hospital.

---

**Were the hospital attorneys right?**

---

**ANSWER**
Refusing to drop the hospital from the lawsuit, the court held that Kolakowski's nurses should have known his signs and symptoms were unusual and demanded immediate attention. Thus, they had a duty to relate those signs and symptoms to a doctor immediately. *When* the doctor decided to treat the signs and symptoms had no bearing on the nurses' responsibility, the court ruled.

## UNDERSTANDING TORT CLAIMS

Like all health-care professionals, you're vulnerable to lawsuits. If a patient feels your nursing care is inappropriate, he might well file a lawsuit claiming one of six torts. The law classifies each of those six torts as either an intentional tort—a direct invasion of someone's legal right—or an unintentional tort—a civil wrong from the defendant's negligence. This chart shows you both intentional and unintentional torts and examples of improper nursing actions that could lead a patient to use each claim in a lawsuit.

| TORT CLAIMS | IMPROPER NURSING ACTION |
|---|---|
| **UNINTENTIONAL TORT** | |
| **Negligence** | • Leaving foreign objects inside a patient following surgery<br>• Failing to observe an ICU patient as the doctor ordered<br>• Failing to ensure a patient's informed consent<br>• Failing to report a change in a patient's vital signs<br>• Failing to report a staff member's negligence that you witnessed |
| **INTENTIONAL TORTS** | |
| **Assault** | • Threatening a patient |
| **Battery** | • Forcing a patient to ambulate without his consent<br>• Forcing a patient to submit to injections |
| **False imprisonment** | • Confining a patient in a psychiatric unit without a doctor's order<br>• Refusing to let a patient return home |
| **Invasion of privacy** | • Releasing private information about a patient to newspaper reporters<br>• Allowing unauthorized persons to read a patient's medical records<br>• Allowing unauthorized persons to observe a procedure<br>• Taking pictures of the patient without his consent |
| **Slander** | • Making false accusations about a patient in front of newspaper reporters |

ordered for a 3-month-old infant, but she accepted 2 attending doctors' mistaken endorsements of the order. (They thought she was referring to an *oral* dosage.) In fact, the dosage ordered was an overdose for injectable digoxin. The nurse administered the medication as ordered and the child died. The nurse, the doctor who originally ordered the medication, and the hospital were found liable.

**Patient precautions**

Don't participate in a surgical procedure unless you're satisfied the patient has given proper informed consent (see Entry 12). Never force a patient to accept treatment he's expressly refused (see Entry 13). And of course, if you're a surgical nurse, *always* check and double-check that no foreign objects (sponges, pins) remain inside the patient after an operation is completed.

(See *Negligence: Who's Responsible?* pages 252-253.)

Don't use any patient-care equipment you're not familiar with or not trained to use (see Entry 22).

Take every precaution to prevent patient falls. (See *Preventing Patient Falls*, page 140.) This is a very common area of nursing liability. Patients who are elderly, infirm, sedated, or mentally incapacitated are the most likely to fall (see Entry 22).

---

## PROTECTING YOURSELF: ALWAYS QUESTION THESE ORDERS

Do you always assume the doctor is right, and follow his orders even if they seem vague or medically inappropriate? If you do, you could be jeopardizing your nursing career. Your responsibility as a nurse is to question *any* dubious order you receive. Some types of orders may actually be detrimental to your patient's health—and legally dangerous for you.

Here are four types of orders you must always question:

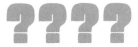

### • AMBIGUOUS ORDERS

Follow your hospital's policy for clarifying ambiguous orders—orders that are vague or have more than one possible interpretation—and document your actions. If your hospital doesn't have a policy covering this situation, contact the prescribing doctor and (as always) document your actions (see "Telephone Orders," below). Then ask your nursing administration for a step-by-step policy to follow in this situation.

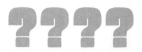

### • ANY ORDER A PATIENT QUESTIONS

A doctor can change his orders at any time, including while you're off duty. So a patient may know something about his prescribed care that no one has told *you*. If a patient protests a procedure, medication dosage, or medication route—saying that it's different from "the usual," or that it's been changed—give him the benefit of the doubt. Question the doctor's orders, following your hospital's policy if one exists.

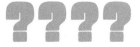

### • INAPPROPRIATE ORDERS

A change in your patient's condition may mean that a standing order is no longer appropriate. When this occurs, delay the treatment until you've contacted the doctor and clarified the situation. Follow your hospital's policy for clarifying the order.

*Note: If you're an inexperienced nurse, you should take steps to clarify all standing orders. Contact the prescribing doctor for guidance. Or tell your supervisor you're uncertain about following the order, and let her decide whether to delegate the responsibility to a more experienced nurse.*

If, after you carry out the order, the treatment is affecting the patient adversely, discontinue it. Then report all the unfavorable signs and symptoms to the patient's doctor. *Resume treatment only after you've discussed the situation with the doctor and clarified his orders.*

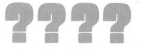

### • TELEPHONE ORDERS

Whenever a doctor gives you an order by telephone, be sure to document all the details. Follow your hospital's policy to the letter. If your hospital has no formal policy, document your conversation and subsequent actions using the following guidelines:
• Write down the time of the call, the date, and the doctor's name; describe the patient's condition and other circumstances that prompted the call.
• Review the patient's condition in detail with the doctor.
• Write down his orders as you listen.
• Read the orders back to him to be sure you've recorded them accurately.
• Document that you've read the orders back and that the doctor confirmed them.

The case of *Stevenson v. Alta Bates* (1937) involved a patient who'd had a stroke and was learning to walk again. As two nurses, each holding one of the patient's arms, assisted her into the hospital's sun-room, one of the nurses let go of the patient and stepped forward to get a chair for her. The patient fell and sustained a fracture. The nurse was found liable: the court stated she should have anticipated the patient's need for a chair, and made the appropriate arrangements, *before* bringing the patient into the sun-room.

## A final word

Here's a malpractice pitfall that can make any of the others much worse: failure to carry adequate professional liability insurance (see Entry 41). This is the Ultimate Pitfall. Remember, if you're ever sued and found liable for damages, your insurance may be all that stands between you and serious financial hardship.

Of course, your constant objective as a nurse is to provide the best possible patient care. Worrying about possible malpractice lawsuits won't help you do this. Instead, use your knowledge of malpractice pitfalls constructively. How? By giving your nursing care with conscious intent to avoid malpractice pitfalls. Doing this will help ensure that your care always meets legal and professional standards.

---

# 40 Understanding the res ipsa loquitur rule

The Latin phrase *res ipsa loquitur* literally means, "The thing speaks for itself." Res ipsa loquitur is a rule of evidence designed to equalize the plaintiff's and the defendant's positions before the court, when otherwise the plaintiff would be at a disadvantage in proving his case—a disadvantage not

of his own making. (Res ipsa loquitur *doesn't* apply when a plaintiff simply fails to prove his case.) Essentially, the rule of res ipsa loquitur allows a plaintiff to prove negligence by circumstantial evidence, when the defendant has the primary—sometimes the only—knowledge of what happened to cause the plaintiff's injury.

The res ipsa loquitur rule derives from a 19th century English case, *Byrne v. Boadle* (1863). In this case, the injured person had been struck by a flour barrel that fell from a second-floor window of a warehouse. In the ensuing lawsuit, the plaintiff wasn't able to show which warehouse employee had been negligent in allowing the barrel to fall. The court applied the concept of res ipsa loquitur to the warehouse owners, who were found liable in the absence of proof that the employees *weren't* responsible for the plaintiff's injury.

## What does this rule mean to you, as a nurse?

Res ipsa loquitur is applied only in malpractice cases involving alleged negligence. As you probably know, in most medical malpractice cases, the plaintiff has the responsibility for proving every element of his case against the defendant; until he does, the court presumes that the defendant met the applicable standard of care. But when a court applies the res ipsa loquitur rule, the burden of proof shifts from the plaintiff to the defendant, who must attempt to prove that the plaintiff's injury was caused by something other than his, the defendant's, negligence.

Obviously, this unusual legal situation must be applicable only in special circumstances. Do you know what they are?

Suppose you're a defendant in a typical malpractice lawsuit. The plaintiff-patient, through his attorney, alleges that you were professionally negligent. Ordinarily his attorney has the responsibility of proving, by a preponderance of the evidence, that you failed to meet an applicable standard of care. But if the plaintiff-patient's attorney can show that three key elements were present when you allegedly harmed the plaintiff, he can ask the court to invoke the rule of res ipsa loquitur. If the court grants this request, then you and your attorney must prove you *weren't* negligent.

The three key elements are:
- The act that caused the plaintiff's injury was exclusively in your control.
- His injury wouldn't have happened in the absence of your negligence.
- No negligence on the plaintiff's part contributed to his injury.

The following case, *Sanchez v. Bay General Hospital* (1981), illustrates typical circumstances in which courts invoke the res ipsa loquitur rule.

In February, 1975, Mrs. Sanchez entered Bay General Hospital for elective surgery—a laminectomy. Following the surgery, the surgeon implanted an atrial catheter to minimize the chance that an air embolism would form in her heart.

When Mrs. Sanchez was transferred to the post-operative ward, her condition began to deteriorate. The nurses there made several initial errors:
- They didn't examine the patient's chart, so they weren't aware that the catheter had been put in place.
- They neglected to perform a neurologic examination.
- They didn't notify a doctor of her deteriorating vital signs.

Eventually, Mrs. Sanchez went into cardiac arrest, and an emergency department doctor ordered immediate administration of medication. The nurses then made the error that sealed Mrs. Sanchez's fate: They mistook the atrial catheter for an I.V. line and administered the medication through it. The medication went directly to Mrs. Sanchez's heart, causing brain death a few hours later. The children of Mrs. Sanchez later sued the hospital for the wrongful death of their mother.

The court, invoking the res ipsa loquitur rule, granted a directed verdict

to the children of Mrs. Sanchez. The court indicated that the hospital had the burden of proving that Mrs. Sanchez's death was caused by something other than the staff's negligence—or, alternatively, that she died even though the staff had given due care to prevent her death. The hospital was unable to refute the court's presumption of negligence. The hospital appealed the directed verdict, but the appellate court sustained the trial court's judgment in favor of Mrs. Sanchez's children.

Courts have been more willing to apply the res ipsa loquitur rule in cases where the defendant was the only one in a position to know what caused the injury, and when the patient knew nothing. Courts *won't* apply the rule when the evidence offered by the defendant explains all the facts of the injury and its cause.

## What other types of cases invite a res ipsa loquitur ruling?

Perhaps the most common case associated with the res ipsa loquitur rule is the so-called foreign-object case. In such a case, the plaintiff alleges that a foreign object—for example, a sponge, a needle, or a pin—was left inside him after surgery.

Courts have also been willing to invoke the res ipsa loquitur rule because of injuries to plaintiffs involving body parts completely unrelated to the plaintiffs' surgery.

Take the Wisconsin malpractice case, *Beaudoin v. Watertown Memorial Hospital* (1966). A patient suffered second-degree burns on the buttocks during vaginal surgery. She brought suit, claiming negligence. The court upheld her attorney's right to request application of the res ipsa loquitur rule on the basis that injury to an area unrelated to surgery results from failure to exercise due care.

## Critics and defenders of the res ipsa loquitur rule

Critics of the rule feel the courts have been too free in letting plaintiffs use it. They call it "the rule of sympathy" and contend that, by invoking it, the plaintiff can quickly catch the sympathetic ears of judge and jury. Health-care professionals particularly contend that the rule puts them at an unfair disadvantage as defendants. They feel that, by making them shoulder the burden of proof, the rule singles them out for more negligence liability than other

---

*"Critics of res ipsa loquitur call it 'the rule of sympathy'."*

---

types of defendants face. Also, invoking the rule usually eliminates the plaintiff's responsibility to introduce expert testimony. Defenders of the rule feel its value lies in drawing the court's attention to the fact that a plaintiff's unusual or rare injury is itself sufficient to cause suspicion that the defendant was negligent.

## How courts in different states apply the rule

In some states, courts cannot apply the res ipsa loquitur rule. Most states, however, do allow courts to apply some form of it. For example, neither Michigan nor South Carolina applies the rule by name but each does apply the rule of circumstantial evidence of negligence, which is the same concept. Until recently, Pennsylvania rejected the rule outright. But in *Gilbert v. Korvette, Inc.* (1974), it adopted the Restatement of Torts, the evidentiary rule of res ipsa loquitur.

## How courts in Canada apply the rule

The Canadian courts formerly applied the rule of res ipsa loquitur infrequently in medical malpractice cases. In most such cases, the courts based their decisions on the "ordinary medical experience of mankind."

Then, in *Holt v. Nesbitt* (1953) and again in *Cardin v. City of Montreal* (1961), the Supreme Court of Canada clearly stated that the rule of res ipsa loquitur applied in malpractice cases. In *Holt v. Nesbitt*, the plaintiff was a patient of the defendant, an oral surgeon. While the plaintiff was under general anesthesia, a sponge lodged in his windpipe, causing death by suffocation. The court decided that failure to invoke res ipsa loquitur would give the health-care practitioner unfair—and therefore unwarranted—protection in a malpractice lawsuit. In effect, the court put the patient's protection from bad medical practice above the health-care practitioner's protection from a difficult malpractice lawsuit.

The Canadian courts progress slowly in mediating malpractice lawsuits. That's because differences in expert opinion are the rule, not the exception, and because many lawsuits present issues not previously resolved. The Canadian courts do, however, seem to want to make sure that the rule doesn't place too heavy a burden on the defendant.

## A final word

Find out whether you're currently working in a state that doesn't apply the res ipsa loquitur rule. If you are, and you're ever sued, at least you won't have to prove you weren't negligent. Many states are expanding their applications of the rule, so stay informed about the status of the rule in your state. Your professional nursing organizations and the nursing literature should help keep you posted.

# 41 How good is your professional liability insurance?

Consider this scenario: You're a surgical nurse responsible for the instrument count in an operating room. During a major surgical procedure on a grossly overweight patient, you hand over various instruments to the surgeon, including an Ochsner clamp (a 9″-long hemostat). After the last suture, you sign off your instrument count list, verifying that all the instruments are present and accounted for. But that Ochsner clamp—it wasn't withdrawn; it remains in the patient's abdominal cavity for 11 months before anyone discovers it. During that time it has rusted, perforated the patient's colon, and caused adhesions.

The patient sues the hospital for malpractice and names you as a defendant for making an incorrect instrument count.

You claim that the surgeon—as "captain of the ship"—had ultimate responsibility; he counters that he's only as competent as those who work with him.

What do you do? Your career and all of the tangible benefits you've worked a lifetime for are now in jeopardy. And the situation could get worse. Consider this: The jury awards the plaintiff a

GLOSSARY

## KEY TERMS IN THIS ENTRY

**"captain of the ship" doctrine** • A legal doctrine that considers a surgeon responsible for the actions of his assistants when those assistants are under the surgeon's supervision. This doctrine is similar to the borrowed-servant doctrine.

**damages** • An amount of money a court orders a defendant to pay the plaintiff, in deciding the case in favor of the plaintiff.

**liability** • Legal responsibility for *failure to act*, so causing harm to another person, or for *actions* that fail to meet standards of care, so causing harm to another person.

**malpractice** • A professional person's wrongful conduct, improper discharge of professional duties, or failure to meet standards of care—any such actions that result in harm to another person.

**professional liability insurance** • A type of liability insurance that protects professional persons against malpractice claims made against them.

million dollars in damages. Cases like this are not unusual. Nurses are being named in malpractice lawsuits more and more frequently. Someday it could happen to you.

Because you're vulnerable, you need professional liability insurance. Insurance for nurses isn't new. What *is* new is that your expanded health-care role makes having insurance crucial. You're at risk, especially if you work in a specialized setting, such as an intensive care unit.

Unfortunately, some nurses are skeptical; they believe that purchasing professional liability insurance makes them a more attractive target for compensation claims and increases their chances of being sued. This is dangerous thinking. Given the legal risks you face on the job, you simply can't afford to be without insurance.

## Buying financial protection

What do you get when you buy professional liability insurance? You get protection for a designated period from the financial consequences of certain professional errors. The type of insurance policy you buy defines the amount that the insurance company will pay if the judgment goes against you in a malpractice lawsuit.

You can buy a policy designated as "single limits" or "double limits." In a single-limits policy, you buy protection in set dollar increments, for example, $100,000, $300,000, or $1,000,000. The stipulated amount will shield you if a judgment goes against you.

In the less common double-limits policy, you buy protection in a combination package, such as $100,000/$300,000, $300,000/$500,000, or $1,000,000/$3,000,000. In a double-

---

*"If the insured nurse has a policy limit of $1 million, her own assets probably will never be at risk."*

---

limits policy, the sums are what your insurance company will make available to protect you if more than one patient sues you for the same alleged error. This happens, for instance, when a nurse administers the wrong medication to several patients. While the single-limits policy will protect you against injuries to more than one patient, the double-limits policy makes considerably more money available to protect you when you're involved in multiple lawsuits.

What if a judgment against you exceeds the policy limits? This is called an *excess judgment* for which you're personally responsible. Depending on the laws in your state, almost everything you own, except for a limited portion of your equity in your home and the clothes on your back, may be taken

to satisfy the uninsured portion of a judgment.

Contrast the uninsured nurse with the nurse who had the foresight to protect herself with adequate professional liability coverage. If the insured nurse has a policy limit of $1 million, her own assets probably will never be at risk.

But how can a nurse afford $1 million worth of insurance? You'll be relieved to know that premiums for insurance coverage of, say, $1 million are not much greater than they are for insurance with a relatively small limit. That's because a substantial part of the premium goes toward the insurance company's willingness to assume the risk in the first place; higher limits don't increase the premium proportionately. You may be surprised at how reasonably a medical-surgical nurse can buy professional liability insurance at group rates. Even for critical care nurses, the American Association of Critical Care Nurses has generous and reasonably priced coverage. (See *Choosing Professional Liability Coverage That's Right for You.*)

## Types of professional liability insurance protection

Professional liability insurance can protect you at the time a patient claims the malpractice occurred (occurrence policy) or when he brings a lawsuit for damages (claims-made policy).

An occurrence policy protects you against an error of omission or commission occurring during a policy period, regardless of when, after the policy ends, the patient makes a claim against you.

The claims-made policy protects you only against claims made against you during the policy period. A claims-made policy is cheaper than an occurrence policy because the insurance company is at risk only for the duration of the policy. However, you can purchase an extended-reporting endorsement, or tail coverage, which in effect turns your claims-made policy into an occurrence policy.

## What does the insurer owe you?

Professional liability insurance supplies you with more than just financial protection. The insurance company also owes you a legal defense and must provide attorneys to represent you for the entire course of litigation. Since insurance companies aren't in business to lose money, they retain highly experienced attorneys with considerable experience in malpractice lawsuits.

When they prepare your defense, they'll secure research on the subject of the lawsuit; obtain expert witnesses; handle motions throughout the case; and prepare medical models, transparencies, and photographs. Your insurance company will pay for preparing such a defense.

During litigation—and indeed even before a lawsuit is actually filed in court—your insurance company actively strives for a settlement with the patient's attorneys, to save time and money. This may not be in your best interests, however. In the United States, if you believe your professional reputation is at stake, you may be able to refuse to agree to an out-of-court settlement. If your policy contains a threshold limit—a stated amount of money—your insurer can't settle a case out of court without your permission. Without a threshold limit, your insurer has total control over out-of-court settlements.

If the lawsuit against you goes to court, the insurer has the right to control how the defense is conducted. The insurer's attorney makes all the decisions regarding the case's legal tactics and strategy.

Of course, you have a right to be kept advised of every step of the case. Most insurers will keep you informed because the insurer knows that:
- A successful defense depends in part on the defendant's cooperation.
- You can sue the insurer if it fails to provide a competent defense.

If you lose a lawsuit, the insurance company will cover you for whatever the jury awards in general and special

---

### CHOOSING PROFESSIONAL LIABILITY COVERAGE THAT'S RIGHT FOR YOU

As you probably know, all professional liability insurance policies aren't the same. To find one with the liability coverage that fits your needs, compare the features each policy offers. Does the policy cover claims made *before* the policy expires (claims-made coverage), or does the policy cover negligent acts committed during the policy period, regardless of when the claim is made (occurrence coverage)?

Also, check for these options:

- coverage when nurses under your supervision are negligent
- coverage for misuse of equipment
- coverage for errors in reporting or recording care
- coverage for failure to properly teach patients
- coverage for errors in administering medication
- coverage in case the hospital sues you
- coverage for professional services you perform in an emergency outside your employment setting.

---

damages. In the United States, the jury awards general damages to relieve:
- pain and suffering
- worsening change in life-style
- present and future medical expenses
- past and future loss of earnings
- decreased earning capacity.

In Canada, the jury awards damages similarly, except that the Canadian courts consider decreased earning capacity to be part of general, not special, damages.

Whether you practice in the United States or in Canada, your insurance company will not cover you for punitive damages. These are damages the jury awards in a civil case usually involving malicious conduct. They're meant to punish the defendant without sending him to prison.

# ENSURING PROTECTION EVEN AFTER YOUR POLICY EXPIRES

*I'm afraid I'm in hot water. I had malpractice insurance for the 5 years I was practicing nursing full time. When I took a year's maternity leave, I let my policy lapse, thinking I'd renew it when I returned to work. During my leave, I found out that a patient I'd cared for 2 years before was threatening to sue the hospital and me for negligent care.*

*I immediately called my insurance agent. He told me that he couldn't help me because I had a "claims-made" policy. This means that even though I was covered by the policy when I cared for the patient, I'm not covered now—because the claim was made after the policy expired.*

*My insurance policy had always been my security blanket. Now, I'm scared. What can I do?—RN, Mich.*

First of all, the patient is only threatening to sue. He may not actually file a lawsuit. And even if he does, the hospital attorneys may be able to make a settlement with him before the case goes to court. (About 80% of all malpractice cases are settled before a trial.)

If the case does go to court and the patient wins, the hospital's insurance coverage may be sufficient to settle the claim.

You're right to be concerned, though. If you lose the case and, under the respondeat superior doctrine the hospital insurance carrier makes a settlement with the patient, the hospital can turn around and sue you for the amount of the settlement. (Providing, of course, that it wasn't actually found liable.) If you have no money, the hospital can deduct from your paycheck. The prospect of years of indebtedness to your employer is frightening indeed, although this seems unlikely from the details you've described.

By all means, when you renew your insurance policy, make sure it's an "occurrence" policy. An "occurrence" policy provides the broadest protection available— it ensures coverage anytime in the future as long as the policy was in force when the incident occurred. Without a doubt, this would be your best security blanket.

*This letter was taken from the files of Nursing magazine.*

Many states are taking steps to decrease malpractice litigation. One widely accepted way is by imposing a statute of limitations, which limits the amount of time a person has to file a lawsuit (see Entry 43). Some states have imposed a maximum limit on how much a jury can award in general damages. This restriction, however, is legally questionable and has been challenged in court as being unconstitutional. Medical associations and insurance companies are also trying to limit malpractice lawsuits, in two ways: by forcing them into arbitration—thus removing them from the province of laymen juries—and by requiring that they be screened by a medical malpractice screening panel. If the panel decides the plaintiff's claim isn't valid, the plaintiff can't file suit unless he posts a bond to cover his defense costs in advance. More than half the states have set up screening panels, although the panels have been criticized by consumer groups and plaintiffs' attorneys and challenged in court as being unconstitutional.

## Indemnification: Who gets it and why

If several insurance companies are representing different parties in a malpractice lawsuit, they'll typically file counteractions against the other parties; what they're seeking, of course, is compensation, that is, indemnification, for all or part of any damages the jury awards. Such cross-suits are common. Let's return to the example cited at the start of this entry. The patient would have sued these parties: the hospital, the surgeon, the assisting surgeon, the anesthesiologist, and any nurse who assisted at the actual operation. Many states now permit damages to be apportioned among multiple defendants, the extent of liability depending on the jury's determination of each defendant's relative contribution to the harm done. For example, suppose you were the nurse responsible for the instrument count and the court held you 75% liable. Your insurance company would pay 75% of the total award. The other insurance companies would be held liable for the remaining 25%, based on the percentage of harm attributed to each remaining defendant. However, if one of the codefendants, say the surgeon, decided that he'd been judged negligent only because of your negligence, he could instruct his insurance attorneys to file a new, separate lawsuit in his name against you.

Suppose you had more than one insurance policy that applied to this patient's claim. For example, you might have malpractice coverage through the hospital where you work and a professional organization you belong to, as well as your own insurance policy. All three insurance companies might well be involved. Who pays how much? That depends on several issues too complex to discuss here. What's important is that you make sure you promptly notify *every* insurance company you have a policy with that you're the target of a malpractice lawsuit. This will prevent any of the companies from using the "policy defense" of lack of notice or late notice. (See Entry 44.)

### Where do you go for insurance?
Insurance companies are numerous and offer a multiplicity of insurance policies. If possible, choose an agent who has experience handling professional liability insurance. If you don't know how to find one, call your local nursing organization. Someone there should be able to give you leads on qualified insurance representatives.

## Applying for professional liability insurance
In applying for professional liability insurance, you have to be meticulous in describing your practice. You can secure insurance protection for virtually every aspect of nursing, so the more precise you are about your responsibilities, the more your policy will be tailor-made to your needs. You can get a policy that covers you in specific areas to supplement a general policy that your hospital or clinic has already provided for you. Or you can get a policy that covers you over and above the coverage you already have, such as a group policy offered by a professional organization.

Such organizations offer group plans at attractive premiums. You'll still want to review the extent of that coverage with *your* insurance agent to make sure it's adequate for your needs. This way you'll avoid duplicating insurance protection and be able to fill any holes in the protection you already have.

### A final word
What do your insurance policy dollars buy you? In a few words, "peace of mind."

At present, most states don't require you to carry professional liability insurance. But someday all states may do just that. Don't wait until it becomes law in your state. You need professional liability insurance now.

# 42 Does your employer's insurance protect you?

If a patient sues you, will your employer's professional liability insurance protect your professional and financial interests? You have a critical

## KEY TERMS IN THIS ENTRY

**damages** • An amount of money a court orders the defendant in a case to pay the plaintiff, in deciding the case in favor of the plaintiff.

**malpractice** • A professional person's wrongful conduct, improper discharge of professional duties, or failure to meet standards of care—any such actions that result in harm to another person.

**professional liability insurance** • A type of liability insurance that protects professional persons against malpractice claims made against them.

**respondeat superior** • "Let the master answer." A legal doctrine that makes an employer liable for the consequences of his employee's wrongful conduct while the employee is acting within the scope of his employment.

stake in knowing the answer to that question, because you can't afford not to have professional liability protection. Of course, most health-care analysts believe you should have your own professional liability insurance as well (see Entry 41). But you can't wisely assess your own insurance needs until you determine how much coverage your employer's insurance gives you.

## Seeing the need for insurance protection

Health-care institutions such as hospitals aren't required to have malpractice insurance, but virtually all of them do. Why? Because an institution is usually liable for an employee's mistakes. And liability imposes the obligation of paying financial damages to injured patients. Without professional liability insurance, your employer would have to pay damages awarded to a patient out of the institution's funds. This, of course, could bankrupt the institution.

What makes your employer liable for your actions? A legal principle called

respondeat superior. The principle means that when you negligently cause injury to a patient while acting within the course and scope of your job, your employer is liable for the damages. The principle applies to all professions, not just to health care. For example, a utility company is liable for injuries that result if one of its on-duty truck drivers runs into a pedestrian.

## Checking a policy's terms and exclusions

Insurance companies that provide professional liability coverage for hospitals and other health-care institutions reduce the risk they assume with that coverage in several ways. One way is by always stipulating a precise coverage period, typically one year. Another way is by carefully defining the type of coverage they'll provide—whether, for example, it's an occurrence or claims-made policy. A third way is by putting exclusions in malpractice policies. These exclusions vary considerably from policy to policy, but all stipulate specific acts, situations, or personnel that the insurance won't cover. For example, most policies won't cover court-ordered punitive damages—money a defendant must pay as punishment for injuring a patient. (Don't confuse this with compensatory damages—the amount the jury decides actually covers the loss or harm—which the policy *will* cover.)

## How an insurer can deny coverage

Besides exclusions, insurers can use other circumstances to deny coverage to you or your employer, such as:

• The insurance policy lapses because your employer failed to pay the premiums.

• Your employer refuses to cooperate with the insurance company, for whatever reason.

• The insurer discovers that your employer made misstatements on the insurance application.

In some malpractice situations, an

insurer could agree to provide you with a defense but refuse to pay damages awarded to a patient. The insurer agrees to defend you in this situation because he doesn't want to be accused of breach of contract. But he must notify you of his intention not to pay damages in a reservation-of-rights letter. This letter informs you and your employer that the insurer believes the case falls outside what's covered by the insurance policy. When your employer and the insurer disagree about whether insurance coverage exists, the dispute may have to be resolved through separate legal action in court. Similarly,

## RESPONDEAT SUPERIOR

If a nurse commits a negligent act and a patient sues her, she's not the only one in legal hot water. The patient may also sue the nurse's employer. According to the doctrine of respondeat superior, the employer—hospital, agency, institution, or doctor—is also liable for the nurse's negligence. Why? Because as long as the nurse is considered an employee, her employer is responsible for her actions.

Take, for example, *Crowe v. Provost* (1963): A mother returned with her child to her pediatrician's office one afternoon after having been there earlier that morning. The mother was frantic. She said her child was convulsing. The doctor was out at lunch, so the office nurse briefly examined the child. Then she called the doctor to

report the child's condition. She told the doctor that she didn't feel the child's condition had changed since he had examined her and that he didn't need to rush back. The nurse then left the office while the mother and child waited for the doctor to return.

Shortly after the nurse left, the child vomited violently, stopped breathing, and died before the receptionist could contact the doctor. The mother filed negligence charges against the nurse. At the trial, the court found the nurse's negligence was indeed the proximate cause of the child's death. However, the doctor was also liable, according to the doctrine of respondeat superior, since the nurse was working as the doctor's employee.

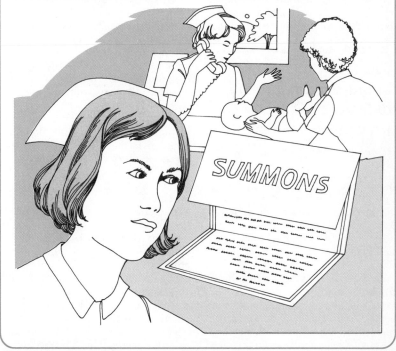

you have the right to bring such action against your employer's insurance company if they refuse to cover you.

## Assessing the limits of a policy

Each professional liability insurance policy has a maximum dollar coverage limit. Your employer can purchase coverage that exceeds the basic limit, and many hospitals do so for extra protection.

Most hospitals also have a deductible provision that makes the employer responsible for damages under a certain figure. The higher the deductible limit, the lower the premium charged by the insurer.

You should pay careful attention to the deductible limit because your employer can settle a claim against you under that figure without ever consulting you or the insurer. Because you won't have a chance to defend yourself and because many people interpret a settlement as an admission of guilt, such an action could tarnish your professional reputation. A tarnished reputation in turn could jeopardize your ability to get your own profes-

---

> *"Most health-care institutions demand having control over when an insurer can settle a case."*

---

sional liability insurance or to get a new job. To minimize this problem, maintain close contact with your employer's legal staff if you're sued, and insist on being informed about each step in the case.

## Why hospitals want a threshold limit

Most health-care institutions demand having control over when an insurer can settle a case. To gain this control, the employer normally sets a threshold limit—usually $3,000. The insurer can settle a case below the threshold without the employer's permission. But to settle a case above the threshold, the insurer must get the employer's permission. Why does the employer want the threshold? To protect its reputation for safety and quality care—the same reason you have for not wanting your insurance provider to settle a lawsuit against you without informing you. If an insurer were allowed to settle cases behind an employer's back, the employer could become more prone to malpractice lawsuits as its reputation sinks.

## How your employer provides for your defense

If you're sued and your employer's insurance covers you, what protection will you get? The insurer has a duty to provide a complete defense, including assigning an attorney to handle the entire case. The insurer will pay the attorney fees as well as any investigation costs and expert witness fees.

The attorney will provide you with an opportunity to confer with him and give your side of the story. If your employer grants written consent to settle the case, the insurer may do so, or it may decide to try the case in court if its legal advisors overrule the employer.

If the plaintiff wins the lawsuit, the insurer is obliged to pay damages awarded to the patient up to the insurance policy's coverage limit.

## Understanding how indemnity works

Can a hospital or another nurse who's been sued claim, in turn, that you're partly or wholly responsible for the patient's injury? Yes. The numbers of such cross-action suits—called indemnification suits—are rising dramatically. Your own hospital, a fellow nurse, or a lab technician—as long as each has individual professional liability insurance—can file an indemnification suit against you even though you're all covered by the same hospital insurance policy. This possibility strengthens the argument for having your own professional liability insurance.

### A final word

Don't assume you're adequately protected if you're covered under your employer's professional liability insurance policy. You have a right to know exactly how your employer's insurance covers you. To find out, get a copy of the insurance policy from your employer and let your own professional liability insurance agent review it. Your agent—usually without a fee—will welcome the chance to determine the extent, limits, and exclusions of your employer's insurance coverage for you. Taking the time to find out how well your employer's insurance protects you could be one of the most legally astute moves you make.

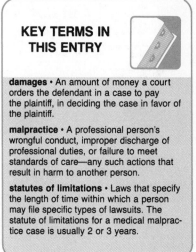

## KEY TERMS IN THIS ENTRY

**damages** • An amount of money a court orders the defendant in a case to pay the plaintiff, in deciding the case in favor of the plaintiff.

**malpractice** • A professional person's wrongful conduct, improper discharge of professional duties, or failure to meet standards of care—any such actions that result in harm to another person.

**statutes of limitations** • Laws that specify the length of time within which a person may file specific types of lawsuits. The statute of limitations for a medical malpractice case is usually 2 or 3 years.

# 43 Understanding statutes of limitations

Suppose a patient sues you for malpractice 5 years after he left your care. Ordinarily, his lawsuit won't be valid, because all states have statutes of limitations that specify a limited period of time when a patient may sue for malpractice. So you don't have to worry? Yes, you do—because the patient's attorney knows about the statute of limitations, and he's filing suit anyway. This means he believes the court will set aside the statute for his client. Under certain specific conditions, the court can interpret the statute of limitations to give a plaintiff-patient more time to seek damages.

As you're probably aware, a statute of limitations is a law that specifies a limited number of years when one person can seek damages from another. For medical malpractice, the statute of limitations is specified in each state's medical malpractice law. (See *Statutes*

*of Limitations,* pages 268 and 269.) Nurses, however, usually aren't expressly covered under these statutes of limitations. This means that when a nurse's defense alleges a patient's malpractice claim is invalid because he didn't file suit until after the statute of limitations had expired, the court must determine which applies: the statute of limitations for state medical malpractice law or the statute of limitations for general personal-injury lawsuits. (The malpractice law's statute of limitations is usually shorter.) The court bases its decision on the two following considerations:

• *how much statute-of-limitations protection the court believes the defendant-nurse's job warrants.* For example, if her job forces her to make many independent patient-care judgments, the court will apply a strict—or short—statute of limitations. A short time limit offers more protection, because the patient has less time to seek damages.

• *the type of negligent act the plaintiff-patient claims the nurse committed.* For example, an injured patient may sue a nurse for any one or for several of the charges that constitute malpractice—

## STATUTES OF LIMITATIONS

Your state laws specify the length of time within which a person may file a medical malpractice charge. This chart will provide you with information on the exact time limits in all 50 states and the District of Columbia.

| STATE | TIME FROM OCCURRENCE | TIME FROM DISCOVERY |
|---|---|---|
| Alabama | 2 years | 6 months |
| Alaska | 2 years | Applicable only to minors |
| Arizona | 3 years | 3 years |
| Arkansas | 2 years | 1 year |
| California | 1 year | 1 year |
| Colorado | Not applicable | 2 years |
| Connecticut | 2 years | 2 years |
| Delaware | 2 years | 2 years |
| District of Columbia | Not applicable | 3 years |
| Florida | 2 years | 2 years |
| Georgia | 2 years | 2 years |
| Hawaii | Not applicable | 2 years |
| Idaho | 2 years | 1 year (applies only to foreign object lawsuits) |
| Illinois | Not applicable | 2 years |
| Indiana | 2 years | Not applicable |
| Iowa | Not applicable | 2 years |
| Kansas | 2 years | 2 years |
| Kentucky | Not applicable | 1 year |
| Louisiana | 1 year | 1 year |
| Maine | 2 years | Not applicable |
| Maryland | 5 years | 3 years |
| Massachusetts | 3 years | 3 years |
| Michigan | 2 years (for doctors) 3 years (for nurses) | 2 years (for doctors) 3 years (for nurses) |
| Minnesota | 2 years | 2 years |
| Mississippi | Not applicable | 2 years |

| STATE | TIME FROM OCCURRENCE | TIME FROM DISCOVERY |
|---|---|---|
| Missouri | 2 years | 2 years |
| Montana | 3 years | 3 years |
| Nebraska | 2 years | 2 years |
| Nevada | 4 years | 2 years |
| New Hampshire | 2 years | uncertain |
| New Jersey | Not applicable | 2 years |
| New Mexico | 3 years | Not applicable |
| New York | 30 months | 30 months |
| North Carolina | 3 years | 1 year |
| North Dakota | Not applicable | 2 years |
| Ohio | Not applicable | 1 year |
| Oklahoma | Not applicable | 2 years |
| Oregon | Not applicable | 2 years |
| Pennsylvania | Not applicable | 2 years |
| Rhode Island | 3 years | 1 year |
| South Carolina | 3 years | 3 years |
| South Dakota | 2 years | Not applicable |
| Tennessee | 1 year | 1 year |
| Texas | 2 years | 2 years (applies only to limited circumstances) |
| Utah | Not applicable | 2 years |
| Vermont | 3 years | 2 years |
| Virginia | 2 years | Not applicable |
| Washington | 3 years | 1 year |
| West Virginia | 2 years | 2 years |
| Wisconsin | 3 years | 1 year |
| Wyoming | 2 years | 6 months |

such as negligence or breach of contract. The patient's attorney, of course, determines which charge has the best chance of winning the most damages for his client, and structures his case accordingly. Then, if a statute of limitations is used as part of the nurse's defense, the court will decide which statute of limitations to apply in relation to the patient's charges.

## How statutes of limitations developed

Why are statutes of limitations necessary? Because as time passes, evidence vanishes, witnesses' memories fail, and witnesses die. A time limit for bringing lawsuit ensures that enough relevant evidence exists for a judge or jury to decide a case fairly.

To define that limit, state legislatures established statutes of limitations for general negligence that usually give a person 3 years to sue another for damages. These are the laws that plaintiffs invoke in general personal-injury lawsuits. Then, in response to pressure from medical and insurance groups, some states went a step further. They established shorter statutes of limitations for professions that require independent and risk-taking judgments. The statutes of limitations of medical malpractice laws, for example, usually give the patient 2 years or less to sue for damages.

You should know, however, that in some states, only doctors are subject to medical malpractice statutes of limitations—not nurses. Why? Because these states view the nurse as someone basically carrying out orders and not making independent, risk-taking judgments. In a Michigan case, *Kambas v. St. Joseph's Mercy Hospital of Detroit* (1973), for example, a heart attack patient lost full use of his arms after receiving anticoagulant drug injections. Because the patient brought the suit over 2 years after the incident, the nurse-defendant's attorneys tried to invoke Michigan's 2-year medical malpractice statute of limitations. The

plaintiff-patient's attorney argued that the state's 3-year general negligence statute should apply. The state supreme court ruled for the patient, concluding that because nurses don't exercise independent judgment, as doctors do, they aren't entitled to the protection of the medical malpractice statute of limitations.

## When does a statute of limitations begin to run?

A statute of limitations sets a limit for filing a malpractice lawsuit, but a patient can sometimes successfully file suit after the time limit expires. In fact, determining when the applicable statute actually begins to run has become the pivotal question whenever a nurse's or doctor's attorney invokes a statute of limitations as a defense in a malpractice case. Normally, the statute begins to run on the date the plaintiff's injury occurred. But what if the plaintiff doesn't *know* he was injured, or doesn't find out he has a basis to file suit because of his injury, until after the normal statute of limitations has expired? Legislatures and the courts—which are continually struggling with this question—have devised a series of rules to help courts decide, in individual malpractice cases, when a statute should properly begin to run. A court can apply these rules, when a plaintiff-patient's attorney requests that it do so, to extend the applicable statute of limitations beyond the limit written in the law. This means that the defendant-nurse's use of a statute of limitations as a defense is invalidated, and the plaintiff-patient's right to sue is affirmed.

## When the statute begins on the date of injury

When legislatures began writing statutes of limitations, many of them decided that short time limits best served the ideal of fairness. So, they passed statutes of limitations that begin to run on the day a patient's injury occurs. Attorneys call this the *occurrence rule;*

it generally leads to the shortest time limit. In several states, the courts have interpreted the occurrence rule strictly, so that even badly injured patients have been prevented from collecting damages once the applicable statute of limitations expired.

## When the statute begins from termination of treatment

When a patient's injury results from a series of treatments extended over time—rather than from a single incident—a court can apply the *termination-of-treatment rule.* This rule says that a statute of limitations begins from the date of the last treatment. In devising this rule, the courts reasoned that for the patient, a series of treatments could obscure just how and when the injury occurred. The U.S. Court of Appeals applied this rule in *Morgan v. Schlanger* (1967). In a lawsuit filed some years after extensive radiation treatment, a cancer patient claimed she suffered radiation-treatment burns. The defendant-doctors argued that the applicable statute of limitations had elapsed. But the court ruled that the statute didn't begin to run until the treatment ended, so the patient's lawsuit was valid.

The termination-of-treatment rule also may apply even after the patient leaves a nurse's or a doctor's care. For example, suppose a patient you cared for is injured later, in someone else's care, and sues. If the subsequent health-care providers relied on decisions you made earlier in caring for the patient, the court can find you liable. This rule—called the *constructive continuing treatment rule*—gives the court another way to extend the statute of limitations in malpractice cases.

## Counting from when the injury is discovered

Another rule a court can use in determining when a statute of limitations properly begins is based on when a patient discovers the injury. (This may take place many years after the injury occurred *and* after the applicable statute of limitations has formally run out.) This rule—called *the discovery rule*—considerably extends the time a patient has to file a malpractice lawsuit.

Two types of cases where the discovery rule is often applied are cases involving foreign objects left inside patients after surgery (so-called foreign-object cases) and cases involving sterilization. When a nurse or a surgeon leaves a foreign object—such as a scalpel, sponge, or clamp—inside a patient, the patient might not discover the error until long after his surgery. Under the discovery rule, the applicable statute of limitations wouldn't begin to run until the patient found out about the error. A court's decision to apply the discovery rule depends on whether it is satisfied that the patient couldn't have discovered the error earlier. If evidence indicates the patient should have recognized that something was wrong (for example, if he had chronic pain for months after the surgery but didn't take legal action until long afterward), the court could apply the termination-of-treatment rule instead.

Time limits for applying the discovery rule in foreign-object cases vary from state to state. Missouri allows a patient to file a foreign-object suit up to 10 years after the negligence occurs, the longest period any state allows. California allows the shortest period, 1 year from discovery of injury.

In some lawsuits involving incidents of tubal ligation and vasectomy, the courts have allowed the discovery rule to apply when a subsequent pregnancy occurs. In these cases, the courts' reasoning is that a patient can't discover

> *"A time limit for bringing a lawsuit ensures that enough evidence exists to decide a case fairly."*

# HOW MISTAKES CAN HAUNT YOU MANY YEARS LATER

*Answer true or false:*
A patient can sue you for malpractice a decade after you've treated him.

*The answer:*
True, because a court can lengthen the statute of limitations in malpractice lawsuits.

In the following case, *Lopez v. Swyer* (1971), the court lengthened the statute of limitations by nearly a decade because a patient's doctors concealed information from her. New Jersey housewife and mother Mary Lopez, age 32, discovered a lump in her right breast. She underwent a radical mastectomy, and several doctors prescribed postsurgical radiation treatments. Mrs. Lopez's family doctor referred her to a radiologist for the treatments.

Mrs. Lopez had radiation treatments six times a week for more than a month. As a result of this excessive treatment, she suffered extremely painful radiation burns over most of her body. When she asked why the complications were so severe, her doctors assured her the complications weren't unusual. They never told her that the treatments could have been too numerous and too strong.

Mrs. Lopez's condition worsened. Over the next several years, she was hospitalized 15 times, including twice for reconstructive surgery made necessary because of the radiation treatment. She didn't file a malpractice lawsuit until she heard a consulting doctor tell other doctors, gathered near her hospital bed, that she'd been a victim of negligence.

A lower court dismissed her suit because the 2-year statute of limitations for filing malpractice lawsuits had expired. But an appeals court ruled that the statute of limitations didn't start until Mrs. Lopez found out that her doctors had concealed the truth about her radiation treatments. That ruling let Mrs. Lopez bring the facts in her case before a jury.

the negligence until the procedure proves unsuccessful—no matter how long after the surgery this proof occurs.

## Putting restrictions on the extension rule

Because the discovery rule is so generous to plaintiffs, some states—notably Texas—have restricted its application in malpractice cases. These states prefer to keep statutes of limitations' time limits short. A number of states have adopted separate statutes of limitations, one for readily detected injuries and one for injuries discovered later. In California and Ohio, for example, a patient must file suit within 1 year after he discovers an injury. But neither state allows the patient to file suit beyond 4 years after the injury occurred. Other states permit statute-of-limitations extensions only in foreign-object cases.

## How proof of fraud extends the statute of limitations

Courts, in most states, will extend an applicable statute of limitations indefinitely if a plaintiff-patient can prove that a nurse or doctor used fraud or falsehood to conceal from the patient information about his injury or its cause. In most concealment cases, the law says that the concealment must be an overt act, not just the omission of an act. The most flagrant frauds involve concealing facts to prevent an inquiry, elude an investigation, or mislead a patient. Such a case was *Garcia v. Presbyterian Hospital Center* (1979). In this case, a patient who sued was operated on for cancer of the prostate gland twice in 1972 and once again in 1973. He'd repeatedly asked his doctor and attending nurses why the third operation was needed, but he hadn't received any explanation. Some time later, he learned that the third operation had resulted from retention of a catheter in his body during the second operation. The court held that the applicable statute of limitations did not prevent the patient from bringing suit.

## When the plaintiff-patient is a minor or is mentally incompetent

Generally, state laws give special consideration in injury cases to minors and mentally incompetent patients because they lack the legal capacity to sue. Some states postpone applying the statute of limitations to an injured minor until he reaches the age of majority—age 18 or 21, depending on the state (see Entry 26). And some states have specific rules about how statutes of limitations apply to minors.

Cases involving mentally incompetent patients who file after statutes of limitations have expired usually follow the discovery rule or a special law. Most of these special laws say that a statute of limitations doesn't begin until the patient recovers from his mental incompetence.

## How long should medical records be kept?

Because, in some instances, a patient can file a malpractice suit years after he claims his injury occurred, you must keep accurate medical records on file for years (see *How Mistakes Can Haunt You Many Years Later*). The complexity of malpractice cases requires you to recall specific clinical facts and procedures. Complete documentation of your care is usually found only in the records. These records provide your best defense. Without them, you're legally vulnerable.

Exactly how long must you maintain medical records? Few states have laws setting precise time periods, but many legal experts urge hospitals and other health-care facilities to maintain medical record files long after patients are discharged. New Jersey requires hospitals to keep medical records for 7 years. Some states have adopted the Uniform Business Records Act, which calls for keeping records for no less than 3 years.

Some states allow microfilm copies of medical records to be admitted as evidence in malpractice cases, but other states insist that only the original records can be used in court.

## Using the statute-of-limitations defense

When a defendant-nurse and her attorney use a statute of limitations as a defense, they're making—in legal jargon—an affirmative defense. This means that the defendant raises the issue of a statute of limitations, and the plaintiff must prove that it is still running (such as by asserting an extension rule). If the court decides the statute has elapsed, the plaintiff-patient's case is rendered invalid.

## A final word

If you're named as a defendant in a malpractice lawsuit, you'll need all the help you can get to defend your professional and financial interests. Statutes of limitations provide you with a defense your attorney won't overlook: the law recognizes the importance of limiting the time when a patient can claim damages against you. But don't forget: No statute of limitations exists on your responsibility to your patients to give them the best nursing care you possibly can.

---

# 44 What to do if you're sued

Imagine you're at the nurse's station, catching up on paperwork, when a stranger approaches and asks for you. When you identify yourself, he thrusts some legal papers into your hands and starts to walk away. Baffled, you manage to ask, "What's this all about?" He replies, "You've just been sued."

As you look over the papers, you realize he's not joking. You recognize the name of a former patient as the suing party (plaintiff), and you see your name listed as the defendant. As you skim through the papers, you learn that you've been accused of "errors and omissions." A nagging worry for most nurses has just become reality for you: you've been sued for nursing malpractice.

What should you do? To do nothing is to invite disaster. Failing to respond could result in a default judgment against you.

Obviously, you must take action. What action? That will depend on whether you have professional liability insurance (see Entry 41). Regardless, *you must take action immediately*.

## What to do if you're insured

If you're covered by your employer's insurance, immediately contact your legal services administrators at work (see Entry 42). They'll tell you how to proceed.

If you have your own professional liability insurance, pull out your policy and read the section that tells you what to do when you're sued. Every policy describes whom you should notify and how much time you have to do it. Immediately telephone this representative and tell him you've been sued. *Document the time, his name, and his instructions*. Then, hand-deliver the lawsuit papers to him and get a signed, dated receipt for them. Or send them by certified mail, return receipt requested, so you're assured of a signed receipt.

If you don't contact the appropriate representative within the specified time, the insurance company can refuse to cover you. So to protect yourself, make sure you *act quickly, document your actions*, and *get a receipt*.

Make no mistake: When you notify your insurance company that you've been sued, it will first consider whether it *must* cover you at all. Your company does this by checking for any policy violations you may have committed. For example, your company will check whether you gave late notice of the lawsuit, gave false information on your insurance application, or failed to pay a premium on time. If the company is sure you've committed such a violation, it will use this violation as a *policy defense,* and it can simply refuse to cover you. If the company thinks you've committed such a violation but isn't sure it has evidence to support a policy defense, it will probably send you a letter by certified mail informing you that the company may not have to defend you, but that it will do so while reserving the right to deny coverage later, withdraw from the case, or take other actions. Meanwhile, the company will seek a declaration of its rights from the court. If the court decides the company doesn't have to defend you, the company will withdraw from the case.

Usually, an insurance company takes this action only after careful consideration. Why? Because this action may provide the insured nurse with grounds for suing the company. If you receive such a letter, find a malpractice attorney to defend you in the lawsuit against you and to advise you in your dealings with the insurance company. If your case against the insurance company is sound, he may suggest that you sue them.

If your insurance company doesn't assert a policy defense, your company representative will select and retain an attorney or a law firm specializing in medical malpractice cases as your *attorney of record* in the lawsuit. Once he's designated as your attorney of record, this attorney is legally bound to do all that's necessary to defend you.

Your employer will almost certainly be named as a codefendant in the lawsuit. But even if this isn't the case, notify your employer that you're being sued. Your insurance company may try to involve your employer as a defendant.

### What to do if you're not insured
If you don't have insurance, your own or your employer's, you'll have to find your own attorney. *Don't even consider trying to defend yourself.* You need an attorney who's experienced in medical malpractice, because the case will be complex and the opposition will be

## KEY TERMS IN THIS ENTRY

**attorney of record** • The attorney whose name appears on the legal records for a specific case, as the agent of a specific client.

**discovery** • A pretrial procedure that allows the plaintiff's and defendant's attorneys to examine relevant materials and interrogate all parties to the case.

**malpractice** • A professional person's wrongful conduct, improper discharge of professional duties, or failure to meet standards of care—any such actions that result in harm to another person.

**policy defense** • Reasons your professional liability insurance company may give—concerning how well you've maintained the policy—for not covering you when you make a claim.

**professional liability insurance** • A type of liability insurance that protects professional persons against malpractice claims made against them.

composed of experienced attorneys. (See *How to Find an Attorney,* page 276.)

Make appointments with a few attorneys who seem qualified to defend you. (Usually, an attorney won't charge you for this initial meeting.) When you meet with each one, ask how long he thinks the lawsuit will take and how much money he will charge. Also, try to get a feeling for the attorney's understanding of the issues in your case. Then choose one as your attorney of record. Do this as soon as possible.

### What your attorney will do
Your attorney will file the appropriate legal documents in response to the papers you were served. Of course, he'll ask you for help in preparing your defense. He should give you a chance to present your position in detail. Remember, all such discussions between you and your attorney are *privileged.* This

means that your attorney can't disclose this information without your permission.

Your attorney will also obtain complete copies of the pertinent medical records and any other documents he or you feel are important in your defense. In addition, he'll use *discovery devices* to uncover every pertinent detail about the case against you. These discovery devices are legal procedures for obtaining information. Some discovery devices your attorney may use include an *interrogatory* (questions written to the other party that require answers under oath), *a deposition* (oral cross-examination of the other party, under oath and before a court reporter), and *a defense medical examination* (a medical examination of the injured party by a doctor selected by your attorney or insurance company).

Of course, the plaintiff-patient's attorney will also use discovery devices,

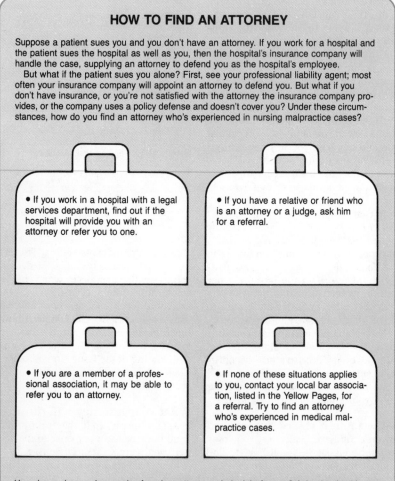

## HOW TO FIND AN ATTORNEY

Suppose a patient sues you and you don't have an attorney. If you work for a hospital and the patient sues the hospital as well as you, then the hospital's insurance company will handle the case, supplying an attorney to defend you as the hospital's employee.

But what if the patient sues you alone? First, see your professional liability agent; most often your insurance company will appoint an attorney to defend you. But what if you don't have insurance, or you're not satisfied with the attorney the insurance company provides, or the company uses a policy defense and doesn't cover you? Under these circumstances, how do you find an attorney who's experienced in nursing malpractice cases?

• If you work in a hospital with a legal services department, find out if the hospital will provide you with an attorney or refer you to one.

• If you have a relative or friend who is an attorney or a judge, ask him for a referral.

• If you are a member of a professional association, it may be able to refer you to an attorney.

• If none of these situations applies to you, contact your local bar association, listed in the Yellow Pages, for a referral. Try to find an attorney who's experienced in medical malpractice cases.

How do you know when you've found an attorney who's right for you? Ask other health-care professionals if they've heard of the attorney you're using, and go by his reputation.

## SETTLING OUT OF COURT

Malpractice attorneys estimate that only 10% of malpractice lawsuits that are filed actually go to court—and of those that go to court only 10% actually end with a final judgment. What happens to the rest—the vast majority of cases? They're settled out of court.

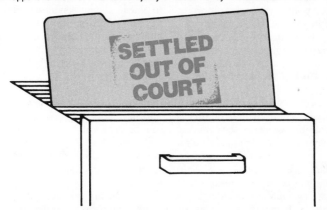

If you're involved in a malpractice lawsuit, there's a good chance that with your help your attorney will settle out of court. When you discuss settlement with him, remember these points:

• If you're covered by professional liability insurance, the terms of your policy will determine whether you and your attorney, or the insurance company, can control the settlement. Most policies do not permit the nurse to settle a case without the consent of the insurance company. In fact, many policies (especially those provided by employers) permit the insurance company to settle *without the consent* of the individual nurse involved. Review your policy to determine your settlement rights. If the policy isn't clear on this point, call the insurance administrator of your hospital or the insurance company, and ask for clarification.

• Offer your insurance company's representative and your attorney all the information you can about the case, so they can not only evaluate your liabilities (and the plaintiff's liabilities) but also figure the best settlement with the plaintiff. As an attending nurse, you may be in the best position to provide crucial observations concerning the patient's state of mind—often the basis of a successful settlement.

• Remember, if you settle your case out of court, that doesn't mean that you're admitting any wrongdoing. The law regards settlement as a compromise between two parties to end a lawsuit and avoid further expense. In other words, you may choose to pay a settlement rather than incur possible greater expense (both financial and emotional) in defending your innocence at a trial.

---

so you may have to answer interrogatories and appear for a deposition as well. Your attorney will carefully prepare you for these procedures. (See *What To Expect at the Deposition*, page 279.)

Your attorney will also prepare you to testify at the trial. He'll tell you how to dress and how to act (see Entry 45). Remember, he wants to win the case, too, so do what he tells you. Remember also that your failure to cooperate with an attorney provided by an insurance company can be used as a policy defense.

This doesn't mean you must say or do *anything* he asks. If you feel you must contradict him, you have the right to state your position and to protect your professional reputation in court. If you feel your attorney is asking you to do or say things that aren't in your best interest, tell him so. You have the right to change attorneys at any time.

If you believe an attorney selected by your insurance company is more interested in protecting the company than in protecting you, discuss the problem with a company representative. Then, if you still feel that he isn't defending you properly, hire your own attorney. If this happens, you may have grounds for suing the insurance company and the company-appointed attorney.

## What to do before your case goes to trial

*Study the copies of the medical records.* Your attorney will ask you to do this as soon as possible. Examine the complete medical chart, including nurses' notes, laboratory reports, and doctors' orders. On a separate sheet of paper, make appropriate notes on key entries or omissions. But *don't* make any changes on the records. Such an action will destroy your case by undermining your credibility. Remember, you're not the only person with a copy of these records (see Entry 37).

*Create your own legal file.* Ask your attorney to send you copies of all documents and correspondence pertaining to the case. Try to maintain a file that's as complete as your attorney's. Also, make sure you understand all the items

> ## "If you feel the insurance company's attorney isn't defending you properly, hire your own attorney."

in your file. If you receive a document you don't understand, ask your attorney to explain it. Maintaining such a file should keep you up to date on the status of your case and prevent unpleasant surprises in court.

*Fill out an incident report.* If the hospital or clinic where you work asks you to fill out an incident report, consult with your attorney before doing so.

Usually, these incident reports can't be used as evidence, but they may influence future prospective employers. So have your attorney help you fill out the report—your career may be at stake.

*Limit talk about the case.* Don't try to placate the person suing you by calling him and discussing the case. Your chances of talking him into dropping his lawsuit are very slim. And every word you say to him can be used against you in court.

In fact, before the trial, don't discuss the lawsuit with *anyone* except your attorney. This will help prevent information leaks that could compromise your case. And to protect your professional reputation, don't even mention to your colleagues that you've been sued.

*Protect your property.* Ask your attorney about the legal devices you can use to protect your property. Many states have *homestead laws* that permit you to protect a substantial part of the equity in your house, as well as other property, from any judgment against you. Such protection is essential if you don't have insurance or if damages exceed your insurance, and you'll be glad you have it if you lose the case and the damages awarded do exceed your insurance coverage (see Entry 41).

## Your day in court

Your case may eventually go to trial. While your attorney prepares your defense, he'll also explore the desirability of reaching an out-of-court settlement. If he decides an out-of-court settlement is in your best interest, he'll try to achieve it in the period before your trial date. (See *Settling Out of Court*, page 277.)

If your case does go to trial (see *The Legal Process: Step by Step*, pages 280 and 281), you'll participate in selecting the jury. During this selection process, attorneys for both sides will question prospective jurors, and your attorney will ask your opinion on their suitability. Either attorney may reject a small number of prospective jurors without

## WHAT TO EXPECT AT THE DEPOSITION

When you think of being sued, you probably wonder what happens, and what you'd have to do. One event that occurs early in a lawsuit—after it's filed—is the taking of depositions.

In this legal procedure, the attorney for the person suing you (the plaintiff) questions you in the presence of *your* attorney and a court reporter. As part of the discovery process, the deposition enables both parties to review each other's cases to see if one is stronger than the other. Remember, most malpractice cases are settled out of court, so the deposition is crucial.

Before you appear for the deposition, review all the medical records in the case. They may help you recall important facts. During the deposition, the plaintiff's attorney has the right to inspect and copy any materials you bring to aid your memory. So show them to your attorney before the deposition for his inspection and approval.

Your attorney will probably advise you to respond to all questions with simple answers and not to volunteer or elaborate on any information. If you have any doubts, avoid absolute answers. Memory fades with time and, even with the aid of medical records, you won't be expected to recall details or actual conversations that took place some time ago. Remember, if the case goes to court, you'll be held accountable for the answers you gave at the deposition.

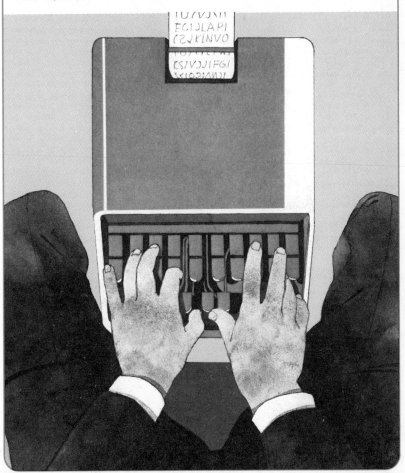

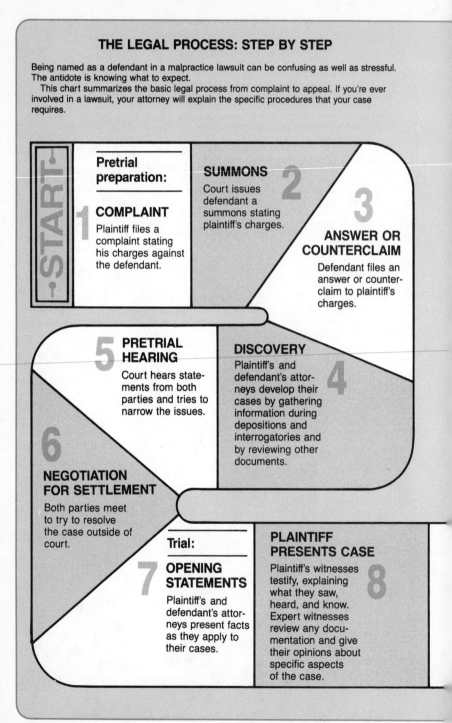

## THE LEGAL PROCESS: STEP BY STEP

Being named as a defendant in a malpractice lawsuit can be confusing as well as stressful. The antidote is knowing what to expect.

This chart summarizes the basic legal process from complaint to appeal. If you're ever involved in a lawsuit, your attorney will explain the specific procedures that your case requires.

**START**

**Pretrial preparation:**

**1 COMPLAINT**

Plaintiff files a complaint stating his charges against the defendant.

**2 SUMMONS**

Court issues defendant a summons stating plaintiff's charges.

**3 ANSWER OR COUNTERCLAIM**

Defendant files an answer or counterclaim to plaintiff's charges.

**5 PRETRIAL HEARING**

Court hears statements from both parties and tries to narrow the issues.

**4 DISCOVERY**

Plaintiff's and defendant's attorneys develop their cases by gathering information during depositions and interrogatories and by reviewing other documents.

**6 NEGOTIATION FOR SETTLEMENT**

Both parties meet to try to resolve the case outside of court.

**Trial:**

**7 OPENING STATEMENTS**

Plaintiff's and defendant's attorneys present facts as they apply to their cases.

**8 PLAINTIFF PRESENTS CASE**

Plaintiff's witnesses testify, explaining what they saw, heard, and know. Expert witnesses review any documentation and give their opinions about specific aspects of the case.

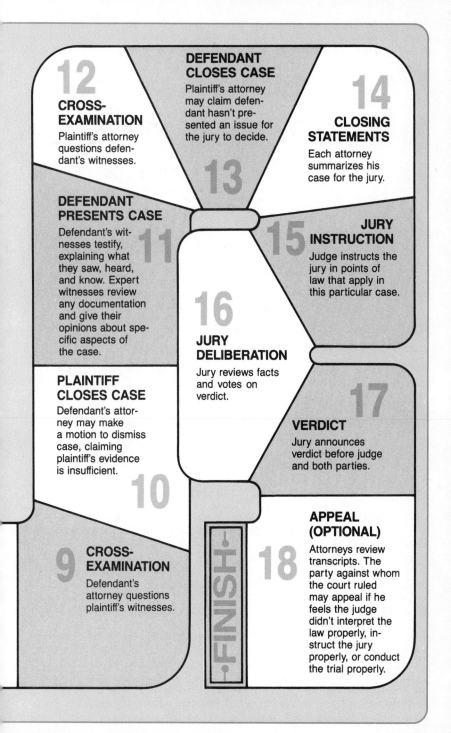

**12**

**CROSS-EXAMINATION**

Plaintiff's attorney questions defendant's witnesses.

**DEFENDANT CLOSES CASE**

Plaintiff's attorney may claim defendant hasn't presented an issue for the jury to decide.

**13**

**14**

**CLOSING STATEMENTS**

Each attorney summarizes his case for the jury.

**DEFENDANT PRESENTS CASE**

Defendant's witnesses testify, explaining what they saw, heard, and know. Expert witnesses review any documentation and give their opinions about specific aspects of the case.

**11**

**15**

**JURY INSTRUCTION**

Judge instructs the jury in points of law that apply in this particular case.

**16**

**JURY DELIBERATION**

Jury reviews facts and votes on verdict.

**PLAINTIFF CLOSES CASE**

Defendant's attorney may make a motion to dismiss case, claiming plaintiff's evidence is insufficient.

**10**

**17**

**VERDICT**

Jury announces verdict before judge and both parties.

**9**

**CROSS-EXAMINATION**

Defendant's attorney questions plaintiff's witnesses.

FINISH

**18**

**APPEAL (OPTIONAL)**

Attorneys review transcripts. The party against whom the court ruled may appeal if he feels the judge didn't interpret the law properly, instruct the jury properly, or conduct the trial properly.

## SUCCESSFULLY CHALLENGING MALPRACTICE CHARGES

Suppose a patient in your care is injured and he sues you. If your attorney can establish one of the following defenses, the court will either dismiss the charges against you or reduce the damages for which you're liable:

| DEFENSES | RATIONALE |
|---|---|
| **FALSE CHARGES** | Does the plaintiff have legally sufficient proof that your actions caused his injuries? If he doesn't, the court may rule that the charges against you are false and dismiss the case. |
| **CONTRIBUTORY NEGLIGENCE** | Did the plaintiff, through carelessness, contribute to his injury? If he did, some states permit the court to charge the plaintiff with failing to meet the standards of a reasonably prudent patient, barring him from recovering *any* damages. |
| **COMPARATIVE NEGLIGENCE** | A few states permit the court to apportion liability—barring the plaintiff from recovering *some,* but not all, of the damages he claims. |
| **ASSUMPTION OF RISK** | Did the plaintiff understand the risk involved in the treatment, procedure, or action that allegedly caused his injury? Did he give proper informed consent and so voluntarily expose himself to that risk? If he did, the court may rule that the plaintiff assumed the risk, knowingly disregarding the danger, and so relieved you of liability. |
| **BORROWED SERVANT** | Were you working under the direct supervision of a doctor, such as in an operating room? If you were, the court may rule that you *and* the doctor share the liability for your negligence. |

any reason (this is called a *peremptory challenge*). And you, the plaintiff, or either attorney may reject an unlimited number of jurors for specific reasons. For instance, you may reject someone who knows the plaintiff or who has any legal interest in the lawsuit. (This is called a *challenge for cause.*)

To help prepare you to testify at the trial, your attorney will ask you to review the complete medical record, your interrogatory answers, and your deposition. In addition, you should review the entire legal file you've been keeping, to make sure you understand all aspects of the case (see Entry 45).

The trial may last several days—or even several weeks. After all the witnesses have given their testimony, the jury—not the judge—will decide if you're liable. If the jury finds you liable, it will also assess damages against you.

### Protecting your professional reputation

During the trial, your professional reputation will be at stake. Project a positive attitude at all times, suggesting you feel confident about the trial's outcome (see Entry 45 for a discussion of techniques for testifying). Never disparage the plaintiff inside or outside the courtroom. Characterizing him as a gold digger, for instance, can only generate bad feelings that may interfere with the settlement. You won't want to speak to him during the trial, but if you do, always be polite and dignified. Remember, you don't want to do anything that suggests you lack confidence in your position or dislike the plaintiff.

As you know, losing a malpractice lawsuit can jeopardize your future. Prospective employers (as well as prospective insurers) will want to know if you've ever lost a nursing malpractice lawsuit or if you've ever been a defendant in one. If you have, you'll probably find job hunting more difficult than it used to be. You'll also pay an increased insurance premium, and you may find that some insurance companies will simply refuse to cover you.

### Looking ahead

Recently, some state legislatures have reformed their laws to limit the number and the impact of malpractice lawsuits. For instance, some legislatures have limited the time allowed for filing suit by amending their states' statutes of limitations (see Entry 43); others have limited the amount a jury can award to a plaintiff. In addition, the increasing use of arbitration procedures is helping reduce the number of these lawsuits that go to trial.

### A final word

As you continue to expand your nursing expertise and to accept greater patient-care responsibility, you'll also accept greater legal risks. So to help protect yourself, you must keep up with changes in the law that affect your practice. And, of course, you must always practice within the limits prescribed in your nurse practice act.

If, despite these precautions, a stranger someday thrusts those dreaded legal papers into your hands, follow the recommendations discussed here. They apply no matter where you practice in the United States or Canada. And they'll help you survive a malpractice lawsuit.

# 45 Techniques for testifying in a malpractice lawsuit

When you're called to testify in a malpractice lawsuit, as a defendant or as an expert witness, you can use a number of techniques to help reduce stress and enhance the value of your testimony. In the courtroom, claims, counterclaims, allegations, and contradictory evidence will probably be coming at you hot and heavy at times. Here's how to keep cool through it all.

### First, the deposition

Before the trial, you'll be called to give a deposition (see Entry 44). (If you've been called to testify as an expert witness, you should be aware that some states don't permit expert witnesses to give pretrial depositions.) Where you give the deposition can vary. It can take place in an attorney's office or in a special room in the courthouse set aside for that purpose. The deposition takes place in a less formal atmosphere than a courtroom provides, but don't forget that a court reporter will be transcrib-

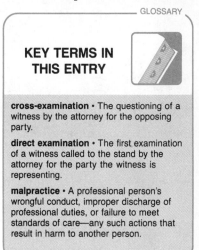

GLOSSARY

**KEY TERMS IN THIS ENTRY**

**cross-examination** • The questioning of a witness by the attorney for the opposing party.

**direct examination** • The first examination of a witness called to the stand by the attorney for the party the witness is representing.

**malpractice** • A professional person's wrongful conduct, improper discharge of professional duties, or failure to meet standards of care—any such actions that result in harm to another person.

## HOW THE COURT SELECTS AND USES AN EXPERT WITNESS

When an attorney looks for an expert witness in a nursing malpractice case, he wants a nurse with two important qualifications: a good educational background and substantial and relevant clinical experience.

Usually an expert witness' credentials have to match or exceed a defendant's. For example, a psychiatric nurse defendant with 2 years' experience may insist that a prospective expert witness have at least comparable experience. Some courts allow an RN to testify about the care an LPN or LVN gives, but not the reverse. Some courts don't allow LPNs/LVNs to testify at all. Others allow an LPN/LVN to testify, but with restrictions.

Before a trial begins, an attorney may call on you, as an expert witness, to review the defendant's file and evaluate the defendant's liability. Then, after the trial begins, the attorney may ask you to testify as an expert witness.

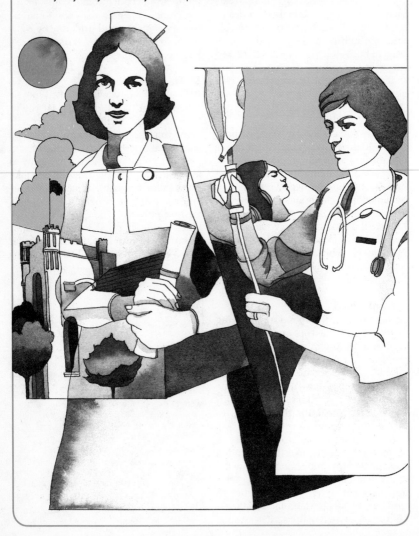

ing everything you and the attorneys say. In a way, it's a rehearsal of what will come later, during the actual trial. At the trial, the plaintiff's and the defendant's attorneys have the right to use your testimony to bolster their respective cases.

## Under oath: Looking and acting your best

How you come across to the jury from the witness stand is very important. This is when the jury forms its first—and sometimes lasting—impression of your credibility. So dress conservatively, and wear little or no jewelry. You want the jury to concentrate on what you say, not on how you look.

Malpractice lawsuits are notoriously slow-moving. The one you're involved in may seem to be in permanent slow motion. Interruptions occur in the form of recesses, attorneys' lengthy arguments in judges' chambers, and calling of witnesses out of turn. Be patient no matter what happens. And when you're asked to appear, be prompt. You may not score points by your punctuality, but you'll definitely lose a few if you aren't in court when you're called to testify.

When you testify, the jury doesn't expect you to be letter-perfect or to have instant—or total—recall. If you don't have an answer, say so. Listen closely to questions, and answer only what the questioner has asked. Always answer the questions simply and in lay terms, and *never* elaborate or volunteer information. If you're going to be describing a piece of equipment that's unfamiliar to a layman, get your attorney's approval to bring it to the courtroom and show it to the jury. And above all, be honest. When your testimony must be critical of a colleague or of your hospital's policies, you may be tempted to bend the truth a little. Don't.

## The cross-examination: Staying the course

During cross-examination, the opposing attorney will try to discredit your testimony. This may take the form of an attack on your credentials, experience, or education—especially if you're testifying as an expert witness. Another way of discrediting your testimony is by the "hired gun" insinuation. The cross-examining attorney may imply that because you accept payment for your testimony, you're being unethical. Just remember that as an expert witness you have the right to expect compensation for the time you spend on behalf of the case in and out of the courtroom. Say so if the matter comes up.

Another ploy the opposing attorney can use to discredit your testimony is the "hedge." He may try to get you to change or qualify an answer you gave previously on direct examination or at the deposition. He may also try to con-

> *"When you testify, always answer questions simply and in lay terms, and never elaborate or volunteer information."*

fuse the issue by asking you a similar—but hypothetical—question with a slightly different—but significant—slant. Just remember that a simple but sincere "I don't know" often reinforces a jury's belief in your honesty and competence. Obviously, your best protection against cross-examination jitters is adequate preparation.

## A final word

In most states, nurses now are recognized as professionals, uniquely qualified to give testimony about how their profession is—and should be—practiced. For example, a Pennsylvania malpractice lawsuit typified the courts' increasingly respectful attitude toward nursing (*Capan v. Divine Providence*

## WHAT MAKES A WITNESS "EXPERT"?

After Cecil Wood died, his wife charged that his nurses had been negligent (*Wood v. Rowland*, 1978).

Mrs. Wood planned to base her case on the expert testimony of a registered nurse named Mrs. Miller. Mrs. Miller had reviewed the pertinent hospital records, and she was prepared to testify that the nurses who cared for Cecil Wood failed to meet a reasonable standard of care in at least four ways:
- One nurse failed to tell the doctor that Cecil Wood had heart disease and was taking medication for it.
- The nurses failed to take Wood's vital signs as ordered by the doctor.
- The nurses failed to take Wood's vital signs before injecting meperidine (Demerol).
- The nurses failed to offer a reasonable standard of care in some tests they performed on Wood.

Mrs. Miller took the witness stand but was never able to give her opinion. The defendant's attorney pointed out that Mrs. Miller had been employed in her work as a nurse by only one hospital. Mrs. Miller had described her qualifications: she'd graduated from a diploma program in 1963 and then had worked at the same hospital for 3 years—until 1966. For the next 2 years, she'd worked as an office nurse. Then she'd been unemployed for 5 years. In May, 1973—one month after Cecil Wood's death—Mrs. Miller had started working again as a float nurse, in the same hospital where she'd worked previously.

Mrs. Miller testified that her education and experience made her familiar with local nursing standards, even though she'd never worked in the hospital where Cecil Wood had been a patient. But the defendant's attorney asked if Mrs. Miller knew the standards of nursing care or procedures in other hospitals. She said no. The defendant's attorney then said that policies may vary from hospital to hospital—that the policies of the hospital where Mrs. Miller worked might have been different from the hospital policies where Mr. Wood died. Finally, he asked the judge to refuse to allow Mrs. Miller to testify as an expert witness and to enter a directed verdict in favor of the hospital. The judge agreed.

Mrs. Wood appealed. If you were the appellate judge, how would you decide?

The appellate judge said the trial judge who refused to accept Mrs. Miller as an expert witness was wrong. According to the appellate judge, Mr. Wood's care didn't concern hospital administrative standards, which *would* require an expert witness familiar with the standards adopted by various hospitals. Instead, the Wood case concerned professional nursing standards—requiring an expert witness in *that* area. Did Mrs. Miller have this expertise? Yes, said the appellate judge; the courts define an expert as someone who has superior knowledge on a subject. Mrs. Miller's education and experience were not common to the average person, so she met this test. The fact that she worked in only one hospital might have affected the weight of her testimony, but it didn't disqualify her from giving it.

*Hospital,* 1980). In this case, the court wouldn't let a doctor testify on nursing standards because he couldn't show that he knew his hospital's nursing standards. In a Georgia-based malpractice lawsuit (*McCormick v. Avret,* 1980), a patient developed a permanent injury from a severe infection and sued. The patient alleged that the injury resulted from a doctor's faulty technique in withdrawing blood. The court allowed a nurse to testify on techniques for maintaining equipment sterility (although not on the standard of care for drawing blood).

The measure of professionalism for nurses includes how much integrity they exhibit while testifying in the courtroom as well as in the settings where they practice their profession. If you're ever called to testify during a malpractice lawsuit, do all you can to represent your profession with honesty and dignity.

# Selected References

Albana, F., and Reig, D., eds. *Negligence Compensation Cases Annotated.* Wilmette, Ill.: Callahan and Co., 1977.

Alton, Walter G., Jr. *Malpractice: A Trial Lawyer's Advice for Physicians.* Boston: Little, Brown & Co., 1977.

Bernzweig, Eli. *The Nurse's Liability for Malpractice: A Programmed Course,* 3rd ed. New York: McGraw-Hill Book Co., 1981.

Cazalas, Mary W. *Nursing and the Law,* 3rd ed. Rockville, Md.: Aspen Systems Corp., 1979.

Creighton, Helen. *Changing Legal Attitudes: The Effect of the Law on Nursing.* New York: National League for Nursing Publications, 1974.

Creighton, Helen. *Law Every Nurse Should Know,* 4th ed. Philadelphia: W.B. Saunders Co., 1981.

Eccard, Walter T. "A Revolution in White: New Approaches in Treating Nurses as Professionals," *Vanderbilt Law Review* 30:839, 1977.

Hemelt, M., and Mackert, M. *Dynamics of Law, Nursing and Health Care,* 2nd ed. Reston, Va.: Reston Publishing Co., 1982.

James, A. Everett. *Legal Medicine with Special Reference to Diagnostic Imaging.* Baltimore: Urban & Schwarzenberg, 1980.

Kinkela, Gabriella G., and Kinkela, Robert V. "Hospital Nurses and Tort Liability," *Cleveland-Marshall Law Review* 18:53, January 1969.

Kraftds, Melvin D. *Using Experts in Civil Cases,* 2nd ed. New York: Practising Law Institute, 1982.

Lesnick, Milton, and Anderson, Bernice E. *Nursing Practice and the Law,* 2nd ed.

Westport, Conn.: Greenwood Press, 1976.

Mackert, M.E., and Hemelt, M.D. "Prescription for a Witness...Learn Your Way Around a Courtroom," *NursingLife,* 2:80, January/February 1982.

*Medical Malpractice Litigation 1982,* Litigation and Administrative Practice Series. New York: Practising Law Institute, 1982.

Miller, Carol. *Nurses and the Law.* Danville, Ill.: Interstate, 1970.

Murchinson, Irene, et al. *Legal Accountability in the Nursing Process,* 2nd ed. St. Louis: C.V. Mosby Co., 1982.

Murchinson, Irene A., and Nichols, Thomas S. *Legal Foundations of Nursing Practice.* New York: Macmillan Publishing Co., 1970.

Pozgar, George D. *Legal Aspects of Health Care Administration.* Rockville, Md.: Aspen Systems Corp., 1979.

Sarner, Harvey. *The Nurse and the Law.* Philadelphia: W.B. Saunders Co., 1968.

Sheridan, Peter N. "Sindell and Its Sequelae—or How to Manage Multiparty Litigation," *Forum* 17(4):1116-38, Spring 1982.

Walker, Dorothy. "Nursing 1980: New Responsibility, New Liability," *Trial* 16(12): 42-47, December 1980.

Wasmuth, Carl E., and Wasmuth, Carl E., Jr. *Law and the Surgical Team.* Baltimore: Williams & Wilkins Co., 1969.

Willig, S. *The Nurse's Guide to the Law.* New York: McGraw-Hill Book Co., 1970.

Wright, Cecil A., and Linden, Allen M. *Canadian Tort Law: Cases, Notes, and Materials,* 7th ed. Toronto: Butterworth and Co., 1980.

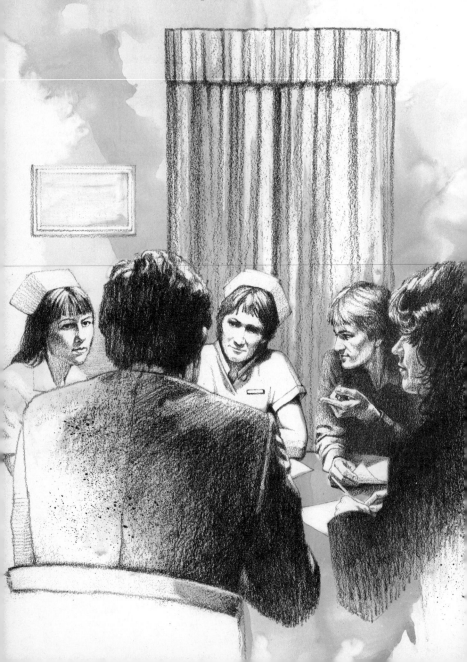

# Contracts and Collective Bargaining

# Introduction

In recent years, more and more nurses have felt the need to join an employee union. On the theory that strength comes in numbers, these nurses have joined forces to bargain with their employers for improved economic and working conditions. And many such groups have achieved their goals.

But for most nurses, the decision to join a union isn't an easy one. They maintain the traditional view that union activity is unprofessional. For them, negotiating for wages and working conditions impedes, rather than assures, quality patient care. Other nurses are reluctant to depend on an organization for their economic and professional well-being. They prefer to deal with their employer on a one-to-one basis. Still others object to the cost of union dues and the commitment of time and effort that unions demand of their members.

If you're one of the nurses who's still wrestling with these issues, this chapter will help you. You'll become familiar with the pros and cons of union membership, the functions of unions, and the legal mechanisms—collective bargaining, grievance procedures, and arbitration—that unions use to achieve their economic and professional objectives.

At some point in your career, you may have to choose whether or not to join a union. Prepare now, so you can make the right decision when that time arrives.

### Getting started
This chapter takes an in-depth look at employment contracts and explores all aspects of the union issue. For example, if you don't know what a valid contract is, read Entry 46, "Contracts—check thoroughly before you sign." This entry defines the elements of a legal contract, discusses its enforceability, lists the steps you must take to terminate it, and tells you how to avoid breaching it.

Would you like to organize a union where you work? Entry 47, "Organizing a union," describes the role of an organizer and discusses the rights and responsibilities of employees and the employer during the organization process.

Have you ever wondered how collective bargaining works? Entry 48, "The legalities of collective bargaining," explores the roles of employer and employees in the collective bargaining process, and reviews the laws giving nurses the right to bargain collectively. The entry also explores the legalities of holding a strike.

How does a union resolve disputes with the employer when negotiations reach an impasse? Entry 49, "Grievances and arbitration," discusses ways to resolve a dispute without going to court. The entry explains the various types of grievance procedures, their purposes, and the steps that each involves. It discusses the legalities of arbitration—when grievance procedures have failed—and the role the arbitrator plays in reaching an accord.

### If you join

State or federal laws determine basic bargaining rights, depending on where you work. Find out what those rights are. Then learn how to exercise them in your best interests.

If you're a nurse at a state, county, or municipal government facility, your state law defines your right to bargain.

If you're employed in a federal institution, the Civil Service Reform Act governs your bargaining rights.

If you work in a private health-care facility, the National Labor Relations Act (NLRA) determines your bargaining rights.

The NLRA also empowers the National Labor Relations Board to decide what's an appropriate bargaining unit. In a few instances, RNs and LPNs/LVNs have been put in the same bargaining unit, with the consent of the RNs. In other instances, RNs have won the right to bargain as a separate professional group, while LPNs/LVNs have been placed in a bargaining unit with technicians and health-care assistants.

### A final word

All nurses are concerned about their economic status and working conditions. Decent wages mean economic security for you and any family members who may depend on you. Optimum working conditions can mean job security, job satisfaction, and the chance to deliver the best possible patient care.

How you ensure that your economic and working conditions meet your personal and professional standards depends on your particular situation. Joining a union may or may not be the best means for you to achieve your goals. To find out, take a close look at the issue of union membership—its advantages, disadvantages, and alternatives. The best decision you can make about whether or not to join a union is an informed one.

# 46 Contracts—check thoroughly before you sign

Did you sign a contract when you began your current job? If so, did you read it carefully before you signed it? Chances are you just glanced at it, then signed your name to it. Even if you took the time to read it, you may not have known what terms to look for or understood all the conditions. For example, was the contract an individual or union contract? Did it contain any implied terms?

*"Knowing what to look for in a contract will help you decide if a job is really right for you."*

Did it adequately define your duties, the extent of your authority, and your benefits? Did it explain the procedure for terminating the contract?

These questions are important for you. Why? Because you're likely to work in more than one hospital during your career. And each time you transfer, you'll enter into some type of contractual agreement with your new employer.

Knowing what to look for in a contract will help you decide if a job is really right for you. And being able to interpret contract terms will help you function within the contract's specified limits.

## Recognizing various types of contracts

A contract is a legally binding agreement that one or more persons or groups makes with another person or group either to do or not to do something. But unlike a simple agreement, which isn't legally binding, a contract can be enforced in court.

According to U.S. and Canadian law, a contract is legally binding if:
• you've accepted an offer from another person or persons either to do or not to do something
• you and the other person are legally competent—of age and without mental impairment
• you and the other person understand the terms of the agreement
• the terms of the agreement are lawful
• you receive something of value, such as money, from the other person for fulfilling the agreement.

In general, agreements regarding conscience, morals, and social activities aren't legally binding. For example, if you break a lunch date with a friend, you can't be fined or taken to court for violating your agreement. But if you violate any term in a legally binding contract, you might face such consequences.

The law protects the parties of an express contract from fraudulent practices by requiring that these contracts, such as mortgages and deeds, be written.

In most cases, the contract you enter into with your employer will also be a formal, written contract. It may be an individual contract (which you negotiate personally with your employer) or a collective contract (which a labor organization or union negotiates with the employer for the employees). Contract terms may differ between the two. In an *individual contract,* wage increases may be awarded automatically and may not be linked to certain criteria, such as merit or experience; in a *collective* or *union contract,* wage increases may be awarded automatically based on merit and seniority.

Other contracts that you make with patients or co-workers will probably be either express or implied contracts. An express contract may be written or oral. Suppose that during an interview at a hospital you're offered a position as a staff nurse for a particular shift at a particular salary. If you verbally agree to the offer, you've entered into an oral express contract. However, if you verbally agree to it and sign the hospital's written draft of the terms, you've entered into a written express contract. If you sign only a *statement* saying you've read and understand the hospital's policies and procedures, this is not an express contract, but rather an implied contract. The specificity of the contract's wording determines whether it's express or implied.

Contracts, of course, do not have to be written to be legal and binding. Most

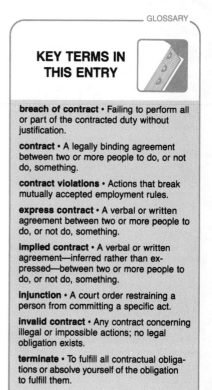

GLOSSARY

### KEY TERMS IN THIS ENTRY

**breach of contract** • Failing to perform all or part of the contracted duty without justification.

**contract** • A legally binding agreement between two or more people to do, or not do, something.

**contract violations** • Actions that break mutually accepted employment rules.

**express contract** • A verbal or written agreement between two or more people to do, or not do, something.

**implied contract** • A verbal or written agreement—inferred rather than expressed—between two or more people to do, or not do, something.

**injunction** • A court order restraining a person from committing a specific act.

**invalid contract** • Any contract concerning illegal or impossible actions; no legal obligation exists.

**terminate** • To fulfill all contractual obligations or absolve yourself of the obligation to fulfill them.

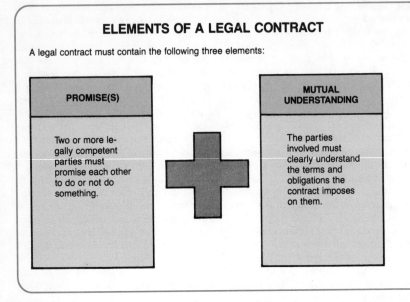

## ELEMENTS OF A LEGAL CONTRACT

A legal contract must contain the following three elements:

**PROMISE(S)**

Two or more legally competent parties must promise each other to do or not do something.

**MUTUAL UNDERSTANDING**

The parties involved must clearly understand the terms and obligations the contract imposes on them.

oral contracts are as legal and binding as written contracts. However, legal problems can arise. To begin with, most state courts don't consider an oral contract valid if its terms cannot be fulfilled within a year. An example is an employment contract, which usually runs indefinitely. In the previous example of an oral express contract, the period of employment would determine the contract's validity.

In addition, since the terms and conditions of oral contracts aren't committed to paper (as written contracts are), oral contracts are subject to each party's memory and interpretation. Changes in hospital policy and personnel, and the passage of time, can blur the original interpretation of the contract and cause disagreements between parties about its correct terms and promises.

Most contracts contain implied conditions—elements of the contract that aren't explicitly stated but are assumed part of the contract. For example, your employer will assume that you'll practice nursing in a safe, competent manner, as defined by your nurse practice act and your professional standards,

and that you'll maintain the hospital's standards and follow its policies and procedures. At the same time, you'll assume, based on implied conditions, that your employer will staff your unit adequately and with qualified personnel, will ensure a safe working environment, and will provide all necessary supplies and equipment for you to do your job.

If you decide to accept the contract, you can verbally agree to it, sign it, provide a written acceptance of it, or simply report for duty. If you fail to respond in any way to the offer, the employer can't interpret your silence as acceptance. But he may withdraw his offer to you, without penalty, at any time before you accept it.

### Breach of contract

When you breach a contract, you've unjustifiably failed to perform all or part of your contractual duty. A substantial breach of contract is never lawful. If you signed a contract which specified that you would work every third weekend and then you refused to do so, you would be breaching your contract. Your employer can either discharge (fire)

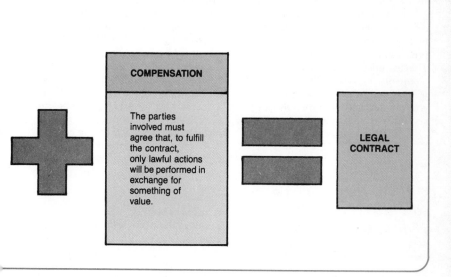

**COMPENSATION**

The parties involved must agree that, to fulfill the contract, only lawful actions will be performed in exchange for something of value.

**LEGAL CONTRACT**

you or seek an injunction against you. An injunction is a court order that would prevent you from working as a nurse for another employer. However, since an injunction is difficult to obtain and expensive, a hospital rarely seeks one against a nurse. But even if your employer doesn't take action against you, your breach of contract may damage your reputation and make it difficult for you to get a job at another hospital.

Your employer can also be guilty of breach of contract. If, for example, your employer fails to give you the vacation time specified in your contract, he has breached your contract. You can attempt to rectify the situation by first discussing it with your immediate supervisor. Show her your paycheck stubs as proof of the hours you worked and the compensation you received for it, and compare the stubs with your assigned work schedule. Then discuss the terms of your contract with her, and give her an opportunity to explain the error. If she offers you no satisfactory compensation and you've exhausted all channels of appeal, you may need to discuss the problem with an attorney

who has contract expertise. Provide the attorney with a written log of your attempts to rectify the situation, including what each person said and the date and time of their statements.

If you work in Canada, instead of seeking out an attorney, you can appeal for help to the provincial government agency that enforces minimum employment standards legislation. They will not charge you a fee.

### Terminating a contract

When you terminate a contract, you've either fulfilled all your obligations under the contract or absolved yourself of the obligation to fulfill the contract's terms.

Most contracts don't specify termination dates for your services. You can terminate them at any time, if you follow proper notification procedures. You can terminate other contracts, including those with termination dates, if your employer agrees to it. Follow the procedures outlined in your contract for giving written notice to your employer of your plans to leave. Most contracts require that you give 2 to 4 weeks' notice. If your contract has an automatic termination date, don't renew the contract after it expires.

Your employer can terminate your contract if he determines that you're incompetent or that you've behaved unprofessionally on the job (see Entry 64). This includes actions such as yelling at a patient, or striking him or a member of his family. Before discharging you, your employer would probably give you several warnings about the quality of

---

## "Your ability...to understand contract terms... can help you protect your rights as an employee."

---

your work. Then he might confront you with several examples of your shortcomings, from previous written evaluations of your performance. If you don't want to lose your job, you should discuss areas of improvement with him. He might be willing to arrange a probation period for you during which you can work to regain his confidence in you.

If you disagree with your employer's charges, you can request an evaluation by someone else who supervised your work, or you can request a transfer to another unit where you'd be reevaluated after an agreed-on length of time. However, your employer isn't obligated to agree to either request. If he doesn't, you can seek written support from your co-workers that will refute your employer's charges. You can also seek support from your employee union, if you have one. It may file a grievance in your behalf.

If you feel you've been unjustly terminated, you should do these things: ask your co-workers to vouch for you in writing; if you belong to a union, seek union support; and if you don't belong to a union, hire an attorney to represent you.

## When is a contract invalid?

A contract is considered invalid when the agreement concerns actions that are either illegal or impossible to carry out. A contract is considered illegal or void when: (1) a person lies to an employer about her qualifications as a nurse and signs a contract with him; (2) a person is forced to sign a contract; (3) the agreement involves theft or other unlawful actions; (4) a minor or mentally incompetent person signs the contract.

A contract is considered impossible to carry out when a party to the contract becomes physically or mentally disabled.

## A final word

Knowing about contracts won't directly improve the quality of your nursing care. But your ability to recognize the various types of contracts, to know what to look for in them, and to understand their limits can help you protect your rights as an employee and also secure benefits that will increase your satisfaction on the job.

# 47 Organizing a union

Since 1974, the number of nurses who've joined unions has increased significantly. Why? In that year, Congress amended the National Labor Relations Act to allow employees of private, nonprofit health-care institutions and agencies to unionize. (The act applies to employees of hospitals and other health-care facilities with an annual revenue of at least $250,000; and to nursing homes, visiting nurses associations, and related facilities with an annual revenue of at least $100,000.)

So if you work in such a place, you have the protected right to join a union and to help organize a bargaining unit. (Before 1974, only nurses in profit-making hospitals or nursing homes

# WHAT HAPPENS WHEN THE UNION WANTS IN:
## THE ELECTION PROCESS

Suppose you're working in a hospital in the United States (election procedures in Canada vary from province to province) where some of the employees want to unionize. Organizers have distributed leaflets and authorization cards. At least 30% of all the proposed union employees must sign these cards to authorize a union election. (If 50% or more sign authorization cards and the employer chooses to recognize the union, the law doesn't *require* an election.)

After the employees sign the authorization cards, the following steps occur:

> The union organizer notifies the National Labor Relations Board (NLRB), and an NLRB representative steps in as a referee and organizes the election.

> The employer may challenge any employee's eligibility. For example, an employee in a supervisory position may not be considered eligible according to the employer's interpretation of the law.

> The NLRB holds a hearing to decide who's eligible to join the union.

> The NLRB determines the place and election date. Then the employer and the union begin campaigning.

> The employer provides the NLRB with a list of the names and addresses of all eligible employees within 7 days after the NLRB announces the election date and place. The NLRB gives this list to the union.

> On election day, employees vote by secret ballot to accept or reject the union. If more than one union is on the ballot, the nurse can select one of the unions or vote for no representation.

> The NLRB representative tallies the votes. The results depend on *the majority of the ballots cast,* regardless of what proportion of eligible employees actually vote. (If only a minority of eligible employees actually vote, those few employees will decide the question of unionization for all the employees.)

| |
|---|
| If a majority of the voting employees choose the union, that union is legally required to represent *all* eligible employees, even those who didn't vote. The NLRB will certify the union as the employees' collective bargaining representative. |
| If a majority of the voting employees reject the union, the law prohibits another election involving any union for one year. |

could join unions and get labor-related protection from the law.)

After nurses won the right to unionize, many unions sought to represent them. The American Nurses' Association (ANA) has supported unionization for nurses since 1946. In fact, state ANA affiliates serve as the bargaining agent for most unionized nurses—representing more than 120,000 nurses. All other unions combined represent only about 50,000 nurses. (See *The ANA and Collective Bargaining*, page 304.)

Although the amendment opened the door for widespread efforts to persuade nurses to join union ranks, many nurses are not sure of their rights and limitations.

If you wanted to join a union or help organize one, would you know what legal protections and limitations you'd have? This entry will give you the information you need to understand how a union can become your representative in a health-care institution.

## The pros and cons of unionization

Many nurses have joined unions to improve their economic status, their working conditions, and their professional status. But some nurses have ambivalent feelings about unionization. You might share those feelings considering unionization's pros and cons.

Union proponents argue that unionization gives you a strong voice in bread-and-butter issues such as wages, benefits, and pensions. They also point out that unionization assures you fair grievance procedures and more influence in patient-care decisons. And it gives you more control over working conditions, such as scheduling and staffing. With these advantages, unionization equalizes the bargaining power between you and your employer.

But critics of unionization point to some disadvantages. Many critics say unionization tarnishes nursing's image by shifting attention from nurses' traditional focus on meeting patients' needs to concern about their economic status. Some nurses fear the potential disruptiveness of picketing and strikes. Other nurses argue that unionization creates an antagonism between them and their employers that prevents effective cooperation.

## Protecting your right to unionize

Who protects your right to unionize? The regulations governing union organizing among nurses come under the jurisdiction of the National Labor Relations Board (NLRB), the federal agency that enforces the national labor laws (see Entry 48). The NLRB will protect you when you want to organize a union or decertify one (vote the union out), protect your right to join a union, or defend you against unfair labor practices. The NLRB will also help an employer by enforcing regulations that control picketing and strikes and by providing remedies for a union's unfair labor practices.

If you want to organize a union, the NLRB will supervise procedures for elections. Election procedures involve the rules that both the union and management must follow when you vote on

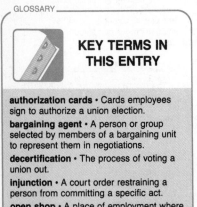

GLOSSARY

### KEY TERMS IN THIS ENTRY

**authorization cards** • Cards employees sign to authorize a union election.

**bargaining agent** • A person or group selected by members of a bargaining unit to represent them in negotiations.

**decertification** • The process of voting a union out.

**injunction** • A court order restraining a person from committing a specific act.

**open shop** • A place of employment where employees may choose whether or not to join a union.

**union shop** • A place of employment where employees must join a union.

## APPEALING TO THE NLRB

Employees, as well as employers, can appeal to the National Labor Relations Board (NLRB) about unfair labor practices. What can you do if you're organizing a union and you feel management is engaging in unfair labor practices? First, tell your union organizer. If she feels your charges are valid, either you or the union can report the charges to the NLRB. The board will ask you for a sworn statement concerning the dates and times of the alleged events, the names and positions of management staff involved, and the names and addresses of other employee witnesses. Your statement will serve as a legal affidavit and will supply the board with the information it needs to carry out an investigation.

Suppose the board finds through its investigation that your charges are valid—that management is engaging in unfair labor practices. Then, it'll issue a formal complaint against the employer.

The employer may appeal the board's finding. However, if the court upholds the board's determination, the employer must comply with the board's penalty—usually reinstating employees, issuing back pay, or restoring other benefits.

Consider this fictional example: While nurses at Good Faith Hospital were organizing a union campaign, supervisors asked them for the names of nurses who attended the meetings sponsored by the organizers. Also, one supervisor suggested to her staff that if a nurses' union was organized, the union might try to force management to increase wages—which, because of the hospital's precarious financial position, could cause layoffs. Several nurses complained about the supervisor's remarks at a subsequent union meeting. The union organizers agreed that management was interfering with union organization—an unfair labor practice—and consequently filed a charge with the board.

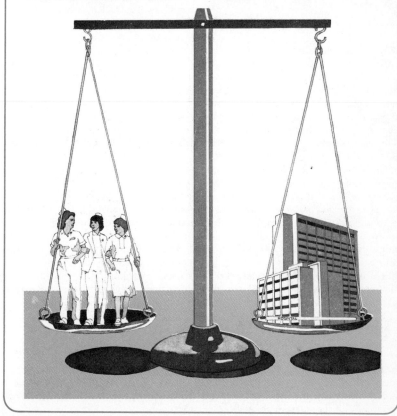

whether to join a union. Unfair labor practices may arise during the election process.

### Following the rules for union elections

If you want to get a union election where you work, the first step involves distributing authorization cards or, sometimes, a petition. Nurses or union representatives may distribute the cards. Nurses who want a chance to vote on the issue (whether they want a union or not) sign an authorization card. In the United States, if at least

---

*"Neither management nor union can interfere with your individual rights."*

---

30% of the eligible nurses sign the cards, you or the union can ask the NLRB to authorize and supervise an election. (If 50% or more of the eligible nurses sign the cards, the law allows the employer to forego the election process and simply recognize the union. This rarely occurs.) In Canada, 35% to 50% of the nurses must sign the cards to authorize an election. (For more on the election process, see *What Happens When the Union Wants In,* page 295.)

The union and management may disagree about which nurses are eligible to vote. Either side can challenge a nurse's eligibility. The NLRB will settle an eligibility dispute by reviewing the nurse's job description, her actual duties and responsibilities, and her supervisory functions, if any.

If you're voting in a union election, you may find more than one union on the ballot. The reason: After the first petitioning union demonstrates that 30% or more of the eligible nurses want an election, other unions can get on the ballot if they can get a show of interest from 10% of the nurse-employees.

### Management's limitations and rights

To protect your right to organize and belong to a union, the NLRB requires management to comply with five major limitations:
- Management can't interfere with your organizing activities.
- Management can't discriminate against you for participating in union activities, for testifying against management, or for filing a grievance.
- Management can't dominate a union by gaining undue influence over it, such as by paying union expenses or giving union leaders special benefits.
- Management can't refuse to bargain in good faith.
- Management must assume responsibility for any unfair labor practice committed by a supervisor.

But management also has rights protected by the NLRB. Under the law, management can:
- tell you the disadvantages of belonging to a union
- explain to you your election rights, such as your right to refuse to sign an authorization card
- encourage you to vote in a union election.

### Limitations placed on the union

The union must also comply with certain limitations. The NLRB ensures that the union:
- bargains in good faith
- assumes responsibility for any unfair labor practice committed by union officials
- doesn't threaten or force you to support the union
- doesn't demand that your employer do business only with companies—such as suppliers—that have unions.

Neither management nor the union can interfere with your individual rights assured by other laws, such as the Fair Labor Standards Act, the Civil Rights Act, the Age Discrimination in Employment Act, or equal rights amendments in states where those laws exist.

## RECOGNIZING UNFAIR LABOR PRACTICES

Like other employees, you have a legal right to participate in union activities. If your employer infringes on that right—through interference, domination, discrimination, or refusal to bargain—you can charge your employer with unfair labor practice. What's an unfair labor practice? Read the following examples to find out.

*Interference* includes:
• unilaterally improving wages or benefits during a union campaign to influence employees to vote against the union
• making coercive statements about participation in union activities
• threatening to close down the facility if a union is elected
• questioning employees about union activities
• spying on—or implying the possibility of spying on—union meetings.

*Domination* includes:
• paying a union's expenses
• giving union leaders special compensation or benefits
• taking an active part in organizing a union.

*Discrimination* includes:
• discharging, disciplining, or threatening an employee for joining a union or for encouraging others to join
• refusing to hire anyone who belongs to a union
• refusing to reinstate or promote an employee because she testified at a National Labor Relations Board hearing
• enforcing rules unequally between employees who are involved in union activities and those who aren't.

*Refusal to bargain* includes:
• taking unilateral action that affects any employment conditions either covered in an existing contract or included among legally mandated areas of bargaining
• refusing to meet with a union representative
• refusing to negotiate a mandatory issue
• demanding to negotiate a voluntary issue.

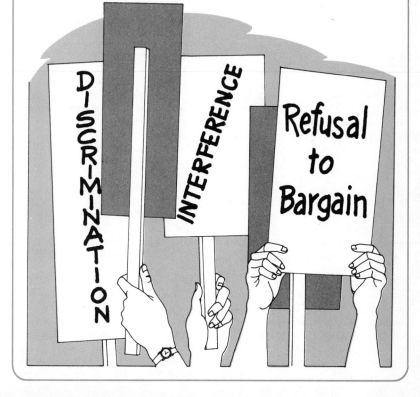

# UNDERSTANDING NURSES' UNIONS

If you're like most nurses, you have many questions about unionization. Here are questions and answers that'll clarify some of the issues:

**Q** *Can I join a labor union?*

**A** Yes. Congress amended the National Labor Relations Act in 1974 to cover private, nonprofit hospitals and health-care institutions. The law covers all private hospitals that provide at least $250,000 worth of health-care services a year and all related facilities that provide services worth at least $100,000. Most hospitals and nursing homes fall in those categories. Before then, the law allowed only nurses in profit-making hospitals and nursing homes to unionize.

**Q** *Can I be forced to join a union?*

**A** If you work under a contract that includes a "union shop," you have to join the union within a specified time to keep your job. If the contract provides for an "open shop," you can choose not to join the union and still keep your job.

**Q** *Can the hospital where I work fire me for helping to organize a union there?*

**A** Federal regulations strictly forbid an employer from firing you or taking any other reprisal against you for union organizing.

**Q** *What consequences do I face if I refuse to participate in my union's strike?*

**A** As long as you continue to work, your hospital or health-care institution will pay your wages and benefits. No union can force you to strike. But you might face some antagonism—even retaliation—from those colleagues who do strike.

## How a union organizer can help you

Nurses may start efforts to organize by asking a union for assistance. The union will assign one of its experienced workers to help in the organizing process. Often this person is a former hospital employee who has worked in a union organizing campaign.

The union can support the effort to unionize by supplying encouragement, stationery, printing, legal advice, organizational guidance, and other services. The union can also arrange for meeting halls and for publicity. And the union can file the proper election petitions with the NLRB.

## After the ballots are counted

The election determines whether the union wins or loses. To win, the union must get votes from a majority of the nurses who voted. If elected, the union will negotiate a contract that will include mutually agreeable wages, benefits, and work rules, devised by the negotiators and ratified by members of the bargaining unit.

Remember that regardless of the election's outcome, everyone will continue to work together. If the union wins, both management and labor will have to adjust to new rules spelled out in the contract. If the union loses, management should correct the problems that led to the organizing campaign, or it will probably face a renewed union effort in the future.

Different bargaining units usually represent different groups of workers in the same hospital. For example, RNs and LPNs/LVNs belong to different bargaining units and belong to different unions.

Be prepared to expend a lot of energy after you commit yourself to helping a unionization drive. A great deal of work is involved.

Don't let your commitment prevent you from maintaining good relations with supervisors and co-workers who oppose the union. When your view-

## PROTECTING YOUR RIGHT TO ORGANIZE A UNION

Who'll protect you if your hospital punishes you solely because you're involved in unionizing activities? The federal government will—in the form of the National Labor Relations Board (NLRB). The board enforces the National Labor Relations Act. This act explicitly sets forth your rights to form and join a union. The scenario that follows illustrates how the NLRB will protect your unionizing efforts:

Suppose you're working as a hospital pediatrics nurse. You support an effort to unionize the hospital's nurses. When asked by union organizers, you agree to distribute union pamphlets to your colleagues. You begin giving out pamphlets in the nurses' lounge, but a hospital administrator orders you to stop. He tells you the hospital's solicitation policy prohibits anyone from distributing literature inside the hospital. You remind him that the hospital has allowed employees to distribute other information. For example, the hospital let hospital nurses put a volunteer informa-

tion booth in the hospital's lobby for the city cancer society. You ignore the administrator's order and resume handing out the pamphlets.

The next day you're called into your nursing supervisor's office and fired. Stunned, you ask for an explanation. The supervisor gives you two reasons: violating the hospital's nonsolicitation policy and disobeying the administrator.

You file an unfair labor practice charge with the NLRB. After a hearing, the board concludes that the hospital can't prevent you from distributing the pamphlets on your own time in a nonwork area. The board also concludes that the hospital was discriminatory in applying the nonsolicitation policy.

In this situation, the board would order the hospital to reinstate you, pay your back wages, and refrain from punishing you or any other nurse who was active in the union drive.

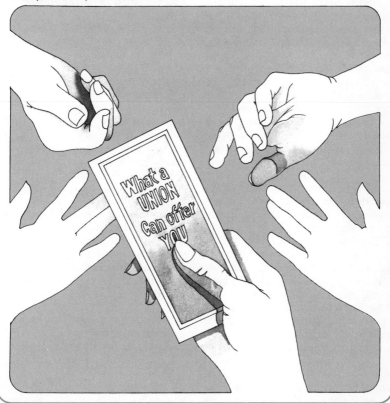

points and those of others compete, heated arguments and feelings of resentment can result. Remember that labor and management don't have to be adversaries.

### A final word

If you believe that organizing a union is necessary to improve the professional or economic status of the nurses who work in your institution, remember: the full force of the law will protect your efforts.

# 48 The legalities of collective bargaining

Collective bargaining is a legal process in which employees, acting as an organized unit, negotiate with their employer about working conditions and economic issues such as wages, hours, and fringe benefits. The process is based on the principle that, in a democracy, all groups have the right to organize. However, nurses and other health-care professionals have been explicitly granted that right only since 1974. Since then, nurses have made great strides in the area of collective bargaining. Today, nurses across the country are improving their professional and economic status through active participation in collective bargaining units.

The first milestone for collective bargaining came in 1935 with the passage of the National Labor Relations Act (NLRA). This act required employers to bargain with their employees, and it provided for the formation of a National Labor Relations Board (NLRB) to enforce the provisions of the act.

A second milestone for nurses came in 1946, when the American Nurses' Association (ANA) launched its Economic Security Program to establish national salary guidelines for nurses.

Together with the NLRA, the ANA facilitated nurses' right to bargain collectively.

In the years between 1946 and 1974, a number of federal and state laws affecting collective bargaining rights were passed—some of them narrowing previous laws.

In 1947, for example, the National Labor Management Relations Act (NLMRA)—known as the Taft-Hartley Act—said nonprofit organizations, including nonprofit hospitals, didn't have to bargain with their employees.

In 1962, an amendment to the NLMRA gave federal employees, including nurses, the right to bargain collectively.

And in 1974, another amendment explicitly granted employees of nonprofit facilities the right to bargain collectively again. (This amendment, officially named the 1974 Health Care Amendments to the Taft-Hartley Act, is commonly called the Taft-Hartley Amendment.)

In the meantime, several states had passed legislation requiring nonprofit hositals to bargain with their employees. So nurses who worked for nonprofit hospitals in Connecticut, Idaho, Massachusetts, Michigan, Minnesota, Montana, New Jersey, New York, Oregon, Pennsylvania, and Wisconsin had some bargaining rights all along.

State laws also define the rights of nurses who work for state, county, and municipal health-care institutions. Some states give these government employees the right to organize and bargain, but not the right to strike. Other states assign a specific arm of the state government to negotiate labor concerns or mandate pay scales for state-employed nurses.

### The National Labor Relations Board's purpose

Congress, in the NLRA, provided for the formation of the NLRB to administer and enforce the act's provisions. (In Canada, the provincial labour relations boards handle local labor issues, and the Canada Labour Relations Board deals with labor issues at the federal level, as in the case of military hospitals.)

The NLRB is specifically responsible for enforcing the NLRA and the NLMRA, determining appropriate bargaining units for employee groups, resolving disputes between labor and management, and conducting elections for employee bargaining representa-

> *"The collective bargaining process is based on the principle that, in a democracy, all groups have the right to organize."*

tives. The NLRB will not assert jurisdiction over labor laws for minimum wages, overtime pay, termination, and discrimination unless those issues have been written into the employees' labor contract and the contract doesn't provide for binding arbitration of alleged violations. If arbitration is provided for, the NLRB usually declines its jurisdiction and defers to the arbitrator.

The NLRB recognizes seven bargaining units within health-care facilities. The units, most recently identified in the NLRB case *St. Francis Hospital and Local 474, International Brotherhood of Electrical Workers* (1982), are: RNs and working nurses with licenses pending; doctors, excluding house staff; all other professionals; technical workers, including LPNs and LVNs; service and nonskilled maintenance employees, such as ward clerks, nursing assistants, aides, and orderlies; skilled maintenance employees, such as plumbers; and business clerical staff. (Such bargaining units don't exist in Canada.)

The NLRB resolves disputes between an employer and any of these bargain-

ing units by interpreting provisions in the NLMRA. For example, according to the law, a hospital *must* bargain with its employees, each party bargaining in good faith, about issues that directly or indirectly affect wages, hours, or working conditions. The NLRB has broadly interpreted the mandatory bargaining issues to include seniority; leaves of absence; work schedules and assignments; time off, including breaks, holidays, and vacation time; benefits; promotion policies; layoff policies; and grievance and discipline procedures. The NLRB also considers employee representation concerns as mandatory bargaining issues. These concerns include arbitration, union dues payroll check-off, and other union security matters.

Bargaining is only necessary for other issues if both the hospital and the employees voluntarily agree to it. For example, the NLRB considers as vol-

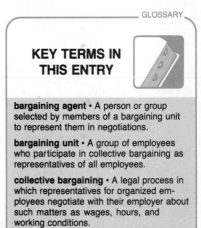

GLOSSARY

## KEY TERMS IN THIS ENTRY

**bargaining agent** • A person or group selected by members of a bargaining unit to represent them in negotiations.

**bargaining unit** • A group of employees who participate in collective bargaining as representatives of all employees.

**collective bargaining** • A legal process in which representatives for organized employees negotiate with their employer about such matters as wages, hours, and working conditions.

**mandatory bargaining issues** • Issues such as wages and working conditions that an employer must address during collective bargaining.

**unfair labor practices** • Tactics used by the employer or union that are prohibited by state and federal labor laws.

**voluntary bargaining issues** • Issues such as non-economic fringe benefits that an employer or union may or may not address during collective bargaining.

# THE ANA AND COLLECTIVE BARGAINING

Since 1946, the American Nurses' Association (ANA) has supported collective bargaining, and most RNs have chosen their state nurses association as their collective bargaining representative. Because state nurses associations are professional associations—not just labor organizations—their role in the collective bargaining process is controversial.

Proponents contend the state nurses associations, with their many professional concerns besides salary and working conditions, are the natural labor representatives for a group of professionals who come to the bargaining table with more than the traditional economic concerns.

Opponents who belong to the associations wonder whether collective bargaining itself is professional, and whether it's an appropriate role for their professional association to play. Members of some state nurses associations say no, and their associations don't engage in collective bargaining.

Employers and other unions challenge the associations' ability to represent staff nurses' interests and needs. These opponents say that so many association members are supervisors and administrators that state nurses associations are management-dominated, and therefore are inappropriate employee bargaining representatives. Some employers exert pressure on their nursing managers not to participate in their state nurses association because of the association's labor activities.

Once a state nurses association gets involved in collective bargaining, its activities are the same as any other bargaining agent's. The association represents its members in contract negotiations and in resolving grievances.

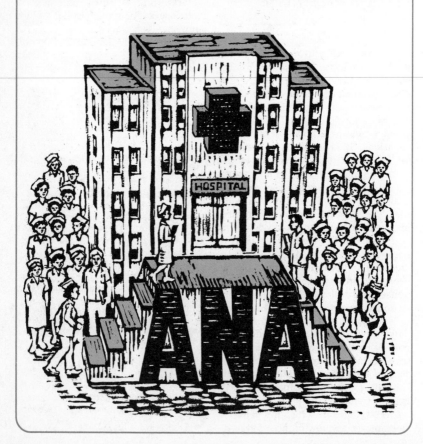

untary bargaining issues all other possible legal employment issues. Illegal issues such as requiring newly hired employees to join a union in less than 30 days, or prohibiting a person from being hired or from receiving benefits or promotions because of his age, race, sex, or religion are prohibited from being bargaining issues.

Since nurses can't force an employer to bargain over voluntary issues, bargaining for professional concerns usually depends on how committed the nurses are to the issues, how willing they are to bargain for them, and how flexible the employer is.

The NLRB interprets the employer's obligation to bargain in good faith as his responsibility to recognize and accept all validly selected employee representatives. And it views an employer's interference with his employees' organized activity as illegal infringement on the employees' right to organize and bargain collectively.

If a hospital or bargaining unit disagrees with an NLRB decision, either party can appeal that decision in a federal appellate court. In Canada, the courts won't interfere with a professional organization's decision unless that organization has acted outside its jurisdiction or has violated common law through its decision.

The NLRB hears many disputes on determining appropriate bargaining units (cases include *Mercy Hospitals of Sacramento, Inc.*, 1975; and *St. Francis Hospital and Local 474, International Brotherhood of Electrical Workers*, 1982), defining the supervisor's role, and protecting the employee's right to picket and solicit (cases include *NLRB v. Baptist Hospital*, 1979; and *Los Angeles New Hospital*, 1981). For example, in *NLRB v. Baptist Hospital*, the NLRB reaffirmed its prohibition of solicitation in upper-floor hospital corridors and sitting rooms that adjoined patient rooms and treatment rooms. However, the board upheld the employees' right of solicitation in first floor lobbies, the gift shop, and the cafeteria, unless the hospital could prove that patients frequented those areas.

## The decision to strike

Collective bargaining doesn't guarantee that the bargaining parties will ultimately reach an agreement. If the parties arrive at a stalemate in which neither party is willing to compromise, employees may decide to strike in hopes of forcing the employer to make concessions. A strike decision is an extreme measure, so labor laws have established provisions that require any curtailment of services to be orderly, thus protecting the employer and the public.

Some Canadian provinces prohibit health-care employees from striking. In these provinces, compulsory arbitration is imposed when employees and employer fail to reach an agreement. The arbitrator can then draft and impose contract terms.

In the United States, negotiating parties must follow this timetable—and series of steps—before a strike can be called:

• The side wanting to modify or terminate the contract must notify the other side 90 days before the contract expires (or labor or management proposes that changes take place).

• If, 30 days later, the two sides don't agree, they must notify the Federal Mediation and Conciliation Service (FMCS), and the corresponding state agency, of the dispute.

• Within 30 days, the FMCS will appoint a mediator and, if necessary, an inquiry board.

• Within 15 days, the inquiry board will give both sides its recommendations.

• If, after 15 more days, the parties don't agree, the employees may plan to strike. If the union didn't have employees vote earlier, it will hold a strike vote at this point.

• If a majority of employees vote to strike, the union must send management a notice at least 10 days before the scheduled strike, specifying the exact date, time, and place of the strike.

CASE STUDY

# THE PERILS OF NOT BARGAINING

Can a hospital avoid collective bargaining by refusing to recognize its staff's union? Of course not. The law—strengthened by court-case decisions—requires a hospital to bargain in good faith with duly elected unions. Here's a key court case, *Eastern Maine Medical Center v. NLRB* (1981), that illustrates this principle:

Nurses at Eastern Maine Medical Center voted 114 to 110 to be represented by the Maine State Nurses' Association, the state's largest nurses' union. In response, the hospital administration adopted a strong anti-union stand, refusing to meet with the nurses for collective bargaining talks. Moreover, the administration gave substantial wage-and-benefit increases to nonunion employees and withheld the increases from the union nurses.

The administration's policy of not bargaining with the union made the union nurses bitter and frustrated. And the union filed unfair labor practice charges against the hospital administration.

The National Labor Relations Board (NLRB) concluded that the hospital had violated the National Labor Relations Act by refusing to bargain in good faith and had discriminated against the union nurses. The board directed the hospital administration to negotiate with the union and to pay the wage-and-benefit increases withheld from the union nurses.

In upholding the board's actions, an appeals court ruled that the hospital's refusal to negotiate violated the nurses' collective bargaining rights.

---

The strike cannot be scheduled before the contract expires.

Employees who ignore the strike provisions and engage in illegal strikes lose the protection of the NLRA. They may be discharged by their employer. Unions that sanction or encourage illegal strikes may have their certification revoked by the NLRB.

## What's involved in delaying a strike

Employees may delay a strike for up to 72 hours if they feel the extra time would enable them to come to terms with management.

To delay the strike, they must give management written notice at least 12 hours before the strike was scheduled to start.

If the initial strike date passes during the negotiations, the union must issue another 10-day strike notice.

If the contract expires during the negotiations, the employer and employees remain bound by the contract.

## A final word

Collective bargaining is relatively well established among nurses in the United States and Canada. But it remains a controversial and often emotional topic. Many nurses who recognize the benefits of a collective voice still wonder whether organized union activity is consistent with their professional philosophies. Unfortunately, no single answer exists, because each nurse's professional and economic situation is unique.

To help assess your particular situation and to make an informed decision about participating in collective bargaining, ask yourself these questions: Will collective bargaining help my professional and economic status? Can I address my professional concerns through collective bargaining? Can I devote the time and effort that such organized activity demands? Can I change my working conditions as an individual, or do I need to organize with other nurses?

Only you can answer these questions. Keep in mind, as you ponder them, that labor laws exist to protect your rights as an employee as well as the rights of your employer.

# 49 Grievances and arbitration

As a staff nurse or a nurse manager, you can appreciate the need for procedures to settle labor disputes. You know what happens when an employee's dispute isn't resolved: Tempers quicken, morale declines, and apparent injustices smolder. That's why union and management officials give grievance and arbitration procedures high priority when they negotiate collective bargaining agreements.

As unions become more common in hospitals and other health-care institutions, you need to understand how grievance and arbitration procedures work. Even if your workplace isn't unionized, understanding these procedures can help you create fair work rules and grievance procedures where you work.

### Filing a grievance: A method of resolving disputes

When unionized employees and management sign a labor contract, they agree to abide by certain rules and policies during the contract's duration. A contract can't cite every dispute that may arise, so it includes grievance procedures. Grievance procedures establish specific steps that both sides agree to follow in trying to resolve disputes in an orderly fashion.

What's a grievance? That depends on the contract. Some contracts define a grievance as any complaint that reflects dissatisfaction with union or management policies. But most contracts define a grievance as a complaint that involves contract violations.

As a staff nurse, you or your union representative can file a grievance against your employer. Your union can file a grievance against management. Management can file a grievance—usually called a disciplinary action—against any employee. Most grievances are filed against management because of management's decision-making role.

### Knowing the types of grievances

Most grievances fall into one of two classifications: unfair labor practices and violations of a contract, a precedent, or a past practice. Unfair labor practices are tactics prohibited by state and federal labor laws. For example, under federal law, an employer who discriminates against you because you're involved in union activities commits an unfair labor practice. Violations of a contract, precedent, or past practice are actions that break mutually accepted work rules. For example, suppose your contract says a supervisor must give you 2 weeks' notice before making you rotate to another shift. If a supervisor assigns you to another shift without giving you notice, you can file a grievance.

### The causes of grievances

Grievances can involve an almost infinite number of complaints, but some occur consistently. Management often takes disciplinary action against employees who:

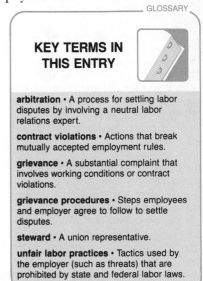

GLOSSARY

## KEY TERMS IN THIS ENTRY

**arbitration** • A process for settling labor disputes by involving a neutral labor relations expert.

**contract violations** • Actions that break mutually accepted employment rules.

**grievance** • A substantial complaint that involves working conditions or contract violations.

**grievance procedures** • Steps employees and employer agree to follow to settle disputes.

**steward** • A union representative.

**unfair labor practices** • Tactics used by the employer (such as threats) that are prohibited by state and federal labor laws.

- allow personal problems to interfere with their jobs
- fail to perform their assigned duties
- show poor work habits, such as tardiness or unreliability
- take an antagonistic attitude toward management in labor relations when serving in union positions.

Employees often file grievances against supervisors who:
- dispense discipline inconsistently
- show favoritism
- treat employees unfairly.

Other common sources of grievances include management's selection policies for promotions, favored shift assignments, disciplinary actions, and merit salary raises. Staff nurses sometimes file grievances when they're temporarily assigned head nurse responsibilities without getting commensurate pay.

Many grievances result from unwitting contract violations (such as poorly thought-out work load decisions) by *first-level* or *mid-level managers*. Personnel and labor relations departments can resolve many actions that would otherwise lead to grievances by answering labor questions and offering advice.

### Grievances follow step-by-step patterns

The elements of a grievance procedure vary from contract to contract. But the key elements always include reasonable time limits for filing a grievance and making a decision, procedures to appeal a grievance to higher union-management levels if the grievance isn't resolved, assigning priority to crucial grievances (such as worker suspensions or dismissals), and an opportunity for both sides to investigate the complaint.

The first step is usually an informal discussion between nurse and supervisor. She may then submit her complaint in writing. If the supervisor doesn't or can't resolve the grievance, the nurse can ask for a union representative, or steward, to assist her. The representative will meet with the supervisor to discuss the grievance's merits. If the supervisor stands firm, the nurse can then file a written complaint within a contract-specified time period. Subsequent hearings move to higher levels of management. The number of steps in a grievance procedure varies with each contract's provisions.

> *"Participants in the grievance procedure need to know when to compromise on a disputed issue."*

### Gripe or grievance: Making the distinction

Smooth labor relations require both sides to honor the contract's terms and to show good will when using the grievance procedures. Participants from both sides need to consider when to compromise or retreat on a disputed issue. For instance, union representatives must often defuse complaints before they become formal grievances. And an effective union representative must distinguish between a grievance and a gripe. What's the difference? A grievance is a substantive complaint that involves a contract violation. A gripe is a personal problem unrelated to the contract.

Sometimes union or management representatives pursue a groundless grievance for political or harassment purposes. A nurse's self-interest or her resentment of authority can lead to a groundless grievance. So can a supervisor's poor decision making or misuse of her authority. And sometimes neither side can work out a settlement on a substantive issue.

Whatever the reason, sometimes the grievance procedure fails to resolve the dispute. That's when arbitration enters the picture.

# WHAT CONSTITUTES A LEGITIMATE GRIEVANCE?

If you're not sure whether you have a legitimate grievance, read these examples of the five types of grievances. If your grievance matches one, it's probably legitimate.

### Contract violations

Your employment contract is binding between you *and* your employer. If your employer violates that contract, you have a valid grievance. In the following examples, assume that the contract prohibits the employer action described:
- You're performing the charge nurse's job 2 or 3 days a week but still receiving the same pay as other staff nurses.
- You've had to work undesirable shifts or on Sundays more often than other nurses.
- Your supervisor doesn't post time schedules in advance.
- Your employer discharges you without just cause.

### Federal and state law violations

Any action by your employer that violates a federal or state law would be the basis for a grievance, even if your contract permits the action. For example:
- You receive less pay for performing the same work as a male nurse.
- You don't receive overtime pay that you're entitled to.
- Your employer doesn't promote you because of your race.

### Past practice violations

A past practice—one that's been accepted by both parties over an extended period but is suddenly discontinued by the employer without notification—may be the basis for a grievance. For example:
- Your employer charges you for breaking equipment when others haven't been charged.
- Your employer revokes parking lot privileges.
- Your employer eliminates a rotation system for float assignments.

A past practice violation often becomes a complicated grievance and can occur even if the past practice isn't specified in the contract. If the practice violates the contract, either party can demand that the contract be enforced. If the practice is unsafe, an arbitrator may simply abolish it.

### Health and safety violations

Grievances in this category most often involve working conditions an employer is responsible for even if the contract doesn't cover the specific complaint. For example:
- You're required to hold patients during X-rays.
- You have no hand-washing facilities near patient rooms.

### Employer policy violations

Your employer can't violate its own rules without being guilty of a grievance, even though it can change the rules unilaterally. For example:
- You haven't received a performance evaluation in 2 years, although your employee handbook states that such evaluations will be done annually.
- Your employer assigns you a vacation period without your consent, contrary to personnel policies.

## Learning the process of arbitration

Arbitration is a process that settles a labor dispute by presenting evidence to a neutral labor relations expert, usually an employee of a private or government agency. Unions and management aren't legally required to include arbitration clauses in their contracts, so arbitration isn't automatic. One side must seek it after the grievance procedure fails to resolve the dispute. The side requesting arbitration gives a written notice to the other side that arbitration has been called for. Then the requesting side contacts one of several national agencies that supply arbitrators, such as the Federal Mediation and Conciliation Service or the American Arbitration Association. Sometimes the labor contract specifies which agency to use. Both sides must agree on a specific arbitrator and the date, time, and place for the arbitration hearing.

The arbitration hearing closely follows a courtroom proceeding, although it's not as formal. The side that requests the arbitration has the burden of proof and must present evidence that the contract has been violated. (However, when a nurse challenges disciplinary action, management must prove its case first by presenting supporting evidence.) In any arbitration hearing, both sides may call and cross-examine witnesses. The requesting side makes a closing summary, followed by one from the opposing side. Each side can submit written briefs instead of making summary statements.

The arbitrator usually renders a written decision weeks or even months after the hearing. But if both sides request an immediate response, the arbitrator can issue an oral decision and withhold a written explanation of the decision unless requested by both sides.

Both sides prefer arbitration to a lengthy court fight because arbitration is speedier and less expensive, and it doesn't require attorneys. But when a dispute goes to arbitration, both sides lose control of the outcome because, in the United States, the arbitrator's decision is binding. The other side can challenge the decision in court, but the court rarely overturns an arbitrator's decision. In Canada, the court may supervise arbitration itself but will never overturn an arbitrator's decision.

## Resolving complaints due to unfair labor practices

Most grievances arising from contract violations follow contract-stipulated grievance and arbitration procedures. But charges of unfair labor practices go to the National Labor Relations Board (NLRB), the federal agency that prosecutes unfair labor practices. The NLRB will conduct a hearing to review evidence and then issue a decision. Either side can challenge an NLRB decision in court.

If a nurse has a complaint involving discrimination on the basis of race, religion, national origin, age, or sex, she can file a charge of discrimination with the federal Equal Employment Opportunity Commission (EEOC) or a comparable state agency in addition to filing a grievance. The EEOC handles violations of laws such as:

• the Equal Pay Act of 1963, which forbids wage discrimination based on an employee's sex
• the Civil Rights Act of 1964, which forbids job and wage discrimination based on an employee's religion, race, sex, or ethnic background
• the Age Discrimination in Employment Act of 1967, which forbids discrimination based on an employee's age.

The EEOC will also prosecute disputes involving sexual harassment. Employees don't have to be union members to file a complaint with the EEOC.

## A final word

Grievance and arbitration procedures exist to ensure that you have recourse when a contract is violated or when disciplinary actions are unfair. Remember, at any time during your nursing career—in a staff or supervisory position—you could become involved in a labor dispute. You might be an employee filing a grievance, a witness in an arbitration hearing, or a supervisor accused of treating an employee unfairly. Your best help *then* will be the knowledge of grievance and arbitration procedures you can start getting *now*.

## Selected References

American Nurses' Association. *Guidelines for the Individual Nurse Contract.* Kansas City, Mo.: American Nurses' Association, 1974.

Bernzweig, Eli P. *The Nurse's Liability for Malpractice: A Programmed Course,* 3rd ed. New York: McGraw-Hill Book Co., 1981.

Cazalas, Mary. *Nursing and the Law,* 3rd ed. Rockville, Md.: Aspen Systems Corp., 1979.

Creighton, Helen. *Law Every Nurse Should Know,* 4th ed. Philadelphia: W.B. Saunders Co., 1981.

Fenner, Kathleen M. *Ethics and Law in Nursing.* New York: Van Nostrand Reinhold Co., 1980.

*The Guide to Basic Law and Procedures under the National Labor Relations Act.* Washington, D.C.: U.S. Government Printing Office, 1978.

Hemelt, Mary, and Mackert, Mary. *Dynamics of Law, Nursing and Health Care,* 2nd ed. Reston, Va.: Reston Publishing Co., 1982.

Klaus, Robert C. "The Ins and Outs of Collective Bargaining," *Journal of Nursing Administration* 10(9):18-21, September 1980.

Rothman, Daniel A., and Rothman, Nancy L. *The Professional Nurse and the Law.* Boston: Little, Brown & Co., 1977.

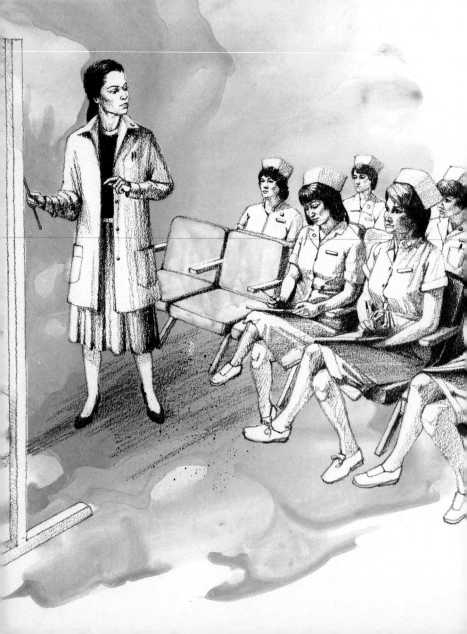

# Your Choices in Nursing Education

## Introduction

You undoubtedly felt a strong sense of accomplishment the day you graduated from nursing school. And the day you passed your licensing examination also gave you the glow that comes from a job well done. Now you're a working nurse, with a whole new set of professional hurdles to clear. And one of the biggest is keeping up with what's happening in your chosen field.

Health-care technology has rapidly and continually advanced in recent years. Sometimes you may feel that those advances are outdistancing your ability to keep pace. Whether you're a newly graduated nurse or a nurse with several years' experience, you're probably wondering how you can best meet the challenge. The most sensible answer is getting more education.

Regardless of your needs, the menu of courses and programs available to help you do your job better is wide and versatile; it ranges from a BSN program for working nurses to continuing education credits to keep you on course in your specialty. This chapter can help you determine your own educational needs and select the best program for you.

The American Nurses' Association has proposed that, after 1985, a bachelor's degree be required for entry into professional nursing. Do you know how this proposal will affect you? Whether you're a student nurse or a working nurse, it can have a major impact on your professional career. Entry 50, "Understanding entry-into-practice issues," defines the proposal for you and explores its significance to the profession.

If you're a nurse who's already decided to pursue a BSN program, you're halfway to your goal. But the other half of the decision—what particular program to enter—can be a tough one. Entry 51, "BSN programs: The advantages and options," describes and discusses the four major types of BSN programs available. It also gives you some guidelines on selecting the program that'll be right for you.

Suppose you're a recent graduate just starting out on your first job. Relating what you learned in school to your new job responsibilities can be difficult. To make the transition smoother, some hospitals use nursing internship programs. Entry 52, "Nursing internship programs: Antidote to reality shock?", tells you how these programs work. This entry also serves as a valuable guide for the experienced nurse who'd like to be a preceptor in an internship program.

All areas of health care are becoming more complex. As a nurse, you need relevant, up-to-date information about specialization in nursing. Before de-

## THE UPS AND DOWNS OF NURSING PROGRAMS

This chart shows you how nursing education's direction has changed over the past 3 decades.

In 1955, almost 85% of nursing schools were hospital-based diploma programs. This chart shows how these program numbers have dwindled: By 1981, almost 80% of nursing schools weren't diploma programs. Why? Because associate and bachelor's degree programs had dramatically *increased* in number. In 1981, more than 50% of the nursing schools in the nation offered associate-degree programs, compared to only about 5% of nursing schools in 1955. Bachelor's degree programs' numbers have swelled, too. Today, better than 25% of nursing schools offer bachelor's degrees. In 1955, only about 10% of them did.

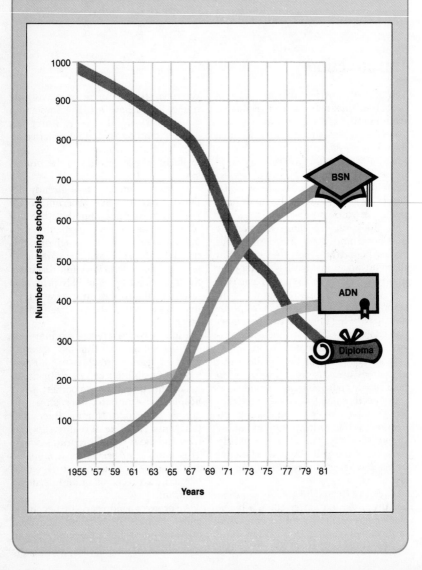

## COMPARING NURSING PROGRAMS

**Diploma**

- Prepares hospital staff nurse
- Affiliated primarily with hospitals; may be associated with a college for supporting course work
- Requires high school diploma or equivalent; also requires college entrance examination for most schools
- Runs 3 years—27 to 36 school months
- Grants nursing diploma

**ADN**

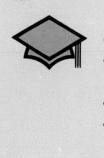

- Combines nursing and sciences with some general education to prepare hospital staff nurse
- Affiliated primarily with community or junior colleges; some, with 4-year colleges
- Requires high school diploma or equivalent; also requires college entrance examination for most schools
- Runs 2 years—18 to 21 school months
- Grants associate degree in nursing

**BSN**

- Combines liberal arts and general education with nursing courses to prepare nurse who can function in various nursing roles and health-care settings
- Affiliated with colleges and universities
- Requires high school diploma or equivalent and college entrance examination; may require prerequisite courses before admission to nursing major
- Runs 4 to 5 years
- Grants bachelor's degree in nursing

ciding on a program of specialization and possibly certification, be sure you know all the alternatives open to you. Entry 53, "Preparing for specialty practice," gives you an informed overview of those alternatives.

You may already be practicing in a state where continuing education for nurses is mandatory. In other states, the debate is still going on. In today's nursing practice, the question isn't "Should a nurse pursue continuing education?" but rather "Should her continuing education be voluntary or mandatory?" Entry 54, "Continuing education—voluntary or mandatory?", looks at both sides of the question. This entry also gives you an update on the continuing education controversy in both the United States and Canada.

Because of the proliferation of continuing education programs, finding out what's available and what's best for you are real challenges. No one wants to spend hard-won time and hard-earned money on a program that's ill-

# STUDENT LOANS:
## WHERE TO GO TO FINANCE YOUR EDUCATION

If you'd like to continue your nursing education or possibly finish a degree, but don't have the funds, student loan programs may offer you the funds you need. The chart below explains three types of programs that lend money to nursing students. Check the financial aid office at the school you plan to attend for more complete information—including the current interest rates on such loans—and for application forms. The demand for student loans is heavy, so apply early.

| LOAN PROGRAM | SOURCE OF FUNDS | LOAN LIMIT | INTEREST RATE | REPAYMENT TIME |
|---|---|---|---|---|
| Guaranteed Student Loan Program (GSL) | Bank or other lending institution | Up to $2,500 per year | 9% per year | Begins 6 months after graduation, leaving school, or dropping below half-time enrollment |
| National Direct Student Loan (NDSL) | Federal government | Up to $3,000 for first 2 years; up to $6,000 for BSN degree programs; more available for graduate and professional programs | 5% per year | Begins 6 months after graduation, leaving school, or dropping below half-time enrollment; payment extended over 10 years |
| Nursing Student Loan | Federal government | Depends on government funding and student's financial need | 6% per year | Begins 6 months after graduation, leaving school, or changing majors |

conceived or that doesn't give what it promised. Entry 55, "Choosing a continuing education program," not only shows you what's available but helps you make a prudent choice.

If you're a nurse who needs help in sorting out educational choices, this chapter is for you. Read on to discover the wealth of educational choices facing you and how to select from among them to enhance your professional growth.

# 50 Understanding entry-into-practice issues

Entry into practice is currently a hotly debated issue among nurses. The issue centers around the position of the American Nurses' Association (ANA) that a bachelor's degree should be the minimum requirement for entry into professional nursing practice.

Some nurses support the entry-level requirement in principle, but feel that it won't work in practice. Others reject the idea outright. Still others feel that the trend toward the bachelor's requirement has already begun and is gaining momentum.

Although debate over the issue divides nurses, most agree on this: The entry-level issue is changing the nursing profession by creating new professional standards that will affect your future as a nurse. You should get involved now in the issue of entry into practice.

## Understanding the trend toward a bachelor's requirement

In 1909, students enrolled in this country's first baccalaureate nursing program. Since then, efforts to increase educational requirements for nurses have become more organized in terms of professional support, more focused in terms of goals, and much broader in scope. In 1965, the ANA published its position paper on education for entry into professional practice. This position paper advocated that nursing education nationwide take place in academic institutions. Professional nursing students would complete a bachelor's degree program, and technical nursing students would complete an associate degree program. The new standards would be implemented gradually, this position paper suggested, over several decades: new bachelor's degree graduates would gradually replace nondegree nurses currently in practice.

Unfortunately, many nurses misinterpreted the ANA's position to mean that all nondegree nurses would either have to return to school to complete a bachelor's program or lose their licenses. After the initial flare-up of emotions, debate over the issue—at least on the national level—reached a standstill.

Then, in 1976, the debate was reactivated: The New York State Nurses Association passed a resolution requiring that, beginning in 1985, nurses would have to earn bachelor's degrees in order to enter the profession. The resolution further stipulated that a waiver, or grandfather clause, would protect the rights and licensure of currently licensed nurses.

Two years later, at the ANA's 1978 convention, the association reaffirmed its position and voted to implement the new educational requirements by 1985. The ANA's 1985 resolution also set deadlines for identifying competencies and titles for the bachelor's and associate degree nurse.

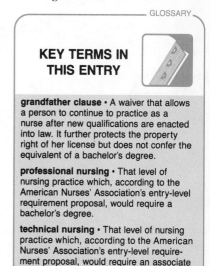

GLOSSARY

### KEY TERMS IN THIS ENTRY

**grandfather clause** • A waiver that allows a person to continue to practice as a nurse after new qualifications are enacted into law. It further protects the property right of her license but does not confer the equivalent of a bachelor's degree.

**professional nursing** • That level of nursing practice which, according to the American Nurses' Association's entry-level requirement proposal, would require a bachelor's degree.

**technical nursing** • That level of nursing practice which, according to the American Nurses' Association's entry-level requirement proposal, would require an associate degree or graduation from a diploma program.

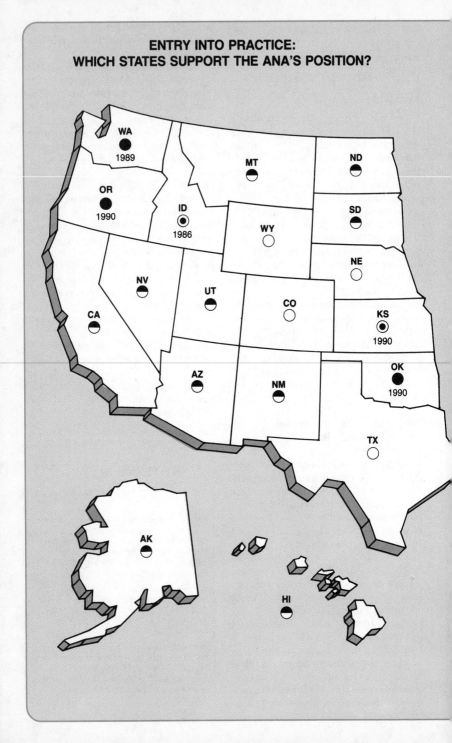

**ENTRY INTO PRACTICE:**
**WHICH STATES SUPPORT THE ANA'S POSITION?**

The following chart shows you which states support the American Nurses' Association's (ANA) position on entry into practice. As you know, a number of states have developed plans to establish a BSN requirement, and some of them have set target dates for when that requirement should go into effect. Other states have no plan but do have entry-requirement target dates. Still other states support the ANA's position but haven't taken any action toward establishing the BSN requirement.

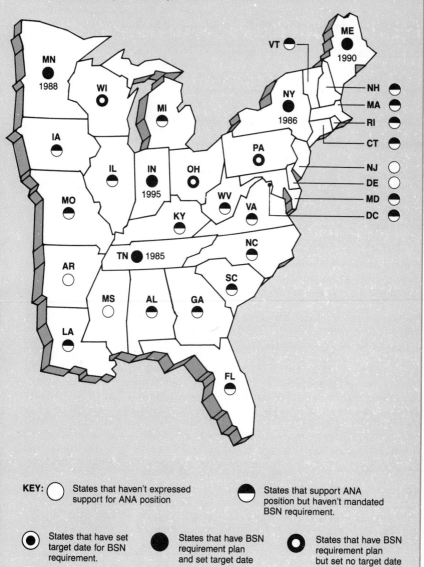

**KEY:** ◯ States that haven't expressed support for ANA position

◑ States that support ANA position but haven't mandated BSN requirement.

◉ States that have set target date for BSN requirement.

● States that have BSN requirement plan and set target date

◎ States that have BSN requirement plan but set no target date

## Conflicting views of the ANA's position

In its 1965 position paper, the ANA stated its continued support for LPN/LVN, diploma, associate degree (AD), and bachelor's degree programs. It endorsed the need for a bachelor's requirement for professional nursing practice; an associate degree or diploma for technical nursing practice; and a certificate in practical/vocational nursing for practical/vocational nursing practice.

Most groups that support the bachelor's degree entry-level requirement feel that the nursing profession would benefit from the requirement in the following ways:
• increased knowledge base and research skills that will better enable the nursing profession to meet society's changing demands
• increased quality of patient care
• improved leadership and management capabilities
• improved accountability and power for the nursing profession
• increased public awareness of nursing roles and capabilities
• improved professional status for nurses
• enhanced educational and professional advancement.

Opponents of the bachelor's degree entry-level requirement, however, question the need for changing basic nursing requirements. They feel that the present system, with four levels of nursing education, adequately meets society's health-care needs.

Organizations of licensed practical/vocational nurses fear that the entry-level requirement may increase the cost of nursing education and possibly eliminate the role of practical/vocational nurses in the future. The National Federation of Licensed Practical Nurses, the National Association for Practical Nurse Education and Service, and some service groups—such as the American Health Care Association—have voiced their opposition to the entry-level requirement. In March 1979, the National Advisory Council on Vocational Education adopted a formal resolution to oppose the ANA's position.

Among the major reasons why these groups oppose the bachelor's degree entry-level requirement are:
• lack of evidence that change is warranted
• projected increased educational and (probably) health-care costs
• a decreased supply of nurses as a result of the increased educational requirements
• decreased access to the nursing profession for minorities and disadvantaged persons as a result of the increased cost of a nursing education
• disruption in the present four-level nursing system
• difficulty with nurses' moving from state to state, and with licensure reciprocity, if entry-level requirements aren't adopted nationwide
• insufficient availability of BSN/RN completion programs.

Until now, the American Hospital Association and the American Medical Association have taken no official positions on the issue.

In Canada, nurses are involved in a similar debate over the entry-level issue. Many Canadian nurses have opposed the Alberta Association of Registered Nurses' resolution to require a bachelor's degree for professional nurses by the year 2000. The Canadian Nurses Association (CNA) has established a Committee on Entry into Practice to study the effects of the requirement on Canadian nursing practice. The CNA plans to appoint a national task force to create proposals for implementing the requirement over a period of 20 years.

## Implementing the entry-level requirement—when and how?

Implementation of the ANA's proposed entry-level requirement by 1985 seems unlikely. But a more gradual implementation, perhaps over a period of 30 to 40 years, will probably occur.

One obstacle to 1985 implementation

# OTHER PROFESSIONAL ORGANIZATIONS SPEAK OUT

Here's what the National League for Nursing has to say about entry into practice in its February 1982 position paper:

> Increased sharing by nurses of accountability for the quality and cost of health care compels greater concern not only for the education of graduates of nursing programs—that they be adequately prepared to make independent decisions based on sound knowledge and experience—but also for their appropriate utilization within the health-care system....
>
> "Nursing as an occupation, in the broadest sense, covers a wide range of activities that may be viewed as a continuum beginning with simple nurturing tasks, progressing through increasingly complex responsibilities and culminating in critical decision-making activities. To meet the reality of this wide range of responsibilities and activities, a corresponding range of nursing practice roles is required; these have come to be referred to as vocational, technical, and professional nursing practice.
>
> "For each nursing role, adequate pre-service preparation must be required.... (P)rofessional nursing practice requires the minimum of a bachelor's degree with a major in nursing. Preparation for technical nursing practice requires an associate degree or a diploma in nursing. Preparation for vocational nursing requires a certificate or diploma in vocational/practical nursing.
>
> "Therefore,...the National League for Nursing supports the education of nurses in programs that differ in purposes and lengths and that prepare for varying kinds of practice entailing different degrees of responsibility.

Here's what the American Association of Critical Care Nurses has to say about the entry-into-practice issue as of January 1982:

> The Registered Nurse is committed to ensuring that all patients receive optimal care. This nurses practice is based on the following:
> - Individual professional accountability
> - Thorough knowledge of the interrelatedness of body systems and the dynamic nature of the life process
> - Recognition and appreciation of the individual's wholeness, uniqueness, and significant social and environmental relationships
> - Appreciation of the collaborative role of all members of the health-care team
>
> "Therefore, be it resolved that the minimal preparation for entry into professional nursing practice should be the baccalaureate degree in nursing;
>
> "Be it further resolved that registered nurses not currently holding a baccalaureate degree in nursing be granted professional status;
>
> "Based upon a recognition and thorough understanding of [the] problems which exist for many of its members [to fulfill the requirements for achieving a baccalaureate degree], be it further resolved that AACN continually address the problems and incorporate mechanisms into organizational activities that will assist the AACN member without a baccalaureate degree in nursing to attain said degree.

For the complete texts of these position papers, see the appendices.

is the lack of unified support from nurses. Also, too few students will graduate from bachelor's degree programs in 1985 to make the entry-level requirement feasible.

However, efforts *are* underway to im-plement the requirement; 11 of the 41 state nurses' associations that support the ANA's position are actively pur-suing implementation plans. The New York and Ohio associations have been unsuccessful, so far, in getting legis-

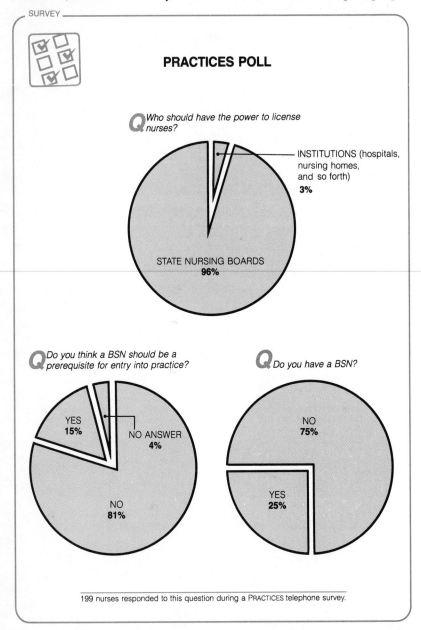

SURVEY

# PRACTICES POLL

**Q** Who should have the power to license nurses?

INSTITUTIONS (hospitals, nursing homes, and so forth)
**3%**

STATE NURSING BOARDS
**96%**

**Q** Do you think a BSN should be a prerequisite for entry into practice?

YES
**15%**

NO ANSWER
**4%**

NO
**81%**

**Q** Do you have a BSN?

NO
**75%**

YES
**25%**

199 nurses responded to this question during a PRACTICES telephone survey.

lation passed for the 1985 entry-level requirement. Other state associations established later target dates for implementation, giving them more time to lobby for support. Still other associations have decided to approach the implementation process in stages. For example, before approaching the state legislature, the Minnesota Nurses Association first passed a resolution that established titles for the two levels of nursing practice. It also approved role descriptions that distinguish the bachelor's degree nurse, or RN, from the RN's assistant, who would be a nursing care technician.

The remaining state nurses associations that support the ANA position have been unable to actively pursue the entry-level issue because of more immediate concerns, such as representation on state boards of nursing, collective bargaining, and third-party reimbursement.

The New Jersey State Nurses Association is the only association in which opponents succeeded in rescinding a resolution that supported the entry-level requirement.

Questions remain as to who will put the entry-level requirement into practice once it becomes law. The state boards of nursing will probably assume that responsibility, because nursing licensure falls under their jurisdiction (see Entry 3). Of course, problems may arise regarding licensure reciprocity if some states remain opposed to the entry-level requirement.

### How will the entry-level requirement affect diploma, AD, and practical/vocational nurses?

If you're a diploma or AD nurse, you may find few opportunities for advancement if the ANA's position on entry into practice is adopted by your state. Even now, certain educational requirements may make you ineligible for certain nursing positions.

For example, a bachelor's degree is currently the minimum requirement for entry into the specialty areas of community-health nursing and school nursing. And in major medical centers, the minimum requirement for nursing management and clinical education staff is often either a bachelor's or a master's degree. So although a grand-

*"A grandfather clause will protect your RN license but it can't guarantee career advancement opportunities."*

father clause will protect your RN license, it cannot guarantee you opportunities for career advancement.

If you're an LPN or LVN, your future is even more uncertain. The very existence of your level of nursing will depend on the ongoing need for LPNs/LVNs in the health-care setting.

### A final word

The entry-level issue has raised a great many questions about the future of the nursing profession. For example, if the ANA entry-level resolution of 1978 is implemented, how will it affect the legal and professional scope of nursing practice? What will be the appropriate roles of the new professional and technical nurses? What official title will each use? How will the new standards for entry into practice affect currently licensed nurses?

Because implementation *will* probably occur, you should familiarize yourself with these basic issues without further delay. Once you understand the issues, you should get involved. Let your state nurses association and your state representatives know where you stand on the entry-level issue. Active involvement in the issue will keep you informed of developments and give you an opportunity to direct the course of those developments—toward the best interests of the nursing profession.

# 51 BSN programs: The advantages and options

Are you a nurse who's considering going back to school to earn a bachelor of science degree in nursing (BSN)? If so, you're not alone. Only about one in five working nurses in the United States and Canada has a BSN—about 200,000 out of 1 million. But more and more nurses—including working nurses who've been out of school for years—are fitting BSN educations into their busy schedules. Why? Because now more than ever, a BSN is a powerful support for a nurse who's serious about a long-term career and professional advancement.

Four key forces are persuading many nurses to get BSNs:

• pressure from nursing organizations and associations that see the BSN as a way to gain undisputed professional status for nurses

• the growing complexity and scope of nursing practice

• the need for increased nursing competency to keep up with technologic advances

• the trend toward requiring a BSN (and higher degrees) for promotion to high-level nursing positions.

You may be wondering, "If I decide to pursue a BSN, what type of program is best for me?" You have more choices than you may imagine. The right choice is critical for your career. Read on to learn how BSN programs differ—and how to choose the one that best fits your needs.

## Understanding BSN degrees and school accreditation

When you're considering working for a bachelor's degree, be sure to choose a school that offers you a BSN. You need to be aware of the difference between a BSN and a bachelor of science degree in a *nonnursing major*.

Some nurses make the mistake of choosing a program that offers only a bachelor's degree with a nonnursing major. A nonnursing degree may sound convenient and attractive, but it has serious limitations for nurses who want to advance. A nonnursing degree program doesn't really prepare you for current nursing practice, offers no nursing courses, and has few or no qualified nurse faculty members.

Some schools don't offer a BSN but do offer a bachelor of science degree with a nursing major, which is virtually the same as a BSN.

A BSN or equivalent degree will prepare you for nursing's modern challenges, for professional advancement, and for entering a master's degree program in nursing—an option you'll want to keep open. A BSN will also give you access to many nursing jobs that specifically require a BSN, such as some military service jobs and community health-service jobs.

When you're choosing a school, make sure that the school and its nursing program are accredited. State boards of nursing set the minimum standards for nursing education, but two other organizations grant accreditation. The Commission on Education (part of the United States Department of Education) grants regional accreditation to a school after evaluating its educational programs, faculty, and facilities, and determining that they meet national

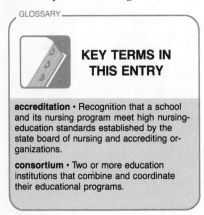

GLOSSARY

## KEY TERMS IN THIS ENTRY

**accreditation** • Recognition that a school and its nursing program meet high nursing-education standards established by the state board of nursing and accrediting organizations.

**consortium** • Two or more education institutions that combine and coordinate their educational programs.

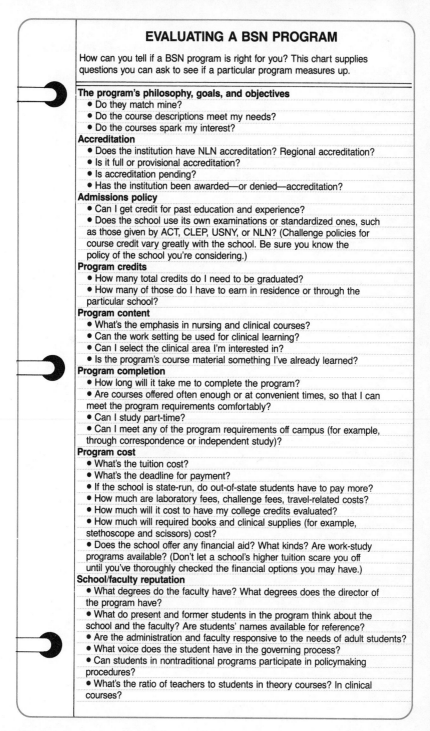

# EVALUATING A BSN PROGRAM

How can you tell if a BSN program is right for you? This chart supplies questions you can ask to see if a particular program measures up.

**The program's philosophy, goals, and objectives**
- Do they match mine?
- Do the course descriptions meet my needs?
- Do the courses spark my interest?

**Accreditation**
- Does the institution have NLN accreditation? Regional accreditation?
- Is it full or provisional accreditation?
- Is accreditation pending?
- Has the institution been awarded—or denied—accreditation?

**Admissions policy**
- Can I get credit for past education and experience?
- Does the school use its own examinations or standardized ones, such as those given by ACT, CLEP, USNY, or NLN? (Challenge policies for course credit vary greatly with the school. Be sure you know the policy of the school you're considering.)

**Program credits**
- How many total credits do I need to be graduated?
- How many of those do I have to earn in residence or through the particular school?

**Program content**
- What's the emphasis in nursing and clinical courses?
- Can the work setting be used for clinical learning?
- Can I select the clinical area I'm interested in?
- Is the program's course material something I've already learned?

**Program completion**
- How long will it take me to complete the program?
- Are courses offered often enough or at convenient times, so that I can meet the program requirements comfortably?
- Can I study part-time?
- Can I meet any of the program requirements off campus (for example, through correspondence or independent study)?

**Program cost**
- What's the tuition cost?
- What's the deadline for payment?
- If the school is state-run, do out-of-state students have to pay more?
- How much are laboratory fees, challenge fees, travel-related costs?
- How much will it cost to have my college credits evaluated?
- How much will required books and clinical supplies (for example, stethoscope and scissors) cost?
- Does the school offer any financial aid? What kinds? Are work-study programs available? (Don't let a school's higher tuition scare you off until you've thoroughly checked the financial options you may have.)

**School/faculty reputation**
- What degrees do the faculty have? What degrees does the director of the program have?
- What do present and former students in the program think about the school and the faculty? Are students' names available for reference?
- Are the administration and faculty responsive to the needs of adult students?
- What voice does the student have in the governing process?
- Can students in nontraditional programs participate in policymaking procedures?
- What's the ratio of teachers to students in theory courses? In clinical courses?

## NEW YORK'S REX PROGRAM: HOW DOES IT WORK?

Suppose you're an RN, age 34, with either a hospital diploma or an associate degree. After 10 years of full-time work, you're eager for a change. Since graduation, you've earned 50 college credits. Now you want to earn a BSN degree and possibly an MSN. Either would open up opportunities for promotion and a salary increase. However, the only BSN program in your area accepts only a few RNs each year, is expensive, and requires attendance in classes and supervised clinical experiences that conflict with your home and work schedules. Furthermore, you already feel equal to BSN graduates because of your clinical experience. You want a chance to prove that competency and earn the degree without having to re-study information and techniques you've already mastered.

Where do you go from here? If you're in this situation, you're the typical candidate for the Regent's External Degree Nursing Program of The University of the State of New York, commonly known as the REX program. This program enables you to earn a BSN degree on your terms because, as an external degree program, REX allows you to take courses and examinations at your own pace, at schools of your choice. Furthermore, as part of the program, you'll periodically take nursing and other related examinations that test your current knowledge as well as your past clinical experience. Because the program is fully accredited by the NLN and fully approved by the New York Board of Regents and the regional academic accrediting body, you'll probably be eligible for conventional tuition assistance and reimbursement programs. What's more, as a REX BSN graduate, you'll be eligible for admission into about 80% of the accredited MSN programs. Interested? For more information and enrollment forms, write to: REX-P83, Room 5D45, Cultural Education Center, Albany, N.Y. 12230.

If you decide to enroll in REX, once you've sent in the proper forms and registration fee, you can expect your education to proceed as follows:

● Within 3 weeks, REX will send a letter of acceptance and other materials telling you how to enroll. They'll ask you to have your college transcripts forwarded directly to the REX registrar. You may submit any credit-bearing college-course grades—regardless of how old they are. You may also submit any credit-bearing courses you took in the military or through the Federal

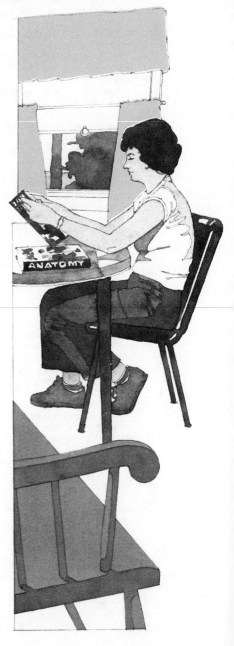

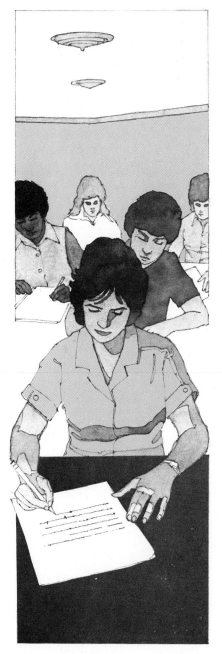

Aviation Agency or Aeronautics Board.
• After the REX registrar evaluates your transcripts, you'll receive a status report indicating the requirements you've met and those you still must meet.
• Next, you'll organize your schedule so you can satisfy the remaining requirements. You may attend classes at a local institution or take examinations to complete either the general education portion or the nursing portion of your degree, or to do both simultaneously. You can write for study guides that'll help you prepare for the nursing examinations. You're responsible for deciding which courses or examinations to take and for writing for the study guides.

You can take all of the written nursing examinations through the American College Testing Program (ACT PEP), at nearly 200 locations throughout the United States and at military bases and embassies around the world. Each time you successfully complete a course or examination, the REX registrar records the score and sends you a new status report indicating what you've accomplished.
• You'll also be required to take three nursing performance examinations at one of the Regional Performance Assessment Centers. You'll find these centers in Albany and Mineola, New York; Atlanta, Georgia; Long Beach and Palo Alto, California; Denver, Colorado; and Milwaukee, Wisconsin. These examinations document, among other things, your ability to administer direct care to hospitalized patients, conduct a health history and physical examination, and teach patients proper health care. They also test your competency in leadership, relating with others, collaboration, patient-care management, research, and decision making.
• After completing all requirements, you can apply for the degree. The nursing faculty will review your records and certify your completion of the program. Then, the New York Board of Regents will award you a BS degree with a major in nursing from The University of the State of New York.

As you may know, New York is the only state that offers a degree based totally on assessment. However, the California State University Consortium has adopted the REX concept and examinations to create its own modified external degree, called the Statewide Nursing Program. Other states, such as New Jersey and Minnesota, have adopted the New York external degree model and soon will make it available.

## FOUR TYPES OF BSN PROGRAMS: ADVANTAGES AND DISADVANTAGES

| | ADVANTAGES | DISADVANTAGES |
| --- | --- | --- |
| **BSN 1** <br> **Post-Licensure Program** | • Takes only 2 years to complete; may offer weekend, evening, or part-time program <br> • All students are RNs | • May use evaluation methods that inadequately assess basic nursing competency <br> • May provide only limited, direct clinical instruction in large classes |
| **BSN 2** <br> **Advanced Placement Program** | • Permits students to earn some credits through examinations or other methods <br> • May offer challenge examinations for a large portion of the nursing major <br> • Offers a structured program of study for those who prefer or need it <br> • Usually integrates RNs with non-RNs in upper-division courses | • May require RNs to begin with the same courses and clinical experiences as beginners, regardless of clinical background <br> • Gives little recognition to special needs of working students <br> • Usually offers only daytime courses <br> • May cost more than other programs, depending on how much course work is required |
| **BSN 3** <br> **Career Ladder (Multiple Entry-Exit) Program** | • Permits students to take courses in a stepped progression, earning credentials at each step <br> • Allows for work periods between earning credentials <br> • Usually gives advanced placement to RNs | • Usually requires students to take courses in exact sequence <br> • Usually offers only daytime, on-campus courses <br> • Gives little recognition to special needs of working students |
| **BSN 4** <br> **External Degree Program** | • Offers a competency-based approach; degree requirements may be satisfied by courses and/or by assessment procedures <br> • Offers self-paced, individualized learning, drawing on past and current experience and coursework <br> • Provides test study guides <br> • Recognizes working students' needs <br> • Imposes no time limit or restrictions on place where learning occurs <br> • Generally costs less than other programs | • Provides limited or no direct instruction <br> • Expects students to establish their own study groups and find their own learning resources <br> • Provides no supervised clinical experience |

## BSN OR BS: WHICH IS BETTER FOR YOU?

**Beware of nonnursing degree programs**

*As an RN, I can enroll in a college BS program with a non-nursing major that will give me 30 semester hours' credit for my nursing experience. Doesn't this make more sense than enrolling in the BSN program and possibly repeating many of the things I've already learned?—RN, Mich.*

According to the National League for Nursing (NLN), BS college degree programs which promise that much of your previous nursing education can be credited toward a degree usually lead to associate or bachelor's degrees in such fields as applied science, biology, education, health science, occupational therapy, psychology, and sociology. Although the programs may provide you with a substantial background in the major, they don't offer any additional preparation in nursing.

Don't be misguided by the programs' publicity. For example, although the program may claim that a major in another field is equal to a major in nursing as preparation for nursing practice, it isn't. And, although the program may claim to be an acceptable base for further nursing education, it isn't. Don't presume that this type of program will lead to job advancement, either. It may not.

Furthermore, if you're planning to enter an MSN program later, you'll find most MSN programs accept only graduates from NLN-accredited bachelor's degree programs or programs with an upper-division major in nursing. So if this is your plan, find out if the NLN approves the degree program you're considering.

This letter was taken from the files of *Nursing* magazine.

standards. The National League for Nursing (NLN) also grants accreditation to a school's nursing education program. The NLN evaluates nursing programs, using national standards established by nurse educators from member schools. Before the NLN will grant accreditation to a nursing program, the college or university must have received regional accreditation.

If you're interested in enrolling in a new program, you should realize that it's not eligible for NLN accreditation until its first class completes the program. Always find out if the school plans to apply for accreditation. If it does, find out its chances for success and the date of NLN review.

### Classifying BSN programs

Educators divide BSN programs into two general groups: generic programs and nontraditional programs. The *generic program* is designed for students with little or no background in nursing, such as students who've graduated from high school or those with no formal nursing background. The program typically requires 4 years of on-campus study, with most nursing courses offered in the junior and senior years, after the student meets arts and science requirements. Some schools begin nursing courses before the student's junior year.

A nontraditional program is sometimes called an open curriculum or educational mobility program. This type of program is designed for diploma nurses, associate degree nurses, LPNs/LVNs, medics, or students with some (and sometimes with no) previous nursing education or experience. Four types of nontraditional programs exist, with only minor variations. Become familiar with these types to better match your educational requirements to your professional goals. (See *Four Types of BSN Programs: Advantages and Disadvantages.*)

## CONSIDERING GRADUATE DEGREE PROGRAMS

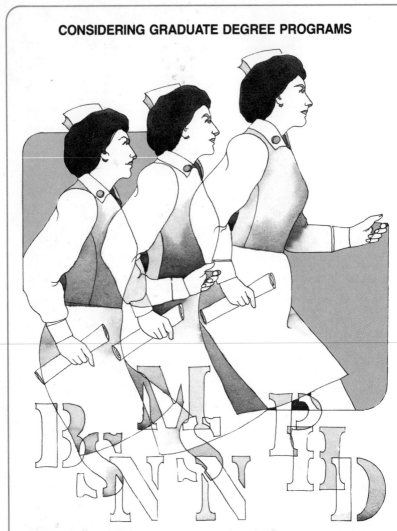

### THE MASTER'S PROGRAM

Many nurses today are assuming leadership positions and entering into collegial relationships with doctors and other health-care professionals. For these nurses, specialized advanced degrees pave the way for success on the job. One advanced degree that nurses are increasingly pursuing is the master's degree in nursing.

*Program Focus*
The traditional master's program in nursing builds on the bachelor's curriculum, which (as you know) prepares nurses for general-

ized nursing practice. A master's program offers nurses a chance to:
• develop clinical expertise in specialized areas of nursing practice.
• acquire skills in conducting research.
• learn to plan and initiate changes in health care.
• acquire a foundation for doctoral study.
NLN-accredited master's programs usually combine the study of a clinical area with study of a functional role. Examples of clinical areas of study include medical-surgical nursing, maternal-child nursing, family nursing, and community-health

nursing. Functional specializations include roles such as clinician, teacher, administrator, consultant, and supervisor. Other master's-degree program courses include an introduction to research methods and the independent study of a research problem using those methods. Some programs require a research-oriented thesis; others require an in-depth case study.

*Admission qualifications*
Most programs require the following qualifications for admission:
• graduation from an NLN-accredited bachelor's program with a major in nursing
• RN licensure
• satisfactory grade point average
• satisfactory scores on the Graduate Record Examination and/or Miller Analogies Test
• (sometimes) work experience.
Most programs require a specific amount of full-time study. However, part-time study, work/study, and evening/weekend programs are becoming increasingly available.

*Degrees offered*
Nursing degrees granted at the master's level include Master of Science in Nursing (MSN), Master of Science with a major in nursing (MS), Master's in Nursing Science (MNSc), Master's in Nursing (MN), Master of Arts with a major in nursing (MA), and Master of Public Health with a major in nursing (MPH). The different degrees reflect schools' differing degree-granting powers as well as different curricula and preparation for different functions, such as practice versus teaching or administration. Certain master's-degree nursing programs accept students with nonnursing bachelor's degrees as well as bachelor's-prepared nurses.

*The Free-Standing Master's Program for Nonnurse College Graduates* at Yale University School of Nursing, and similar programs at Pace University and other schools, offer both basic and advanced preparation in a single 3-year curriculum. This curriculum includes 1 year of sciences and basic nursing skills and 2 years of specialty preparation. The school's granting of an MSN degree is contingent on the student's obtaining an RN license. Students can qualify for the National Council Licensure Examination after four semesters and one summer of study.

*Information Sources*
Over 70 U.S. colleges and universities currently offer accredited master's programs in nursing. The NLN publication, "Master's Education in Nursing: Route to Opportunities in Contemporary Nursing" (updated annually), lists all accredited programs with information about the clinical and functional areas each one covers, curriculum length, degree granted, approximate cost, and availability of financial assistance.

**THE DOCTORAL PROGRAM**
You may feel that earning a doctoral degree is beyond your professional needs. The fact is, though, that more and more nurses are moving in this direction. They're coming to recognize that a doctoral degree can be the springboard to greater career success and personal enrichment. Whether your strength or preference is in clinical practice, research and teaching, or administration, you can reap a multitude of dividends from a doctoral degree. A doctoral degree can:
• strengthen your competency by increasing your knowledge and developing your problem-solving abilities.
• give you greater opportunity to upgrade the quality of your patient care by improving your chances of participating in policymaking.
• increase your job options not only in traditional health-care settings but also in a variety of public and private institutions.
• improve your chances for promotion or for tenure.

The doctoral program you may choose to enter depends on your professional and personal goals. For example, as your career takes shape, you may decide that you derive greatest job satisfaction from research tasks. In that case, you should look into a program that awards a Doctor of Philosophy (PhD) degree. The PhD program prepares you to conduct research by teaching you problem-solving methods. Or you may find administrative, teaching, or consultant duties most appealing. If you do, consider a program that awards a Doctor of Nursing Science (DNS) degree. This program prepares you for the role of administrator, teacher, or consultant by emphasizing the application of research findings and existing knowledge to patient care. What if you most enjoy providing hands-on care to patients? Then you should look into a program that awards a Doctor of Nursing (ND) degree. This program prepares you for entry-level practice in a hospital setting as part of a multidisciplinary health-care team.

## Type I: post-licensure program for RNs only

This type of BSN program has a variety of names: *second step, RN only, BSRN, RN completion, or upper two* program. This type of program is designed to build on the diploma or associate degree you must have before being admitted. The program usually requires some theory testing to validate your prior learning.

You must have a designated number of arts and science credits as well as nursing credits for admission, usually equivalent to 2 years of study. Many schools will allow you to transfer your college credits. You must take most of the remaining courses on the college campus, and within a specified time period.

## Type II: advanced-placement program

Most generic BSN programs offer an opportunity for a limited number of RNs to enroll. If you're admitted, you may be able to transfer some college credits and to earn advanced standing through the school's challenge examinations. Schools use these examinations to determine the number of credits you should receive and your placement level in the program. A school may use nationally standardized examinations or those written by the school's nursing faculty. Schools usually allow the examinations only for the program's lower-division (freshman and sophomore) courses. You'll have to take the same upper-division courses as those required for all generic students. Although most schools won't allow you to bypass upper-division courses by taking examinations, some do have a rapid-progress option that enables you to move through courses quickly.

## Type III: career ladder programs

Also known as *multiple entry-exit programs,* career ladder programs offer a step-by-step educational progres-

sion. In this program, you receive a degree (such as an associate or bachelor's degree) when you complete each step of the ladder. And, unlike other degree programs, this one permits you to leave the program at the completion of any segment, without penalty. Later, you can pick up where you left off. One school or a consortium of schools can offer the program's different steps. Here's how some career ladder programs work:

● When a student completes the first year, she's prepared for practical nurse licensure.

● When she completes the second year, she receives an associate degree and is eligible for RN licensure.

● When she completes the final 2 years, she receives a BSN degree.

## Type IV: external degree program

All three previously discussed types of nontraditional BSN programs require you to take specific courses at specific campuses. But the external degree program (currently offered only by the University of the State of New York) offers you something very different—a degree based on an assessment of your knowledge and skills, no matter where, how, or when you acquired them. An accredited educational institution administers the program. Its faculty members determine the degree requirements, develop theory and performance examinations in nursing, and assess applicants' competency. Such a program lets you learn anywhere, use any available resources, set your own pace, and pay as you go. The programs accept proficiency tests, special assessments and courses from accredited colleges. After you enroll, you request the study guides to prepare for tests. When you're ready, you apply to take tests at designated testing centers. Written tests are offered six times a year, and you can make an appointment to take a performance test. When you pass a test, you'll receive academic credits toward your degree (see *New York's REX Pro-*

gram: *How Does It Work?* pages 326-327).

## Checking a program's essentials

The time and money you'll spend to earn a BSN should compel you to learn all you can about a program before you enroll. Make sure you know which bachelor's degree programs the school offers and what its accreditation standing is. Schools that don't list accreditations in their catalogs may not have sought them or met the required standards yet.

Next, make an appointment with a faculty advisor in the school's nursing program. Be sure to prepare for this appointment so you can ask specific questions about the program's requirements, scheduling, challenge examinations, expenses, and credit for your work experience, as well as any other topics you're concerned about. When you've investigated the program (or several) thoroughly, you'll be ready to make the decision to enroll.

## A final word

The number of generic BSN programs continues to grow slowly, owing in part to national economic uncertainties and the present decline in the college-age population. So colleges and universities have started to look elsewhere for students—mainly to adults, such as nurses. They've become more responsive to the educational needs of nurses who want to earn BSNs. This is why, in the past few years, the number of nontraditional BSN programs has grown dramatically.

How can this turn of events help you? For one thing, you can expect an increasing number of colleges and universities to offer more flexible options, more advanced placement, and more external assessment programs to attract working nurses. And that means you have more opportunity than ever before to earn a BSN. But remember, investigate *all* your options before you decide.

# 52 Nursing internship programs: Antidote to reality shock?

Many nurses experience a transitional jolt when they leave the academic setting of the classroom and enter the real-life world of the hospital. Nurses call this *reality shock*. It's related to the disparity between what nurses *learn* in school and what they are called on to *do* when they start working.

What are the causes of this disparity? For one thing, medical technology is advancing so rapidly that keeping up with it is increasingly difficult. Studies have shown that much of what a nurse learns in school is obsolete within several years. For another thing, nursing education has changed over the last 20 years. The increasingly popular bachelor's programs sponsored by colleges and universities normally span 4 years—yet the time a nursing student spends in basic nursing courses is still about what it was under the earlier system. So although nursing study programs today are broader and cover more subject areas than a student had to learn about to graduate from a hospital-affiliated school, she gets *less*—and sometimes *no*—exposure to concepts and methods she'll need once she's on the job.

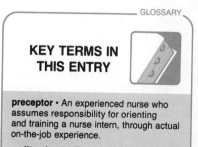

GLOSSARY

## KEY TERMS IN THIS ENTRY

**preceptor** • An experienced nurse who assumes responsibility for orienting and training a nurse intern, through actual on-the-job experience.

**reality shock** • The transitional jolt many nurses experience when they leave the academic setting and enter actual nursing practice.

## UNDERSTANDING THE INTERNSHIP PROGRAM

If you're considering enrollment in an internship program, you probably have a lot of questions about how it works. Here are some of the most frequently asked questions, with their answers.

**Q** *What specific admission criteria, such as education and experience, do internship programs require?*

**A** Most internship programs usually require either an associate degree or a bachelor's degree in nursing. Most programs will admit you with up to 1 year of experience.

**Q** *Is the internship program optional or required?*

**A** This varies with the sponsoring hospital.

**Q** *Will the hospital sponsoring the program require a service commitment following the program? If so, for how long?*

**A** Most likely, yes. The length of the commitment varies with each program.

**Q** *Are program objectives and staff nurse job descriptions usually in agreement?*

**A** Since the program's goal is to prepare the intern for the clinical duties of a staff nurse, objectives and job descriptions are generally comparable and specific.

**Q** *Do the program objectives accurately spell out what the intern should know when she's completed the program?*

**A** Generally, yes; the program objectives relate specifically to the responsibilities outlined in the intern's job description.

**Q** *Who supervises the program's clinical experience?*

**A** Usually a staff nurse with proven clinical competency.

**Q** *Does an intern earn the same salary as other new, nonintern graduates?*

**A** Yes, most sponsoring hospitals pay the nurse intern the same starting salary as they pay other new graduates.

**Q** *Are internship programs available for the LPN/LVN or an RN with more than one year of experience?*

**A** No, not at this time.

## How hospitals are dealing with reality shock

Most hospitals have orientation programs to introduce new staff nurses to their duties. But too often an orientation program is inadequate: it's either too short or too shallow. That's where a nursing internship program can play an important role. It can bridge the gap between classroom theory and the practical know-how a nursing job demands: knowing how to care for many patients at once, meeting tight—or even unrealistic—work schedules, resolving peer-related conflicts, and providing proper nursing care to acutely ill patients.

Nursing internship programs differ from the traditional hospital orientation programs in that they're longer and more clinically intensive. Unlike tra-

ditional orientation programs, which generally last only a few weeks, most nursing internship programs last between 3 and 6 months. A few hospitals sponsor programs that last as long as a year. In this time, a program can provide a lot of clinical instructions. This strengthens the new nurse's caregiving skills and increases her self-confidence.

Typically, an experienced nurse, called a *preceptor*, gives clinical instruction in an internship program. Virtually every internship program has such a preceptor to work one-on-one with new nurse interns. This arrangement assumes that a nurse who's already functioning effectively in a particular hospital setting is the best person to orient a new nurse to that setting.

## Internship programs in Canada: 2 + 1 = success

A Canadian nursing-school graduate is just as vulnerable to reality shock as her American counterpart. Like hospitals in the United States, Canadian hospitals also provide orientation programs for their new nurses. Most of these programs are only a few weeks long, but the merits of extending them to 4 weeks are currently being assessed.

Besides the hospital orientation programs, Canada has two independent nursing internship programs. Called *2 + 1*, these programs consist of 2 years of basic nursing training followed by a year of internship. In that third year, the nurse intern becomes a regular— although temporary—member of the hospital staff. And she draws a salary commensurate with the nursing responsibilities she assumes. These programs seem to be very effective in helping recent graduates meet their institutions' expectations of new nurses' clinical work.

## Weighing the pros and cons

Are nursing internship programs better than typical hospital orientation programs? Supporters claim that internship programs have the following advantages:
- They upgrade patient care by giving the intern a better grounding in how to perform more effective patient assessments and interventions.
- They provide an opportunity to discuss contrasting schools of thought about nursing through program-sponsored seminars.
- They strengthen peer relationships with regular staff members.
- They cut down on duplication of teaching on the unit.

Critics of the internship programs, however, cite the following problems:
- The programs are a quick-fix remedy, not a long-term solution to resolving the gap between classroom theory and clinical experience.
- They remove the intern from a realistic conflict setting by placing her under the protective wing of a preceptor, possibly further delaying her adjustment to reality.
- They provide rotations to only a few specialty units for too short a time to be instructive.
- They prolong the intern's dependence on her preceptor when a program continues for a year or more.

## Becoming a role model

Is preceptorship right for you? Obviously, a sense of commitment is essential. Also important are your clinical competency and support from both your supervisor and administration.

Working alongside a nurse intern can give you a unique opportunity not only to develop your teaching skills but also to hone your clinical ones. Being a preceptor makes it easier for you to reevaluate your own nursing efficiency and standards of care. And don't overlook the prestige involved. Becoming a clinical preceptor can enhance your standing with your co-workers.

Keep this in mind if you become a preceptor: You may assume increased liability. Why? Because acting as a preceptor takes time that you might otherwise take to ensure that your patient care meets all professional and legal standards. If you do decide to become a preceptor, make sure you're not in any way lowering your patient-care standards so you can fit this extra work into your schedule.

Finally, consider if you want the extra responsibility a preceptorship entails—especially if you're doing it for no extra pay. Can you temporarily relinquish some of your other duties when you take on a preceptorship, or will you have to assume the responsibility in addition to your existing duties?

Before you decide, observe a preceptor and intern working together. Find out how they feel about the benefits and burdens of the program. Ask your head nurse and supervisor for their opinions. Get in touch with your hospital coordinator—usually the in-service education coordinator—to find out about the program and its requirements. If you then think a preceptorship is right for you, let the coordinator know you're interested.

**A final word**
If your hospital doesn't have an internship program, consider offering to help plan or implement one. You may want to talk to your director of inservice education or staff development. This will give you insight into what such a program involves and a feel for whether or not you have the necessary motivation to participate.

# 53 Preparing for specialty practice

As you're probably aware, specialization and certification in nursing have grown like Topsy, mainly because of the increasingly sophisticated and complex nature of nursing practice. Many nurses today are choosing to concentrate their nursing skills and knowledge within a particular area of nursing, instead of concentrating on the broad spectrum.

This trend toward specialty practice

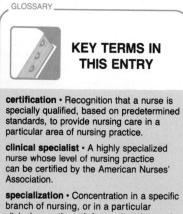

GLOSSARY

### KEY TERMS IN THIS ENTRY

**certification** • Recognition that a nurse is specially qualified, based on predetermined standards, to provide nursing care in a particular area of nursing practice.

**clinical specialist** • A highly specialized nurse whose level of nursing practice can be certified by the American Nurses' Association.

**specialization** • Concentration in a specific branch of nursing, or in a particular clinical area, through focused work experience or formal education, or both.

seems likely to continue and expand. So if you haven't yet, start preparing yourself to answer some new questions about the future of your nursing career. For example:
• "Should I specialize?"
• "What area should I specialize in?"
• "How important is certification?"
• "Will certification advance my professional status and economic standing?"

Answering these questions involves taking a close look at the past, present, and future of specialty nursing practice.

## Development of specialization
The concept of specialization in nursing isn't new: it's been around since at least the turn of the century. Since then, however, specialization has taken on a new meaning for the nursing profession.

In the early 1900s, a nursing specialist was a nurse who either had graduated from a specialized hospital (for example, a children's hospital) or who had worked with specific kinds of patients (for example, pediatric patients). In the 1950s, the title was changed to clinical specialist, and colleges and universities assumed responsibility for providing postbasic education to prepare nurses to practice in particular clinical areas. As these programs became more sophisticated and as colleges began to upgrade their requirements for clinical specialists, graduate schools became responsible for offering clinical specialist programs.

Today, you can specialize in a *specific branch of nursing*, such as community health, or in a *particular clinical area*, such as intensive care. You can qualify as a clinical specialist through focused work experience or formal education. For example, if you've worked on an obstetrics unit for a number of years and taken continuing education courses in obstetrics, your nursing specialty is obstetrics. If you've completed a master's degree program

## CERTIFICATION FOR NURSING ADMINISTRATORS

Maybe you think certification is available only in the clinical specialties, such as medical/surgical nursing, pediatrics, and the like. Not so. The American Nurses' Association (ANA) offers certification to nursing administrators, too. Like a clinical specialist's certification, an administrator's certification attests to her knowledge and ability in her specialty.

If you're an administrator, you can earn certification in nursing administration (CNA) or in nursing administration, advanced (CNAA).

To take the certification examination in nursing administration (CNA), you must:

• be licensed to practice as a registered nurse in the United States or its territories
• hold a middle-management or executive-nursing administrative position
• have worked in an administrative position for 2 of the last 5 years
• have compiled a summary of your administrative responsibilities and experience.

To qualify for the examination in nursing administration, advanced (CNAA), you must:

• be licensed to practice as a registered nurse in the United States or its territories
• hold a master's or higher degree
• hold an executive-level nursing administration position, as defined by Characteristics of Nursing Administrative Levels from the ANA publication *Roles, Responsi-*

*bilities, and Qualifications for Nurse Administrators*
• have been in an executive-level nursing-administration position for at least 3 of the past 5 years
• have submitted a summary of your administrative responsibilities and experience.

If you meet these criteria, you can request an application for certification from the ANA, Dept. N81, 2420 Pershing Rd., Kansas City, Mo. 64108.

After returning the completed application with the required fee, you'll be notified if you're eligible to take the certification examination. Then you must pay an additional fee to take the examination.

You can take the examination at 21 different sites across the nation. It covers these subjects: nursing care delivery; program planning and implementation; personnel management; financial management; management styles and techniques; community and societal concerns of nursing administration. (Candidates for certification in nursing administration, advanced, are required to complete an additional test section.)

If you pass the examination, you'll receive a certificate and can use the designation *RN, CNA,* or *RN, CNAA* after your name. You'll also be listed in the ANA's directory of certified nurses. But most important, you'll have proved that you excel in your specialty—that you're indeed a top-notch administrator.

---

in maternal and child health, the American Nurses' Association (ANA) considers you a clinical specialist in this area.

### Is specialization right for you?
Before you decide whether or not to specialize, you should carefully assess your particular situation, including your work experience and education. Identify your personal and professional goals, too; then ask yourself if specialization will help you achieve them. Next, identify a specialty area that interests you, and research it. Find out the requirements for specializing in that area, whether you must become

certified before you can practice in the specialty area, what your responsibilities would be, and whether hospitals are currently hiring nurses with that specialty. To obtain such information, talk with nurses who are currently practicing in the specialty area you're interested in, or write to the particular specialty organization. (See *National Certification Programs,* pages 338 to 341.)

### Should you become certified?
If you've decided to specialize in a particular area of nursing, you should also explore the requirements for becoming certified. Certification is a prerequisite

## NATIONAL CERTIFICATION PROGRAMS

| ORGANIZATION | TYPE OF CERTIFICATION AND PURPOSE | ELIGIBILITY |
|---|---|---|
| American Association of Critical Care Nurses (AACN) Certification Corporation | Critical Care Registered Nurse (CCRN); recognizes nurse's expertise in critical care | Experience required |
| American Board of Occupational Health Nurses | Certified Occupational Health Nurse (COHN); recognizes nurse's expertise in occupational health practice | Experience required |
| Association of Operating Room Nurses (AORN) National Certification Board | Certified Nurse, Operating Room (CNOR); recognizes nurse's expertise in operating room practice | Experience required |
| Board of Nephrology Examiners, Nurses, and Technicians | Community Health Nurse (CHN); recognizes nurse's expertise in nephrology care | Experience required |
| American Board of Neurosurgical Nursing | Certified Neurosurgical Registered Nurse (CNRN); recognizes nurse's expertise in neurosurgical care | Experience required |
| Council on Certification of Nurse Anesthetists | Certified Registered Nurse Anesthetist (CRNA); recognizes nurse's ability to perform as a nurse anesthetist | Education required |

| CERTIFICATION PROCESS | CERTIFICATION TERM | CERTIFICATION MAINTENANCE |
|---|---|---|
| Multiple choice question (MCQ) examination: 4 hours, given twice a year | 3 years | Reexamination or 100 points in CEARP program during 3-year certification period |
| MCQ examination: given once a year | 4 years | Continuing education, 60 hours during 5-year certification period |
| MCQ examination: 4 hours, given once a year | 5 years | Reexamination |
| MCQ examination: given if at least 25 people request | 6 years | Reexamination or 30 contact hours within 2 years combined with clinical experience |
| MCQ examination: 4 hours, given once a year | 5 years | Reexamination |
| MCQ examination: 4 hours, given twice a year | 2 years | Active practice and continuing education |

*(continued)*

**CERTIFICATION PROGRAMS** *(continued)*

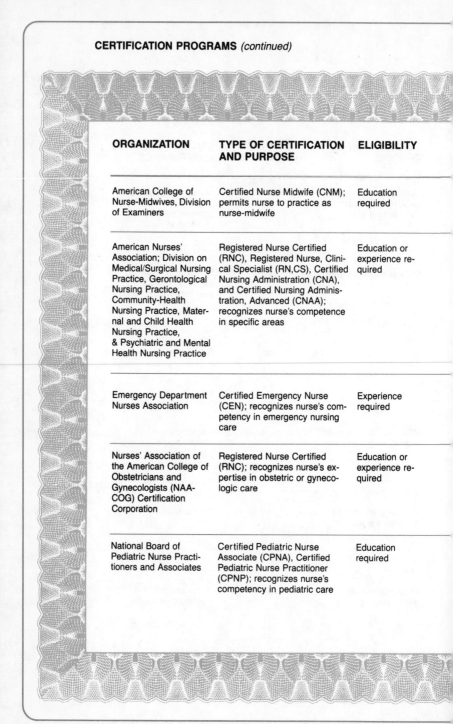

| ORGANIZATION | TYPE OF CERTIFICATION AND PURPOSE | ELIGIBILITY |
| --- | --- | --- |
| American College of Nurse-Midwives, Division of Examiners | Certified Nurse Midwife (CNM); permits nurse to practice as nurse-midwife | Education required |
| American Nurses' Association; Division on Medical/Surgical Nursing Practice, Gerontological Nursing Practice, Community-Health Nursing Practice, Maternal and Child Health Nursing Practice, & Psychiatric and Mental Health Nursing Practice | Registered Nurse Certified (RNC), Registered Nurse, Clinical Specialist (RN,CS), Certified Nursing Administration (CNA), and Certified Nursing Administration, Advanced (CNAA); recognizes nurse's competence in specific areas | Education or experience required |
| Emergency Department Nurses Association | Certified Emergency Nurse (CEN); recognizes nurse's competency in emergency nursing care | Experience required |
| Nurses' Association of the American College of Obstetricians and Gynecologists (NAA-COG) Certification Corporation | Registered Nurse Certified (RNC); recognizes nurse's expertise in obstetric or gynecologic care | Education or experience required |
| National Board of Pediatric Nurse Practitioners and Associates | Certified Pediatric Nurse Associate (CPNA), Certified Pediatric Nurse Practitioner (CPNP); recognizes nurse's competency in pediatric care | Education required |

| CERTIFICATION PROCESS | CERTIFICA- TION TERM | CERTIFICATION MAINTENANCE |
|---|---|---|
| Essay examination: 6 hours, given as requested | Indefinite | Not determined |
| MCQ examination: given twice a year | 5 years | Reexamination or continuing education |
| MCQ examination: 4 hours, given twice a year | 4 years | Not determined |
| MCQ examination: 3 to 4 hours, given once a year | 3 years | Reexamination or 45 contact hours in 3-year certification period |
| MCQ examination: 1 day, given once a year | 6 years | Reexamination or three self-assessment exercises within 5 years |

Adapted with permission from NAACOG Certification Corporation, *Newsletter,* July 6, 1982.

## NURSING SPECIALTIES AT A GLANCE

| | Salaries | | Job Characteristics | | |
|---|---|---|---|---|---|
| | 1981 Average annual salary | Good/flexible hours | Expertise in one nursing skill | Travel | |
| Critical-care nurse | $14,000 + | | | | |
| Home-care coordinator | $14,000 + | ◐ | | | |
| Industrial consultant | $20,000 + to start | ◐ | | ✈ | |
| Infection-control nurse | $18,000 | ◐ | | | |
| Insurance physical examiner | $7 to $10/hr ($20 to $25/hr)* | ◐ | | | |
| Nurse I.V. therapist | $14,000 + | | ★ | | |
| Nurse enterostomal therapist | $14,000 + | | ★ | | |
| Nurse health educator | $14,000 + to start | ◐ | | | |
| Nurse recruiter | $16,000 + | ◐ | | ✈ | |
| Occupational health nurse | $16,000 + | | | | |
| Operating room nurse | $14,000 + | | ★ | | |
| Quality-assurance coordinator | $17,000 + | ◐ | | | |
| Utilization-review coordinator | $14,000 + | ◐ | | | |

*Self-employment rates

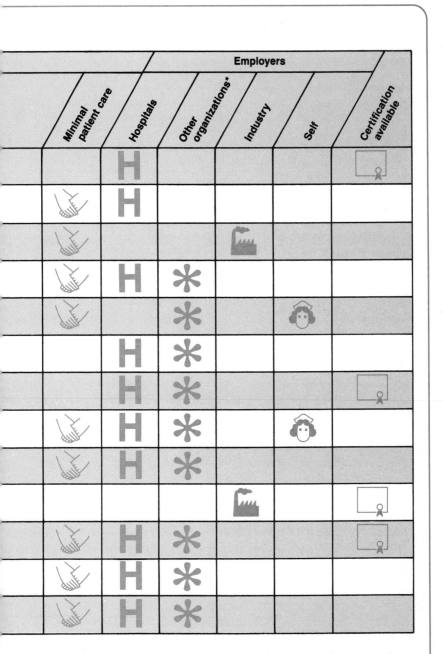

| | Minimal patient care | Hospitals | Other organizations* | Industry | Self | Certification available |
|---|---|---|---|---|---|---|
| | | H | | | | 🏵 |
| | ✋ | H | | | | |
| | ✋ | | | 🏭 | | |
| | ✋ | H | ✳ | | | |
| | ✋ | | ✳ | | 👩‍⚕️ | |
| | | H | ✳ | | | |
| | | H | ✳ | | | 🏵 |
| | ✋ | H | ✳ | | 👩‍⚕️ | |
| | ✋ | H | ✳ | | | |
| | | | | 🏭 | | 🏵 |
| | ✋ | H | ✳ | | | 🏵 |
| | ✋ | H | ✳ | | | |
| | ✋ | H | ✳ | | | |

*Health maintenance organizations, extended-care facilities, outpatient clinics, paramedic organizations, doctors' offices.

in certain clinical areas, such as anesthesia. In other areas, the choice is yours. To make a sound decision on whether or not to become certified, you should know about certification's advantages and disadvantages.

One advantage is the validation it provides that you're specially qualified,

---

*"Nurses must agree on the meaning of certification and set standard requirements for it."*

---

based on predetermined standards, to give nursing care in a particular area of nursing practice. Other advantages include the personal satisfaction and fulfillment that motivate many nurses to seek certification.

Originally, many nurses hoped that certification would increase their professional status and their salaries. But it hasn't worked out that way. Why? In part, because no standardized requirements exist for certification. This means that in some specialties a diploma nurse with a certain amount of experience can be certified, while in other specialties a nurse needs a master's degree to be certified. This lack of standardization has tended to undercut certification's significance.

If you decide to become certified, you can apply to the ANA or the appropriate specialty nursing organization. The ANA can certify you in broad functional areas such as maternal and child health, medical/surgical nursing, and nursing administration. It can also certify you in more specialized areas and roles, such as clinical specialist in adult psychiatric and mental health nursing, high-risk perinatal nursing, and gerontologic nurse practitioner. To date, the ANA has certified more than 15,000 nurses.

Specialty organizations offer certification in prescribed areas of nursing,

such as critical care, enterostomal therapy, and operating room nursing. Requirements for certification vary among the specialty organizations. But like the ANA, most specialty organizations require nurses to pass a certification examination.

If you do become certified in a specialty area of nursing practice, remember that your certification isn't permanent. You'll probably have to obtain recertification from time to time according to your certifying organization's requirements. Requirements for recertification vary among the organizations, but in most instances you'll either have to take another certification exam or provide proof that you obtained a certain number of continuing education units within a specified length of time (see Entry 54).

## What's the future of specialization and certification?
The number of nursing specialties will undoubtedly continue to increase, which will also increase the number of new specialty organizations. Many of these will prepare and offer their own certification examinations. Exactly what this trend toward increased specialization will mean for you, and how it will affect your future in nursing, depends on the actions of the ANA and the various specialty organizations. Hopefully they'll be able to reach an agreement about the meaning of certification and to establish standardized requirements for it. Then specialization and certification can play major roles in shaping the future of the nursing profession and in helping to assure the quality of its practice.

The Canadian Nurses Association is currently studying the issues of specialization and certification. It hopes to gather information that will help define specialization and aid development of guidelines for certification.

## A final word
The nursing profession must speak with one voice on the issues of spe-

cialization and certification. Nurses must agree on their meanings and establish standard requirements for them. Only then will specialization and certification bring increased professional status and compensation.

# 54 Continuing education—voluntary or mandatory?

You might be surprised and, perhaps, dismayed to discover that half of what you learn this year will be obsolete in less than 7 years. So the fact that you've graduated from a school of nursing, completed a nursing degree program, or received certification in a specialty area doesn't guarantee career-long professional competency. To meet the ever-evolving standards of your profession, you must continually update your nursing knowledge through continuing education (CE).

The American Nurses' Association (ANA) defines continuing education as all organized learning experiences that enhance your nursing practice and education, contribute to nursing administration and research, and improve health care offered to the public. You should be able to apply the knowledge and skills that you gain through continuing education to any job you hold at any health-care institution.

In about two thirds of the United States, continuing education is voluntary, which means that you can choose to take CE courses or not take them without any professional or legal consequences. In states where CE's mandatory, you're required to earn a minimum amount of CE credits (established by state law) to renew your nursing license.

## How continuing education works

CE programs can take many forms: lectures, workshops, seminars, symposiums, classroom series, computer-assisted instruction, multimedia presentations, or planned clinical experiences. Many states also recognize independent study as an acceptable way to satisfy continuing education requirements. This means you learn on your own through home study; then you complete a test to prove that you've met the learning goals.

Providers of CE programs include hospitals and nursing homes, colleges and universities, private professional education groups, professional nurses associations, national specialty nurses associations, national health-related associations, the federal nursing services, and commercial companies, such as publishers.

In most states, before a provider can offer a CE program for credit, he must apply to an appropriate CE approver. Approval is recognition that a CE program meets predetermined educational standards. Without such approval, the provider can still offer its program, but you may or may not earn CE credit for taking it.

Some providers of voluntary continuing education can also apply for accreditation. The ANA both approves CE programs and accredits providers of CE programs for RNs. To date, the ANA has

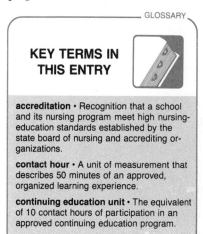

GLOSSARY

## KEY TERMS IN THIS ENTRY

**accreditation** • Recognition that a school and its nursing program meet high nursing-education standards established by the state board of nursing and accrediting organizations.

**contact hour** • A unit of measurement that describes 50 minutes of an approved, organized learning experience.

**continuing education unit** • The equivalent of 10 contact hours of participation in an approved continuing education program.

# MANDATORY CONTINUING EDUCATION FOR RN AND LPN/ LVN RELICENSURE: HOW IT WORKS

| STATE | CONTACT HOUR REQUIREMENTS | APPROVAL BODY | SPECIAL CONSIDERATIONS |
|---|---|---|---|
| **California** | • 30, every 2 years | • For RNs and LVNs*: California Board of Registered Nursing, 1020 N. St. Sacramento, Calif. 95814<br><br>• For LVNs only: Board of Vocational Nurses and Psychiatric Technician Examiners, 1020 N. St., Room 406, Sacramento, Calif. 95814 | • No more than 6 hours home study per licensing period for RNs (no limitations for LVNs)<br><br>• 3 hours course-related clinical practice = 1 contact hour<br><br>• Instead of earning contact hours, RNs may take a comprehensive exam on nursing developments since the previous renewal period<br><br>• Approval of nonapproved offerings not possible |
| **Colorado** | • 20, every 2 years | • Any of over 20 credentialing agencies approved by Colorado Board of Nursing | • No more than 5 hours home study per licensing period<br><br>• Approval of nonapproved offerings not possible |
| **Florida** | • 24, every 2 years | • Florida Board of Nursing, 111 E. Coastline Dr., Jacksonville, Fla. 32202 | • For home study approval, submit approval form including: reason for study, title and description of content, learning objectives, study methods, evaluation method, and number of hours for study<br><br>• For approval of nonapproved offerings, submit the board's approval form. Attach copy of attendance certificate if submitted after the offering |

*California and Texas recognize licensed vocational nurses (LVNs); all other states recognize licensed practical nurses (LPNs).

| DOCUMENTATION REQUIREMENTS | REQUIREMENTS FOR MAINTAINING LICENSE ELSEWHERE | THOSE EXEMPT FROM LICENSURE | CE REQUIREMENTS TO REACTIVATE LICENSE |
|---|---|---|---|
| • Complete an application renewal statement listing each offering by title, date, provider number, and contact hours earned<br><br>• Keep attendance certificates or grade slips from academic courses for at least 4 years | • Take academic courses or participate in CE offerings approved by: national nursing, medical, and hospital associations; regional specialty groups; other state boards of nursing; or nurses associations whose offerings meet California standards | • New graduates (for first renewal)<br><br>• Nurses overseas at least 1 year<br><br>• Nurses totally disabled or with a totally disabled dependent for at least 1 year<br><br>• Federal RNs, military RNs, and LVNs working out of state | • Same as to renew |
| • Fill out license renewal notices listing CE courses | • Meet Colorado requirements; take courses approved by credentialing agency | • Inactive nurses | • 2 contact hours earned during preceding 2-year license period |
| • In state: For academic courses, send official transcript with license number to board; for board-approved offerings, the provider will forward proof of attendance to the board<br><br>• Out of state: For academic courses, send official transcript with license number to board; for offerings, send a copy of attendance certificate, and (if not included on certificate) a brochure or other program literature that specifies the accrediting organization | • Participate in an accredited CE offering | • New graduates (for first renewal)<br><br>• Military personnel<br><br>• Inactive nurses | • If inactive for more than 1 year: 12 contact hours earned within preceding 24 months<br><br>• If inactive for 1 year or less: 24 contact hours earned within preceding 24 months |

*(continued)*

## MANDATORY CONTINUING EDUCATION FOR RN AND LPN/LVN
## RELICENSURE: HOW IT WORKS *(continued)*

| STATE | CONTACT HOUR REQUIREMENTS | APPROVAL BODY | SPECIAL CONSIDERATIONS |
|---|---|---|---|
| **Iowa** | • 15, every year; earned by 3/31 in renewal year | • Iowa Board of Nursing, 300 4th St., Des Moines, Iowa 50309 | • No more than 5 hours home study allowed<br><br>• Approval of nonapproved offerings possible only for out-of-state offerings |
| **Kansas** | • 30, every 2 years | • Kansas State Board of Nursing, P.O. Box 1098, 503 Kansas Ave., Ste. 300, Topeka, Kan. 66601 | • No more than 20% of required contact hours may be earned through home study<br><br>• For approval of nonapproved offerings, fill out board's approval and nonapproval courses form before CE offering begins. Submit to board of review |
| **Kentucky** | • 15, every year | • Kentucky Board of Nursing, 4010 Dupont Circle, Ste. 430, Louisville, Ky. 40207 | • Home study approved after 1984<br><br>• Staff development activities, but no inservice education, accepted<br><br>• 2 hours of planned, supervised clinical practice designed to meet educational objectives = 1 contact hour |

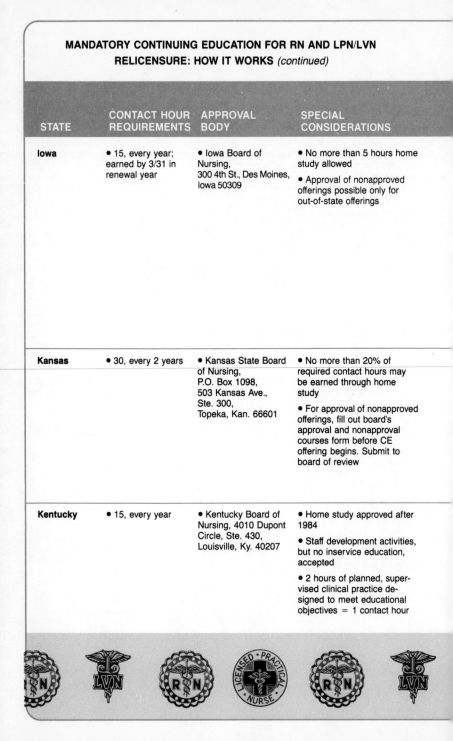

| DOCUMENTATION REQUIREMENTS | REQUIREMENTS FOR MAINTAINING LICENSE ELSEWHERE | THOSE EXEMPT FROM LICENSURE | CE REQUIREMENTS TO REACTIVATE LICENSE |
|---|---|---|---|
| • Complete CE report form and send to board with renewal application<br><br>• Keep attendance certificates and transcripts for at least 4 years | • Take academic courses or participate in out-of-state Iowa-approved offerings; if the other state has mandatory CE, meet that state's requirements; develop an individualized plan with that state board | • Residents of another mandatory CE state who meet that state's requirements<br><br>• Active-duty military members<br><br>• Overseas government employees<br><br>• Some mentally and physically disabled nurses<br><br>• Inactive nurses<br><br>Note: Licensees must apply for an exemption each year | • 15 contact hours earned within 1 year prior to reactivation |
| • Submit an *Individual Nurse Participant Record Form* within 4 weeks after participation: if in state, get form from the instructor with his signature; if out of state, get form from the board<br><br>• When renewing license, list offerings by titles, provider number, date, location, and contact hours earned | • Participate in offerings approved by the ANA or the National Federation of LPNs; for other offerings, contact board before attending | • Inactive nurses | • Same as renewal requirements for year in which nurse applies for reactivation |
| • Send transcripts, a copy of attendance certificates with a description of the offering, and the provider's seal or signature with renewal application | • Participate in CE offerings approved by NLN; State Board of Nursing; CEARP; the National Federation of LPNs; the National Association for Practical Nurse Education and Service; or ANA-approved agencies | • New graduates (for first renewal)<br><br>• Inactive nurses | • 30 contact hours; if inactive for more than 5 years, also complete a refresher course<br><br><br>*(continued)* |

**MANDATORY CONTINUING EDUCATION FOR RN AND LPN/LVN
RELICENSURE: HOW IT WORKS** *(continued)*

| STATE | CONTACT HOUR REQUIREMENTS | APPROVAL BODY | SPECIAL CONSIDERATIONS |
|---|---|---|---|
| **Massachusetts** | • RNs only: 10 in 1984 to 1985; 15 in 1986 and every 2 years thereafter; earned by 12/31 of year before renewal<br><br>• LPNs only: 15 in 1984 to 1986; 15 in 1987 and every 2 years thereafter | • Massachusetts Board of Registration in Nursing, 100 Cambridge St., Room 1509, Boston, Mass. 02202 | • Nursing offerings must include a qualified licensed nurse as a planner or instructor<br><br>• For approval of nonapproved offerings, complete and submit board's approval and nonapproval courses form, 60 days before or 30 days after completing the offering |
| **Minnesota** | • RNs only: 30 every 2 years, earned by 5/31 in renewal year<br><br>• No requirements for LPNs | • No prior approval necessary. Nurse must evaluate program to make sure it meets criteria established by Minnesota Board of Nursing, 717 Delaware St., SE, Minneapolis, Minn. 55414 | • None |
| **Nebraska** | Three options:<br>• 200 hours nursing practice and 20 contact hours CE or inservice education within last 5 years<br><br>• 75 contact hours of CE within last 5 years<br><br>• Graduation from basic nursing program approved by Nebraska board within last 4 years | • No prior approval necessary. Nurse must evaluate program to make sure it meets criteria in board's CE manual: Nebraska State Board of Nursing, Box 95065, State House Station, Lincoln, Nebraska 68509 | • No limit on contact hours, but courses must be nursing-related<br><br>• Courses must have an evaluation device, such as a final test |

| DOCUMENTATION REQUIREMENTS | REQUIREMENTS FOR MAINTAINING LICENSE ELSEWHERE | THOSE EXEMPT FROM LICENSURE | CE REQUIREMENTS TO REACTIVATE LICENSE |
|---|---|---|---|
| • Complete statement on renewal application, listing offerings by title, provider, provider number, date, and contact hours earned | • Participate in CE offerings approved by the ANA, NLN, or National Federation of LPNs; offerings of other Massachusetts-approved providers, or approved academic nursing programs; for all other offerings, follow regular approval procedures | • New graduates (for first renewal)<br><br>• Inactive nurses | • Same as to renew license, earned within the 12 months preceding application for reactivation; if inactive for more than 5 years, also complete a refresher course |
| • When renewing license, complete a board-provided *Evidence Form*<br><br>• Keep records for 2 years after renewal period ends | • Same as in state | • Only inactive nurses, but new graduates can obtain credit for course work completed within 2 years before licensure | • 30 contact hours earned within 24 months before applying for reactivation |
| • Complete and send CE form with license renewal notice | • Meet Nebraska requirements; make sure courses meet criteria in Nebraska's CE manual | • None | • Same as to renew |

*(continued)*

### MANDATORY CONTINUING EDUCATION FOR RN AND LPN/LVN
### RELICENSURE: HOW IT WORKS *(continued)*

| STATE | CONTACT HOUR REQUIREMENTS | APPROVAL BODY | SPECIAL CONSIDERATIONS |
|---|---|---|---|
| Nevada | • 30, every 2 years | • Nevada Board of Nursing, 1135 Terminal Way, Ste. 209, Reno, Nev. 89502; or an ANA-accredited approver | • No more than 6 hours of home study allowed <br><br> • Courses given by an accredited college or university need not be approved <br><br> • For approval of nonapproved offerings, send all required information for board review with license renewal form; no guarantee of approval |
| New Mexico | • 30, every 2 years | • New Mexico Nurses Association, 303 Washington, SE Albuquerque, N.M. 87108; or an approver accredited by the ANA or recognized by the board | • For approval of nonapproved offerings, complete a New Mexico Nurses' Association approval form before participating in offering |

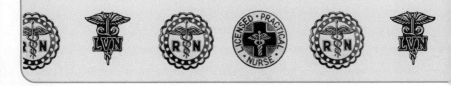

accredited most state nurses associations, several national specialty nurses associations, some federal nursing services, and one state board of nursing, in Nevada. The ANA also has accredited numerous college and university CE programs and certificate programs for nurse practitioners. The National Federation of Licensed Practical Nurses approves continuing education programs for LPNs.

An LPN or LVN wanting to earn CE credits should only take National Federation–approved programs. However, the National Federation will usually approve any ANA-approved course for LPN/LVN CE credits.

Agencies and organizations don't have to be ANA-accredited to offer CE programs. But you should check their credentials carefully before you enroll

| DOCUMENTATION REQUIREMENTS | REQUIREMENTS FOR MAINTAINING LICENSE ELSEWHERE | THOSE EXEMPT FROM LICENSURE | CE REQUIREMENTS TO REACTIVATE LICENSE |
|---|---|---|---|
| • Send a board-provided form with renewal application<br><br>• Keep grade slips, transcripts, and attendance certificates at least 4 years | • Take academic courses; or participate in ANA or ANA-accredited offerings, or home-study courses | • Inactive nurses (however, the board is asking for a legislative change to exempt new graduates for the first renewal) | • 30 hours in the preceding 2 years (or as negotiated with board) |
| • Send an association-provided notarized form with renewal application | • Participate in offerings approved by organizations listed under *Approval body* column at left | • Inactive nurses | • If inactive for less than 5 years, and reactivated in first year of licensure biennium, meet CE requirements by time of renewal; if reactivated in second year of biennium, meet CE requirements by time of second renewal<br><br>• If inactive for 5 years or more, also complete a refresher course |

in one of their programs. Programs not accredited by the ANA may have drawbacks: since they're not necessarily planned by nurses, they may be too simple, too complex, or irrelevant for nurses.

When you enroll in a CE program, you're expected to complete all required exercises and activities within a stated amount of time and to submit an evaluation of the experience. You accumulate a contact hour for every 50 minutes that you participate in the approved program. That block of time consists only of the activities that specifically contribute to the learning experience. When you've accumulated 10 contact hours, you're awarded a continuing education unit (CEU) or, as they're called in some states where continuing education is voluntary, CEARP points. CEARP stands for Continuing Education Approval and Recognition Program. (See *Understanding CEARP*, page 356.)

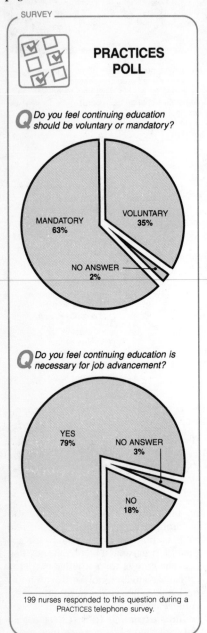

**PRACTICES POLL**

**Q** *Do you feel continuing education should be voluntary or mandatory?*

MANDATORY
63%

VOLUNTARY
35%

NO ANSWER
2%

**Q** *Do you feel continuing education is necessary for job advancement?*

YES
79%

NO ANSWER
3%

NO
18%

199 nurses responded to this question during a PRACTICES telephone survey.

If you work in a state where continuing education is voluntary, you're free to accumulate as many contact hours as you like, whenever you like. However, if you live in a state that requires mandatory continuing education, you must complete the number of contact hours that state law specifies to renew your nursing license, whether you're an RN, LPN, or LVN. In some states, RNs and LPNs/LVNs are required to complete the same number of contact hours. In other states, RNs may be required to complete more contact hours than LPNs/LVNs.

Most providers of continuing education have developed record-keeping systems to keep track of all continuing education offerings, the individual learners who participate in continuing education, and the learners' CEUs. The systems are designed to store information for at least 5 years and to allow learners and providers to retrieve information quickly and efficiently.

Records of course offerings usually include a description of the course, its objectives, teaching strategies, criteria for completion, and a plan for evaluating the participants. Other information that's usually included is the faculty's professional credentials; a roster of participants who received contact hours; the number of contact hours awarded; and a summary of the participants' evaluations.

Individual learner records contain the learner's name and address, the name of the course he participated in, the place where it was held, the course's starting and ending dates, and the number of contact hours the learner earned.

### The controversy—voluntary or mandatory continuing education?

Continuing education is a nurse's professional responsibility. Today, because many states have enacted mandatory CE legislation, it's now a legal responsibility for many nurses as well (see Entry 2). But the nursing profes-

## EVALUATING AN EMPLOYER'S CONTINUING EDUCATION PROGRAM

Before you decide to enroll in a continuing education (CE) program sponsored by your employer, you may want to ask some of these questions:

Is it a program that will earn you CE units (CEUs), or just an orientation to your institution?

What are the prerequisites, if any? For example, must you work in a clinical specialty area to attend a program on that topic?

Are you released from on-duty work to attend these programs, or must you attend before or after work?

Do you have to pay for the program?

Does your employer require you to earn a given number of CEUs? Is CE tied to the employee-evaluation process?

If you attend an in-house CE program, are you expected to file a report or hold a conference to discuss the program with co-workers?

sion is divided on the issue of mandatory continuing education. Some nurses object to the legal obligation that mandatory continuing education imposes on them. They prefer to set their own goals for keeping up to date in nursing. Other nurses feel that mandatory requirements are the only way to assure that nurses will keep their nursing knowledge current and that employers will encourage continuing education.

Mandatory continuing education is an outgrowth of the consumer movement of the 1960s. During that period, the public, concerned about the quality of health care, began to ask for proof that the health professionals who cared for them were truly competent practitioners. Many nurses who shared the public's feelings communicated their concern to the federal and state legislatures. The result: Many states passed laws mandating continuing education for nurses.

California was the first state to enact mandatory CE legislation. Other states have profited from California's example when developing their own legislation. Under California's legislation, the state board of nursing interprets the terms of mandatory law and establishes rules and regulations to ensure that nurses meet its requirements. RNs and LVNs must submit proof of CE partic-

ipation to their licensing board. They must show that they completed the required number of CE contact hours during the 2 years immediately preceding their license renewal date. The law grants military nurses practicing overseas more time to fulfill the CE requirement. And it exempts new graduates from the requirement for 2 years.

Today, 20 states have laws that require some form of continuing education; 11 states require continuing education for all RNs, LPNs, and LVNs; 7 states require continuing education for certain classifications of nurses; and 4 states have legislative power to require continuing education. (See *Mandatory Continuing Education for RN and LPN/LVN Relicensure: How It Works,* pages 346 to 353.)

But other states are unlikely to pass

## UNDERSTANDING CEARP

In states where continuing education (CE) is voluntary, the Continuing Education Approval and Recognition Program (CEARP) helps to ensure that you don't waste your time taking poor-quality CE courses. In these states, providers of CE programs—state nurses' associations, national specialty associations, and federal nursing services—have established their own methods for offering and approving CE mutually accepted programs. Each method meets minimum, mutually accepted standards. Because all the methods

share common objectives, the providers have identified them collectively as CEARP. CEARP's objectives are:
● to record your participation in CE activities
● to make sure that CE offerings meet identified needs in nursing education
● to encourage you to regularly update your knowledge, skills, and attitudes about nursing care
● to keep you informed of available CE programs and offerings.

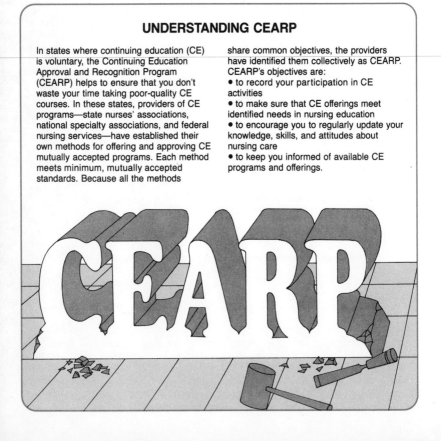

mandatory continuing education laws for several reasons. Many nurses oppose mandatory continuing education because getting required contact hours costs time and money. For example, fulfilling a 30-contact-hour requirement can cost you several hundred dollars every 2 years. In addition, your hospital may not reimburse you for the course fees, travel costs you may incur, or time that you had to take off from work.

If you're in a specialty area of practice, you may have few continuing education offerings to choose from. And if you work in a rural area, you may have few opportunities to attend continuing education programs. In either situation, you'd have difficulty fulfilling your continuing education requirement.

Some states recognize independent study as acceptable mandatory continuing education. But because you can't always document this kind of learning experience accurately, most states limit the amount of independent study that they'll accept.

Some hospitals have tried to remedy some of the problems of time, cost, and availability of continuing education offerings by providing on-site continuing education courses. (See *Evaluating an Employer's Continuing Education Program,* page 355.) But you should be aware of the drawbacks. Hospitals may not have personnel who are qualified to teach continuing education in certain areas of specialization and management. And on-site continuing education deprives you of contact with peers from other work settings.

Because criteria for approving mandatory continuing education programs vary from state to state, continuing education courses that may be acceptable in one state may be unacceptable in another. Consequently, if you decide to move to another state, you may be unable to transfer your contact hours.

These problems and others have dampened the enthusiasm many health-care professions had for mandatory continuing education in the 1970s. In fact, the mandatory continuing education trend is already waning: new mandatory CE legislation hasn't been introduced in any state in the past 2 years.

## A final word

The ANA is currently studying the issue of credentialing for all nurses, from licensure to certification to requirements for continuing education. The ANA hopes to use the study's findings to establish a center for credentialing that the entire nursing profession will recognize as the official accrediting body for both voluntary and mandatory continuing education. The public would be better served by such a system. And nurses would be able to move freely from one state to another, confident that licensing boards and other official agencies would recognize their participation in continuing education, no matter where it occurred.

# 55 Choosing a continuing education program

You've probably taken some continuing education (CE) programs to learn new ideas and skills. But have you always felt as though you've gotten your money's worth? Chances are good that you've been disappointed at least once.

Attending a program that doesn't help you in your practice probably leaves you feeling frustrated—you've wasted time and money. Perhaps you've vowed not to let it happen again. How can you prevent it?

As you know, choosing the program that's best for you isn't always easy. That's because you have such a wide variety of continuing education providers and programs to choose from, and you have to consider each program's cost.

Checking out the many programs to find one that meets your needs will take time. But the time you spend doing this will ultimately *save* you both time and money.

## Where to get information on CE programs

Begin your CE investigation by collecting information on CE programs available in your area. One of the best ways to start is to get on the mailing lists of several CE providers. How do you do this? Ask your co-workers which CE fliers they receive. Get the names of those providers and write to them. Also ask your co-workers if they've attended any CE programs that were particularly helpful. If they have, get the names of the providers of those programs, and write to them as well.

Check with the nursing service administration, the inservice or staff development department, the library, and the personnel department where you work to see which CE fliers they receive. Review these fliers to see if specific programs or providers interest you. Then write to as many of the providers as you wish and ask to be put on their mailing lists.

Check back occasionally with the appropriate departments so you can review the newest offerings.

You can also find out about CE programs by checking nursing journals. Often they list CE programs offered at the local, state, regional, and national levels. If a program looks interesting, contact the provider to get all the details you'll need before deciding whether to attend.

Your state board of nursing may be another valuable source of information on CE programs. In fact, in states with mandatory continuing education, the board of nursing may be the best source of such information (see Entry 54).

Here's another tip: call the universities in your area and find out which ones have CE departments for nurses. Ask any that does to send you a catalog or fliers of its offerings.

As you probably know, many state nurses associations (and their local district associations) provide CE programs. If you're a member, you'll receive information about these programs regularly. If you're not, you can write for a calendar of CE programs, although you may have to pay for it.

If you belong to a nursing specialty organization, you'll be able to find out about CE programs from the national organization or its local chapter. Some local chapters even review and formally recommend CE programs.

## How to evaluate CE programs

Before you can evaluate CE programs, you must determine what your CE needs are and identify exactly what you want from a CE program. To begin, decide what aspects of nursing practice you need to be competent in to do your job. Identify them specifically, in terms of nursing actions. For example, if you're beginning to work in a critical care unit, you may need to learn more about managing arterial lines. Then, after identifying your needs, read the program brochures, analyzing the following components:

*Purpose.* The brochure should state the program's purpose in general terms. Make sure this purpose matches your reason for seeking a CE program. For example, the program's purpose might be "To gain competence in life-support techniques."

# COMPARING HOSPITAL-BASED AND COLLEGE/UNIVERSITY-BASED REFRESHER COURSES

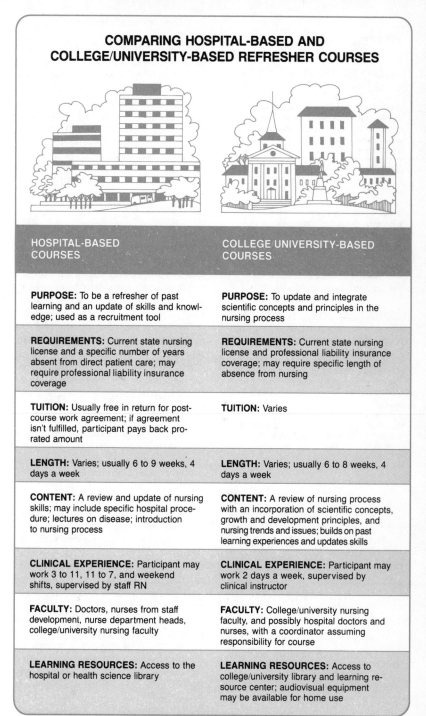

| HOSPITAL-BASED COURSES | COLLEGE/UNIVERSITY-BASED COURSES |
|---|---|
| **PURPOSE:** To be a refresher of past learning and an update of skills and knowledge; used as a recruitment tool | **PURPOSE:** To update and integrate scientific concepts and principles in the nursing process |
| **REQUIREMENTS:** Current state nursing license and a specific number of years absent from direct patient care; may require professional liability insurance coverage | **REQUIREMENTS:** Current state nursing license and professional liability insurance coverage; may require specific length of absence from nursing |
| **TUITION:** Usually free in return for post-course work agreement; if agreement isn't fulfilled, participant pays back pro-rated amount | **TUITION:** Varies |
| **LENGTH:** Varies; usually 6 to 9 weeks, 4 days a week | **LENGTH:** Varies; usually 6 to 8 weeks, 4 days a week |
| **CONTENT:** A review and update of nursing skills; may include specific hospital procedure; lectures on disease; introduction to nursing process | **CONTENT:** A review of nursing process with an incorporation of scientific concepts, growth and development principles, and nursing trends and issues; builds on past learning experiences and updates skills |
| **CLINICAL EXPERIENCE:** Participant may work 3 to 11, 11 to 7, and weekend shifts, supervised by staff RN | **CLINICAL EXPERIENCE:** Participant may work 2 days a week, supervised by clinical instructor |
| **FACULTY:** Doctors, nurses from staff development, nurse department heads, college/university nursing faculty | **FACULTY:** College/university nursing faculty, and possibly hospital doctors and nurses, with a coordinator assuming responsibility for course |
| **LEARNING RESOURCES:** Access to the hospital or health science library | **LEARNING RESOURCES:** Access to college/university library and learning resource center; audiovisual equipment may be available for home use |

## GETTING YOUR EMPLOYER TO FINANCE YOUR CONTINUING EDUCATION

Most employers offer some kind of financial assistance if you attend a continuing education (CE) program. But what if your employer has no financial assistance policy? Follow these steps to negotiate with your employer. If you can clearly show how what you learn will make you a more valuable employee, he may decide to pay for all or at least part of your CE program.

• Assemble the necessary information—course content, cost, location, time.

• Put your request in writing, including a rationale for why your employer should send you to this particular activity.

• Be prepared to negotiate for what you want *most*—course fees, travel expenses, time off—and possibly to forego some less important items in your request.

• Emphasize the benefits that your patients and colleagues will gain because of what the CE program will teach you.

• Present your proposal far enough ahead of time so that schedules and paperwork can be arranged.

• Anticipate your employer's possible objections and develop a contingency plan. (Can a colleague substitute for you at work? Can you attend another conference instead?)

• Report to your employer afterward about the program and its benefits, and express support for the system that made your attendance possible.

• Share your program materials and information with anyone who's interested.

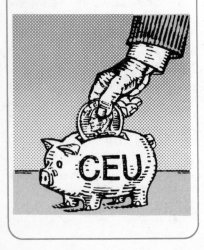

*Objectives.* Although the purpose statement will be general, the objectives should be specific. Be wary of objectives couched in vague or general language. For example, an objective such as "To improve the quality of patient care" doesn't tell you much. So look for objectives that tell you exactly what you'll learn. An objective such as "To perform assessment of the respiratory system" lets you know what the program will teach you. Of course, you also want to make sure that the objectives match your learning needs.

*Audience.* Check the brochure's statement on the intended audience to make sure the program is geared to your professional level.

*Content.* Read the outline of the program's content. Ask yourself if the content seems appropriate to the program's objectives, and consider whether it fits your learning needs. Finally, ask yourself if the CE provider has allowed sufficient time for you to learn the information outlined.

*Teaching methods.* As you may know, people learn best when they're allowed to participate in the learning process. So find out if the program uses participatory methods, such as small group discussions or simulated or real clinical practice. Also, check the enrollment limit. If the class is large, the instructor probably won't be able to give any individual help.

*Faculty credentials.* Read the credentials of the faculty members to see whether they seem qualified to teach the program. Be sure to check the description of their work experience. Remember, you want to learn things you can use in your practice, so you'll want an instructor whose work experience seems most appropriate.

*Program approval.* Make sure that an appropriate organization, such as a state board of nursing or nurses association, has approved the program for contact hours or continuing education units (CEUs). Usually, such approval indicates a quality program. If the brochure says that such approval is pending, call the provider *before* you register, to ensure that it's approved.

*Provider reputation.* Ask a few people who've attended previous programs offered by the provider if they'd recommend the program.

*Cost.* When comparing the costs of programs, consider how long they'll last and who's teaching them. Usually, the longer the program or the more well known the speaker, the higher the cost will be. Also, determine what the program fee includes. For example, does it cover handouts, textbooks, meals, or social activities? Don't forget to add the cost of necessary travel and lodging to the program fee before making your comparison. Also, see if the provider has a refund policy in case you can't attend or the program is canceled.

*Program evaluation.* Check the brochure to see if you'll be asked to evaluate the program after you've completed it. The sponsor should want to know what you think to improve the program. If it doesn't, you have reason to question the program's quality.

## Financing continuing education
Financing your continuing education is your responsibility. However, your employer may share this responsibility with you, since the knowledge and skills you gain benefit not only you but your patients and the institution as well. Find out if your employer will share the cost of your continuing education. (See *Getting Your Employer to Finance Your Continuing Education.*) Whether he will or not, you should try to obtain quality continuing education at the most reasonable cost possible.

## A final word
Choosing a CE program that's best for you will take time and thought. But think of this evaluation and selection process as an education in itself. If you use it carefully, you'll choose CE programs that are right for you—and you'll also learn to be an efficient continuing-education consumer.

## Selected References

American Nurses' Association. *1983 Certification Catalog.* Kansas City, Mo.: American Nurses' Association, 1983.

American Nurses' Association. "A Social Policy Statement," *American Nurse* 13:3, January 1981.

"Clinical Experience Proposed for Ontario," *AORN Journal* 29(7):1364, June 1979.

Hinsvark, Inez G. "Credentialing in Nursing," in *Current Issues in Nursing.* Edited by McCloskey, Joanne C., and Grace, Helen K. Boston: Blackwell Scientific Publications, 1981.

Jones, Faith M. "ANA's Certification for Specialization," in *Current Issues in Nursing.* Edited by McCloskey, Joanne C., and Grace, Helen K. Boston: Blackwell Scientific Publications, 1981.

Lenburg, Carrie B. "The External Degree in Nursing: An Alternative Ready for Adoption," in *Current Issues in Nursing.* Edited by McCloskey, Joanne C., and Grace, Helen K. Boston: Blackwell Scientific Publications, 1981.

Lewison, D., and Gibbons, L. "Nursing Internships: A Comprehensive Review of the Literature," *Journal of Continuing Education in Nursing* 11(2):32-38, 1980.

Minor, M.A., and Thompson, L. "Nurse Internship Program Based on Nursing Process," *Supervisor Nurse* 12:28-32, January 1981.

Morgan, D. "Upgrading the Work of New Graduate Nurses," *Dimensions in Health Service* 55:28, November 1978.

Plasse, N. J., and Lederer, J.R. "Preceptors: A Resource for New Nurses," *Supervisor Nurse* 12:35, June 1981.

Putney, J.C. "Specializing Without Going Back to School," *NursingLife* 1:30-35, July/August 1981.

Spicer, J.G. "Pitfalls in Developing Nurse Internship Programs," *Nursing Administration Quarterly* 3:69-73, Spring 1979.

Weiss, S. J., and Ramsey, E. "An Interagency Internship: A Key to Transitional Adaptation," *Journal of Nursing Administration* 7:36-42, October 1977.

# Your Choices About Your Job

## Introduction

You're looking for a job. Perhaps you're just entering the job market or reentering it after taking time off for school or to raise a family. Or maybe you're relocating or moving up the career ladder. Maybe you're just dissatisfied with your present job.

Whatever your reason for seeking a job, you need to give careful thought to the job choices available to you, to your legal rights when you're applying or being interviewed for a job, and to your rights as an employee when you're hired—or fired. You also need to be aware of your options on the job: the potential salary as well as benefits, such as health and life insurance.

But practical issues aren't your only concern. You also need to know if this job will match your professional goals. For instance, if you've had special preparation to develop assessment skills, you probably want a job in which those skills will be used and valued. If acute care is your preference, you'll steer clear of jobs in chronic geriatric settings.

This chapter will help you sort out these practical and professional job issues, and it will help you to make beneficial job decisions.

### Nurses' job options—then and now
The whole issue of job choices and options is fairly new in the nursing profession. Nurses traditionally have been given little choice in their job situations. If you worked in the 1950s, you may have been given a choice about where you worked, but you probably had no voice in such matters as what shift you worked or your pay scale. This all changed in the 1960s. With the women's movement highlighting the neglected job status of all women, nurses became increasingly vocal in their demands for determining their own professional destinies. In 1966, for example, 2,000 nurses in 33 San Francisco–area hospitals resigned during a dispute over salary demands. Soon afterward, the California Nurses' Association endorsed the use of strikes for gaining nurses' economic objectives. In June of 1974, when their contract talks broke down, 4,400 members of the California Nurses' Association walked off their jobs.

These were historic actions. They paved the way for you and for all nurses to be more assertive in negotiating—not only for better working conditions and fair wages but also for greater professional autonomy. Currently, the high demand for nursing services in many parts of the country puts you in a favorable position. You can demand more from employers in areas such as wages and flexible (nontraditional) staffing patterns.

As you know, choosing a job is a major decision. The wrong choice can leave you feeling unfulfilled and discontented. The right choice gives you satisfaction and fulfillment and puts you on the path to achieving your professional and your personal goals. Entry 56, "Should you change jobs?" offers guidance toward making the right job choice.

Few nurses find perfect jobs right away. Finding the right job can be very interesting and challenging, but it can also be frustrating and demoralizing. What can make all the difference? Forming a career plan and acquiring job-hunting skills. Entry 57, "Job hunting made easy," tells you where and how to look for a job, what resources are available, and how you can best utilize those resources.

## The ins and outs of interviewing and negotiating

But this is only a beginning. You need to be able to write a résumé that will pique a prospective employer's interest and make him want to know more about you. The résumé presents a summary of your employment history, your skills, and your talents. Entry 58, "Writing a winning résumé," shows you how to do just that.

Once you've successfully attracted an employer's attention, the next step is to consider how you'll handle the job interview. This is the best opportunity you'll have to convince an employer to hire you, and it requires careful preparation. In Entry 59, "Making the most of your job interview," you'll find the guidance you need.

If an interview is successful, you and a prospective employer are ready to negotiate the terms of your employment. You need to know which factors will help you negotiate successfully and which options you can choose when negotiating with an employer. Entry 60, "Learning negotiation techniques," and Entry 61, "Salary and benefits options you can bargain for," tell you what you need to know.

## Coping with the new job

Once you've decided to accept a job, a new challenge awaits you: starting off on the right foot. Every job involves expectations—yours, patients', co-workers', and supervisors'. Sometimes these expectations will clash and cause conflict. How you handle these conflicts will often determine whether you become a satisfied, productive employee or an employee who's disgruntled and ready to move on. Read Entry 62, "What to expect in a new job," for helpful insights that will improve your prospects for job satisfaction.

## Leaving the job

Leaving your job is a serious matter. Once you've made the decision (or if you know you'll be asked to leave), you want to handle yourself well and preserve the possibility of a good future reference from your employer. Entry 63, "The professional strategy of resigning," offers instruction in writing your letter of resignation and in handling the exit interview. Entry 64, "Surviving being fired," will help you avoid the personal and professional scars that so often result from this unpleasant experience.

Taken together, the entries in this chapter describe methods for coping with all phases of the job cycle. With this information, you'll be prepared to make job choices that will keep your nursing career bright and fulfilling.

# 56 Should you change jobs?

As you probably know, changing jobs is a fact of life for nurses:
• Annual turnover rates are as high as 50% in some hospitals.
• National nursing-career studies indicate that a typical staff nurse moves in and out of the labor force several times in her career.

• Nurses also frequently move from full-time to part-time work, or the reverse.

Changing jobs can be a rewarding growth experience when your decision to make a change and your choice of a new job reflect a well-thought-out career plan. But if you make these decisions hastily, changing jobs may become an upsetting, depressing, and self-defeating experience. To make your next job change a positive experience, use the guidelines that follow.

### Planning: the basis for any job change

A job change should be part of an overall career plan. If you haven't made such a plan, begin now to think about where you are, where you're going, and what your short and long-term goals are—in your personal life as well as in your career. (See *Knowing What You Want,* page 366.) Consider where you'd like to be and what you'd like to be doing 1 year, 5 years, as much as 20 years from now (see Entry 65).

Here's an idea some nurses have used to examine their career choices: Start a diary. Write down what you'd like to do and the setting you'd like to do it in, up to 20 years from now. Your feelings might change from week to week, but over time, a pattern will develop. This is the first stage in formulating your personal and professional goals.

You also need to do some long-range, lifetime planning. What goals do you want to accomplish in your lifetime? Consider how many of these goals are job related. To help you organize and direct your thinking about your nursing career, you may wish to read career-planning guides, attend a career-planning workshop, or discuss your interests and ideas with a career counselor.

Take the time to decide what's really important to you. Then list what your goals are now. Check this list frequently as you continue your career planning, and update it as necessary. Remember, your nursing career is *you.*

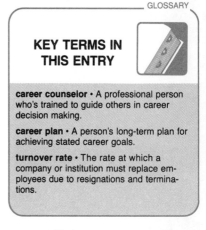

## KEY TERMS IN THIS ENTRY

**career counselor** • A professional person who's trained to guide others in career decision making.

**career plan** • A person's long-term plan for achieving stated career goals.

**turnover rate** • The rate at which a company or institution must replace employees due to resignations and terminations.

You wouldn't want someone else to make snap decisions about your life—be sure you don't do this yourself.

### Taking stock of yourself

If you're thinking of a job change, you need more than a set of goals. You need to match up your goals with realistic self-analysis. Why? To help you decide whether your goals are realistic. One method of self-analysis involves listing your strengths, preferences, weaknesses, limitations, and interests. Using some pages in the diary you've already started, write down your answers to the following questions:

• What kinds of patients have you cared for successfully in the past? List such characteristics as types of illnesses (and whether acute or chronic), patients' ages, and complexity of care. Why do you think your care was successful?

• What kinds of activities do you do best, and why?

—independent activities, such as primary care, clinic work, patient education?

—direct patient-care activities?

—highly structured activities, such as intensive care, where the demands are immediate and require high levels of technologic skills?

—supervisory activities, such as those of a charge nurse or team leader?

—teaching activities, such as staff de-

## KNOWING WHAT YOU WANT

Before you change jobs, be sure you know what you're looking for. Ask yourself: "Which job factors are important to me? And which are *more* important than others?"

Those same questions were asked of 581 nurses. Job factors are listed below in the order of their importance to the nurses polled.

To develop your own profile, take the test yourself. Check the job factors important to you, and put them in order: most important to least important. You'll then have a profile of your preferences in a new job.

| JOB FACTOR | RATING |
|---|---|
| | **(Percent of RNs rating factor *very important* or *somewhat important*)** |
| Reputation of hospital | 98% |
| Salary | 98% |
| Shift and scheduling policies | 97% |
| Nurse:patient ratio | 96% |
| Educational benefits | 95% |
| Fringe benefits | 95% |
| Continuing-education assistance | 94% |
| Advancement opportunities | 94% |
| Personal safety | 94% |
| Type of hospital | 86% |
| Number of specialty units | 77% |
| Hospital size | 76% |
| City hospital | 66% |
| Rural hospital | 53% |
| Internship program | 51% |
| Social/recreational opportunities | 36% |

velopment and inservice orientation?
—patient-advocate activities?
—departmental liaison activities?
• Do you like to work alone or in groups? This can be critical.
• Which areas of health care do you enjoy working in the most? Do you prefer working as a hospital staff nurse, as a community health nurse, or in a specialty, such as pediatrics, obstetrics, or intensive care?
• Do you prefer to work with individuals, families, or large groups—such as in the community, a school, or a factory?
• Are you active on hospital committees or in professional organizations? Describe your involvement and how you

feel about the work.
- Do you like to guide and assist new staff members and watch them grow professionally?
- Do you like to initiate well-thought-out plans, or do you prefer to carry out others' plans?

After answering these questions, write a summary of your professional strengths and interests. Reread it, then discuss it with friends, a counselor, or a mentor. Think about the type of job that would permit you to use these strengths and interests and develop them further.
- What are your weaknesses and limitations? In what areas do you need more experience, more information, or a change of attitude? What limitations do you have that must be factored into any decision about a new job? Identifying your own weaknesses and limitations isn't easy. But because it takes special effort, doing it is a kind of strength you can feel good about. Listing your limitations doesn't mean you need to try to change each one. In fact, accepting your limitations is an important part of the job hunt. If, for example, you've listed as one of your limitations "inability to work outside of scheduled hours because of child-care responsibilities," considering a job that requires flexible hours would be unrealistic for you. Analyzing your weaknesses helps you avoid taking a job that emphasizes something that ranks high on a list of your limitations instead of on the list of your skills.

Even if you feel you'll have difficulty overcoming your weaknesses, recognizing their existence will help you choose a job that capitalizes on your strengths. If you do want to try overcoming some of your weaknesses, take a continuing-education course to supplement your knowledge and maybe change your outlook.

## Reviewing your present job
Before making any definite plans for a job change, take a good look at your current job. What does it provide? Answer the following questions as completely as possible:
- Does your present job offer you career mobility? Where can you go, how can you grow in your hospital (or other health-care institution)?
- Is your job challenging?
- Are you given recognition for a job well done? Are you encouraged to speak up? Are your opinions considered important?
- Is your job compatible with your lifestyle? With your biorhythms?
- Does it provide you with support and friendships that you would hesitate to leave?
- Are your fringe benefits good? Consider your tuition reimbursement, organizational memberships, retirement contributions, dental insurance, free health care.
- Is your present salary competitive

---

### "Are you being paid a salary that's proportionate to your growing skills and responsibilities?"

---

with the pay in similar jobs in other institutions? (Professional organizations can usually provide you with information about average pay scales. Other sources of information you may find useful include newspaper ads and colleagues in other institutions.)
- Are you being paid in proportion to your growing skills and responsibilities? Has your salary kept pace with the cost of living? (Make a graph of your salary increases over the past 5 years. Compare the results with the annual rate of inflation; in recent years it has ranged from 5% to 15%.)
- Do you like your current geographic location, or would you rather live someplace else?

Reviewing the answers to these questions will give you a clear idea of what your present job offers and what it lacks. After you've reviewed your answers, list 10 negative aspects and 10 positive aspects of your job, arranging each list in the order of your personal priorities.

## What don't you like about your present job?

Look at the 10 negatives you listed. Begin with your first item—the worst aspect of your current job. Can you do anything to change the situation, or is it totally controlled by others? If, for example, the first negative listed is "working all three shifts," ask yourself if you can do anything about changing your work schedule. Can you negotiate with your supervisor for a better schedule? Will an opening for working straight shifts occur soon? Could you arrange to transfer to another station? Or are all three options out of your control?

Next, think about each of the other negatives on your list in terms of who controls the situation and whether you have any influence. Be sure that those things you believe others control totally really *are* out of your sphere of influence. Often, an honest, open discussion with your supervisor will change your perception of your ability to influence your job environment. After you've determined which of the negatives you can change and which you can't, decide how important such changes would be to you. Would you keep your job if you could change all or some of them? This analysis will give you added information with which to make a job-change decision.

In your list of negatives, one or more items may relate more to personal unhappiness than to on-the-job factors. For example, your feelings about family members may influence how well you get along with your colleagues at work. Consider whether you have unresolved personal problems that need your attention. If you don't resolve them, you may carry these personal problems to a new job. Don't blame your job for problems you bring to it.

## What would your "dream job" be?

After you've taken inventory of yourself and your current job, spend some time thinking about your "dream job." Look at your goals list again. Change it if some of your ideas have changed. Now—if you could have any job in the world, what would you choose? How would you describe your "dream job"?
• Do you want responsibility, accountability, and authority in patient care? If this is more than you want, describe your preferences in as much detail as possible.
• Do you want a fast pace? A slow one?
• What kinds of people do you most want to work with?

Now, look at your current job in light of all you've learned from your self-inventory, your analysis of your present job, and your description of your "dream job." Weigh all the pros and cons of a job change before you make a final decision. Talk with nurses who have jobs like yours in different institutions. Compare your experiences and assessments with theirs. You may find you have benefits and opportunities in your current job that other jobs wouldn't offer. And you may be surprised to find that what you've learned by your fact-finding efforts gives you confidence as well as information for making decisions about your job.

## Making your decision

Is a job change the answer for you? You've stated your goals; assessed your strengths, preferences, interests, and weaknesses; examined your present job; and envisioned your dream job. These are the basic tools for career planning. Before you decide on your next career move, you may repeat the steps suggested here several times. Remember, job environments change, and your needs and goals will also change as you grow in your area of nursing practice.

If you plan to change jobs—or change fields—you should be able to state clearly why the change is necessary and

# CONSIDERING A NEW JOB?

*I got my BSN 2 years ago and since then have worked steadily as a staff nurse on a medical-surgical unit of a teaching hospital. I like my work generally, but it's not what I'd want to do for the rest of my life.*

*My problem is, I don't know what I want to do. Should I specialize in something? And if so, what? Sometimes I think about community health nursing. Then sometimes office work sounds the best. Like I said, I just don't know what I want.—RN, Mich.*

First think of the job that will give you the most opportunity to do what you appear to like best—is it a hospital nursing specialty, community health, office nursing, or something else? Then, before you make any firm decisions, try to figure out whether your personality fits in with the "personality" of the setting—unit, office, hospital—of the new job you're considering.

To do this, start by analyzing your own personality. For example, do you like independence and responsibility, or do you feel more comfortable under close supervision?

Next, try to assess the personality of the new job setting you're envisioning. Is it fast-paced or slow-paced, modern or old-fashioned? Would you be working as part of a team, or alone?

To avoid a mismatch between you and your new job, try to determine if you'll probably fit in, if your personality will make you compatible with your future colleagues. After considering these factors, you should be in a better position to get the kind of job you're looking for.

This letter was taken from the files of *Nursing* magazine.

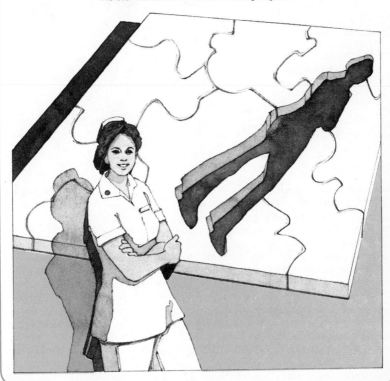

## OPPORTUNITIES OVERSEAS

*I'm an RN with an associate degree, and I'm interested in practicing in England. I've heard the U.S. Air Force (USAF) offers opportunities abroad, but I wonder what chances I'd have of being stationed in England. Should I enlist?*—RN, Iowa

According to the U.S. Air Force, opportunities in USAF hospitals overseas vary from country to country and year to year, depending on staffing needs. The higher your education level, the more likely you are to have your choice of locations. But you'll probably be stationed where you're needed the most.

Before joining, you might ask a recruiter if he can give you an idea of your assignment location. Make sure you get any promises in writing.

For more information on working overseas, here are several civilian organizations that offer opportunites abroad:

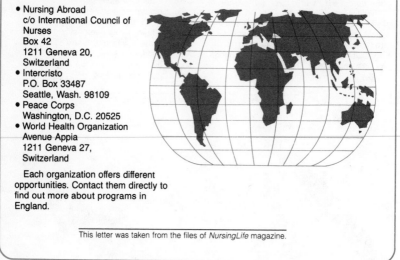

- Nursing Abroad
  c/o International Council of
  Nurses
  Box 42
  1211 Geneva 20,
  Switzerland
- Intercristo
  P.O. Box 33487
  Seattle, Wash. 98109
- Peace Corps
  Washington, D.C. 20525
- World Health Organization
  Avenue Appia
  1211 Geneva 27,
  Switzerland

Each organization offers different opportunities. Contact them directly to find out more about programs in England.

This letter was taken from the files of *NursingLife* magazine.

how it fits with your career goals. Review your goals regularly. Evaluate them, and use them to help you set job priorities. How will a particular job change help you meet your goals?

Before making a final decision to change jobs, consider the timing of the change. How many major changes are happening in your life now? If you're involved in deciding about such matters as marriage or divorce, a new house, or a new baby, this may not be the right time to change jobs. Coping with too many changes—even positive ones—can create unnecessary stress

and weaken your decision-making capability.

## A final word

Don't be afraid to make a job change, but do be sure that any change you make is well thought out and advantageous to you. Even if you decide not to change jobs, you'll find that your analysis and planning provide insight about yourself and about new opportunities in your current job. You just may come to realize that the grass on your side is as green as you want it to be.

# 57 Job hunting made easy

You've decided you need or want to change jobs. For successful job hunting, you'll need a thoughtful, thorough, and purposeful plan. Remember, looking for another job can be exhilarating—and exhausting.

As a nurse, you're not alone in your desire to change jobs. Current statistics are difficult to interpret because of recent fluctuations in the economy, but long-standing evidence suggests that up to 50% of the nation's nurses leave their hospital jobs each year. Indeed, many leave nursing altogether. In the 1970 census, 20% of formerly registered nurses had not maintained their licensure.

Unfortunately, many nurses who decide to change jobs end up frustrated and self-defeated in their search for new employment. Here's how you can avoid this fate and end up with the job you want.

## How to start looking for a new job

The first place to start looking is in your present location—in fact, in your present job! Make sure you've exhausted all the opportunities available to you (see Entry 56). Maybe you're looking for more responsibility or for different rewards. Start by examining your present job's potential. Would a few changes make all the difference? Are those changes possible? Then negotiate for alterations in your present job description, and perhaps for the opportunity for further education that will give you what you want. For example, if the reason you're looking for a new job is because you want to learn to care for critically ill patients, you can negotiate for tuition for coronary-care nursing courses, and for certification-exam fees, in return for accepting increased patient-care responsibilities. Or perhaps your desire for a new job stems from your interest in working with families of pediatric patients—helping them understand their children's illnesses, growth and development problems, or medical therapy. If so, why not ask your supervisor and your medical colleagues to help you write these responsibilities into programs that you can provide? These responsibilities also involve some daytime duty for program development and implementation.

Keep in mind that a successful job change starts with a positive approach to looking for the right job. (See *Changing Jobs: Finding the Right Type of Hospital*, page 372.) To avoid developing a negative attitude that could undermine any efforts you make, analyze your situation before you begin. Make sure you're willing to expend the necessary time, energy, and money for the job hunt. Remember that changing jobs incurs some monetary losses, such as loss of vacation time, sick leave, and retirement benefits. And that job-hunting entails expenses, such as telephoning, traveling, and preparing résumés.

You'll also have to spend personal

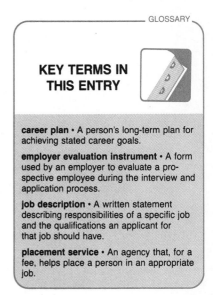

GLOSSARY

**KEY TERMS IN THIS ENTRY**

**career plan** • A person's long-term plan for achieving stated career goals.

**employer evaluation instrument** • A form used by an employer to evaluate a prospective employee during the interview and application process.

**job description** • A written statement describing responsibilities of a specific job and the qualifications an applicant for that job should have.

**placement service** • An agency that, for a fee, helps place a person in an appropriate job.

## CHANGING JOBS: FINDING THE RIGHT TYPE OF HOSPITAL

You're an academically qualified, currently licensed, and highly motivated nurse ready for a new nursing job in a hospital setting. What type of hospital is best for you? Here's a chart that details some important characteristics you should consider in choosing where you want to work.

| TYPE OF HOSPITAL | CHARACTERISTICS |
|---|---|
| **Services:** | |
| General | • Offers a variety of general health services, such as surgery, medicine, obstetrics, and pediatrics |
| Specialty | • Provides care for patients with a particular type of illness. Some admit only patients of one sex or children of a specific age group. |
| Combined general/specialty | • Offers both general health services and care for patients with particular types of illnesses |
| **Type of care:** | |
| Acute | • Treats acutely ill patients. Patient may stay up to 30 days; after 30 days, patient is transferred to an extended-care hospital. |
| Extended | • Treats chronically ill patients of all ages and patients who no longer require acute-care medical attention but still require medical and nursing care |
| **Size:** | |
| Under 100 beds | • Provides general services. Nurses assume more responsibilities in addition to direct patient care. |
| 100 to 300 beds | • Provides general health services and one or two specialties. Nurses may assume greater responsibilities in addition to direct patient care. |
| Over 300 beds | • Offers several specialties. Nurses assume limited responsibilities. Offers nurses progressive salary and benefit packages; provides in-depth inservice and continuing education programs along with opportunities to gain advanced technologic experience |

energy, at least an hour or two a day, for a thorough job hunt. Keep in mind that you may search from 6 months to a year to find the right job. Decide on a realistic time limit for your job hunt, and begin with an honest self-analysis to find out why you want to look for something else (see Entry 56). Remember that not all your strengths are job related. For example, having interper-

sonal communication skills and good family support systems are especially helpful when you're job hunting. And you must also draw on reserves of personal energy.

### How to find out about new job opportunities

The first place to look for new job opportunities is your present place of employment. Read bulletin boards and personnel office newsletters; ask about any upcoming vacancies. You can also telephone other organizations or institutions, such as hospitals, clinics, and public health services, to find out if any jobs are available.

If you want to change your geographic location, begin looking in professional journals that list job advertisements. These advertisements also can give you a broader idea of the kinds of jobs you're qualified for. Look in big-city newspapers, too.

Remember, if you're looking in unfamiliar areas of the country, you'll also have to locale-hunt. *Locale hunting* refers to gathering information about an area's cost of living, life-style, cultural and professional opportunities, and even climate conditions. Remember, a good job in an area you don't like usually doesn't work out. So don't respond to an area's newspaper ads if you already know you won't like it there.

If you've selected a city or town where you want to work, contact employment agencies there. If you can get the area's local newspapers, check them for job openings. And don't forget that civil service agencies also employ nurses. City and state public health departments, hospitals, penal institutions, and clinics often list their positions with central personnel offices.

Sometimes the quickest way of obtaining information about available jobs is through the grapevine. Information seems to pass through the grapevine faster than through ads or any other medium. Remember, though, that these leads may be inaccurate or incomplete, so you may be disappointed when you follow them up.

You may also use a placement service (employment agency), especially if you're looking for a specialty unit or administrative job. Placement services are companies that gather information about employment opportunities and set up job interviews for client nurses (See *Placement Services: Considering the Sources,* page 374.) When you use a placement service, you don't have to do all of the legwork in finding out about openings. However, the placement service may not have access to all the openings you may be able to discover on your own. Remember that placement services usually charge fees for their services. Sometimes the employer will pay the fee if you're hired, but you should be sure what the placement service's fee policy is *before* you sign up for interviews.

### Making the initial contact

Follow up every job lead, no matter what its source is. The first step, of course, is the initial contact with the employer or with the individual advertising the position. The initial telephone conversation is important; you want to make a good impression as well as obtain more information about the position. *You want to get as much information as you can over the telephone.*

> ## "Often the quickest way of obtaining information about available jobs is through the grapevine."

Often the first contact will be with a secretary or some other person not involved in the actual hiring. Begin the conversation by stating your name, the title of the position you're interested in, and your interest in receiving more information. If you're in luck, the organization or institution will have printed materials to send you—information on job requirements, evaluation methods, salary scale, benefits package, and so forth.

If you're invited to come for an employment interview, you'll obtain more information at that time to help you decide whether the job is right for you. Usually, the prospective employer will ask for your credentials prior to the interview—such as your résumé and the completed application form. (See Entries 58 and 59.)

### "Maybe this job's the one"— how to decide

An important part of your job hunt involves analyzing what a potential new job offers. Compare what you like about your present job with the job you're investigating. Would the new job be as interesting and rewarding? What benefits does the new job offer compared to the old?

Be sure you also review the job description and related employer-evaluation instrument for any job you're interested in. The job description should detail specific, day-to-day tasks that you'd be performing. And the evaluation instrument will tell you what job requirements are considered most important. Make sure you also understand how your job performance would be rated.

Summarize the job requirements and list them. These requirements should roughly correspond—positively or negatively—to the personal strengths, weaknesses, and limitations you've previously listed (see Entry 56). Matching the job requirements with your own characteristics will help identify any mismatches. For example, if one of the job requirements is supervision of nursing-assistant personnel, and one of the evaluation items is "appropriately assigns nursing assistants to patient care," you can add the corresponding strength, "2 years' team leader experience with LPNs and aides." Or maybe you don't have primary care experience to correspond with the job requirement

---

OPINION

## PLACEMENT SERVICES: CONSIDERING THE SOURCES

How do you learn about nursing job openings? Probably through hospital recruiters and word-of-mouth referrals from colleagues. But what if these sources don't turn up what you want? You may want to consider using a placement service. This is an agency that knows what jobs are available and will try to locate the one that's right for you. Before you decide whether or not to try a placement service, consider these pros and cons:

| PROs | CONs |
|---|---|
| • Placement services have access to far more job openings than you'd uncover on your own. <br> • They can give you good advice: not only on how to prepare an effective résumé but also on how to make the best impression at the interview. <br> • They'll do the necessary legwork for you, such as arranging interviews with prospective employers and forwarding your résumé. <br> • They may be able to guide you to other nursing-related jobs you haven't considered. <br> • They usually don't charge a service fee or commission if you accept the job they find for you (but make sure of this *before* you sign anything). | • Placement services are only as good as the agents representing you. They may be more interested in filling a job than in finding the one that's right for you. <br> • Since the employer usually pays the placement fee, the salary he offers through a placement service may be less than what he would have paid if you'd negotiated for the job on your own. <br> • Placement services don't offer you a bonus for accepting a job referral. Hospital recruiters frequently do offer a bonus as an incentive to accept the job offer. |

of initiating a total patient-family nursing care plan for primary patients. Then you know you can't meet the evaluation criterion, "develops 24-hour cardex nursing care plan." You may decide not to pursue the job any further, or you may sign up for continuing-education workshops on primary care. This type of comparative analysis will give you good insight into whether a new job is appropriate for you, and it will show you whether you need more preparation in some areas. Comparative analysis can also help you identify when you're overqualified for a position.

Scheduling is another area where personal limitations may restrict your new job choices. For example, suppose one job-description item says, "teaches, once yearly, the 6-week, evening prenatal classes to mothers-to-be," and the evaluation item says, "mothers admitted after instruction have been well-prepared for labor and delivery room procedures." You may be quite pleased about the teaching and accountability involved, but you may be unable to schedule 6 evenings in a row because of personal or professional commitments. If so, this job isn't the one for you right now.

If you have more strengths listed than the number of job-description requirements and evaluation items, you may well have more preparation and skill than the position requires. (Before deciding against the job, however, find out if it actually involves more than the job description shows.)

Here's a way to compare two or more potential new jobs to see which one's better for you: List the requirements and evaluation criteria for each, in separate columns, and then see how your strengths and weaknesses match up.

Remember, comparing various jobs can help you recognize your own potential in today's competitive job market. When you list requirements of jobs, you'll sometimes find you have some required skills that you haven't included in your list of strengths. You can

add these strengths to your résumé and include them when you're considering other new jobs.

## A final word

If you understand and use the job-hunting strategies described in this entry, you'll be able to plan for career advancement based soundly on self-analysis and job analysis. The job-hunting plan you develop will serve you well every time you change jobs as you continue to pursue your career in nursing.

# 58 Writing a winning résumé

A résumé is documentation of your career, useful for self-analysis and vital to your career advancement. A well-written résumé is essential to a successful job search. A winning résumé—one that helps get you the job you want—must effectively highlight your expertise and experience. When you've developed a winning résumé, you'll have written evidence of your achievements as well as a job-application tool.

Certain basic components should be included in every résumé. Other items of information may or may not be included. Before writing your résumé, you'll need to decide what kind of information should go into it, how you want to organize the information, and what writing style you want to use.

## Understanding résumé formats

As you know, your résumé is the summary of your qualifications and experience that you use in applying for a job. Three aspects of this definition are worth extra emphasis:

• Your résumé is a *summary*, and a brief one at that. It should be a concise presentation that will interest prospective employers in learning more about

GLOSSARY

## KEY TERMS IN THIS ENTRY

**cover letter** • A letter that a person seeking employment sends, together with his résumé, to a prospective employer. The cover letter states the applicant's interest in applying for a particular job.

**employment interview** • An exploratory meeting between a job applicant and a prospective employer.

**résumé** • A written summary of a person's work qualifications and experience, used in applying for jobs.

you and your experience. How will they learn more about you? By inviting you in for an interview. Your résumé is the key to further contact with employers (see Entry 59).

• Your résumé is an account of your qualifications and experiences, usually including relevant nonwork experiences.

• Your résumé is often the first impression of you a potential employer receives. So it's very important!

The two most-often-used résumé-organization plans or formats are the chronologic format and the achievement-oriented format. (See *The Achievement-Oriented Résumé.*) The chronologic format, in which a person's education and work history are presented in reverse chronologic order, is used more frequently. You're probably familiar with this type of résumé. In an achievement-oriented résumé, the person's most impressive achievement is presented first and followed by other achievements in descending order of importance.

## What are a résumé's standard components?

Certain basic information should always appear in your résumé:

• identifying data, such as your name and address

• your educational qualifications
• your employment background
• your professional activities and achievements, such as association memberships, publications, and honors you've received.

*Identifying data.* Every résumé should contain your full name (no nicknames), address, and the telephone number where you may be reached. (Make sure that you're readily available at the number you give or that someone will politely and accurately take your messages.) Other identifying information, such as your age, marital status, and number of dependents, may be included, but it's not required. If you consider it an invasion of your privacy, leave it out.

*Educational qualifications.* This section should include, first, credentials related to your highest level of education, followed by the others in reverse chronologic order. Explain any degrees or credentials that have only local or regional significance. Remember, include information about your continuing education, too. (You may want to spell this out in detail in another section of your résumé.) The following paragraphs show how you can briefly describe your educational experiences:

"Diploma in Nursing, Home Town Hospital, 9/78 to 6/81.

"This 3-year, NLN-accredited school of nursing afforded me the opportunity to learn in a large medical center affiliated with a local college. The psychiatric rotation was made available through the state mental health center. During this time I was active as an officer in the Student-Nurse Association.

"B.S. in Nursing, Home Town University, 9/72 to 6/76.

"This NLN-accredited baccalaureate program included clinical experiences at numerous hospitals and public health agencies. I was able to take a clinical elective in the coronary care unit for 5 weeks. My extracurricular activities included work on the university newspaper.

"A.D. in Nursing, Home Town Hospital, 9/80 to 6/82.

"This NLN-accredited, 2-year program included practice in two hospitals and a mental health center. The 5-week pediatric rotation took place in the local children's hospital. I graduated with honors from the college and with a recognition award from the pediatric nursing staff."

You'll have to decide whether to include information related to your educational record—your professional license or registration number, any certificates you've earned, or your class rank or standing. Certificates, such as the cardiopulmonary resuscitation certificate awarded by the Red Cross, and specialty certificates, given by the American Nurses' Association and the American Association of Critical Care Nurses, should be highlighted; these are very desirable credentials to have.

You should *not* include your state-board test results or school grades, although these may be discussed in the interview.

*Employment background.* You'll normally present your employment history in reverse chronologic order in your résumé. This means you put your most recent or current position first, the one before that one next, and so on. Be sure to be specific about your title. A charge nurse and a unit manager, or an assistant nursing director and a nursing supervisor, may or may not be synonymous in various parts of the country. Don't forget to write "charge nurse duties" after "staff nurse" if taking charge was part of your job. To give your résumé that winning edge, you may want to describe, in a short paragraph, the major responsibilities each job involved. The following paragraphs show how to highlight these jobs.

## THE ACHIEVEMENT-ORIENTED RÉSUMÉ

Awards and honors, education and experience. The sum of your nursing career so far. You want to make the most of it on your résumé. You can simply list your achievements within each major category. But to make your résumé more effective, try listing them according to their importance or relevance. Here's a sample résumé that uses this *achievement-oriented format:*

Health: Excellent
Marital Status: Married

Joan Brown, RN, MS
609 Hillside Drive
Anderson, Tex. 59847

AWARDS AND HONORS
Received Merit Raise, General Hospital, 1982
Elected Delegate to State Nurses Convention, 1980
Sent by Orthopedic Association to National Seminar, 1981

EDUCATION
MS, Anderson University, 1983
20 credits toward MSN, State University, 1980-82
BS, Northern State University, 1976
Continuing Education Certificate as Orthopedic Technician, 1974

EXPERIENCE
Head Nurse, Orthopedic Unit, General Hospital, 1978-1980
Staff Nurse, Orthopedic Unit, General Hospital, 1976-1978
Staff Nurse, Part-time, General Hospital, while obtaining MS degree, 1980-present

"Staff Nurse, Emergency Room, Home Town Hospital, 9/80 to 10/82.

"As a staff nurse in this trauma center emergency department, I was often assigned triage duty. I also developed written instructions for patients who were sent home with casts or with sutures. In addition, I specialized in intervening with parents who were suspected of child abuse.

"Staff Nurse, Medical Floor, Home Town Hospital, 8/79 to 10/82.

"As a staff nurse on this 36-bed oncology/cardiovascular floor, I became comfortable in caring for adults with these chronic disorders. I often had charge duty and would delegate care responsibilities to five or six other nursing-staff members. I instructed all the new employees on our unit in our discharge planning procedure.

"Nurse Technician, Surgical Floor, Home Town Hospital, summer 1979.

"The technician position included nursing-aide duties as well as expanded responsibilities for patient care under an RN's guidance. On this surgical floor, I was able to work with the enterostomal therapist in teaching ostomy patients."

Information in this section of your résumé can vary in format, depending on how much you want to say. For example, you need to decide whether you will list, or list and describe, your previous jobs and whether you will give your reasons for leaving those jobs. (This information is not required, although you may be asked about it in an employment interview.)

Another decision relates to salary. Should you include in your résumé your present salary, your salary history, or the salary you're looking for? As a general rule, salary information isn't included in résumés; salary negotiating is more appropriate during an interview.

*Professional activities.* The final section of your résumé focuses on your professional affiliations. Your memberships reflect your interest in various organizations and your support for their work toward improving the profession. These memberships may also reflect your interest in maintaining your own competence, because many of these organizations are known for providing continuing education for their members. Membership in health-related organizations that aren't specifically nursing organizations, such as heart, cancer, or arthritis associations, shows your support for research and public education.

Membership in these organizations isn't all you should list in this section of your résumé, however. Include volunteer work you've done, committee work you've done, offices you've held, and any honors you've received, such as certificates of recognition or attendance. You should also list honors from educational institutions, community groups, your church, and your fellow

---

*"A winning résumé includes optional information that may be very effective in getting an employer's attention."*

---

nurses, because these honors reveal the esteem others have for you.

Along with professional memberships and honors, list any professional articles or books you've written and published and any research you've done. Publication reflects your concern for your profession and your ability to communicate.

## What else may a résumé include?

Although every résumé should contain the standard components discussed above, a *winning* résumé may include information that's considered optional but that sometimes is very effective in getting an employer's attention. Optional information that may enhance your résumé includes dates of professional licensure or certification, references, continuing-education activities, and personal hobbies or interests.

*References.* Under this heading, you should state, "Available on request."

Have the list handy when you go to an interview, however, so you can give it to your prospective employer if he asks for it.

This list should include the names, addresses, titles, and telephone numbers of individuals who can personally

## PREPARING A WINNING COVER LETTER

Your cover letter, along with your résumé, should catch a prospective employer's attention and convince him that you're qualified to interview for the job. Follow this example to prepare your cover letter correctly:

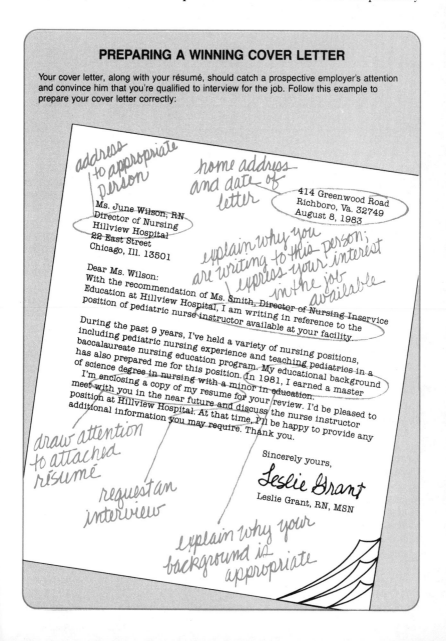

endorse your professional and personal qualifications. Be sure to contact these individuals in advance to get permission to use their names—and their assurance that they not only can recommend you but also have time to write a reference.

Keep the list short, preferably four to six people. Two or three references should be professional people who've worked with you. The other references should be personal references—people who can attest that you are mature, responsible, and trustworthy. You might include as references a previous supervisor, a school instructor, and professional colleagues. Sometimes a prospective employer will ask you to contact your references to request that they send him letters of recommendation.

*Continuing-education activities.* You can also add a list of your continuing-education experience to your résumé. Consider organizing these activities by topic to enhance your background. For example:

"Clinical Workshops
Workshop on EKGs, State University, 6/1980.
Interpreting Laboratory Studies, Inservice Home Hospital, 9/1980.
Management Workshops
Time Management and Delegating, Nurse Managers 7/1979.
Staffing Patterns, Home Community College, 4/1978."

*Personal activities.* Some search committees consider how well-rounded a person's background is. So you may want to include hobbies, volunteer work, and church or political activities in your résumé. When you're making decisions about what to put in or what to leave out, try putting yourself in the place of the person who'll be reading it. What information would make the best impression?

### The cover letter
When you're responding to an employment advertisement or sending your résumé to the personnel office of an institution where you'd like to work, include a cover letter. (See *Preparing A Winning Cover Letter,* page 379.) The cover letter concisely explains why you wish to apply for a job. For example, you might say, "I wish to be considered for employment in the trauma center of your hospital. I'm seeking employment at your center because it has always been cited as a leader in trauma nursing." You may also indicate the title of the position you are seeking.

Your résumé is often the first impression a prospective employer has of you. Be sure it—and your cover letter as well—are well written and neatly typed.

### A final word
Remember to keep your résumé brief and to read through it before your interview. You don't want any surprises! If you've prepared it carefully, your résumé should help you win the job you want.

# 59 Making the most of your job interview

After you've updated your résumé (see Entry 58) and sent it to a prospective employer, you're ready for the next step—the job interview. This is a step you may take many times during your nursing career. Your well-written résumé has gotten your foot in the prospective employer's door. How successful you are at the interview will depend on how well you've prepared yourself to talk about your accomplishments and the job you want.

Employment interviewing is a mutual exchange of information. The employer seeks information to determine your qualifications for the job. You need information to determine whether the job is right for you. If you're overqualified for the job but you take it anyway, you may become bored, dissatisfied, and negative. What if you're under-qualified? Then you'll need prolonged training and extra supervision; you could create a burden on the institution and a morale problem as well. Remember, a nurse who accepts a job she's unsuited for hurts herself as well as the institution or organization that hires her.

## Preparing for the interview

A job interview provides your prospective employer, who knows your professional background from your résumé and job application, with new information about your personal *qualities,* those traits that you demonstrate when you interact with others. The job interview gives you the opportunity to put your best foot forward—to make your good qualities known.

Before going to the interview, review the following points once more (see Entries 56 to 58):
• your work experience
• your attitudes toward your work, yourself, and other people
• your education
• your interests
• your goals.

Once you've completed this self assessment, you'll be ready to work on how you'll present your qualifications at the interview. (See *ABCs of a Job Interview,* page 384.) You need to be able to speak comfortably about your accomplishments and show how they contribute—directly or indirectly—to your work. For example, your ability to make long-range plans shows your maturity and organizational ability. Your involvement in community affairs shows a commitment to society. Your social activities show a diversity of interests and an ability to relax and get away from your work. Think about ways you can create these and similar impressions as you talk with the interviewer.

Do some homework, too, on the institution or organization that will be interviewing you. Get copies of the an-

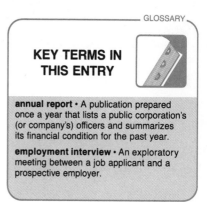

GLOSSARY

## KEY TERMS IN THIS ENTRY

**annual report** • A publication prepared once a year that lists a public corporation's (or company's) officers and summarizes its financial condition for the past year.

**employment interview** • An exploratory meeting between a job applicant and a prospective employer.

nual report, the newsletter, and any other materials available from the public relations department or personnel office. These items will provide you with background information and other material for discussion. They'll also enable you to ask pertinent questions at the interview. Remember, your degree of self-confidence during the interview will be in direct proportion to your preinterview preparation. A high degree of self-confidence and a positive attitude about the interview will help mask any feelings of excitement, nervousness, or apprehension you may have. You'll also increase your confidence if you're neatly dressed and well groomed.

## At last! The interview

The interviewer will set the interview's tone. It may be formal and structured, so that you only discuss your previous job performance and your skills, or it may be an informal conversation laced with discussion of your personal and social activities. Be alert to the interviewer's conversational direction at the start of the interview, and follow it.

Regardless of the interview's format, the focus is on you. As you know, first impressions are lasting. So ensure a positive first contact with your prospective employer by being alert, pleasant, and enthusiastic.

Arrive at the interview 10 minutes ahead of schedule. Be sure you know the name and title of the person who'll

## USING LETTERS TO YOUR PROFESSIONAL ADVANTAGE

Here are some sample job-applicant letters. Use them as guides to help you land a job and start it on the right note.

**Setting up the interview**

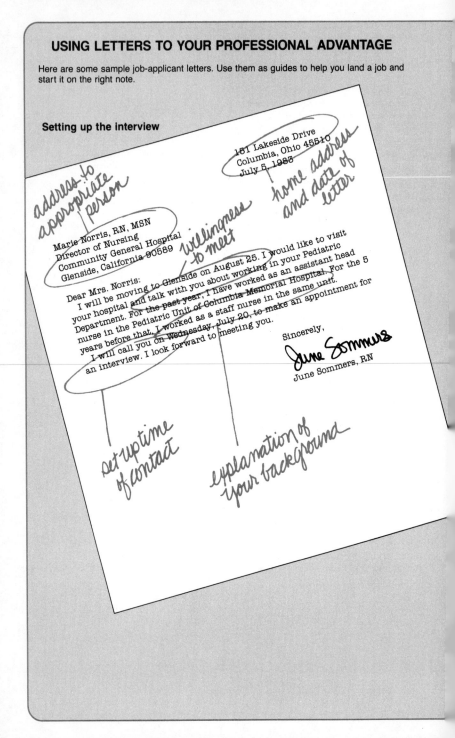

*address to appropriate person*

*willingness to meet*

*home address and date of letter*

151 Lakeside Drive
Columbia, Ohio 45510
July 5, 1983

Marie Norris, RN, MSN
Director of Nursing
Community General Hospital
Glenside, California 90589

Dear Mrs. Norris:

I will be moving to Glenside on August 25. I would like to visit your hospital and talk with you about working in your Pediatric Department. For the past year, I have worked as an assistant head nurse in the Pediatric Unit of Columbia Memorial Hospital. For the 5 years before that, I worked as a staff nurse in the same unit.

I will call you on Wednesday, July 20, to make an appointment for an interview. I look forward to meeting you.

Sincerely,

June Sommers

June Sommers, RN

*set up time of contact*

*explanation of your background*

**Following up the interview**

*address to appropriate person*

151 Lakeside Drive
Columbia, Ohio 45510
August 8, 1983

*home address and date of letter*

Marie Norris, RN, MSN
Director of Nursing
Community General Hospital
Glenside, California 90589

Dear Mrs. Norris:

I enjoyed meeting you and discussing the current opening in your Pediatric Department. I was particularly impressed with both the facilities and the opportunities for professional growth at the hospital. Please keep me in mind for this current opening.

Thank you again for taking the time to discuss my potential employment and to show me your Pediatric Department. I am looking forward to hearing from you soon.

Sincerely,

June Sommers

June Sommers, RN

*expression of interest and appreciation for the interview*

*expression of your gratitude and interest*

---

**Accepting the offer**

*address to appropriate person*

Marie Norris, RN, MSN
Director of Nursing
Community General Hospital
Glenside, California 90589

151 Lakeside Drive
Columbia, Ohio 45510
August 18, 1983

*home address and date of letter*

Dear Mrs. Norris:

I gladly accept the offer to be a staff nurse in the Pediatric Department at Community General Hospital. I will report on September 12 at 8 a.m., as you requested.

I am looking forward to joining your excellent staff and to working in the challenging environment of your Pediatric Department.

Sincerely,

June Sommers

June Sommers, RN

*acceptance of offer*

*confirmation of plans*

*expression of interest*

## ABCs OF A JOB INTERVIEW

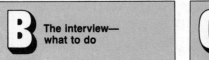

### A  The interview preliminaries

To go to a job interview feeling composed and confident, you have to do a lot of advance planning. Before any interview, take these steps:
• Respond to an employer's ad—send a cover letter and your résumé to your prospective employer.
• Ask for a personal appointment with the director of nursing or whoever is in charge of hiring.
• Practice the interview. Rehearse the answers to foreseeable questions about your education, your nursing experience, why you want to change jobs or left your previous job, your duties in your last job, and your nursing philosophy.
• Be prompt on the day of the interview: arrive 10 minutes ahead of the scheduled time, if possible.
• Look your best for the interview. Dress conservatively, and make sure you're neatly groomed.

### B  The interview— what to do

When you walk into the interviewer's office, follow these tips:
• Stand until the interviewer invites you to sit.
• Place any personal belongings beside you or on the floor.
• Address the interviewer as Ms. or Mr. unless you're asked to use a first name.
• Don't slouch or fidget; sit upright and be attentive.
• Don't chew gum or smoke cigarettes.
• Answer the interviewer's questions with confidence.

### C  The interview— what to ask

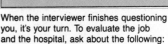

When the interviewer finishes questioning you, it's your turn. To evaluate the job and the hospital, ask about the following:
• patient-care assignments
• staffing policies
• advancement opportunities
• continuing education
• salary
• working conditions and work shifts
• employee benefits

---

be interviewing you. When you meet your interviewer, shake hands, smile, and make eye contact. Sit down when you're invited to do so. The interviewer will start the conversation; listen carefully and respond appropriately to the formal or informal tone he sets for the conversation. Then relax and answer the questions that are an integral part of any job interview. Speak clearly so that your enthusiasm and sincerity are evident. Before the interview, you studied the essential requirements of the job; now, explain how your experience and abilities can fulfill them.

Here are some questions employment interviewers commonly ask, along with suitable answers to them.
Q. *Why did you apply here for a job?*
A. The hospital is clinically and educationally progressive, and I feel my abilities will be an asset to it.
Q. *What are your long-range goals?*
A. After I broaden my clinical experience, I intend to take courses so I can teach in a clinical setting.

Q. *What is your greatest strength?*
A. I think it's my ability to organize and manage people. I developed this ability as a Girl Scout leader, a camp counselor, and an officer in the Student Nurses' Association.

Q. *What are your limitations?*
A. I'm not aware of any limitations that will prevent me from doing a good job for your hospital.

Q. *Why are you changing jobs?*
A. To broaden my experience and test my skills in a new environment.

Q. *Why did you choose your specialty?*
A. In working with children, I've found that I can contribute to their growth and development. I find that very satisfying.

Q. *What do you know about our organization?*
A. [Tell the interviewer what you have learned about the organization from their annual report, particularly information about its latest accomplishments.]

Q. *What hobbies do you enjoy most?*

A. Hobbies that involve interaction with other people. I like to hike and play tennis, and I belong to bowling and swimming clubs.

These are the kinds of questions that an interviewer usually asks. You should be aware that the interviewer is forbidden, by law, to ask other specific questions. (See *The Job Interview: What the Interviewer Can and Can't Ask.*) You're protected against such questioning by Title VII of The Civil Rights Act of 1964, amended by the Equal Employment Opportunity Act of 1972, and the Age Discrimination and Employment Act of 1967, amended in September 1978. (Detailed information about these acts may be obtained from the Equal Employment Opportunity Commission in Washington, D.C.) If you're asked any of these illegal questions, you may give the information, if you think it won't jeopardize your job prospects. Or you can just tactfully change the subject. Or you can simply say, "I know you'll understand if I choose not to an-

---

## THE JOB INTERVIEW:
## WHAT THE INTERVIEWER CAN AND CAN'T ASK

In interviewing for a job, you'll be answering a host of questions. You can expect most of them to be fair and proper. Some questions, however, are inappropriate or even prohibited by law. If you're asked such a question, don't feel obligated to answer. You can discreetly refuse or turn the conversation to another subject.

| Valid subjects | Inappropriate or illegal subjects |
|---|---|
| • Education | • Nationality |
| • Work experience (where, when, how long) | • Race |
| • Reason(s) for leaving your previous job | • Creed |
| • Reason(s) for applying for prospective job | • Color |
| • Reason(s) you think you're qualified | • Religious beliefs |
| • Strengths and weaknesses as they pertain to the prospective job | • Age |
| • Future professional goals | • Marital status |
| • Participation in community or social activities | • Sexual preference |
| • Hobbies and avocations | • Financial or credit status |
| • Job-related criminal convictions | • Criminal arrests or non-job-related criminal convictions |

swer that question."

While the interviewer is evaluating your potential *for* the job, you should be evaluating the potential *of* the job, trying to determine whether it's the one for you. Is the work setting fast-paced or slow-paced? Does it encourage independent nursing judgments, or are most nursing functions of the dependent type? Is the nursing management autocratic, democratic, or laissez-faire? Will the work environment meet

## KEEPING SCORE OF YOUR INTERVIEWS

Chances are you'll talk with a number of interviewers at different hospitals before deciding on the position that's right for you. While you're making the rounds, keeping track of each possible job's working conditions, career opportunities, salary, and fringe benefits won't be easy.

## CAREER INTERVIEW SCORECARD

| | HOSPITAL | | | |
|---|---|---|---|---|
| 1. Were you given a written description of the responsibilities for the nursing position? | | | | |
| 2. Will you be responsible for a reasonable number of patients? | | | | |
| 3. Does the position offer opportunities for administrative and clinical advancement? | | | | |
| 4. Is the chain of command such that you'll report to a nursing administrator (for example, director of nursing), or to a nonnursing administrator? | | | | |
| 5. Does the hospital specify standards of nursing practice? | | | | |
| 6. Will you receive what sounds like adequate orientation for the position? | | | | |
| 7. Is the hospital's policy for department transfers fair? | | | | |
| 8. Does the hospital provide adequate professional liability insurance? | | | | |
| 9. Is the starting salary for the position acceptable? | | | | |
| 10. Does the hospital offer shift and weekend differentials? | | | | |
| | | | | |
| **TOTAL** | | | | |

all or most of your needs? (Don't put the interviewer on the spot by asking for help in determining your needs or making your decision. You should know your needs in advance of the interview. Remember, an interview *is* an interview—not a counseling session.)

Be ready to ask questions about the job at any pause in the interview. Near the end, reaffirm your interest in the job and ask when you can expect to learn the interview's outcome. Don't

To help you do this, here's a handy career interview scorecard. Use it to rate each hospital position you investigate. Give each hospital a plus ( + ) or minus ( − ) for each question. When you've concluded your interviewing, add up the scores for each hospital you've visited and compare your totals. The hospital with the highest score (the most pluses) is probably the right hospital for you.

| HOSPITAL | | | | |
|---|---|---|---|---|
| 11. Is shift rotation or floating required? | | | | |
| 12. Is the benefits package (health/life/disability insurance, vacations, holidays) good? | | | | |
| 13. Are there other benefits such as pharmacy discounts and child-care services? | | | | |
| 14. Is continuing education available at the hospital? | | | | |
| 15. Does the hospital offer tuition reimbursement for continuing-education courses at colleges/universities? | | | | |
| 16. Are there special benefits for working weekends, holidays? | | | | |
| 17. Is flexible scheduling available (for example, work 3 days, off 3 days)? | | | | |
| 18. Does the area offer adequate and acceptable housing accommodations? | | | | |
| 19. Is hospital-subsidized housing available? | | | | |
| 20. Is transportation to and from the hospital provided for all shifts? | | | | |
| 21. Does the hospital have patrolled parking facilities and escort services for late-night shifts? | | | | |
| **TOTAL** | | | | |

discuss salary and benefits at this first interview unless the interviewer brings them into the conversation. The proper time for this discussion is at a later interview, when you're seriously being considered for the job.

### Actions you should take after the interview

Professional etiquette requires that you send a thank-you letter to your interviewer. This gives you the opportunity to remind the interviewer of your qualifications and your interest in the job. Send a letter, too, when you formally accept or decline a job offer. (See *Using Letters to Your Professional Advantage,* pages 382 and 383.)

### A final word

When the interview is over, critique it. Think about your rapport with the interviewer, the amount of information exchanged, and the degree of self-confidence you exhibited. Each successive interview will yield valuable information that will help you measure your job strengths, weaknesses, and needs. (See *Keeping Score of Your Interviews,* pages 386 and 387.) The ultimate goal of an interview, of course, is to be selected for the job (presuming you want it). But don't become discouraged if you're not selected. Whether you get a particular job or not, the self-knowledge you gain from your interview experiences will ultimately help you land the job you want.

# 60 Learning negotiation techniques

When you negotiate with someone, you discuss or bargain to reach agreement. *Discussion* means talking about something in a deliberate fashion, offering opinions in a constructive and (usually) friendly manner. *Bargaining* involves both parties' identifying what should be given or done by each and then mutually agreeing to those terms. Negotiating the terms of a job is something like building a bridge—from what you know, and want, to what the prospective employer knows and wants. The most difficult part of building that bridge is laying the foundations.

### Preparing to negotiate

As with most situations, doing your homework—planning—*before* negotiation will pay off *during* negotiation. You may consider planning time-

---

## "In every negotiation, both the other party and you want something."

---

consuming but don't give this task short shrift. You'll be spending 2,000 hours per year in whatever job you get, so a few hours of planning are hours well spent.

What's involved in planning? Finding out what you want. To help you do this, ask yourself the following questions:

• Why am I looking for another job? What aspects of my old job did I like? What aspects did I dislike? Is the job change for personal reasons? Or have I found that a certain field in nursing isn't for me?

• What's most important to me? Is it salary, hours and scheduling, quality of patient care, time off, assignment load, working comfortably with peers, or getting recognition?

• What types of patients give me the most satisfaction to work with?

• Where would I like to live—in what state or geographic region? In a city, in a small town, or in the country?

• What about the setting? Do I want to work in a medical center, a clinic, a community hospital, or a public health agency?

Learn from your answers to these

questions. Know what type of job you're looking for. Know what aspects of your work are important to you. Doing this will allow you to negotiate from a position of strength and certainty and will enhance your chances of getting a job that best suits your needs.

## Learning tips and techniques for negotiating

When you've decided what kind of job you want and why, write down in a list the points you want to cover—the aspects of the job important to you—*prior* to negotiation time. (For example, what is the salary range? (See *Comparing Nurses' Salaries,* page 391.) What is the weekend rotation? What about shift rotation? What is the number of patients per normal assignment? What about benefits, such as medical and dental insurance? (See *Comparing Job Offers: A Salary Checklist,* page 392.)

This list will guide you during negotiations and allow you to concentrate on what's being said, not on what you want to ask next.

Now you're ready to negotiate. Use the following tips and techniques to maintain a position of negotiating strength:

• Recognize that, in every negotiation, both the other party and you want something. Therefore, you're as potentially important to the other person as he is to you. If you've done your homework, you'll know what you want. Find out what the other party wants. Get specifics. The institution is expecting to fill its needs, and you'll negotiate more effectively if you identify what those specific needs are. Ask about long-range planning, about the institution's philosophy, and about how institutional policy is implemented. Many unit supervisors, for example, are looking for mature nurses to balance their unit staff. Suppose you've been out of work for a few years. You've just taken a refresher course and now you're looking for a job. If the institution considers maturity an asset, your lack of current experience could be considered a trade-

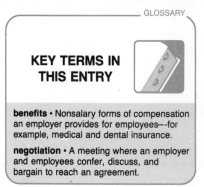

## KEY TERMS IN THIS ENTRY

**benefits** • Nonsalary forms of compensation an employer provides for employees—for example, medical and dental insurance.

**negotiation** • A meeting where an employer and employees confer, discuss, and bargain to reach an agreement.

off for your maturity and previous experience.

• Be positive about what you have to offer—you're very good at what you do and you have the credentials to prove it. Don't be afraid to tell the interviewer what you do well. How else will he know? But also be realistic. For example, if you have a diploma background and 6 months of experience, don't think you're qualified to fill a head nurse position.

• Learn about any "challenges" (problems) the institution is encountering in its delivery of care. Decide how you could best help the institution meet those challenges, and share your ideas with your interviewer. What skill, experience, and enthusiasm do you have that would indicate you're fit for the job? If, for example, the interviewer tells you that care plans are a problem, let him know about the weekly patient-care conferences you initiated on your last job—conferences that helped with this very problem. Your prospective employer will be more amenable to negotiating salary, benefits, and working conditions with you if you show the negotiator that you can help the institution in specific areas.

• Avoid dead-end situations. Don't get sidetracked by differences of opinion or feeling. To establish a battleground over a difference of opinion is to lose the negotiation. Suppose, for example, you feel strongly that charting on progress notes is preferable to charting on nurses' notes, but the interviewer feels

## SHOULD THE CERTIFIED NURSE RECEIVE A RAISE?

*As a career-oriented nurse, I've recently become certified in my specialty, geriatric nursing. The hospital where I work offers a pay increase to nurses once they've earned a BSN degree, but doesn't compensate for certification. Should I ask for an increase in recognition of my certification?*—RN, N.Y.

Your hospital isn't the only one not automatically giving a pay increase for certification. Since certification is still comparatively new in nursing, you may have to wait some time before employers compensate with pay increases for the expertise your certification attests to.

But this shouldn't stop you from *trying* to get an increase in recognition of your certification. Begin by photocopying all pertinent information and placing it in your personnel file. Since certification is an expensive process, include a record of the expenses and time involved in getting it. Then approach your director of nursing and your personnel manager and request a pay increase. You may have to try more than once. But even if you *don't* get more money, you'll still have the satisfaction of your expertise in your specialty. You can't put a price on that.

---

This letter was taken from the files of *Nursing* magazine.

---

otherwise. So what? Charting isn't a negotiation issue, so don't make it one.

• Avoid making the other person feel he's wrong. Your aim is to promote agreement, not argument. Phrases that can help you get past areas of disagreement include: "That's a good point." "It's interesting that you bring that up." "I can see why it would be important for you do it this way." If you're asked a direct question about a specific subject, say how you feel, but if you don't agree and you're not asked to comment, allow the discussion to move on.

• Ask questions and *listen* to the answers. Since your questions are all written down, you won't have to worry about forgetting what you want to ask. Concentrate on what's being said. If something doesn't sound right to you, ask for clarification. For example, if the interviewer says, "You'll be required to work a double shift occasionally," ask how often. How often are double shifts required now? How will you be compensated? Don't be unpleasant—you'll get a better response and more information by being cordial—but remember, these are legitimate questions that you have every right to ask.

If you anticipate feeling uncomfortable about asking key questions like these, practice beforehand with a friend. Say out loud what you want to say to the interviewer. "What is the salary range of this position?" "How soon do increases occur?" Run through all of your questions. If you practice, you'll be more comfortable. If you're more comfortable, you'll project confidence. And if you're confident when you're negotiating, you'll get better results.

• Don't let a negotiation become a confessional. When you can, help the interviewer consider your weaknesses in a positive light. You might say, "I'm a terrible workaholic. I tend to get so caught up in following a patient that I forget to go to lunch." Stay away from any form of negative admission. However, if there are specific negatives—in your references, for example—discuss them honestly.

• Don't fall into the trap of thinking of yourself as unequal, of thinking the doctors and administrators are in control. Temerity in negotiating only perpetuates these feelings of inferiority. So negotiate for your own good. You're worth it! Know what you do well. Know why you're special. Figure out how you'll be an asset to the organization, and communicate it.

A last word of advice: Don't go into a negotiation acting as if your life depended on it or as if the outcome was cast in stone. One bad interview or one bad job selection doesn't have to blight your entire career.

### A final word
As the negotiating session comes to a

close, be sure to recap the important points you covered, such as salary range, working hours, shifts, and benefits. This recap will help clear up any erroneous impressions either of you had during the exchange. Pin your interviewer down about when he'll contact you or when you should contact him.

What if things don't work out exactly as you planned? Perhaps you:
• got what you wanted but the job is disappointing
• had to compromise more than you

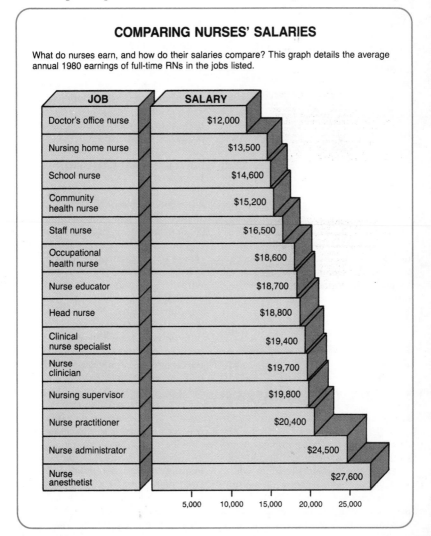

## COMPARING NURSES' SALARIES

What do nurses earn, and how do their salaries compare? This graph details the average annual 1980 earnings of full-time RNs in the jobs listed.

| JOB | SALARY |
|---|---|
| Doctor's office nurse | $12,000 |
| Nursing home nurse | $13,500 |
| School nurse | $14,600 |
| Community health nurse | $15,200 |
| Staff nurse | $16,500 |
| Occupational health nurse | $18,600 |
| Nurse educator | $18,700 |
| Head nurse | $18,800 |
| Clinical nurse specialist | $19,400 |
| Nurse clinician | $19,700 |
| Nursing supervisor | $19,800 |
| Nurse practitioner | $20,400 |
| Nurse administrator | $24,500 |
| Nurse anesthetist | $27,600 |

5,000    10,000    15,000    20,000    25,000

## COMPARING JOB OFFERS: A SALARY CHECKLIST

Comparison shopping for your best salary deal isn't hard. First consider these *income* factors:

- Hourly rate
- Weekday E/N shift differential
- Weekend differential
- Charge differential
- Others (such as critical care differential, BSN or MSN differential)

Then, consider these *expense* factors:

- Health insurance deduction
- Life insurance deduction
- Dental insurance deduction
- Retirement plan deduction
- Disability insurance deduction
- Professional liability insurance premium
- Parking/transportation fees
- Others (such as child-care costs, local taxes, recreation facility fees, car maintenance)

By comparing these factors for each employer you're negotiating with, you can see at a glance who's offering the best "real" salary.

---

expected to get the job

- didn't get what you wanted, and didn't take the job.

Don't give up. Instead, continue to use your negotiating skills to bargain for what you want, step by step or job by job. If your goals are sound, you'll eventually achieve them.

---

# 61 Salary and benefits options you can bargain for

As you probably know, monetary compensation for professional nursing services rendered is on the high side in the 1980s. Why? Because of nursing-staff shortages in the 1970s that led to a sizable jump in the average income of today's nurse. But you and your nursing colleagues have no guarantee that your salaries will continue to increase at the same rate. In fact, cost-containment pressures and government cutbacks may cause a considerable slowdown in salary increases for nurses. If this happens, your benefits package and your negotiable options will become increasingly important in your overall financial picture.

Do you know the total amount of your compensation from your employer? Keep in mind that compensation is not simply your hourly rate, but your hourly rate *plus* the various benefits your employer offers. Almost every employer offers both salary and benefits—but the benefits package may vary greatly from one institution to another. When you choose a job, be sure you understand the salary and benefits options open to you so you can make the decision that best fits your financial and professional needs.

## Salary: Looking beyond the hourly rate

Because basic salary is so important, it's a good place to begin this discussion. No doubt about it, your hourly rate is important. It serves as the foundation of your annual income. A nurse's hourly rate is usually computed on the basis of her experience—type and amount—with consideration given to her educational background. (Some employers pay more for a bachelor's or a master's degree.) But beyond the hourly rate, the differential rates—different rates paid because of differing working conditions—are also important. Some common types of differentials are shift, holiday, and on-call.

*Shift differentials* can add a sizable amount to your annual earnings. They usually represent a set percentage over your base rate (for example, 15% for evenings/nights and 20% for weekend evenings/nights) or a dollar increment (for instance, $1.25/hour Monday through Friday for evenings/nights and $2.25/hour for Saturday or Sunday evenings/nights). If your new job calls for you to work on *holidays,* find out if you'll be paid time and a half for the holidays actually worked, in addition to straight time for the holiday itself. *On-call duty* is defined in different ways in different institutions. If you're considering a job that requires on-call duty, ask about the rate you'll be paid while you're on call at home, as well as the rate you'll be paid if you're called in to work.

*Overtime* can also add a hefty amount to your annual earnings. Be sure to ask how much weekly overtime a typical staff member usually works. The answer will also give you a good idea of the hospital's staffing levels. In evaluating the effect of overtime on your overall earnings, of course, you need to know the number of hours in the basic work week—35, 40, or 80? You also need to know the scheduling pattern used. For example, some employers using the "three 12-hour shifts" scheduling will pay overtime only after you've worked 40 hours.

Another salary-related factor you should consider is *profit sharing.* It has the potential for making a substantial contribution to your annual income or to your pension fund. Obviously, profit sharing is available only in for-profit (as opposed to not-for-profit) institutions. Profit-sharing plans give employees the opportunity to purchase stock in the corporation that owns the institution, or to have money placed in an investment fund for their retirement.

Because profit-sharing plans vary, you should ask several questions about the plan a potential employer offers:
● What would your out-of-pocket costs—if any—be?
● When would you become eligible to participate in the plan?
● Are there limitations on the amount of stock you could buy?
● When are dividends paid?
● Is there a payroll-deduction plan?

## Health insurance: examining the plans

As a nurse, you're surely aware of the importance of health insurance. But do you know what to look for in a health insurance plan for yourself? Health insurance, of course, is offered by almost all employers. Here's a description of some of the health insurance options you will encounter:

The *basic* plan covers hospitalization and medical/surgical costs and may be supplemented by a major medical plan. Under the basic plan, you may be given the option of choosing between two methods of compensating your health-care providers.
● The *fixed-fee method* is based on a schedule of amounts the insurance company wil pay for specific procedures. If your doctor charges more than the fixed fee, you pay the difference.
● Under *the UCR plan,* the insurance company will cover actual costs deemed "customary" and "reasonable."

The *major medical* plan covers expenses beyond those the basic plan covers. You should be familiar with two terms important in major medical health insurance plans: deductible and coinsurance. The *deductible* is a set dollar amount that you must pay before the plan takes over payment. Once you've met the deductible, the plan begins to pay a percentage (usually 80%) of the remaining costs it covers. This is referred to as *coinsurance.*

The *comprehensive* plan essentially

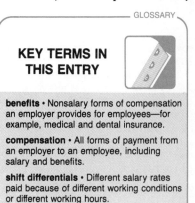

GLOSSARY

## KEY TERMS IN THIS ENTRY

**benefits** • Nonsalary forms of compensation an employer provides for employees—for example, medical and dental insurance.

**compensation** • All forms of payment from an employer to an employee, including salary and benefits.

**shift differentials** • Different salary rates paid because of different working conditions or different working hours.

## CHECKING OUT THE EXTRAS

Fringe benefits—those "extras" a prospective employer sometimes offers in addition to the standard wage and benefits package—may not be central to your decision to take or turn down a particular job. But if you're deciding between two jobs that are otherwise equally attractive, fringe benefits might tip the scales. The following chart lists some common and less common benefits, their basic features, and questions you should ask about each.

| BENEFIT | BASIC FEATURES | QUESTIONS TO ASK |
|---------|----------------|------------------|
| **Relocation/ moving expenses** | • Employer reimbursements paid either when you move or periodically during your first year | • Must you promise to work a specific period to receive this benefit? |
| **Free housing** | • Free housing—for example, in a hotel—usually limited to 60 days | • Will employer help you find suitable, permanent housing, or are you on your own? |
| **Subsidized** | • Subsidized housing—in which you share the cost—usually for more than 60 days | • Must you promise to work a specific period of time for this benefit? |
| **Employer-sponsored credit union (CU)** | • Accounts similar to those offered by savings & loans or thrift institutions, but with higher interest rates on savings accounts and lower interest rates on loans. Some CUs will make automatic deductions from your payroll check. Some CUs also offer checking accounts. | • Do you have to be a CU member for a specific period of time (for example, 1 year) before you can obtain a loan? <br> • Does the CU have an annual membership fee? <br> • Is the CU's location convenient for you? |
| **On-site child care center** | • Supervised day-care center | • Is this service free, or do you have to pay for it? <br> • Does the center have any age restrictions for the children? (For example, does it only allow children between ages 3 and 6?) <br> • What are the center's hours of operation? |

combines the basic plan and the major medical plan.

A *health maintenance organization (HMO)* provides comprehensive health care for a fixed monthly fee, usually paid through payroll deductions. The HMO provides full medical services, including routine preventive health care as well as hospitalization. The provision for preventive care is the main difference in coverage between HMO services and the services that basic and major medical health-care insurance provide.

*Health-related* insurance—becoming more and more popular—may be dental or vision insurance, or both. Dental plans usually cover only routine dental care. Some plans, however, cover more complex work—for example, orthodontics. Vision plans usually cover the cost (with limitations) of eye examinations, glasses, and contact lenses.

If an employer offers you several health-plan options, think carefully about the one that will be best for you. Review the plans' summaries, which your employer (or potential employer) should be able to give you, before you make a decision.

In evaluating any health insurance plan, note the extent of the coverage provided. Note, too, the limits of the coverage you'd receive:

• How many inpatient days are paid for?

• What outpatient services, if any, are covered?

• Does the plan cover services in extended-care facilities?

• What coverage do you have if you become ill or injured outside of the plan's geographic area?

• When—once you're employed—do you become eligible to participate in the plan?

• If you wish to change to it from another plan, or from it to another plan, are open enrollment periods scheduled during the year?

• If you leave your job and don't immediately have group health insurance on another job, is your present group policy convertible to an individual policy?

After reviewing the provisions of the employer's health plan or plans, evaluate the cost-effectiveness of each. In addition to looking at the total annual cost of the premium, look at how much of the premium you'll have to pay out-of-pocket and at how much the employer pays. (Some employers pay the entire amount.) You may also want to explore the costs and benefits of family coverage.

If you're thinking of selecting an HMO, consider the following questions:

• Is an HMO health-care center located near where you work or live?

• Are you willing to forego being cared for by your present doctor and willing to be cared for by the HMO's team of doctors?

• Would you be satisfied to be cared for in the hospital(s) the HMO has contracts with?

• How does the cost of this plan compare with those of the other plans you've considered?

• Do your present dentist and ophthalmologist or optometrist participate in the plan being offered?

## Understanding employer-offered life insurance and disability plans

Now let's talk about life insurance. Health insurance is considered the most valuable employer-offered insurance— you might need it at any time—but life insurance is also important. The reason to buy life insurance, of course, is to ensure that your survivors will be cared for after your death.

An employer may offer either of two types of group life insurance:
• group term insurance
• group whole-life insurance.
Because the whole-life plan, which features savings and the build-up of cash values, is less common, this discussion focuses on the term plan.

Essentially, the *term plan* pays benefits only at the time of death. However, the amount of coverage will vary. Coverage usually represents a multiple of your annual earnings. You may have the option, for example, of choosing coverage of one, two, or three times the amount of your basic annual salary. If that is $20,000 a year, your insurance coverage could be for $20,000, $40,000, or $60,000. Some plans include clauses that provide double coverage in the event of accidental death and dismemberment insurance to cover loss of limbs or body functions as the result of an accident. Premiums for life insurance may be either contributory or noncontributory. Under a *contributory plan*, you share the cost of the premium with your employer. Under a *noncontributory plan*, your employer pays the total amount.

Some life insurance plans include *disability benefits*. Many employers, however, prefer to offer separate disability benefits designed to provide income when illness or accident takes the employee off the job. Disability plans vary in the length of time they cover you. Some coverage is short-term, some is long-term. Regardless of whether the plan covers you for 90 days or until retirement, the amount paid usually represents a percentage of your base salary. Consider the usefulness of this benefit in light of your own financial situation. If you were off the job for several months because of disability, would you have enough savings and enough sick-leave time to tide you over? Disability insurance can provide peace of mind at relatively minimal (or no) cost.

One final note on life insurance. Be sure to find out if you can continue the plan in case you leave your job. Can you convert it from a group plan to an individual plan? If so, what is the projected cost and what are the limitations? (Most plans permit you to switch to an individual plan, but not to increase your original coverage.)

## The importance of professional liability insurance

Professional liability insurance is a vitally important form of insurance. As a nurse, you must make sure that your coverage is adequate to pay today's high malpractice damages/awards. (For a thorough discussion of professional liability insurance, see Entries 41 and 42.)

## Your personal and professional development: Options your employer may offer

When you change jobs, you're usually planning to stay in the new one for at least a couple of years. So with any prospective employer, you'll probably want to explore the possibilities for continuing your education.

If you're planning to get a *degree*—either now or later—you'll need to know the answers to some or all of the following questions:

• Does the employer offer any tuition benefits covering degree-granting programs? If so, what requirements must you meet, and what requirements must the program meet, for you to be eligible for tuition benefits?

• How much tuition coverage are you entitled to? Is it paid up-front, or is it reimbursable only after you successfully complete the course?

• When are you eligible to receive tuition benefits?

• Would you have to commit yourself to a specific period of employment in order to be eligible?

• What would the consequences be if you left your job while you were receiving tuition benefits?

• Are benefits offered to part-time employees? To spouses or dependents of employees?

• What opportunities for *continuing education* does the employer offer?

• Does the institution have a staff-development department or an in-service department?

• If so, what kind of programs does it offer? How often are they offered?

• Will you receive continuing-education units if you take the in-house programs? (This is important even if continuing education is not mandatory in your state.)

Here's one more matter to consider—the employer's policies governing *participation in educational activities.* Will you be paid while attending workshops and seminars? Is the number you can attend limited? Is the amount the institution will spend on such activities limited? The employment interview is a good time to find out the answers to all these questions. By reviewing your personal goals and priorities in terms of the benefits offered, you should be able to make the best possible selection where educational benefits are concerned.

## Paid days off: Reaping the rewards

Of course you're aware of the importance of knowing how many paid days off you will have. But do you know how to evaluate their actual worth? Most employers offer a set number of paid days for vacation, illness, holidays, and (sometimes) so-called personal days. To evaluate the actual benefits of these paid days off, you need to know the answers to the following questions:

• Do vacation days accrue? Do you, for example, receive an additional day of vacation for each added year of service? Can you carry unused vacation days over to the following year?

• If you don't use all your sick-leave days, can they be carried over and added to the next year's paid sick days?

• Can you cash in (be paid for) unused vacation and sick-leave time? If so, when can you do it? At the end of each year, or when you leave your job?

• What rate is paid for the holidays you work?

• Would you be penalized for taking a sick day the day before a holiday?

Some employers provide a lump-sum number of days off that the employee can use as she sees fit—for vacation,

> *"Carefully examine what's being offered to you so that you pick the package that comes closest to meeting your particular needs."*

sick leave, or personal time. This plan offers flexibility, but it also makes responsible use of the time a must. Obviously, if you use up all your time for vacation and personal days, you'll have a problem if you become ill.

## Considering job staffing and scheduling

Although they're not really bargaining options, job staffing and scheduling patterns are important concerns of every staff nurse. (For in-depth coverage of these topics, see Entries 102 and 103.)

## Remembering the extras

Some institutions offer additional fringe benefits that you'll find are worthwhile for you to explore. (For some examples of these benefits, see *Checking Out the Extras*, page 394.)

## What every nurse needs to know

Most nurse recruiters can attest that nurses do take time to assess their professional priorities. Early in job interviews, nurses ask questions about the professional environment, such as: Is primary care practiced here? What is the institution's nursing philosophy? What is nursing's relationship with the house staff? How is the institution organized? Are there chances for advancement?

You should just as carefully consider the salary and benefits that will best meet your particular needs. To make this a little easier, you may want to develop a salary-and-benefits checklist, which you can use to compare the compensation packages of the employers that interview you. This checklist will also make it possible for you to evaluate your annual income.

## A final word

As you know, not all employers offer the same benefits or offer them in the same way. You need to examine each employer's benefits carefully. That way, you'll be able to evaluate the cost-effectiveness of each package and the extent to which it meets your particular needs. You should also be alert to changes being made in benefit programs. Some employers, for example, are experimenting with cafeteria-style benefit packages. Employees select, from the benefits offered, those they believe are essential or desirable for them—and receive cash for those they don't select.

If you're beginning to give serious thought to the importance of the various components in your compensation package, and wondering whether you should make or request changes, remember that the information presented here is only an overview. If you want to know more, ask more questions to increase your knowledge of the different options. Above all, be sure you've got the best compensation package available to you.

# 62 What to expect in a new job

When you accept a new nursing job, you're joining a professional team that has specific patient-care goals and standards you need to know about. But your success on the new job will depend on more than the soundness of your nursing judgment and the proficiency of your technical skills. The health team and others in your new work setting are a social group who know each other and know what to expect in their relationships with each other. This means that your degree of success on the job will also depend on your sensitivity and responsiveness to group attitudes and needs. Forming and maintaining pleasant and productive working relationships is crucial to success at *any* job.

GLOSSARY

## KEY TERMS IN THIS ENTRY

**change agent** • A nurse or health-care professional who works to bring about beneficial change for co-workers or patients.

**preceptor** • An experienced nurse who assumes responsibility for orienting and training a nurse intern, through actual on-the-job experience.

**turnover rate** • The rate at which a company or institution must replace employees due to resignations and terminations.

## Starting the new job: Orientation and adjustment

Your initial employment period will include orientation to the institution's policies and procedures along with indoctrination and clarification concerning the institution's values—many of them unstated and not part of formal policy. This is a very important period. As you learn the ropes and become accustomed to the group, the group also becomes accustomed to you. Remember, the relationships that form during this period will affect your work style, your loyalty to the institution, and your dedication to your own practice values.

Current turnover rates among hospital-employed nurses are high. This means that many (if not most) nurses are in the position of being newcomers several times during their careers. At any given time, probably several nurses on a single unit's staff will be relative newcomers. You may find that the senior nurses who welcome or orient you have not been on the unit for very many months themselves. They may not be completely familiar with the ways of the unit yet, let alone the institution. What does this mean to you, as a newcomer? It means you can't expect to sit back and *become* oriented. Orientation must be a very active process in which you assume individual responsibility, recognizing that this period will set the stage for your nursing practice during your employment at this institution. Your orientation period will either produce a feeling of accomplishment or a feeling of frustration on the job. If this period is unsatisfying, you may turn to another new job. But if you haven't learned how to work with others in the delivery of health care, and haven't recognized your ability to influence the outcome, you're destined to find the same frustrations elsewhere.

## Two nurses' stories

After working for 2 years on a general medical/surgical floor in a small community hospital, Jane Gibbons and

## REALITY SHOCK

What's reality shock? It's the stunned feeling newly licensed nurses sometimes experience when they first try to apply "book learning" to what's expected of them on the job. Too often, the values formed in school and through reading professional literature seem to be at odds with the values these nurses observe in the practice setting. The gap between their expectations and reality can be very wide. Even their expectations of the work environment and their basic responsibilities may differ from reality. So instead of feeling confident, a newly licensed nurse may feel unsure, confused, even stupid. She may also feel angry and depressed that her student experiences, license, and degree (if she has one) don't automatically make her proficient.

Experienced nurses can suffer from reality shock, too, in starting a new job. If this happens to you, remember that forewarned is forearmed. Avoiding reality shock involves preparing yourself for the differences you'll encounter and arming yourself with constructive ways of coping. Expect differences, and allow yourself time to adjust to them. Set up a support system for yourself as soon as possible. If you prepare yourself for new challenges, you'll be able to reduce the potentially devastating effects of reality shock.

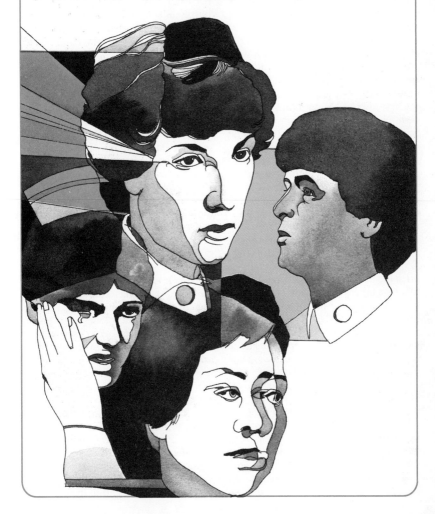

Nancy Jones, both RNs, moved to a nearby city and took jobs in a large regional health-care center. They were both eager to get involved in specialty practice, and they believed that their 2 years' general nursing experience had given them the grounding for dealing with a variety of patient problems. Jane got a job in the pediatric oncology unit; Nancy chose the cardiac surgical intensive care unit (CSICU).

After 3 months' orientation, Nancy felt comfortable amid the bleeping monitors of the CSICU. Although she'd been forewarned about the stress of working in critical-care units, she was happy with her choice. Jane, however, wasn't so sure about her job choice. She complained that established routines were "set in stone," and that innovation would be unlikely. She began to echo the litany of gripes she heard from her co-workers. As friends back home listened to Jane and Nancy talk about their new jobs, they wondered how working in two units in the same hospital could cause such different reactions.

True, each unit had its own composite personality, which for the most part reflected the values and attitudes of the individuals in it. And working on each unit entailed anxiety and pressure. But relationships with co-workers could be expected to provide a support base for coping with work assignments. A newcomer's adjustment depended largely on how she interacted with other members of the staff, not on the way she dealt with specific patient problems.

When Nancy started her new CSICU job, she didn't hide her enthusiasm or her trepidation. She asked others for their suggestions and about *their* first experiences on the unit. Instead of identifying with the gripes of her co-workers, Nancy got them to identify with *her* situation. When she read articles suggesting ideas different from those practiced in the unit, she shared the articles and asked for her colleagues' opinions. After some weeks, she identified various strengths among the staff. She then knew whom to ask for help and counsel in various situations. She could select role models, and she did. Her relationships with co-workers were forming a basis for mutual goal setting and achievement. The proportion of time she spent on nonproductive griping was minimal. Co-workers recognized Nancy's influence in focusing them on patient care, even though her expertise paled next to their proficiency.

Jane's orientation was very different from Nancy's. When Jane first came onto the pediatric oncology unit with her staff-development instructor, she hardly talked to the other staff nurses. Instead, she directed all of her inquiries to the instructor, the head nurse, or the head nurse's assistant. Day after day, Jane questioned unit protocols and frequently commented about better ways of doing things—ways she'd read about in journals.

One of Jane's major professional goals was to be a change agent in improving patient care. As her patient-care assignments increased, she had less supervision from senior staff, yet she seldom discussed patient-care issues with her co-workers. What she *did* do was listen to others' griping during coffee breaks and chime in with further criticisms of the way things were. She offered pat solutions to long-standing problems. Soon she was "part of the system," expressing her dissatisfaction with the way things were but not coming up with anything better, even in specific patient situations—her special interest.

What made these two nurses' situations different? Could Jane have made her orientation outcome more like Nancy's?

## The challenge of a new job

Learning to fit in, to meet others' expectations at the same time you're working toward your own goals, is the challenge a new job offers. So the first step in your new job is to assess expectations—yours and theirs—and find ways to mesh them.

A new job is challenging and, of course, you're probably excited. But you probably also have feelings of self-doubt, insecurity about your skills, and anxiety about your social acceptance. All these feelings are normal. If you've recently graduated, or if you're new to a specialty, you may be even more nervous—you'll be testing new skills in your new job. Or maybe you've been promoted into your new job. This means you'll be faced with new role expectations—as a supervisor, a head nurse, a clinical specialist, or an instructor—and new ways of dealing with your co-workers. This change may

---

*"The challenge of any new job is learning to fit in and to meet others' expectations."*

---

be even more stressful because you're adjusting to a new job in your old work setting, where established relationships may have to change.

If you're an experienced nurse who's been out of the work force for a while, you may be worried about rusty skills and unfamiliar technologies.

### What do *you* expect?

Do you know exactly what you're looking for in a job? Can you put it into words? Or do you just take it for granted that you'll know it when you see it or miss it if it's not there? (See Entry 56.)

If this isn't your first job, compare what you expect the new job will be like with jobs you've had in the past. Use your former experience as a rehearsal for how you think your co-workers will respond to you on the new job. In thinking this way about your old job, can you see how you might do some things differently this time around to get a more positive response?

Be sure to consider whether your expectations are realistic. You set yourself up for disappointment if you dream the impossible dream. The better you are at putting your ideas and job expectations into words, the more likely you are to form them realistically and pursue them successfully in your new job.

As you think about your expectations, consider how much your performance counts in meeting them. Your expectations shouldn't be passive—completely dependent on the job environment or the institution's expectations *as they existed before you arrived.* Be prepared to work hard to achieve your expectations. You have to initiate action to achieve the results you want. If you haven't been working toward your goals day by day, right from the beginning, you can't expect to wake up after several weeks or months and find you've achieved them. Remember, the path of least resistance always beckons, especially when the work load is heavy (and when isn't it?). Unfortunately, this path seldom leads you where you want to go. Caution: Getting on this path is easy in the early days of a new job, when your initial efforts are aimed at feeling comfortable in the new environment and getting to know the people. Make a conscious and deliberate effort to keep from falling into an unproductive routine focused on socializing.

Success on the job requires daily assessment of how you're doing, including assessment of how specific situations could have been handled differently. For example, if you don't assess and adjust your interactions with patients right from the beginning, you'll find these interactions tend to be influenced by the way things *are,* not by the way you want them to be. (See Entry 76.)

You can assess how your expectations mesh with a prospective employer's, to some extent, even before you take a new job. (See Entries 56 and 57.) Assessment methods you can use include carefully reading the job description (see Entry 57), listening closely to the interviewer's questions and responses during your job interview (see Entry 59), and learning about the institution's reputation in the nursing community and among consumers. If you tour the hospital or unit, don't just look at the equipment and physical facilities; watch how people interact with each other.

At the job interview, find out how many staff members are pursuing degrees, and what kinds of degrees. This will give you some idea of your potential co-workers' interests and, to some extent, career orientations. It will also give you an idea of how well you'd fit in, in terms of education and experience.

As you formulate your expectations, be realistic about your own skills. You may envision yourself as a crusading change agent. However, if you're not well versed in the basics yet, you're probably not ready to write proposals for newer and better ways of doing things. Key your expectations to your own communication and management styles, too.

## What do *they* expect?

First of all, "they" goes beyond the manager who writes your job description. Many other persons' expectations are involved in your work. For example, patients' expectations are often determined by preconceptions—appropriate or not—of what nursing and nursing care are all about. (They may get these preconceptions from television.) You know that patients need to be educated so they can become full partners in planning for their care. But this doesn't always happen, so some patients may ask for nursing services unrelated to their nursing-care needs. Their expectations are unrealistic, yes—but they're also *real* expectations that call for a response from you. (Patients' very real discomforts, anxieties, and fears may also make their expectations unrealistic.)

What about the employing institu-

tion's expectations? No matter how much lip service professional goals receive, the necessity of accomplishing the institution's goals comes first. You know that modern health care is heavily bureaucratized, and that cost-containment is high on the list of institutions' priorities. The level of an institution's staffing will help you assess its level of practice and whether you'd fit in. For example, if the staffing level barely allows time for basic nursing care and medical treatment, then no matter what the institution's stated philosophy is, teaching and counseling will be considered luxuries.

But maybe you don't plan to pursue another degree, and you don't want more interactions with patients and their families than basic nursing care calls for. If so, you'd probably be wise to steer clear of a hospital that:
• boasts about its primary nursing practice
• has staff nurses serving as preceptors for students and graduates
• is implementing an aggressive patient-teaching program on all its medical and pediatric units.

These institutions probably wouldn't meet your expectations, and you probably wouldn't meet theirs.

Remember, again, to carefully consider the health-team colleagues you'll be working with. What do you think their expectations of you will be? As mentioned above, a work situation is a social situation. Established ways of relating are part of the professional environment in every institution. Some institutions are more formal, and some institutions have more interdisciplinary collaboration, than others. Sometimes a health team's interpersonal expectations are related to social interactions after hours. How comfortable you are with the health team's established social traditions will be an important influence in your adjustment to your new job.

## When your orientation's over

Soon you'll become a fully productive

member of your institution's staff. Then your job won't be new anymore. You'll be a resource person—for better or worse—for those who join the staff after you. Remember, even the most junior old-timers are in a unique position to identify newcomers' needs and suggest better ways of helping them adjust. Many hospitals have developed preceptor programs, in which experienced nurses work with less-experienced nurses. If you become a preceptor, you'll do more than teach newcomers practice skills. You'll be a person to whom newcomers can turn to test their job expectations and receive guidance, reassurance, and realistic evaluation. Our medical colleagues have a long history of preceptor relationships. In nursing, such relationships may one day extend beyond the orientation period; this would facilitate consultative practice and enhance patient care.

### A final word

In the past, many nurses had only one or two jobs in their entire careers. Today, for a number of reasons, nurses are mobile. Whether you take a new job because you're pursuing specialization or advancement (or both) or for personal reasons, you'll have the most success if you make a sincere effort to fit in with your new colleagues. To do this, you'll need flexibility, openness to others' ideas and values, and the ability to cope with interpersonal differences.

# 63 The professional strategy of resigning

When you must resign, careful planning can fashion a positive approach to your future opportunities. If you don't plan—well, consider Jennifer Bryant, RN:

Jennifer arrives for her appointment with the head nurse feeling anxious and apprehensive. She plans to inform this supervisor that she has accepted a

GLOSSARY

## KEY TERMS IN THIS ENTRY

**exit interview** • A formal meeting between an employee and his immediate supervisor, his supervisor's supervisor, or a member of the personnel department, where the employee offers his perspective on the circumstances that prompted his resignation.

**personnel file** • The compilation of an employee's records, including his job application, résumé, continuing-education records, and employment record with that company.

**resignation** • The formal notification a person gives to terminate his employment.

job at another hospital, where she'll work as an assistant head nurse. Jennifer's career goal is to work in nursing administration, so she believes this new job will give her an excellent opportunity to develop her management skills. Still, she's nervous, and she feels an unsettling sense of guilt.

Sound familiar? This scenario occurs often in hospitals throughout the country. The reasons why it occurs, and the resignees' methods of coping, vary widely. But the experience is inevitably stressful.

In the past, many people worked for the same employers throughout their working careers. Today, we live in a dynamic and mobile society. Job changes are common. Yearly turnover rates within the nursing profession average between 35% and 60%. So you can be pretty sure that you'll be confronted with the resignation process several times in your nursing career.

The term *resignation* refers to the act of voluntarily relinquishing a job. The actual act of resigning, of course, is voluntary, but the person resigning doesn't always want to. So this entry discusses two categories of resignation: voluntary and involuntary.

*Voluntary resignation* occurs when the employee makes an unpressured

## WRITING YOUR LETTER OF RESIGNATION

Your letter of resignation should contain all the elements identified in the following sample letter:

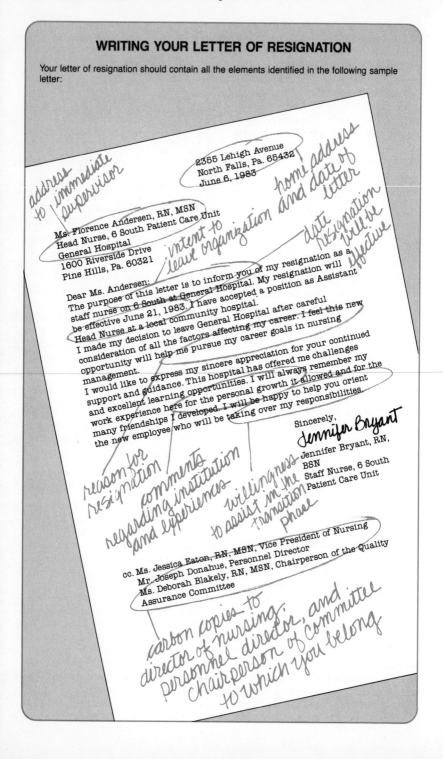

*address to immediate supervisor*

2355 Lehigh Avenue
North Falls, Pa. 65432
June 6, 1983

*home address and date of letter*

Ms. Florence Andersen, RN, MSN
Head Nurse, 6 South Patient Care Unit
General Hospital
1600 Riverside Drive
Pine Hills, Pa. 60321

Dear Ms. Andersen:

*intent to leave organization*

The purpose of this letter is to inform you of my resignation as a staff nurse on 6 South at General Hospital. My resignation will be effective June 21, 1983. I have accepted a position as Assistant Head Nurse at a local community hospital.

*date resignation will be effective*

I made my decision to leave General Hospital after careful consideration of all the factors affecting my career. I feel this new opportunity will help me pursue my career goals in nursing management.

*reason for resignation*

I would like to express my sincere appreciation for your continued support and guidance. This hospital has offered me challenges and excellent learning opportunities. I will always remember my work experience here for the personal growth it allowed and for the many friendships I developed. I will be happy to help you orient the new employee who will be taking over my responsibilities.

*comments regarding institution and experiences*

*willingness to assist in the transition phase*

Sincerely,

*Jennifer Bryant*

Jennifer Bryant, RN, BSN
Staff Nurse, 6 South Patient Care Unit

cc. Ms. Jessica Eaton, RN, MSN, Vice President of Nursing
Mr. Joseph Donahue, Personnel Director
Ms. Deborah Blakely, RN, MSN, Chairperson of the Quality Assurance Committee

*carbon copies to director of nursing, personnel director, and chairperson of committee to which you belong*

choice to leave a particular job. Resigning to move to another geographic location, to pursue further education, or to accept a better job are examples of free-choice resignation situations.

*Involuntary resignation* occurs when an employee is more or less forced to leave a job. In such situations, something is occurring that's beyond the employee's control, something that compels the individual to resign. Involuntary resignations happen for a number of reasons. These include being continually asked to perform tasks that violate personal values and working in an environment that stifles personal growth and well-being. When an employee has no control over such a situation, the only solution may be to leave her job. (If overwhelming pressures or other compelling reasons force you into an involuntary resignation, check Section 402 of the Unemployment Compensation Act for useful information on obtaining compensation.)

One example of involuntary resignations involved a Philadelphia hospital where, in 1975, nurses at all levels were concerned over doctors' and administrators' interference in their right to practice professional nursing. Following a management decision to fire the director of nursing, many nurses protested, then resigned on the basis of their own principles and values. In this situation, the forced choice was between their consciences and their jobs. The nurses had no control over the hospital environment, so their decision was to resign.

Resigning involuntarily isn't the same as being fired. A nurse who's fired doesn't initiate the action; she *does* do this when she resigns, even involuntarily. Sometimes a fired nurse's reason for termination goes into her record as resignation, but because the fired nurse hasn't initiated the action, this *isn't* a true involuntary resignation.

Nurses resign their jobs for many reasons. Why a particular nurse resigns often influences what she does next, as well as her future prospects.

## Making the decision to resign

Suppose you're thinking about resigning from your staff nurse position in Hospital X to work in a similar position in Hospital Z. What must you consider in making this decision?

Your first step is to sit down with a piece of paper and list the pros and cons of both your present position and the one in Hospital Z. Comparing these lists will help you decide whether the change is advantageous at this time. Next, consider what you want from your job and career, and what type of job can best help you achieve these goals (see Entry 56).

If you're concerned with specific problems in your job or in your work environment, speak with your head nurse before you consider resigning. She may be able to offer suggestions that will help you deal with the problems. For example, if you're interested in nursing education and feel unchallenged in your job, she may suggest that you develop a teaching project for your unit.

Talk to your nursing colleagues, too, about why they chose to work at your hospital and whether the hospital is meeting their needs and expectations. Do some reality testing. Try to discover if others share your assessment of your situation.

If you possibly can, remain in any permanent job for a minimum of 1 year. You need this much time to adjust to the job and make a well-thought-out decision to stay or leave. Remember, employers are reluctant to hire people who change jobs frequently; this suggests instability and irresponsibility.

After considering how much you value your present job, you'll be ready to make an informed decision about your next step. If you decide your present job isn't meeting your needs, begin thinking about how you'll manage resigning.

## Getting ready to resign

Knowing how to resign from a job may well be as important as knowing how to get one. A resignation must be well planned, well executed, and appropriately timed. Remember, professionalism, consideration for others as well as for yourself, and tact should be foremost in your mind when you resign.

You've made the decision to resign. Before you do, review your hospital's policies regarding health insurance, vacation time, pensions, life insurance, tax-sheltered annuities, holidays, tuition reimbursement, and bonuses. If you have any questions about your status regarding any of these, contact the hospital personnel department.

Here are some questions to ask about benefits:

• How long will you be covered by your health and life insurance after you resign? Can you convert the policies to individual coverage after you leave?

• Are your pension benefits vested? Request a complete record of your account.

• Can your money be left in the tax-sheltered annuity, or must it be transferred to another account?

• How much vacation, holiday, or personal time have you accrued? Can you elect to be paid for this time? Did you take any of this time in advance (so you owe the hospital money)?

• Have you been reimbursed for any college courses in the past? Check to find out if your hospital specifies how long you must remain employed as a condition for tuition reimbursement. If by leaving the hospital now you'll fail to fulfill this requirement, you may be responsible for paying the tuition money back to the hospital.

• Does your present employer pay bonuses for shift work? Must an employee work for a specific period of time before receiving such a bonus? Should you consider continuing in your present job until you receive one?

• Are you eligible for any other termination benefits?

When you've gathered all the facts, you're ready to plan your timetable for effective resignation.

You need to evaluate many factors before you set the time of your departure. Your first consideration is to avoid resigning, if at all possible, until you have another job. Otherwise, you'll have to answer questions about your unemployment. Employers often rate you higher if you're employed, and you may also be in a better bargaining position if you have a steady income.

The customary length of notice for resigning from a hospital is between 2 and 4 weeks. Check your hospital's policy manual or your employment contract to determine the length of notice you should give. This time span is often based on your job level and how difficult the task of replacing you is expected to be. Here's a general guideline: Give notice equivalent to the amount of vacation time you receive. For example, if you have three weeks' vacation, give three weeks' notice.

What if you don't want to, or can't, give the required length of notice? Suppose you've applied to graduate school late in the summer, so you weren't accepted until 2 weeks before the fall semester. Your hospital requires three weeks' notice of resignation, but you have a legitimate reason for being unable to fulfill this requirement. Do you know what action to take in this situation?

First, tell your head nurse about your problem. You may need to discuss it with your supervisor or with your director of nursing. Depending on the situation, your nursing administration may agree to waive the length-of-notice requirement for you.

In various parts of the country, hospitals have refused to pay accrued vacation time to employees who fail to give proper notice. Some employees have challenged this policy in court; disagreement has centered around whether vacation pay is a wage or a gift. Legal decisions have varied. In a recent decision, the court ruled that improper notice of resignation could not affect the payment of accrued vacation pay. In another case, however, the court ruled that because the time frame for

# THE EXIT INTERVIEW: PREPARING TO KEEP CALM

Depending on your reasons for resigning, your exit interview can become an emotionally charged situation—if you let it. To keep calm and avoid an unprofessional exit, take some time before the interview to think about how you'll answer these inevitable questions:

- What are your reasons for leaving the hospital?
- If you could change anything at the hospital that would alter your decision to leave, what would it be?
- What do you dislike about the hospital?
- Do you feel you were treated fairly?
- Do you feel the nursing salaries are fair?
- How do you feel about the benefits program?
- [If you've found a new job] What makes it more attractive than your present one?
- [If you haven't found a new job] What are your future plans?
- Would you ever return to this hospital to work? Why? Why not?

With advance preparation, you'll be able to answer these questions calmly and tactfully. Keep your answers brief and free of personal criticism. Handling yourself well in the exit interview will increase your confidence in your professionalism—and on your next job.

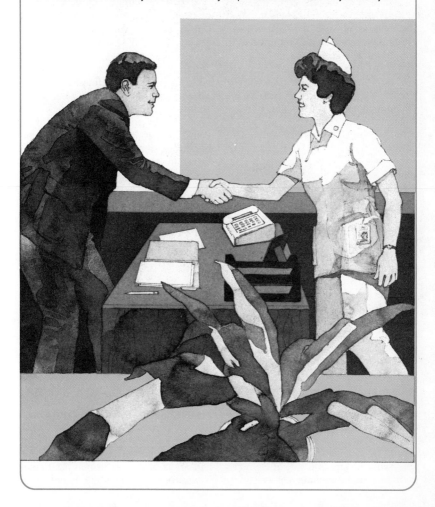

giving proper notice of resignation was agreed on prior to employment, the employee had no inherent right to a vacation or to payment of unused vacation time. Because decisions concerning length of notice differ from state to state, you should discuss this issue with an attorney if it's important to you and you're planning a job change on short notice.

## Understanding resignation procedures

The formal procedure for resigning is submission of the resignation letter. (See *Writing Your Letter of Resignation,* page 404.) Present this letter in person to your immediate supervisor. Send courtesy copies to the director of nursing, the chairmen of committees to which you belong, and the hospital personnel department. The head nurse will process your resignation through the hospital's established channels.

The resignation letter should briefly discuss the following:

• your intention to leave your present job

• the date your resignation will become effective

• your reason for resigning. If you've already accepted another job, you can identify the institution and job without detailing the terms of your employment there.

• sincere comments regarding your appreciation for the opportunities, challenges, learning experiences, and satisfactions you gained in the job you're resigning. (Another thoughtful statement concerns your willingness to assist the hospital in transferring your responsibilities.)

Your resignation letter will become part of your personnel file. Never express negative feelings, such as hostility, resentment, animosity, or bitterness, in your letter. This isn't the appropriate time or place to air old problems. Instead, stress the positive aspects of your job. Tell your colleagues about your resignation only after you've notified your immediate supervisor.

## Getting through the exit interview

Exit interviews are good administrative practice. The purpose of an exit interview is to get the employee's perspective on the circumstances that prompted her resignation. When you resign, your exit interview may be conducted by your immediate supervisor, by the director of nursing, or by a member of the hospital's personnel department.

For staff nurses, anticipation of the exit interview often provokes anxiety. But if you prepare for the interview, you can turn it into a learning experience and remain calm, confident, and in control. (See *The Exit Interview: Preparing to Keep Calm,* page 407.) Prepare yourself by planning ahead.

How honest should you be during the exit interview? The answer depends on your situation. Sometimes an exit interview is kept confidential, and sometimes it becomes part of your personnel file. Sometimes it will be shared with your supervisor. To make the best lasting impression, remain positive during the exit interview. No matter how disenchanted or angry you are now, re-

> *"During the exit interview, giving criticism is appropriate when the intent is to help rather than to retaliate."*

member that someday you may wish to return to this hospital. Think before you speak. Hostility and animosity will serve no constructive purpose. Instead, they may create a barrier to future employment. Don't burn your bridges behind you.

If you trust the interviewer, you may want to constructively criticize problem areas of the institution. Criticism is appropriate when the intent is to help rather than to retaliate. In a tactful and objective manner, state facts and point out alternatives or suggest solutions to problems you've identified. You'll gain the interviewer's respect by conducting yourself in a professional manner.

You have a legal right to see your personnel file: you may want to arrange to do this at your exit interview. (Contact the interviewer in advance, so he can obtain your file and have it ready to show you.) Your personnel file usually includes your original job application, résumé, initial interviewer's notes, salary increases, evaluations, position changes, attendance records, commendations, continuing education record, and resignation letter. When you examine your file, make sure that it's complete and that it details your job history accurately. If disciplinary notes are in the file, make sure that any follow-up regarding improvement is also there. If it isn't, ask your interviewer what method you should use for seeing that this information gets into the file. Remember, having this information on file will be important if you ever want to return to the hospital or if you request references.

Find out about the hospital's policies regarding telephone reference requests. You may want to ask that a personal reference letter from your immediate supervisor be placed in your file. This will expedite telephone references for future employment, because supervisors also change jobs and yours may be difficult to locate at a later date.

### After you resign: Looking back

Your updated résumé needn't include the reasons for your resignation. Be prepared, however, to discuss them in future employment interviews. Remember, remain positive about your past employment. Making negative comments and giving unsolicited criticism reflect a generally negative attitude and will decrease your chances of being hired.

### A final word

When you resign, leave your job amicably and without showing anger. The period between your resignation and your departure is not the time to resurrect old grievances.

As you can see, the ending of a job is just as important as the beginning. Be as prepared for your resignation as you were for your initial employment interview. You'll be glad you behaved in a professional and mature way during these crucial events in your career.

# 64 Surviving being fired

Discharged. Dismissed. *Fired.* Although this doesn't happen to nurses very often, when it does happen it's always an emotional shock. A traumatic experience. If it ever happens to you, you can keep your equilibrium if you've previously considered how to respond to being fired, what to do after being fired, and how to turn being fired to your benefit.

### The termination process: Stage 1

The most common reasons why staff nurses are fired include:
- poor job performance
- chronic tardiness
- excessive absenteeism
- substance abuse
- inappropriate behavior.

Usually the termination process involves several steps, beginning with a verbal warning followed by a written confirmation. If you receive such a warning, heed it. Correct the behavior that prompted it. At this point, you can still act to avoid being fired.

If the warning you receive cites poor job performance as the reason, now's a good time to talk things over with your employer. Ask for specific infor-

GLOSSARY

## KEY TERMS IN THIS ENTRY

**career counselor** • A professional person who's trained to guide others in career decision making.

**career plan** • A person's long-term plan for achieving stated career goals.

**exit interview** • A formal meeting between an employee and his immediate supervisor, his supervisor's supervisor, or a member of the personnel department, where the employee offers his perspective on the circumstances that prompted his resignation.

**grievance procedure** • Steps employees and employer agree to follow to settle disputes.

**job placement officer** • An employee of a job placement agency who works with a person seeking a new job.

**termination process** • The procedure an employer follows to fire an employee.

process may help you realize that you don't want to stay in the job you have. One way to find out if this is true for you is to do some further career planning (see Entry 56). Review your long-range career goals, reconsidering the type of work you like best and the places you'd most like to live and work. If your present job isn't meeting enough of your goals, then make plans that will get you where you want to go. At this point, and for solid professional reasons, you can resign voluntarily (see Entry 63)—and avoid being fired.

## The termination process: Stage 2

If you repeat the offense—whatever it is—you're likely to receive a written warning, followed by an interview with your supervisor or someone else in a position to help you get back on the track in your job. At this point, you may decide you don't want to stay in your present job. Consider resigning (see Entry 63), or plan how to handle being fired. If you resign, you probably won't be eligible for unemployment benefits, but resignation will look better on your résumé.

Prior to your termination, consider your insurance coverage. How long will the institution's health, life, and dental insurance policies cover you after you're fired? Are you covered by other policies? How long will it take you to find another job and get insurance coverage through that institution? Can you take out some temporary insurance or convert your group policies to individual ones, for which you'd pay the entire premium? Does your present employer owe you vacation time or accrued holidays? The more you anticipate and plan before you're fired, the better equipped you'll be to handle the situation.

You may want to contact your state nurses' association for counseling. Call for assistance *before* you agree to termination and *before* you sign any termination-related letters. (You can expect more help if you're a member of

mation about what's expected of you. Were you ever taught how to do what you're expected to do? If not, ask for instruction and the opportunity to practice, so you can improve your performance.

If tardiness is the problem, ask yourself why you're frequently late. What can you do about it? If the problem is excessive absenteeism, consider why you're often absent. What is the underlying problem, and how can you correct it? Perhaps you're unconsciously resisting going to work. Figure out why, and what you can do about it. Are family problems interfering with your attendance? An appropriate referral service may be able to help you with those problems.

Sometimes, as we all know, a so-called political situation is behind a termination warning. If you're caught in a political situation, ask yourself if keeping your job is worth the effort that may be required.

This first stage in the termination

the association than if you aren't.) Nurses' association practices vary among the states. Association staff members who work with economic and general welfare programs may be able to inform you about state laws regarding access to personnel records, how to file for unemployment, and use of grievance procedures, and may give you other useful information. If the nurses in your institution are working under a union contract, the institution must follow the contract's provisions when firing you (see Entry 48).

## How to respond at the time you're being fired

If your supervisor calls you in and tells you she's firing you, listen carefully to what she says. Take deep breaths and exhale slowly to help you relax. Think about what you're going to say before you speak. Then acknowledge that you heard what she said. For example, "I understand that you're firing me because I'm frequently late." You may want to express your disappointment if that seems appropriate. Try hard to maintain your composure. If you know in advance that this interview is coming, try practicing what you'll say and how you'll act. (See *The Exit Interview: Preparing to Keep Calm*, page 407.)

You'll need your composure to carry you through discussion of termination policies, insurance coverage, accrued vacation, accrued holidays, and whether or not the employer will give you a reference for future jobs or help you find one. You want to leave the institution in as good standing as possible. Focus your discussion on the benefits you've gained from working at the institution. Thinking this way may be difficult for you at this time, but in fact you *have* gained additional knowledge and skills on this job that should be useful for other jobs.

If the pronouncement that you're fired catches you by surprise, collect your thoughts as quickly as possible to maintain your composure. If you feel able to discuss it, do so. If you need time to absorb the shock, make an appointment to ask questions and to clarify the termination process or the grievance procedure.

## What to do after you've been fired

After you've been fired, think about whether your employer had good cause to fire you and whether you want to contest the action. If you decide to contest it, familiarize yourself with grievance procedures at your institution. Discuss your potential for reinstatement with your immediate supervisor. If that doesn't get results, write to the department head and, if necessary, to the person the department head reports to. If these efforts don't get the results you're hoping for, you can request a fair-treatment committee hearing, where your alleged violation of the institution's policy will be objectively evaluated. Be sure to keep all documentation that relates to your firing to present to the fair-treatment committee.

If you know that you deserved to be fired, if you do not want to go through a grievance procedure, or if you wouldn't want to stay at this institution under any circumstances, make plans to move on. A clean, fast break is best.

Talk with a supportive person who can help you analyze your situation and plan how to prevent being fired in the future. Ventilate your feelings about being fired. You need to work through them before you start looking for another job, and you'll do this faster if you talk about them.

Once you've worked through your feelings, you can assess your situation more clearly. Again, career planning is the key. Even if being fired helped you escape from a miserable situation, you won't want to get into *another* miserable situation. Ask yourself:

• What kinds of work do you like to do?
• What work don't you like to do?
• What nursing tasks are you good at?
• What tasks *aren't* you good at?

• Did the last job fit you? (A psychiatric nurse, for instance, is likely to be frustrated in an intensive care unit.)

## What to do to get another job — and *until* you get one

Once you've worked through your feelings and objectively assessed your situation, you need to make realistic plans—to cover your financial situation, your search for another job, and your personal well-being. Talk to your spouse and good friends about your problem, and tell them what kinds of help you need from them. They can be very supportive and helpful. Talking to a career counselor and a job placement officer may also be helpful.

Plan your short-term and long-term career goals (see Entries 56 and 57). Consider the relative importance—to you—of salary, fringe benefits, retirement plans, work hours, and opportunities for advancement. Ask yourself which area of nursing attracts you and which climate or geographic location you prefer. Once you've decided what you want to do and where, check professional journals, employment agencies, and college placement services for advertised jobs. Check with friends, relatives, and professional acquaintances about other openings. Contact prospective employers directly, whether they've advertised openings or not. (See Entry 57.)

The availability of jobs and the length of time before you get a job will affect your financial arrangements. If, for example, your previous employer covers your health insurance premium for a month, you won't have to buy temporary insurance if you're employed within the month by a company that provides immediate coverage.

You can't count on getting a new job quickly, however. To protect yourself, plan to stretch your present (postfiring) income and financial resources as far as they will go. How long can your savings last? Find out if you're eligible for unemployment benefits, food stamps, or welfare payments. Figure out ways

you can cut expenses. Don't buy things you don't need, and stop using credit cards.

This is not the time to purchase a new wardrobe—except for a job-interview outfit—or appliances. The grocery list may be one of the easiest places to trim expenses. Don't eat out. (Carry your lunch.) Cut back on expensive meats and prepackaged meals. Clip coupons and buy the supermarket's weekly specials. Cut back on liquor and cigarettes, too.

Conserving energy can also help you cut costs. Turn off lights and electrical appliances when you aren't using them, and try not to run the dishwasher, clothes washer, or clothes dryer with less than a full load. Turn the thermostat down in the winter (and put on a sweater). Keep the air conditioner off or on "low" in the summer.

Most of your personal energy now should be put into getting a new job. When interviewing for a job, don't offer the information that you were fired. But if the interviewer asks your reason for leaving your other job, don't lie. Simply say that you were fired. If you can also say that you've taken action to correct the behavior that caused you to be fired, so much the better. Here are some examples:

• "I was fired because of an alcohol problem. I missed work often because I was hung over. Sometimes I reported to work intoxicated. But since I was fired, I've been attending Alcoholics Anonymous regularly, and I've been dry for 2 months."

• "I was fired because I made several medication errors. Since then, I've taken a pharmacology course and a refresher course on passing medications."

You should be as positive as possible about your last job. Don't criticize your former employer.

## A final word

Surviving being fired is tough. In fact, *everything* about being fired is tough. But you can handle it if you're honest with yourself and if you treat being fired as an opportunity for growth. Sure, you'll be upset at first. But well-focused career planning plus self-corrective action should add up to a new job—maybe a better job—for you.

## Selected References

Aiken, Linda H. "The Nurse Labor Market," *Health Affairs* 1:30-40, Fall 1982.

Althaus, J.N., et al. "Nurse Staffing in a Decentralized Organization: Part I," *Journal of Nursing Administration* 12(3):34-39, March 1982.

Bernzweig, Eli. *The Nurse's Liability for Malpractice: A Programmed Course,* 3rd ed. New York: McGraw-Hill Book Co., 1981.

Bolles, Richard. *What Color is Your Parachute? A Practical Manual for Job Hunters and Career-Changers,* rev. ed. Berkeley, Calif.: Ten Speed Press, 1982.

Brownstone, David M., and Hawes, Gene R. *The Complete Career Guide.* New York: Simon & Schuster, 1980.

Calvert, Robert, Jr., and Steele, John E. *Planning Your Career.* New York: McGraw-Hill Book Co., 1963.

Coulson, Robert. *The Termination Handbook.* New York: Free Press, 1981.

Cowle, Jerry. *How to Survive Getting Fired—And Win!* New York: Warner Books, 1980.

Dickhut, Harold W. *The Professional Resume and Job Search Guide.* Englewood Cliffs, N.J.: Prentice-Hall, 1981.

"For New Nurse: Bigger Role in Health Care," *U.S. News and World Report* 88:59-61, January 1980.

Gulack, R. "Are Your Fringes a Waste?" *RN* 45(7):32-37, July 1982.

Hagberg, Janet, and Leider, Richard. *Inventurers: Excursions in Life and Career Renewal.* Reading, Mass.: Addison-Wesley Publishing Co., 1978.

Heschong, Naomi H. *Get the Job You Want,* 3rd ed. Woodbury, N.Y.: Barron's Educational Series, 1983.

Huckabay, L.M.D., and Skonieczny, R. "Patient Classification Systems: The Problems Faced," *Nursing and Health Care* 2:89-102, February 1981.

Jaquish, M.P. *Personal Resume Preparation.* New York: John Wiley & Sons, 1968.

Kelly, Lucie Y. *Dimensions of Professional Nursing,* 4th ed. New York: Macmillan Publishing Co., 1981.

Kleiner, Brian. "How to Give and Receive Criticism Effectively," *Supervisory Management* 24:37-41, March 1979.

Kleiner, Brian. "Managing Your Career," *Supervisory Management* 25:17-21, March 1980.

Knopf, L. "Registered Nurses Fifteen Years After Graduation: Findings From the Nurse Career-Pattern Study," *Nursing and Health Care* 4(2):72-76, February 1983.

Kroner, Kristine. "Changing Jobs: Take the Gamble Out of It," *NursingLife* 2:50-53, March/April 1982.

Kurman, Annette. "Moving Up the Nursing Ladder," *NursingLife* 2(1):40-43, January/February 1982.

Lotit, Mary Sue, and Kostenbauer, Joyce. *Advance: The Nurse's Guide to Success in Today's Job Market.* Boston: Little, Brown & Co., 1981.

Metzger, Norman, ed. *Handbook of Health Care Human Resources Management.* Rockville, Md.: Aspen Systems Corp., 1981.

Moses, E., and Roth, A. "Nursepower: What Do Statistics Reveal About the Nation's Nurses?" *American Journal of Nursing* 79:1745-56, October 1979.

Morin, William J., and Yorks, Lyle. *Outplacement Techniques: A Positive Approach to Terminating Employees.* New York: American Management Association, 1982.

Nierenberg, Gerard I. *Fundamentals of Negotiating,* rev. ed. New York: Dutton, 1977.

*Resume Preparation Manual.* New York: Catalyst, 1978.

Trandel-Korenchuk, D.M., and Trandel-Korenchuk, K.M. "Current Legal Issues Facing Nursing Practice...Summary of State Law Treatment of the Expanded Nursing Role," *Nursing Administration Quarterly* 5:37-55, Fall 1980.

Underwood, A.B. "What a 12-Hour Shift Offers," *American Journal of Nursing* 75:1176-78, July 1975.

**ENTRIES IN THIS CHAPTER**

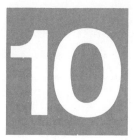

# Working Toward Job Satisfaction

## Introduction

As a nurse, you know about stress. Maybe you can identify with this nurse's situation:

Just as Angie Lacey, RN, was nearing the end of her shift, she heard familiar cries coming from the treatment room. "No, not Harry, not now," she muttered. Harry, a vagrant, visited the emergency department (ED) often with nonspecific complaints of pain. Now he was back, complaining of abdominal pain—so loudly that Angie could hear him through the closed door.

She'd already had a long, hectic shift in the ED. She'd been so busy she hadn't even eaten. Just when she thought she might have a chance to eat, a husky man had staggered in, clutching his chest. Angie had done what she had to do: taken him to the cardiac room, assessed him, started him on oxygen, and put him on a cardiac monitor. When the doctor had started examining him, she'd walked out of the cardiac room—and heard Harry's cries reaching a piercing crescendo. That did it. Angie entered the treatment room, shook Harry by the shoulders, and cried, "Stop it! We've got sick people here!"

If you're like most nurses, you've probably worked long, tiring shifts like Angie's. Have you ever reacted to stress as she did? Stress is inevitable in nursing. If you can't cope with it, you can easily become dissatisfied with your job and your career. But if you learn to cope with it, you can grow both personally and professionally.

During the last few years, stress and job dissatisfaction have become major problems for nurses. Why? A number of social and professional changes have contributed. For example, the high attrition rate among nurses, and reduced enrollments in nursing schools, have helped produce a shortage of working nurses in some regions. And because of the many technologic advances in health care, today's nurses are expected to possess more knowledge and specialized skills than ever before. This often requires additional education but doesn't bring an increase in salary. Finally, the patient population now has an increased percentage of elderly patients with chronic and debilitating diseases. These three trends mean that, in many hospital units, an insufficient number of nurses must provide a wide range of care to many seriously ill patients. Obviously, working conditions like these can produce stress and dissatisfaction.

### Attaining job satisfaction

This chapter can help you make your professional life less stressful and more fulfilling.

In Entry 65, "Career planning: Your guide to job satisfaction," you'll learn

## DON'T LET STRESS CAUSE YOU UNNECESSARY WORK

Stress can make your work harder and less enjoyable. Of course, your job will always involve some stress. But you can manage it—even make it work for you—if you learn to work smarter, not just harder, to keep up. This chart shows how you can plan ahead to minimize the agitating effects of stress on the job.

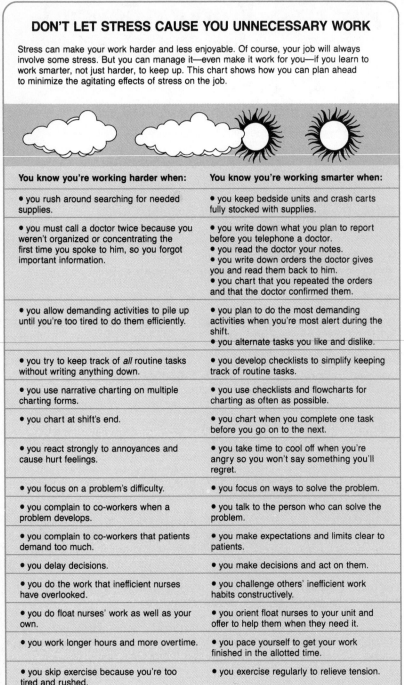

| You know you're working harder when: | You know you're working smarter when: |
|---|---|
| • you rush around searching for needed supplies. | • you keep bedside units and crash carts fully stocked with supplies. |
| • you must call a doctor twice because you weren't organized or concentrating the first time you spoke to him, so you forgot important information. | • you write down what you plan to report before you telephone a doctor.<br>• you read the doctor your notes.<br>• you write down orders the doctor gives you and read them back to him.<br>• you chart that you repeated the orders and that the doctor confirmed them. |
| • you allow demanding activities to pile up until you're too tired to do them efficiently. | • you plan to do the most demanding activities when you're most alert during the shift.<br>• you alternate tasks you like and dislike. |
| • you try to keep track of *all* routine tasks without writing anything down. | • you develop checklists to simplify keeping track of routine tasks. |
| • you use narrative charting on multiple charting forms. | • you use checklists and flowcharts for charting as often as possible. |
| • you chart at shift's end. | • you chart when you complete one task before you go on to the next. |
| • you react strongly to annoyances and cause hurt feelings. | • you take time to cool off when you're angry so you won't say something you'll regret. |
| • you focus on a problem's difficulty. | • you focus on ways to solve the problem. |
| • you complain to co-workers when a problem develops. | • you talk to the person who can solve the problem. |
| • you complain to co-workers that patients demand too much. | • you make expectations and limits clear to patients. |
| • you delay decisions. | • you make decisions and act on them. |
| • you do the work that inefficient nurses have overlooked. | • you challenge others' inefficient work habits constructively. |
| • you do float nurses' work as well as your own. | • you orient float nurses to your unit and offer to help them when they need it. |
| • you work longer hours and more overtime. | • you pace yourself to get your work finished in the allotted time. |
| • you skip exercise because you're too tired and rushed. | • you exercise regularly to relieve tension. |

how to plan your career so you can achieve your professional goals.

Would you like to advance professionally without giving up bedside nursing? Entry 66, "Clinical ladders: Rewarding clinical competence," shows you how. This entry helps you understand clinical ladders and shows you how to advance in your job by moving up the steps.

Do you sometimes think you'll scream if you have to cope with one more patient, doctor, or co-worker? Do you snap at people? Do you sometimes feel too frazzled to function? If these words describe you, you may be headed for burnout. Read Entry 67, "Recognizing the signs and symptoms of stress." It helps you identify your own stress profile and prevent burnout.

Once you know how to spot the causes of stress, you need to know what to do about them. Entry 68, "How to reduce stress and avoid burnout," tells you. This entry explains how—and how *not*—to cope with stress.

Do you know your rights as a nurse? Do you know how to exercise them without infringing on the rights of patients and co-workers? In Entry 69, "Becoming an assertive nurse," you'll learn how to use assertiveness techniques to communicate with others calmly and authoritatively. This approach can be very effective in helping you protect your rights and control your professional (and personal) life.

You know that job satisfaction is the key to a successful nursing career. Each of the entries in this chapter is planned to help you become a more satisfied and productive nurse.

# 65 Career planning: Your guide to job satisfaction

Nursing offers a wide variety of satisfying career options, but you know that

GLOSSARY

## KEY TERMS IN THIS ENTRY

**career plan** • A person's long-term plan for achieving stated career goals.

**long-term goal** • A broad or complex achievement to be accomplished over a relatively long period of time, such as 1 year or more.

**short-term goal** • A simple achievement to be accomplished in a short period of time, such as less than a year; may be one step in achieving a long-term goal.

job satisfaction isn't automatic. You must plan your career carefully so that, from the many career options available, you can select the one that will bring you the most satisfaction.

As a nurse, you're aware that career planning isn't something you do only at the time you get your license and your first nursing job. Your life, your job, and your profession change constantly, so your career planning must be a day-to-day process of assessing yourself and your job, setting career goals and achieving them, and evaluating your progress.

As you know, everyone responds more favorably to self-initiated change than to forced change. Initiating the changes that *you* want is what career planning is all about. If you fail to plan your career, you'll be at the mercy of external forces that could propel you in a career direction you don't want to go. Consider the following example.

Sally Williams, RN, has worked in a medical-surgical unit for 7 years—the last 5 years only part-time. Now, because of financial pressures, Sally must return to nursing full-time. But she's returning to work she doesn't enjoy, and she's dissatisfied with most of her duties.

How did this happen? Well, for Sally, the most rewarding aspect of her nursing experience has been helping patients with terminal cancer and their families to cope. About 6 months ago, when she realized she'd be returning to full-time work, she thought about the rewards of caring for patients with cancer, and she considered joining the hospital hospice team. But then she found she didn't have the necessary experience in cancer nursing. So she gave up her first-choice career goal and settled for a more routine job.

Sally took only the first step in career planning. She knew what she wanted—but she didn't make plans to get it. Now, her nursing career is just drifting along.

To avoid a situation like Sally's and to take control of your career, use a

---

*"Keep in mind that the job that best suits your talents may allow you only limited professional growth."*

---

structured career development strategy (see *How Well Does Your Job Meet Your Goals?*). Here are some strategy steps you can take:
• Assess your strengths and weaknesses, as well as your interests.
• Develop a career plan with short-term and long-term goals.
• Evaluate your progress periodically and, if necessary, reassess your goals.

### Assessing yourself
First, determine what your strengths and weaknesses are. Think about the tasks you handle well and enjoy. Don't overlook tasks you perform outside of nursing. For example, your enthusiasm for organizing church activities may point you toward a job in nursing management. Evaluate what qualities and skills you have that these tasks demonstrate. Next, identify the career options where you'd make frequent use of these strengths. Make a similar eval-

uation, emphasizing weaknesses, to identify jobs you're probably *not* suited for.

Consider the kind of life-style you want, too. Make a list of your personal interests and assign a priority to each.

Next, assess how you respond to changes in your routine and environment. Do some types of changes typically make you feel threatened, anxious, fearful, or impatient? Once you've identified these responses, you can begin to control them. For example, think about past changes in your life, particularly changes that made you alter your personal or work activities. How did you respond? Knowing how you respond to change, and planning change instead of just letting it happen, should minimize your negative reaction.

Evaluate your self-management skills—the skills that help you plan and manage your daily life. Do you have personal habits that could stop you from meeting your goals? For example, suppose you often procrastinate. To break this habit, you'll need to organize a daily planning schedule and abide by it. Remember, breaking old habits requires effort and determination.

### Developing a career plan
Once you've identified your strengths and the kind of life-style that suits you, choose a nursing job that incorporates them. Remember, however, that a job you're very well suited for may allow only limited professional growth. Why? Because you won't be as challenged as you would be in a job that requires you to develop new strengths and overcome old weaknesses. Try to choose a job that will allow you to work with people who have strengths and skills you'd like to develop. Learning from them may help you to convert some of your weaknesses into strengths. Naturally, this professional growth will also make more career options open to you.

Remember, every important career decision involves risks. Taking on a challenging new job means learning

## HOW WELL DOES YOUR JOB MEET YOUR GOALS?

Does your job meet all or most of your professional and personal goals? Taking this survey will help you answer that question. First, check the goals that are important to you. Then, place a 3 rating next to each goal that your job meets exceptionally well; a 2 next to each goal it meets adequately; a 1 next to each goal it meets inadequately; and a 0 next to each goal it doesn't meet at all.

| GOAL | RATING |
|---|---|
| ☐ To work in a specific-size hospital | _____ |
| ☐ To work in the system of nursing care (such as primary care) you prefer | _____ |
| ☐ To work in the specialty area you prefer | _____ |
| ☐ To work the time schedule you prefer | _____ |
| ☐ To have the opportunity to develop long-term relationships with patients | _____ |
| ☐ To have the opportunity to learn and practice advanced clinical skills | _____ |
| ☐ To be given the chance to perform research | _____ |
| ☐ To have the opportunity for advancement | _____ |
| ☐ To have well-defined responsibilities | _____ |
| ☐ To be able to make independent decisions | _____ |
| ☐ To be creative | _____ |
| ☐ To have a voice in policymaking | _____ |
| ☐ To have doctors treat you as a professional | _____ |
| ☐ To have management treat you fairly | _____ |
| ☐ To get the salary you feel you deserve | _____ |
| ☐ To get the fringe benefits you want | _____ |
| ☐ To be given the opportunity for further education | _____ |
| ☐ To be reimbursed for education costs | _____ |

To evaluate your score, first multiply the number of goals you selected by 3. This number represents an ideal score for you. Next, add up all your actual scores. Now divide the second number by the first to come up with a percentage. If it's less than 60%, your job isn't meeting your goals very well, and you may be ready for a job change. If it's between 60% and 80%, your job is generally meeting your goals. If it's over 80%, you should feel fortunate, because your job is meeting a significant number of your goals.

ADVICE

## SMOOTHING OUT A ROUGH START IN A NEW CAREER

*I'm 22 and have my BSN. I started out with energy and high hopes, but now I'm an unhappy nurse, wondering if I'm in the right profession.*

*In a little more than a year, I've had two jobs. My first was in a coronary care unit, where I felt altogether unprepared for the overwhelming responsibility thrust upon me. My second job is in psychiatric nursing. I enjoy the work thoroughly and feel comfortable in this milieu. But I don't enjoy the disorganization of the staff or bearing the brunt of a severe nursing shortage.*

*I'm seriously considering changing fields. But first I think I should try to find some career counseling in nursing. Where can I get the guidance I sorely need?*—RN, Ohio

There *are* organizations set up to counsel nurses who are disenchanted and thinking of leaving nursing. One of the first such organizations in the country was started in 1977 at the University of Texas (Houston) M.D. Anderson Hospital and Tumor Institute. As a result of this program, the average tenure of a nurse at M.D. Anderson

has increased from 8 to 17 months.

If you can't locate a comparable counseling service near you, call your school of nursing. Ask if a faculty member (perhaps one you remember with special respect) would talk with you.

Inquire about a career counselor in your area who's *not* solely involved with nursing. Use his services to explore other options and other careers open to you.

Consider psychotherapy for yourself. If you continue working in a psychiatric area, therapy will be important both for your insight into everyday dealings with patients and for your increased self-knowledge.

Even within your present work setting, you can try several things. For example, hold weekly staff meetings with small groups rather than with the whole staff. The group meetings give everyone a chance to talk about the frustrations of handling the work load and the scheduling, of dealing with patients, and of working with each other. In a small group, staff members can give each other support and positive feedback. Remember, the staff you work with and the relationships that develop can make or break your job in nursing.

This letter was taken from the files of *Nursing* magazine.

new skills that you may or may not master. And if you choose a nontraditional nursing role, such as family nurse clinician, you risk getting other health-care professionals' disapproval. But often your willingness to take career risks can lead to a sense of deep satisfaction in your job. (See *Smoothing Out a Rough Start in a New Career.*)

*Getting the job you want now* is one step in your career plan. But even more important is the long-term planning you should do to establish a career *goal*—a job that will represent real advancement and achievement in your profession. After you've chosen a career goal, you'll need to identify the short-term goals that will mark your progress toward reaching it. For example, if you

want to become a cardiovascular clinical specialist, you must first achieve these short-term goals:

- gaining experience by transferring to a cardiovascular-care unit
- gaining needed education credentials by taking appropriate courses
- meeting practitioners in the field and joining the specialty's professional organizations.

Identify the resources available to help you accomplish your short-term goals. For example, does your employer encourage staff nurses to take college and continuing education courses? When you're identifying resources, don't overlook people, such as educators and professionals established in the field you want to enter. Contact these people—they can help you in your pursuit of your overall goal.

Before you try to implement a career plan, *always make sure the necessary resources are available.* If you don't, you'll be setting yourself up for failure.

Your next step is to set up a firm schedule of short-term goals. Begin by setting some time limits for short-term goals you know you can achieve. For example, if your career goal is to become a member of the hospice team specializing in care of patients with cancer, you might set the short-term goal of taking a course, starting immediately, to learn cancer-care procedures. Then you might set another short-term goal of transferring to the oncology unit within 1 year. After setting time limits for your short-term goals, you can set a tentative time limit for your long-term goal—becoming a member of the hospice team. Remember, when you're setting your goals and your time limits, be realistic. Don't set yourself up for failure.

### Evaluating your progress

Before you implement your long-term career plan, decide how often you'll evaluate your progress and on what terms. Establish some objective standards for judging how well you accomplish each of your short-term goals. (For example, did you achieve satisfactory grades in the specialty course you selected?) But don't make achieving each short-term goal *on time* a critical objective standard. As you make progress, you'll learn things and encounter situations that require you to revise your plan. (For instance, if your family situation changes, you may have to give up attending a specialty course and plan to take it again at a more convenient time.) If you need more time to attain your career goal, that doesn't mean you've failed.

### A final word

Job satisfaction isn't guaranteed. But by staying in control of your career, you can minimize dissatisfaction and get a satisfying sense of growth. The key? Don't let external forces dictate the direction of your professional life. To take control, establish a stepwise career plan, set specific times to reevaluate it, and make any changes that are necessary to keep your career on track. As you achieve your short-term career goals, your confidence and job satisfaction will increase. And so will your chances of achieving your long-term goal—a job that represents significant advancement in your profession.

# 66 Clinical ladders: Rewarding clinical competence

Your job satisfaction won't amount to much if your skills aren't recognized and rewarded with salary increases and promotion opportunities. You know that job satisfaction's important to maintain your enthusiasm for nursing. Because nurses don't always get that sense of job satisfaction, too many of them eventually seek non-nursing jobs. Health-care administrators and nurse managers have recognized this problem and responded by developing clinical ladders—a system for promoting nurses based on how well they demonstrate

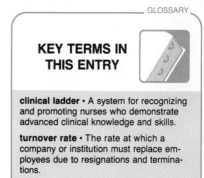

GLOSSARY

## KEY TERMS IN THIS ENTRY

**clinical ladder** • A system for recognizing and promoting nurses who demonstrate advanced clinical knowledge and skills.

**turnover rate** • The rate at which a company or institution must replace employees due to resignations and terminations.

## UNDERSTANDING CLINICAL LADDERS: SAMPLE QUALIFICATIONS AND RESPONSIBILITIES

**QUALIFICATIONS**

**Step 5**
Clinical
nurse
specialist
- graduation from an accredited nursing school
- current license
- master's degree in nursing with 5 years' experience and at least 2 years' specialty clinical experience

**Step 4**
Clinical
coordinator
- graduation from an accredited nursing school
- current license
- associate degree with 5 years' clinical experience, including at least 1 year in a specialty, and demonstrated leadership qualities; or, diploma with 5 years' clinical experience, including at least 1 year in a specialty, and demonstrated leadership qualities; or, a bachelor's degree with 4 years' experience including 1 year in a specialty; or, a master's degree with 3 years' clinical experience, including at least 1 year in a specialty

**Step 3**
Senior
clinician
- graduation from an accredited nursing school
- current license
- associate degree with 3 years' clinical experience; or, diploma with 3 years' clinical experience; or, bachelor's degree with 2 years' clinical experience; or, master's degree in nursing with 1 year of clinical experience

**Step 2**
Clinician B
- graduation from an accredited nursing school
- current license
- associate degree with 2 years' clinical experience; or, diploma with 2 years' clinical experience; or, bachelor's degree with 1 year of clinical experience; or, master's degree with minimal clinical experience

**Step 1**
Clinician A
- graduation from an accredited nursing school
- current license
- associate degree with 1 year of clinical experience; or, diploma with 1 year of clinical experience; or, bachelor's degree with 6 months' clinical experience

**Pre-ladder**
Staff
nurse
- graduation from an accredited nursing school
- current license
- no experience required

Every hospital or health-care institution with a clinical-ladder scheme for career advancement will tailor each job's qualifications and responsibilities to the institution's needs. So no single clinical-ladder scheme will apply to every hospital or institution. This sample, however, is representative of clinical ladders in the United States and Canada.

## RESPONSIBILITIES

- provides nursing care for a patient caseload she selects herself
- conducts nursing research and helps implement the results
- serves as a role model and consultant for other nurses
- evaluates patient teaching effectiveness and revises policies when needed
- initiates planned changes and evaluates outcomes
- helps set criteria for care in conjunction with other disciplines

- identifies and helps solve recurring problems in specific patient groups
- evaluates and monitors patient care
- collaborates with other health-care professionals in planning care
- acts as a resource person for patient-care problems
- provides staff guidance in areas such as patient teaching
- serves as a role model for other nurses

- gives nursing care to a specific patient group
- manages patient-care problems
- teaches patients and families about health care
- performs complicated nursing procedures
- takes independent action in giving nursing care
- serves as a role model for nurses with less experience

- directs care for patient groups
- initiates patient and family teaching
- shows leadership skills in directing care
- performs complicated nursing procedures

- shows beginning expertise in patient care
- identifies patient teaching needs
- sets nursing care priorities
- is accountable for her own practice

- demonstrates basic clinical skills in patient care
- evaluates patients' response to care delivered
- works under close supervision

their clinical knowledge and skills. They're designed to improve your job satisfaction by enhancing your career possibilities.

Hospitals began developing clinical ladders in the 1970s, after the National Commission on Community Health Services (1967) and the National Commission on Nursing and Nursing Education (1970) urged nursing leaders to implement a system for clinical advancement. Why? Because staff nurses who became skilled at caring for patients traditionally could not advance professionally *in that field*. They could receive higher pay and job status only by leaving the bedside and moving into management or teaching positions. When staff-nurse promotions did occur, administrators usually based them on length of service rather than demonstrated clinical ability. So if a nurse chose to continue giving direct patient care, the only tangible motivation she had for growing professionally on the job was the traditional tuition benefit. This sytem didn't encourage staff nurses to strengthen or supplement their clinical skills. Clinical ladders were developed to offer staff nurses a new way to achieve career goals.

### Can a clinical ladder benefit you?

Usually, a clinical ladder forms one part of an overall promotion system called a *career ladder*. The typical career ladder has three tracks, like three ladders standing side by side: clinical, administrative, and educational. If you're working toward promotion, you climb up one career-ladder track—or you can move to another if your career goal changes.

If you're a staff nurse, here's how a clinical ladder can benefit you:
- It can reward your clinical skills through promotions, pay raises, and peer recognition.
- It can allow you to continue bedside nursing and still advance professionally.
- It can give you the opportunity to increase your clinical skills.
- It can allow you to say when you're ready for new clinical challenges.

### How clinical ladders work

Clinical ladders vary in the number of steps available for climbing, although a typical ladder has four or five. Qualifications for each step include requirements for education and work experience (see *Understanding Clinical Ladders: Sample Qualifications and Responsibilities*, pages 422 and 423). As you climb a clinical ladder, each step signifies that you've mastered new and increasingly complex clinical skills. Most clinical-ladder systems

*"The clinical ladder system allows you to say when you think you're ready to advance professionally."*

place a new graduate on the bottom step, but some require that a new graduate achieve minimum skills before she can begin climbing the ladder. The most experienced and skillful nurses, with additional formal education, may reach the clinical ladder's highest step, as clinical nurse specialists.

If you're an experienced but newly hired nurse, you can expect your nursing management to place you on a clinical-ladder step that they feel corresponds to your skills, education, and career goals. After a customary probationary period of 3 to 6 months, you, a peer, and a supervisor will usually evaluate your performance. If this evaluation indicates that you belong on a higher clinical-ladder step, you may be moved to that step.

### How to achieve clinical-ladder promotions

The clinical-ladder system offers you

this critical advantage over traditional nursing promotion systems: *You* determine when you're ready to advance to the next step. By doing the necessary preparation—such as attending seminars, courses, and clinical workshops, and getting additional clinical experience—you master the required skills to move up the ladder. When you think you're ready for a promotion, you must ask for an evaluation. (Be prepared to submit a self-evaluation that documents your additional nursing skills and education.) Then a committee of peers, clinical experts, and managers will review your self-evaluation, evaluate your clinical performance, and either approve or deny the promotion. If it's approved, your promotion will take effect once a vacancy occurs at the right clinical-ladder level. But keep this in mind: The committee can demote you to a *lower* clinical-ladder step if the evaluation indicates that you haven't performed satisfactorily at your present level. (Most clinical-ladder systems will give you a conditional time period to correct deficiencies and avoid demotion.)

Once you're in a clinical-ladder system, you have to expect to climb the ladder slowly, perhaps over 5 to 10 years. Why? Because you'll need a lot of time and work to acquire the skills and education you need for moving up. Also, sometimes employers must limit the numbers of higher clinical positions available, because of economic constraints or the way their institutions are organized.

Because a clinical ladder gives *you* the responsibility for initiating movement, you can stay on one step as long as you wish. Even if you stay on the same step for a number of years, you can still get salary increases through scheduled merit reviews.

## Overcoming resistance to clinical ladders

A clinical ladder can't solve every nurse's job satisfaction problems. No one system can. In fact, some nurses may resist the clinical-ladder concept, particularly very experienced nurses and specialty nurses.

To overcome this resistance, some nursing administrators will:
• phase in the clinical ladder gradually, using a definite plan that everyone knows about
• avoid making other major organizational or staff changes at the same time
• provide continuous, accurate information about the system to keep nurses fully informed and to avoid misconceptions
• emphasize that the system will not jeopardize any nurse's job.

## Look before you climb

Whether your institution's clinical ladder is well established or new, you'll want these important questions answered so you know exactly how the system works:
• Are the clinical ladder's steps equal in status and pay to the corresponding administrative and educational steps on the career ladder?
• What's the chain of command in the clinical ladder?
• Does the ladder include developmental programs to help you acquire skills you need for promotion?
• Does the ladder *require* you to advance?
• What's the specific promotion procedure?
• How are you evaluated, and by whom?

## A final word

Hospitals and other health-care institutions that have implemented clinical ladders report a lower turnover rate among their nurses. And they report that more nurses are choosing to continue giving direct patient care. If you're a staff nurse, these results clearly document that clinical ladders can improve your job satisfaction. Because of clinical ladders' success so far, don't be surprised if they become much more common.

# 67 Recognizing the signs and symptoms of stress

Have you ever felt like leaving nursing because of your job's stresses? Most nurses have that disturbing feeling at one time or another, as stress-induced exhaustion threatens their personal and professional equilibrium. Most of these nurses recover their composure quickly. But too many nurses let stresses continually pile up, making them feel trapped and disillusioned. Some of these nurses *do* leave nursing, because of a condition called *burnout*.

A recent survey indicated how years of stress can affect nurses' job satisfaction. This survey found that the nurses who reported the most job satisfaction had been in the profession less than 1 year.

How can you avoid becoming one of stress's casualties? One way is to learn about stress—the many kinds and causes of stress that exist, and the times when stress can become excessive.

## Characterizing stress

Stress can be a product of your job or personal life, or both. It can be acute or chronic. Acute stress is temporary and noticeably affects a person's ability to cope. Chronic stress is persistent and may go unrecognized as the person adapts to heightened anxiety and tension. A sudden upsurge in critical admissions to your unit could cause acute job-related stress. A persistent shortage of qualified staff on your unit, in contrast, could cause chronic job-related stress. Other examples: acute personal stress is a natural response to a family member's death; chronic personal stress is a natural response to unrelenting financial pressures.

## Work habits as signs of stress

Besides physical responses, certain work habits can indicate when you're under too much stress. One of the earliest signs of stress is a tendency to work harder than your job demands. For example, have you ever found yourself staying at work late every day and working extra shifts? Or skipping meal breaks because you're convinced you're too busy to stop?

Here's another work habit that's a clue to stress: keeping patients at a distance. Do you avoid talking to them, show little emotional response to their needs, or tend to stereotype them? (See *How to Measure Your Stress Level.*)

## What causes job-related stress?

You've experienced long, demanding days at work, so you can probably reel off nurses' most common stressors easily (see *Listening to Yourself to Control Stress*, page 431). You won't be very surprised to learn that *interpersonal conflict* is the *most* common. Anytime you clash with colleagues on the job, you feel sharp stress. And conflicts with doctors and supervisors can cause even more stress than conflicts with your peers.

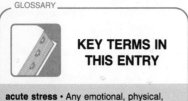

GLOSSARY

### KEY TERMS IN THIS ENTRY

**acute stress** • Any emotional, physical, social, or economic change that produces *temporary* physical or mental tension and sometimes may contribute to the onset of illness.

**chronic stress** • Any emotional, physical, social, or economic change that produces *persistent* physical or mental tension that, if not relieved, produces exhaustion and is likely to contribute to the onset of illness.

**nursing burnout** • The condition of no longer caring about practicing nursing, resulting from chronic, unrelieved, job-related stress. Characterized by physical and emotional exhaustion, sometimes by illness and/or abandonment of a nursing career.

## HOW TO MEASURE YOUR STRESS LEVEL

You may not be aware of just how harmful stress can be to you. To measure your own stress over the past 24 hours, take this easy test, which lists 20 work events. In a survey, staff nurses rated these work events the most stressful. Each of the events has been assigned a validated stress value. Check the events you've experienced in the past 24 hours, then total up those events' stress values. After you've taken the test, read how to interpret the scores.

| Stressful work event | Experienced in past 24 hours | Stress value |
| --- | --- | --- |
| Assuming responsibilities you're not trained to handle | _____ | 67 |
| Working with unqualified personnel | _____ | 64 |
| Dealing with nonsupportive supervisors or administrators | _____ | 61 |
| Working with an insufficient staff | _____ | 58 |
| Caring for a patient who's having a cardiac arrest | _____ | 55 |
| Experiencing conflict with co-workers | _____ | 52 |
| Dealing with a dying patient's family | _____ | 49 |
| Caring for a dying patient | _____ | 46 |
| Working with broken or faulty equipment | _____ | 44 |
| Working with inadequate supplies | _____ | 42 |
| Working an inconvenient shift or schedule | _____ | 38 |
| Assuming responsibilities without thanks or recognition | _____ | 36 |
| Dealing with a difficult doctor | _____ | 34 |
| Trying to communicate with a bureaucracy | _____ | 31 |
| Discharging a patient unprepared for discharge | _____ | 28 |
| Caring for a seriously ill patient | _____ | 25 |
| Spending long periods of time on paperwork or telephone duties | _____ | 22 |
| Having a problem over salary or promotion | _____ | 19 |
| Working with a demanding or noncompliant patient | _____ | 16 |
| Coordinating supplemental personnel | _____ | 13 |

Your total _____    **Total possible score 800**

Obviously, the higher your score, the more stress you've experienced in the past 24 hours. You can estimate your present stress level as follows:

**0-133**   You're under minimal stress, not enough to cause you many problems.

**134-266**   You're under moderate stress. This is the highest level of stress you should permit on a day-to-day basis.

**267-532**   You're experiencing high-level stress. You have trouble relaxing, and you easily become annoyed. Do what you can to reduce your stressors at work, and try relaxation techniques, exercise, and pursuing outside interests to relieve your stress.

**533-800**   You're under extreme stress. Get help quickly. You're a prime candidate for burnout and serious physical or emotional problems if you let this level of stress continue.

The second most common source of nurses' job-related stress is *patient care*—particularly care of patients who are either dying, in critical condition, chronically ill, very demanding, or in need of emergency care.

*Insufficient staffing*, another source of job stress, makes you work longer and harder to make up for the lack of help and adds to your perception that your work load is never-ending.

Many nurses cite *poor nursing leadership* as a job-related stress. If your supervisor doesn't understand the pressures of your job, or isn't clinically competent enough to help relieve it by doing some of your work at peak stress times, you can feel significant stress. For example, if you're a staff nurse, you expect front-line supervisors to pitch in and help with patient care during emergencies, extra-heavy work loads, and staffing shortages. If your supervisor is clinically incompetent, she may not offer help when you need it—or if she does, her inefficiency and mistakes will only increase your stress level.

*Inadequate salary* can lead to another common job-related stress for nurses. Surveys show that approximately 85% of the public believes that nurses aren't paid adequately. For example, although you play a critical role in a patient's recovery, the average doctor's salary is about five times greater than yours.

*Inadequate professional knowledge and skills* can readily produce job-related stress. In nursing's highly technologic environment, you must act decisively in complex patient-care situations, especially emergencies. You need to update your nursing knowledge and skills constantly, but lack of time or money can make this difficult. When you worry that you're not doing your job well, diminished self-confidence can cause stress.

## What causes personal stress?
If job-related stresses don't usually affect you, you must still be wary of personal stress, which can stem from major life changes or your own personality traits.

*Major life changes*—such as divorce—can cause you considerable stress in the form of apprehension, worry, and uncertainty about the future. And if you've ever had to work during a major life change, you know how it can deplete your energy.

Some *personality traits* can cause considerable stress; for example, continually having unrealistic expectations. If you feel responsible for others' work, or if you always assume responsibility when anything goes wrong, you're harboring unrealistic expectations of yourself that will increase your stress. You're also inviting stress if you believe you can accomplish anything if you just try hard enough, or if you believe you can prevent suffering and death.

Other personality traits that lead to stress include:
- *unclear goals*—not knowing where you're headed or what you want to do in life
- *a sense of alienation*—feeling cut off from those around you
- *Type A behavior*—the most prominent personality trait that leads to stress.

## Identifying the Type A personality
A nurse with a Type A personality tries to achieve more and more in less and less time. Do you have a Type A personality? You may, if your behavior is regularly marked by:
- a strong sense of urgency, even about trivial matters
- constant awareness of the passing of time
- easily aroused hostility
- a lack of flexibility
- intolerance of mistakes—yours and other people's
- quick movements and rapid speech
- a tense appearance
- impatience with delays
- a tendency to do two or more things at once

## HOW YOUR PROFESSIONAL LIFE AFFECTS YOUR PERSONAL LIFE

In 1980, a study of over 2,000 people who were successful in business showed that success doesn't have to destroy a healthy private life. A great many of these people had successful, fulfilling professional and personal lives.

But the study did uncover a number of people with frustrating, unfulfilling private lives—people who considered their home as a place to recharge for the next day's work, not as a place for personal accomplishment and satisfaction.

The culprit? Letting negative feelings from work spill over at home. The study showed that this spillover of negative feelings took two forms: psychological withdrawal and inappropriate anger.

Do you bring your negative feelings home? Possibly, if one of these descriptions fits you:

• You're physically present at home, but you're emotionally withdrawn. When family members approach you with problems or demands, you close up like a clam.

• You express yourself through anger. If your husband or your children make minor mistakes, you explode.

In the study, researchers found two major work factors that caused these angry scenes at home:

• A new job is the most common cause. Many people who accept new jobs underestimate the massive amounts of tension the change can create. You probably won't be able to avoid all spillover when you change jobs, so *expect it and warn your family to expect it*. It may last for a long time.

• A misfit situation—the wrong person in the wrong job—is the second most common cause. If you find after a year on the job that you're bringing angry feelings home from work increasingly often, you may simply be in the wrong job. You owe it to yourself and your family to consider changing jobs. Whatever the reason, don't let your professional life ruin your private life. Work to make them both fulfilling.

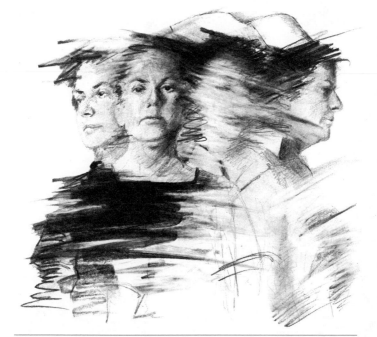

• a negative attitude toward life in general.

The Type A personality is rampant in American society, especially in high-stress professions. This personality's possible rewards include prestige, a sense of accomplishment, admiration from others, and financial gain. Its possible risks include job dissatisfaction, poor interpersonal relationships, and increased likelihood of illness—such as heart disease, hypertension, migraine headaches, and gastrointestinal disorders.

### Nursing jobs that increase the risk of stress

You know that certain nursing jobs are more stressful than others; examples include work in burn units, critical and intensive care units, oncology units, and emergency departments (EDs). These work areas' persistent stress level requires constant coping. Nancy Graham, a traumatologist who works with ED patients and staff, has written: "Most nurses can identify with me when I describe how my body feels after arriving home from work: like a car whose driver has one foot on the accelerator and the other foot on the brake. The result is a feeling of being both completely exhausted and incredibly hyped up." (See *How Your Professional Life Affects Your Personal Life*, page 429.)

### Recognizing nursing burnout

When a nurse isn't able to adapt to all the stresses of her job or life, she may slide into burnout. (See *Are You Heading Toward Burnout?*.)

---

## ARE YOU HEADING TOWARD BURNOUT?

Do you suspect you're on the way to burning out because of stress? If you do, decide how many of the following statements apply to you. More than two "yes" answers means that you're at risk and you've got to begin handling stress better.

| Yes | No | |
|-----|-----|-----|
| ———— | ———— | I'm always exhausted. |
| ———— | ———— | I can't get much sleep. |
| ———— | ———— | I can't seem to relax. |
| ———— | ———— | I'm becoming more cynical. |
| ———— | ———— | I'm often impatient and irritable. |
| ———— | ———— | I feel unappreciated. |
| ———— | ———— | I don't seem to care about my job anymore. |
| ———— | ———— | I don't feel well much of the time. |
| ———— | ———— | I often feel depressed. |
| ———— | ———— | I feel overburdened with work. |

# LISTENING TO YOURSELF TO CONTROL STRESS

Do you know that certain psychological factors can increase job-related stress? By making problems on the job seem bigger than they really are, these factors aggravate the stress you feel. To make matters worse, recognizing these factors is often difficult, because they're personality characteristics that we're used to in ourselves. This chart will help you recognize whether you have the potential to aggravate your stress this way.

| PSYCHOLOGICAL DISTORTION | EXAMPLE |
|---|---|
| **Filtering:** Selectively eliminating some details of a conversation or event to find fault with yourself | You've just finished a detailed care plan for a difficult patient when your supervisor compliments you and says, "I wish you'd write care plans like that for all your patients." You bristle and say to yourself, "She's always criticizing me. Nothing I do is good enough." |
| **Overgeneralizing:** Thinking in absolute terms and exaggerating, drawing a broad conclusion from a shred of evidence | Your supervisor asks you to float to an intensive care unit. You set the rate on a monitor incorrectly and have to write an incident report. You tell your supervisor, "I'll never accept a float assignment again." |
| **Polarizing:** Thinking in extremes, seeing everything in black and white, with no gray areas | A postoperative renal patient on your unit puts on his call light several times a day. Even though you know he's in pain, you remark to a friend, "He complains all the time about nothing." |
| **Using "shoulds":** Using inflexible rules about how you and others should act, disallowing any deviation from the rules | You firmly believe that patients should cooperate with their care. So when Mr. Boughton refuses to take his medication, you become angry and delay answering his call light each time he rings it that afternoon. You think, "Why should I work so hard when he won't cooperate?" |
| **Externalizing:** Blaming only others for your problems, never yourself | Your supervisor asks you to work a couple of hours overtime to help care for an obese cardiac patient whose condition has deteriorated. When you get home, your family is angry because you didn't call to say you'd be late. You think, "It's all her fault—this never would happen if she'd staff properly." |
| **Internalizing:** Blaming yourself for every problem, feeling that everyone at work depends on you, and feeling guilty for not doing work you think is expected of you | As you check a despondent patient at the end of your shift, he accuses you of not spending enough time with him. You've worked hard and well to apportion your time to all your patients, but driving home, you think, "He's right; I should have talked to him more about his problems." |
| **Catastrophizing:** Magnifying a problem until it becomes a disaster in your mind | A young drug addict is admitted to your unit, and you immediately begin to worry: "What if my son starts taking drugs and ends up like this patient?" |
| **Needing to be right:** Thinking that you're always right and that anyone who disagrees with you is wrong | "I've been catheterizing patients since before you were born," you tell a new graduate nurse who wants to show you a new technique. "I don't need a new technique." |

Burnout progresses in three phases; each of them has physical and emotional dangers you must understand. In *phase one,* burnout consists of emotional and physical fatigue progressing to exhaustion. You could be in phase one of burnout if you're tired all the time, if you have trouble sleeping, if you get frequent headaches or body aches or colds, or if you become emotionally depleted and depressed just thinking about going to work.

In *phase two,* a nurse who's burning out develops a negative, cynical attitude. If this happens to you, you may express this attitude by making such comments as, "The floats the nursing office sends us are useless...and the new graduates are worse. They don't teach them anything anymore!" Or you may blame your patients for getting sick or for not following professional advice. Your anger with patients may become more open, so that when you hear another nurse describe a dirty patient as a derelict, you agree instead of defending his rights. Finally, your negative attitude may turn against *you,* making you feel incompetent and unliked. You'll put in just enough work to get by, and you'll probably avoid helping other nurses with their work.

In the *third and final phase* of burnout, a nurse typically feels bitter about everything and everybody, trapped, and completely unable to cope with problems. She also feels that her work makes no difference in improving her patients' care, no matter how hard she tries. As a result, she feels defeated and incapable of continuing her work. Her job satisfaction is probably nil. If she doesn't recognize the danger signs of burnout, she can end up quitting—or being fired.

If you recognize yourself in any part of this description, get help *fast.* If you don't find a way to reduce your stress level, you're risking your health as well as your job.

**A final word**
Don't let job-related or personal stresses accumulate (See Entry 68). Instead, learn to recognize when stress begins to throw your physical and emotional equilibrium out of kilter. How? By learning to raise your *stress consciousness*—your alertness to stress's warning signals. By continually monitoring your stress level, you'll find that you can be kinder to yourself and to others. By avoiding stress, you can replenish the deepest source of every nurse's job satisfaction—the sense of joy in caring for others.

# 68 How to reduce stress and avoid burnout

Of the approximately 1.4 million nurses currently registered in the United States, only about half work full-time in nursing. Of this number, about 330,000 work outside the hospital setting—in clinics, public health departments, doctors' offices, nursing schools, and research laboratories. Why are such large numbers of nurses leaving the profession in general, and the hospital specifically? The major reason is excessive, prolonged stress—*burnout.*

Burnout is a serious problem that can devastate your personal and professional life. It can cause physical or mental illness or extreme emotional pain. And it can lead to serious job dissatisfaction, which can have negative effects on the quality of care that you provide.

Because you—and every practicing nurse—are potential burnout victims, you need to stay alert to burnout's signs and symptoms and become aware of its negative effects. And you need to learn about the preventive measures you can take to reduce or prevent stress in your personal and professional life. Coping effectively with stress is the key to safeguarding yourself from eventual burnout.

## Choosing mechanisms for coping with stress

The first step toward reducing stress and avoiding burnout is to identify the stresses in your personal and professional life (see Entry 67). The next step is to develop coping mechanisms to either eliminate or deal with these stresses effectively. The mechanisms you choose will depend on your particular life-style and outlook on life. But you should keep these points in mind:

*Explore various solutions.* If you can simply eliminate the stress, you've already won the battle. But because stressful situations often involve family members, health-team colleagues, or patient-care problems you face each day, you won't often be able to eliminate the stress they cause. Instead, you'll have to develop mechanisms to cope with your stresses.

*Choose adaptive coping mechanisms.* Adaptive coping mechanisms

---

## *"Coping effectively with stress will safeguard you from burnout."*

---

are constructive actions that you take to change a stress-producing situation. To select actions that will work, you'll need to apply your problem-solving skills as follows:
• Assess the problem.
• Identify its cause.
• Plan and implement a course of action.
• Evaluate your results.

You'll know you've arrived at an adaptive coping mechanism if your actions reduce your stress so you can make progress toward resolving the problems that caused it.

However, if you continue to feel anxious, angry, frustrated, or abused, you're probably using a *maladaptive coping mechanism.* These ineffective and unhealthy actions fail to change the

situation that's causing your stress. Consequently, stress continues to take its toll on you. You may even begin to respond to the stress-causing situation in maladaptive ways. For example, when you feel stress, you may overeat and gain weight. Besides not solving the original problem, your added pounds may create new health problems for you.

• *Keep trying.* You may not succeed at reducing the stressful situation on your first try. But perseverance can make the difference.

• *Don't be afraid to change your tactics.* After several attempts, you may find that a particular coping mechanism is maladaptive, or decide that you'd simply like to try a different approach. Just reinitiate the problem-solving process of assessment, planning, implementation, and evaluation. When you come up with a new approach, give it a try.

• *Proceed slowly.* You can't immediately reduce all the stressors in your life. Concentrate on one or two initially. Once you've begun to manage *them* adequately, start tackling others.

• *Reward yourself.* Plan ahead of time to reward yourself in some way when you've achieved your goal. Then, when you succeed, treat yourself to it.

Besides the acute stress you feel in

# HOW MANAGEMENT CAN HELP PREVENT BURNOUT

"An ounce of prevention is worth a pound of cure" is an adage that certainly applies to burnout. Prevention is the best way to combat burnout, and your hospital's management can contribute. Of course, as a professional, you know you must make every effort on your own to avoid burnout. But you can also suggest that management take these steps to help:

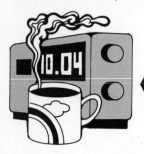

provide relief periods—such as a 15-minute break or even a transfer to a different unit for a few days—to help you recover from particularly stressful situations

rotate assignments to avoid boredom and prevent you from continually working in a highly stressful situation

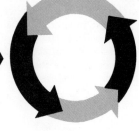

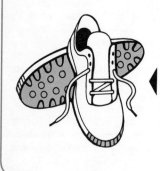

organize peer support groups to let you and your nursing colleagues discuss your professional problems

offer continuing education programs that serve dual purposes: giving you time away from your job's stresses and increasing your ability to handle the job

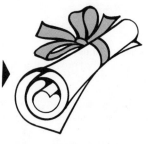

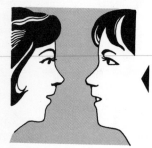

provide you with the chance to learn and use such stress-management techniques as meditation, yoga, relaxation, and jogging and other exercises

particular stressful circumstances, you may sometimes experience general, or chronic, stress in your personal or professional life. To reduce this chronic stress, try to incorporate certain stress-reducing activities and attitudes into your personal and professional routine. Regardless of what's causing your particular stress, this advice can help you lead a healthier, more satisfying, and more productive life.

## Reducing stress in your personal life

How well you maintain your mental and physical well-being can be a major factor in how stress affects you. Keep the following tips in mind:

● *Eat well.* A well-balanced diet, one that provides you with sufficient amounts of calories from the four basic food groups, supplies all the nutrients you need to look and feel healthy. To decide whether you're eating well, analyze your diet and your eating habits. Do you eat to excess? Are you overweight or underweight? Do you eat out of habit, or only when you're hungry? Do you eat more when you're under stress? Are you consuming empty calories, chemical additives, excessive salt or fat?

If you decide that you should improve your eating habits, try to adopt new ones that will meet your particular nutritional needs. But proceed slowly, and set realistic goals. For example, if junk foods are your downfall, try to cut down on them this month. Next month, try to increase your intake of fresh fruits and vegetables. Proceeding step by step, you can permanently change your eating habits—and reduce your vulnerability to stress.

● *Exercise regularly.* A regular exercise program can relieve stress by increasing your cardiac output, respiratory capacity, and blood flow to tense muscles. Choose an exercise program that you'll enjoy, and make sure it will increase your oxygen consumption and raise and sustain your heart rate to its optimal level. Jogging, brisk walking, aerobic dancing, racquetball, and softball are beneficial exercises. (If you need motivation to exercise, think about enrolling in a group program.) Try to exercise four times a week for at least 20 to 30 minutes per session. Proceed slowly, and build up your endurance gradually.

● *Relax.* Effective relaxation reduces your heart and respiratory rates, improves your skeletal muscle tone, and briefly "turns off" your mental/emotional processes, providing you with both a physical and mental break from stress. Relaxation exercises involve a systematic tightening and relaxing of various muscle groups in the body. You can usually perform relaxation exercises anywhere, because most are inconspicuous. If you do them at the first sign of stress, you can quickly dissipate its negative effects.

● *Play.* Allow some time from *each* day to have fun. If the demands of your job have obscured your enjoyment of leisure-time activities, take time to rediscover what's fun for you. Explore and experiment. Don't feel guilty about it. You need play time as much as food and oxygen to maintain a state of healthy balance.

## Reducing stress in your professional life

As a nurse, you know that stress is always a factor in your work. But you can keep stress to a minimum by keeping the following tips in mind:

● *Maintain realistic expectations of your relationships on the job.* At various times in your nursing career, you'll probably have conflicts with nursing administrators or colleagues. Remember, no person is perfect, including you. Accept other people's faults—and be kind to yourself, too.

● *Set realistic job goals.* Don't try to accomplish more than you humanly can. Pushing yourself beyond your limits will create unnecessary stress.

● *Continue your education.* To keep current with the latest nursing developments, enroll in some continuing education courses that are appropriate to your needs. Read professional nursing journals regularly. Get involved in a professional association. You'll gain new knowledge that you can apply to your nursing practice. And you may be relieved to discover that other nurses share your problems and concerns.

• *Learn to say "no."* If you can't oblige your supervisor or a colleague who requests that you work overtime or change your days off, say no politely, and don't feel guilty about it. You're entitled to a personal as well as a professional life.

• *Look for new challenges.* If you're bored with your job, try to make it more challenging. Ask yourself how you can change it to better meet your patients' needs. Try to set new goals for yourself. Assume a new responsibility, if your nursing administration agrees.

• *Cultivate a supportive friendship, or join a support group.* Discuss your concerns with an understanding, supportive friend who will listen and keep the conversation confidential. This simple act can relieve much of your stress. And your friend may even be able to give you new insights into coping with your particular stressful sit-

uation. Or join a nurses' support group. Most are conducted by a mental health clinical specialist, a psychologist, or a psychiatrist, who guides the group in its discussions of job-related concerns.

• *Establish a "decompression routine."* Get involved in some activity, *immediately following the end of your shift*, that will help you forget about the job and relax before arriving home. Chatting with a friend over a cup of coffee before leaving work, or walking home (if possible), may provide you with a relaxing transition from work to home. Experiment to discover what works for you.

• *Take a vacation or leave of absence.* Like anyone else, you have a limit to the amount of stress you can tolerate. If the pressures become too great, take a vacation or leave of absence. Don't feel guilty about it. You can use the time to regenerate your coping abilities.

• *Ask for help from management.* If your job stresses are extreme and can't be reduced, you may need some professional help to cope with them. Find out if someone from your nursing management or hospital administration can refer you to a resource person for help. (See *How Management Can Help Pre-*

---

## TRANSFERRING TO ANOTHER UNIT: ONE WAY TO RELIEVE STRESS

Sometimes the only way you can relieve the relentless stress of a particular job is to transfer to another unit. Here's how to do it properly:

• Put your request in writing, specifying the unit and shift you want. Then briefly list your reasons, keeping the tone positive. Make three copies and keep one for yourself.

• Tell your current supervisor about your request and give her a copy. Maintain rapport with her, even though you hope to leave.

• Make an appointment with the person who initiates transfers in your hospital, and give her your request personally. Explain why you want to transfer—for example, for new or different challenges.

• Follow up on your request in a few weeks to show the supervisor in charge of transfers that you're serious about your decision.

• If you get administrative approval, don't expect the transfer immediately. Administration will need time to consider your request, and, of course, you may have to wait for an opening. Even after your request is approved, you may have to wait for management to find a replacement for you on your current unit.

*vent Burnout,* page 434.)
• *Change your job.* If you've tried to deal with your job stresses constructively, but have been unsuccessful, ask for a transfer to a new nursing unit, or request a shift change. (See *Transferring to Another Unit: One Way to Relieve Stress.*) Remember, prolonged excessive stress will take its toll on you as a nurse and affect the quality of your nursing care.
• *Value yourself.* You may forget that you need to care for yourself as much as for your patients. Stay alert to the warning signs of stress and burnout. If you detect any, don't hesitate to do something about them.

### A final word
Excessive and prolonged stress can have serious consequences in your work as well as in your personal life. If stress is affecting you, start taking measures to reduce it before it progresses to burnout. Reducing stress in your personal and professional life can improve your health, help you become a more confident and productive nurse, and banish burnout.

# 69 Becoming an assertive nurse

Nursing couldn't have shed its confining handmaiden image in recent years without the increasing assertiveness of more and more nurses. For too long, entrenched social customs forced nurses to take a subservient role with other health-care professionals, especially doctors. These customs discouraged nurses from being direct and open in confronting their profession's issues.

Gradually, these customs' grip on nursing began to loosen. Why? Because nurses realized that their image and their professional effectiveness could improve significantly if they asserted

themselves. And, perhaps just as important, nurses realized that assertiveness often results in better patient care. Do you understand the benefits of assertiveness? Here's some practical advice on how to become more assertive.

### Understanding communication styles
When you assert yourself, you're using one of three general communication styles. The others are passive (nonassertive) and aggressive. The best way to understand the benefits of assertive communication is to understand the shortcomings of passive and aggressive communication.

*The passive nurse* is generally hesitant and unsure of herself. She doesn't express her opinions or feelings, because she fears hurting someone or being criticized by others. For example, a passive nurse who sees a colleague using an unsterile technique to change a dressing is unlikely to point out the colleague's error. Instead, she'll just ignore it and hope the colleague won't repeat it. Generally, the passive nurse feels frustrated and may explode into aggressive behavior when she finally does express herself.

*The aggressive nurse* is usually excessively forceful in expressing her feelings, often at the expense of others. She accuses, blames, and demeans her colleagues. For example, she might con-

# ARE YOU AN ASSERTIVE NURSE?

How assertive are you? Here's a questionnaire that will help you find out. Just check **YES**, **NO**, or **SOMETIMES** next to each question. Then read how to evaluate your answers.

| | YES | NO | SOME-TIMES |
|---|---|---|---|
| Do you lack confidence in your nursing judgments? | ☐ | ☐ | ☐ |
| Do you hesitate to express what you're thinking or feeling? | ☐ | ☐ | ☐ |
| Do you feel self-conscious if someone watches you while you work? | ☐ | ☐ | ☐ |
| Do you hesitate to call a doctor about a patient problem? | ☐ | ☐ | ☐ |
| Do you avoid questioning a doctor's order? | ☐ | ☐ | ☐ |
| Do you often use the phrases, "I hate to bother you, but..." or, "This may not be important, but..."? | ☐ | ☐ | ☐ |
| Do you avoid speaking up at nursing staff meetings? | ☐ | ☐ | ☐ |
| Do you fly off the handle when the pressure builds? | ☐ | ☐ | ☐ |
| Do you dissolve into tears when the pressure builds? | ☐ | ☐ | ☐ |
| Do you feel people take advantage of you because you can't say no? | ☐ | ☐ | ☐ |
| Do you have trouble starting a conversation? | ☐ | ☐ | ☐ |
| Do you find it hard to compliment a co-worker on a job well done? | ☐ | ☐ | ☐ |
| Do you find it hard to correct a co-worker who performs a job incorrectly? | ☐ | ☐ | ☐ |
| Do you get flustered when you receive a compliment? | ☐ | ☐ | ☐ |
| Do you vent anger by using obscenities or by name-calling? | ☐ | ☐ | ☐ |
| Do you hesitate to protest if your supervisor gives you an evaluation you consider unfair? | ☐ | ☐ | ☐ |
| Do you accept unreasonable requests to work overtime or double shifts? | ☐ | ☐ | ☐ |
| Do you tend to complain to the nearest person instead of speaking to the one who could actually help solve your problem? | ☐ | ☐ | ☐ |
| Do you tend to criticize new nurses for doing things their way instead of yours? | ☐ | ☐ | ☐ |
| Do you tend to avoid problems rather than solve them? | ☐ | ☐ | ☐ |

A nurse practiced in assertiveness skills should answer **NO** to all or almost all of the questions. If you answered **YES** or **SOMETIMES** to 10 or more questions, you could probably benefit from assertiveness training.

front a medical resident at the nurses' station and bark at him, "I'm tired of cleaning up after you and having to cover for your mistakes!" Such behavior doesn't improve her relationship with the resident or her image as a mature and reasonable nurse. Aggressive behavior may succeed sometimes, but it usually has a negative effect on working conditions.

## Assertiveness: Communicating your confidence

*An assertive nurse* strikes a balance between passivity and aggressiveness. When you're assertive, you feel an important sense of self-confidence. And because you're self-confident, you can express a full range of feelings—including affection, justified anger, and compassionate caring—openly and directly. You respond to situations promptly. You feel you can influence your working conditions.

Surely you can recall a situation when you knew you should speak up— but didn't. Because you held back, you felt frustrated. Assertiveness eliminates that reluctance to state your case, allowing you to reduce anxiety and resentment. As an assertive nurse, you can say no without feeling guilty when you're given an unreasonable assignment. You can say, "I disagree with you" as easily as you can say, "I like what you did." By being assertive, you forthrightly project your own values and judgments. But your self-confidence never becomes aggressive, because you respect others' opinions.

Assertiveness enhances patient care by giving you the confidence to ask questions—even of doctors who dislike interruptions—and to challenge information you suspect may be wrong. (See *Communication Styles: Attitudes and Reactions,* page 440.)

## How assertive responses help you get what you want

Assertive communication gives you a wider variety of responses than passive or aggressive communication provides.

The passive nurse usually makes no comment, and the aggressive nurse usually makes only critical, negative responses. As an assertive nurse, you can make such positive responses as, "I want you to know how much I learned at the inservice." You can also make negative responses, such as, "I don't like you shouting at me." And you can offer a response that sets limits, such as, "Cussing bothers me and I prefer not to hear it." All three types of responses let you express feelings appropriate to the situation, and they're likely to get the results you want. (See *Are You an Assertive Nurse?.*)

## Knowing nurses' rights

An assertive nurse is careful not to infringe on her colleagues' rights. To accomplish this, you must be sensitive to the rights that every nurse can legitimately claim in the workplace. Chenevert, a nurse educator and author, suggests 10 basic nurses' rights that emphasize the need to balance responsibilities and rights. According to Chenevert, you and your nursing colleagues have these rights:

- the right to respectful treatment from colleagues and superiors
- the right to a reasonable work load
- the right to a fair wage
- the right to choose your own priorities outside your job's responsibilities
- the right to ask for what you want or need to do your job
- the right to refuse to work unscheduled overtime or extra shifts
- the right to take personal responsibility for mistakes
- the right to give and receive patient information
- the right to act in the patient's best interest
- the right to express emotions, such as grief and joy, at appropriate times.

These rights reflect expectations about how you want to be treated. But assertive communication must be two-way to be successful, so these rights apply to other people, too. For example, your right to a reasonable work load

## COMMUNICATION STYLES: ATTITUDES AND REACTIONS

The communication style you adopt tells a lot about your personality. Each of the three principal styles—assertive, passive, and aggressive—reflects how you feel, and affects how you act in your working relations with others. This chart describes the behavior or attitude traits for each style, and how others typically react to those traits. As the chart makes clear, if you're an assertive nurse, you command more respect from your peers and have more self-esteem as a result.

| YOUR COMMUNI-CATION SYTLE | HOW YOU ACT | HOW OTHERS REACT TO YOU |
|---|---|---|
| **Assertive** | You clearly express your needs and feelings. | Others know how their behavior affects you. |
| | You stand up for your rights without violating other people's rights. | Others respect you and appreciate your fairness. |
| | You face problems promptly and suggest solutions. | Others acknowledge your efforts in problem solving. |
| | You feel confident about your skills and yourself. | Others recognize your leadership abilities. |
| **Passive** | You feel inadequate to express needs and feelings. | Others are confused about the effect of their behavior on you. |
| | You fail to stand up for your rights. | Others feel guilty, or lose respect for you. |
| | You avoid problems and fail to suggest solutions. | Others conclude that you can't contribute to improvements. |
| | You lack confidence in your skills and yourself. | Others question your clinical abilities. |
| **Aggressive** | You insist that your feelings and needs take precedence over other people's. | Others feel offended or victimized. |
| | You demand your own rights but ignore other people's rights. | Others feel threatened and mistrustful. |
| | You blame others for problems instead of offering solutions. | Others attack your accusations or withdraw in anger. |
| | You feel self-righteous and egotistical about your skills and yourself. | Others learn to avoid contact with you. |

recognizes that if you frequently work weekends and double shifts with few days off, you'll soon experience fatigue, stress, and possibly burnout. This right acknowledges that your anger and resentment build, and patient care suffers, when you're constantly subjected to an unreasonable work load. A passive nurse usually won't talk with her supervisor to resolve staffing problems; instead, she may decide that leaving her job is the only solution. As an assertive nurse, you'll take action. You'll approach your supervisor and say, "I'd like to talk with you about my work load. It's affecting my ability to give good, safe care and I'm physically and mentally exhausted. I'd like to resolve the problem, and I have some suggestions about how to do it." If the supervisor doesn't respond, you'll then go to the director of nursing and calmly restate your problem and your willingness to help resolve it. Even if the director doesn't respond, and you conclude that a transfer or a new job is your best option, you'll have the satisfaction of knowing you actively tried to find a solution.

The right to ask for what you want doesn't guarantee that you'll get it, but you'll feel better when you make your wishes known. Maybe you want orientation to a new procedure, or a special day off. If you keep silent, you'll have no hope of getting what you want and you'll increase your own frustration. But asking may get you what you want. When you do ask, take a mature, straightforward approach, speaking clearly, calmly, and honestly.

### How to become assertive
To become assertive, if you've tended to be passive or aggressive in communicating with others, you must make a conscious decision to change not only what you say, but also how you say it. And you must commit yourself to learning assertiveness skills through observation and practice. Here are some methods for learning these skills:
● Observe how others communicate, noting whether their styles are mainly assertive, passive, or aggressive.
● Practice making assertive comments—first to a mirror, then in actual situations. When doing so, always look directly into someone's eyes. Choose situations where you have a good chance of success.
● Talk with a friend about situations that make you feel passive or aggressive. Ask her to evaluate your behavior.
● Offer constructive solutions to problems instead of criticism.
● Experiment and be persistent. You *can* grow more assertive over time.

You can use other resources to help you learn assertiveness. Reading articles and books can prove helpful. So can attending consciousness-raising groups and workshops. But the best way to learn is to *practice* communicating assertively until you feel comfortable *being* assertive.

### A final word
Assertiveness makes you feel increasingly good about yourself and about being a nurse. Assertiveness won't solve all your work problems, but it *will* help you communicate more effectively and get what you want in many situations. Assertiveness will also help you deal more calmly with stress and act more firmly in your patients' behalf. When you feel more in control of yourself and your work, you'll also feel more satisfied with your job—and your life.

## Selected References

Bakdash, D.P. "Becoming an Assertive Nurse," *American Journal of Nursing* 78:1710-12, October 1978.
Chenevert, M. *Special Techniques in Assertiveness Training for Women in the Health Profession.* St. Louis: C.V. Mosby Co., 1978.
Cohen, S. "Assertiveness in Nursing, Part I," *American Journal of Nursing* 83(3):417-34, March 1983.
Edwards, Barbara J., and Brilhart, John K. *Communications in Nursing Practice.* St. Louis: C.V. Mosby Co., 1981.
Gassert, Carole, et al. "Building a Ladder," *American Journal of Nursing* 82(10):1527-30, October 1982.
Kinzel, Sharon L. "What's Your Stress Level?" *NursingLife* 2(2):54-55, March/April 1982.
O'Brien, Maureen. *Communications and Relationships in Nursing,* 2nd ed. St. Louis: C.V. Mosby Co., 1978.
Stevens, Kathleen R. *Power and Influence: A Sourcebook for Nurses.* New York: John Wiley & Sons, 1983.
Storlie, Francis J. "Burnout: The Elaboration of a Concept," *American Journal of Nursing* 79:2108-11, December 1979.

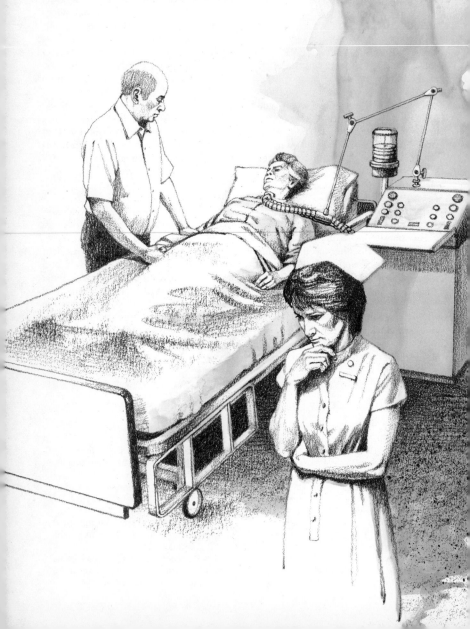

# Ethical Problems

**11**

## Introduction

How do you fulfill your professional obligation to provide adequate care and treatment when a patient exercises his right to decline life-supporting measures?

How do you meet your ethical and legal responsibilities when you suspect a colleague of professional incompetence?

These are the kinds of ethical questions you face. Modern technology has given you the ability to maintain life with artificial means. But modern society has given the consumer-patient the right to refuse such treatment. Modern professional standards have given you the responsibility to make independent ethical decisions. But modern laws are vague and confusing.

In deciding how to handle the ethical questions you face so often, you'll draw on your own experience and moral principles, of course.

But you'll also need to know how society views such questions, and how those views have shaped professional standards (such as the American Nurses' Association Code of Ethics), laws, and court decisions.

The University of Colorado Medical Center offers a course in medical ethics that suggests you use a nine-step procedure for making ethical decisions. Here's what you should do:
● Identify the health problem.

● Identify the ethical problem.
● State who's involved in making the decision (such as the nurse, the doctor, the patient, the patient's family).
● Identify your role. (Quite possibly, your role may not require a decision.)
● Consider as many possible alternative decisions as you can.
● Consider the long- and short-range consequences of each alternative decision.
● Weigh all of these considerations, and make your decision.
● Consider how this decision fits in with your general philosophy of patient care.
● Follow the situation until you can see the actual results of your decision. Use that information to help you make future decisions.

### In this chapter
The entries in this chapter *won't* give you simple answers to perplexing ethical questions in nursing today. Rather, they're intended to identify basic issues, encourage further research, and enhance ethical behavior.

The entries, along with some key questions they address, are as follows:
● Entry 70, "Life support for brain-dead or terminally ill patients." What is your proper role in caring for terminally ill patients? To prolong their lives, or ease their deaths?

• Entry 71, "Patients who want to die." What should you do when a patient asks you to help him die? Is euthanasia ever ethical?

• Entry 72, "Organ donation and transplantation." How does a person become an organ donor? And what are your responsibilities in caring for a donor or recipient?

• Entry 73, "Abortion." What's the

SURVEY

## PRACTICES POLL

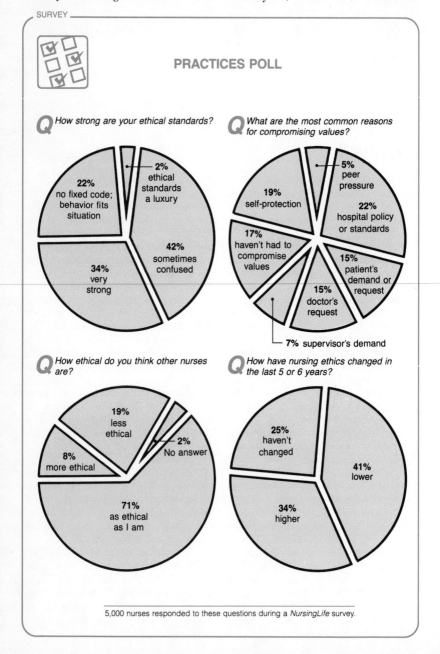

**Q** How strong are your ethical standards?

- 22% no fixed code; behavior fits situation
- 2% ethical standards a luxury
- 42% sometimes confused
- 34% very strong

**Q** What are the most common reasons for compromising values?

- 19% self-protection
- 5% peer pressure
- 22% hospital policy or standards
- 17% haven't had to compromise values
- 15% patient's demand or request
- 15% doctor's request
- 7% supervisor's demand

**Q** How ethical do you think other nurses are?

- 19% less ethical
- 2% No answer
- 8% more ethical
- 71% as ethical as I am

**Q** How have nursing ethics changed in the last 5 or 6 years?

- 25% haven't changed
- 41% lower
- 34% higher

5,000 nurses responded to these questions during a *NursingLife* survey.

# DISAGREEING WITH A DOCTOR'S DECISION TO WITHHOLD INFORMATION

Suppose a doctor decides to withhold information from your patient and, in your opinion, he has no therapeutic basis for his decision. How can you best serve your patient's interests in such a situation? You know the patient has a legal right to be told about his condition (see Entry 12), but you don't want to interfere with the doctor-patient relationship. Here's what to do:

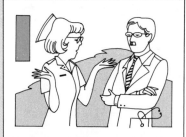

First, discuss the situation with the doctor. Ask him to clarify his reasons for withholding the information. Tell him your feelings and, if you still disagree with him, inform him, as a courtesy, that you intend to discuss the matter with your supervisor.

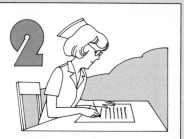

Inform your supervisor, in writing, that you disagree with the doctor's decision. Give her the facts about the patient's condition and explain why you feel the patient should be informed. She'll either handle the matter from that point or tell you why she thinks the doctor is right. If you still feel you're right, tell your supervisor, again as a courtesy, that you intend to take the matter up the nursing chain of command.

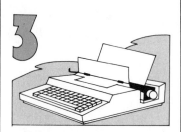

Submit a written explanation of your disagreement with the doctor and what steps you've taken so far to your supervisor's superior, probably the director of nursing. She'll tell you whether or not she intends to pursue the matter herself. If she isn't going to pursue it, tell her, as a courtesy, that you will on your own.

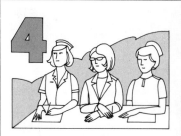

Submit your disagreement, in writing, to your institution's committee on multidisciplinary practice. The committee will issue a ruling on the matter.

# HOW DIFFERENT GROUPS OF SURVEYED NURSES FEEL ABOUT THEIR ETHICS

| WHO'S MORE LIKELY? | YOUNGER NURSES | or OLDER NURSES |
| --- | --- | --- |
| To think ethics are much lower today than they were 5 or 6 years ago? | ◆ | |
| To question doctors' orders if they appear unsafe? | | ◆ |
| To feel doctors are the best judges about how much a patient should know? | ◆ | |
| To say they haven't deceived patients about their medications? | ◆ | |
| To have taken supplies for personal use? | | ◆ |
| To say they're asked to cover up mistakes more often? | | ◆ |
| To worry less about "looking bad" in their notes? | ◆ | |
| To call a code for a terminally ill patient in the absence of specific orders? | | ◆ |
| To say they wouldn't give substandard care to a welfare mother having an illegitimate child...or to a suspected rapist? | ◆ | |

| WHO'S MORE LIKELY? | STAFF NURSES/ TEAM LEADERS | or SUPERVISORY NURSES |
| --- | --- | --- |
| To consider leaving nursing if they had the chance? | ◆ | |
| To feel doctors are often dishonest with patients? | | ◆ |
| To refuse passing medications if they had to float to an unfamiliar unit? | | ◆ |
| To fill out a med error form only if their error is serious? | ◆ | |
| To excuse themselves from doing a job evaluation of a friend? | ◆ | |
| To say they wouldn't offer information about a patient's injury in a hospital? | | ◆ |
| To call a code for a terminally ill patient in the absence of specific orders? | ◆ | |

| WHO'S MORE LIKELY? | LPNs/LVNs or | RNs |
|---|---|---|
| To worry that ethical compromises *might harm patients*? | | 🩺 |
| To worry that ethical compromises *might get them into legal trouble*? | 🩺 | |
| To say doctors are rarely dishonest with patients and their families? | 🩺 | |
| To say doctors have asked them to cover up mistakes? | | 🩺 |
| To be less tolerant of nurses' abusing patients? | 🩺 | |
| To be less tolerant of drug/alcohol abuse on duty? | | 🩺 |
| To discuss cases with others, using discretion to protect patients? | | 🩺 |
| To be comfortable caring for criminals? | 🩺 | |

| WHO'S MORE LIKELY? | NURSING HOME NURSES or | HOSPITAL NURSES |
|---|---|---|
| To view nursing as their lifelong career? | 🩺 | |
| To feel they're conscientious all or most of the time? | | 🩺 |
| To worry most about a guilty conscience if they have to compromise standards? | | 🩺 |
| To have taken supplies for personal use? | 🩺 | |
| To avoid discussing patients with others? | | 🩺 |
| To give patients placebos more frequently? | | 🩺 |
| To call a code for a terminally ill patient in the absence of specific orders? | 🩺 | |
| To assist a man who collapsed in a hospital parking lot, though they aren't covered by professional liability insurance? | 🩺 | |

## IS THE ANA CODE FOR NURSES A LAW?

*Does the American Nurses' Association (ANA) Code for Nurses carry any legal weight? Could I lose my nursing license if I violated that code?*—RN, Mo.

No. You won't lose your license if you violate the 11-point ANA code. Membership in the ANA is voluntary, so you can't be bound by the ANA code. Keep in mind, however, that the code sets *ethical* standards of conduct and practice for the nursing profession. And it can be cited as a guideline for professional conduct and your relationships in a malpractice lawsuit. So you should be aware of the code's provisions, and how they apply.

Of course, you can lose your license for violating your state's nurse practice act, which sets *legal* practice standards for nurses in your state.

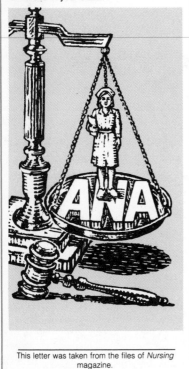

This letter was taken from the files of *Nursing* magazine.

current legal status of abortion? And what are your responsibilities in caring for a patient who's having an abortion?

● Entry 74, "No-code and slow-code: The legalities and ethics." Under what conditions can a written policy regarding orders not to resuscitate patients safeguard doctors and nurses? What's the legal status of so-called slow-code orders?

● Entry 75, "When a colleague is incompetent." How do you decide whether a colleague is incompetent? And what should you do if she is?

### A final word

A study of the ethical issues in this chapter offers several benefits. It will increase your effectiveness as a care giver and decision maker by helping you understand the value systems and legal standards that operate in clinical situations. It will help you recognize situations with a potential for conflict, enabling you to work through them before a conflict develops.

Above all, this chapter will help you understand your own moral code—and how it serves as a basis for your nursing actions and decisions.

# 70 Life support for brain-dead or terminally ill patients

When you help resuscitate terminally ill patients or provide care to replace their vital functions (such as kidney function) with machines, are you prolonging life—or prolonging dying?

This question isn't just an exercise in semantics. It's a question that goes to the very heart of your professional ethics. It's really asking: What are the proper roles of medicine and nursing in caring for the dying?

The technology that prompts these questions is only a few decades old. Until then, little could be done to prolong a dying patient's life. Today, death can often be significantly delayed. But should it be?

Holding death at bay requires a great deal of skill on your part. Not only do you have to develop technologic expertise and the confidence to apply it quickly, but you also have to deliver that expertise in a way that makes prolonged life bearable for your patient and his family.

And holding death at bay takes time. Dying patients receiving extraordinary life support—such as artificial respirators, resuscitators for cardiopulmonary arrests, and dialysis—require extraordinary amounts of your time, keeping you away from other patients.

Meanwhile, the ethical questions keep nagging at you. Should you ignore the needs of patients whose conditions are improving but who will soon deteriorate no matter what you do? Should you do all you can to keep a comatose patient alive without knowing what he'd *want* you to do? Should you abide by a family's plea to "do all you can" when the whole situation is so remote from their daily lives that they can barely understand what you're doing or why?

You've seen the same confusion in your co-workers' attitudes toward maintaining or withdrawing life support, so you can't even look to them for guidance.

In fact, the confusion exists in all levels of our society—among professionals and lay people, in our legislatures, and in the institutions we've traditionally depended on to give us ethical and legal guidance: our churches and our courts.

## Society's view of life-support measures

Extraordinary life-support measures themselves are generally accepted. Most people in our society favor using these measures when a patient has a temporary or reversible threat to his life. Ongoing debate, however, centers on the uses of extraordinary life-

GLOSSARY

## KEY TERMS IN THIS ENTRY

**brain death** • Generally, the cessation of brain wave activity. The legal definition of this condition varies from state to state.

**extraordinary life-support measures** • Resuscitative efforts and therapies done to replace a patient's natural vital functions.

**living will** • A witnessed document indicating a patient's desire to be allowed to die a natural death, rather than be kept alive by heroic, life-sustaining measures.

**quality of life** • A legal and ethical standard that's determined by relative suffering or pain, not by the degree of disability.

**resuscitative life-support measures** • Actions taken to reverse an immediate, life-threatening situation; for example, cardiopulmonary resuscitation.

**right-to-die law** • A law that upholds a patient's right to choose death by refusing extraordinary treatment when the patient has no hope of recovery. Also referred to as a *natural death law* or *living-will law*.

**substitutive judgment** • A legal term indicating the court's substitution of its own judgment for that of a person the court considers unable to make an informed decision, such as an incompetent adult.

support measures with the dying.

Some people propose that such measures are appropriate only when they will improve the quality of a person's life. But they can't agree on a definition of quality. Does improving the quality mean diminishing the suffering? Or does it mean increasing the patient's cognitive awareness, mental competence, productivity, or social worth?

Before allowing for extraordinary measures—such as transplants—to be used, medical ethics boards add two more considerations: Will the patient be able to cope with the results? And will society have the resources to support them?

People generally favor extending life in some situations and letting it end in others. You may have found that your

## WITHDRAWING LIFE SUPPORT: WHO DECIDES?

Who has the legal right to decide whether to withdraw life-support treatment? Usually, the patient alone.

The terminally ill adult who's legally competent has the right to refuse any treatment, including life-sustaining treatment.

If a patient becomes unconscious or incompetent but his wishes are certain, your hospital may withdraw or withhold life support without applying to the courts for a ruling. A patient's wishes are considered certain if he's previously expressed his views or his desires on the matter of life

support in a living will or less formally to his family.

If the patient has been judged incompetent and no one knows what his wishes were when competent, then you can't withhold life-support treatment without a court order. This is also true if the patient is a minor or if he's never been competent. And, except in states with natural death acts, a court order is needed to withdraw life-support treatment once it's been initiated.

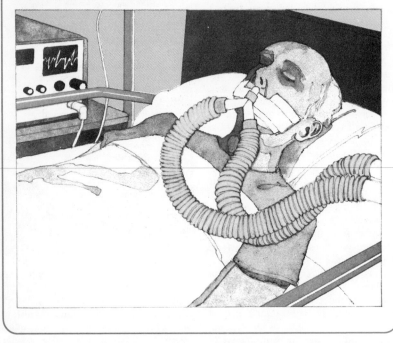

own beliefs vary with different situations. For example, you may believe in withdrawing or withholding intervention to let death occur naturally, in theory. But you may favor extraordinary measures for patients who request them—because you don't think you have a right to try to influence patients' decisions.

Religious beliefs also play into the debate. Some religious groups, such as Christian Scientists, emphasize their reliance on God, not medical interven-

tion. Others accept most forms of medical intervention but seek to define their limits. The Jehovah's Witnesses define limits on *specific kinds* of intervention, forbidding blood transfusions even in life-threatening emergencies. The Roman Catholic church, on the other hand, defines limits on *specific situations* in which intervention is used. For example, in 1980, the Catholic Church upheld the patient's right to refuse extraordinary treatment to protect "both the dignity of the human person and the Christian concept of life against a technological attitude that threatens to become an abuse."

In the midst of this debate, you must contribute and carry out decisions regarding terminally ill patients—when to provide life support and when not to; when to switch on mechanical equipment, and when to turn it off; when to resuscitate, and when not to. Inevitably, many of these decisions have legal as well as ethical dimensions. So you must protect yourself and your patients by finding out how the legislatures and the courts have viewed such decisions in the past.

## U.S. and Canadian laws on treatment of the terminally ill

Unfortunately, current state and provincial laws governing treatment of the terminally ill vary—in large part because no one can define a satisfactory point where a terminal illness becomes terminal.

The Canadian Criminal Code, for example, says that doctors and nurses have a legal duty to perform an act if the omission of that act is or may be dangerous to life. Does this mean that health-care professionals have a duty to use all extraordinary means available to keep all patients alive? Well, the answer depends on your definitions of "alive" and "dead."

As you know, the traditional definition of death—cessation of cardiopulmonary functions—has been outdated by technology. (See *Defining Brain Death*, page 108.) With mechanical support, cardiopulmonary functions can be artificially maintained for long periods of time. This obviously creates a double-bind situation: we have to keep treating the patient until he dies, but he can't die as long as we keep treating him.

One response to this dilemma was a more sophisticated definition of death, based on the concept of brain death. Although a few states have adopted laws defining brain death, most states haven't, evidently accepting the Amer-ican Medical Association's position that "death shall be determined by the clinical judgment of the physician using the necessary, available, and currently accepted criteria."

But some states have supported the belief that patients themselves should play a major role in deciding whether—and when—extraordinary measures are appropriate.

## Right-to-die laws

In 13 states and the District of Columbia, the responsibility for deciding whether to provide or continue life support is shared by the patient. These states are the states that have right-to-die or living-will laws. (See *Living-Will Laws*, pages 186 to 189.)

According to the earliest of these, the 1977 California Natural Death Act, a patient with a terminal illness may sign a "directive" asking his doctor not to use life-prolonging measures. The patient must sign the directive while he's emotionally and mentally competent. He must have two witnesses—and neither witness can be involved in his care. And he must wait for 14 days after the diagnosis of his terminal illness to make such a directive. Once made, however, it's legally binding on the health-care team, unless the patient revokes it.

Similar provisions are found in the right-to-die laws of 12 other states and the District of Columbia (see Entries 13 and 30). All emphasize the voluntary aspect of the patient's decision, and all permit only the withholding or withdrawing of treatment.

Worth noting, too, is the legal status of living wills (see Entry 30). Even in states without right-to-die laws, the wills provide a record of the patient's wishes at a time when he was competent, and they may serve as a basis for later court decisions about terminating treatment.

Because patients have the right to refuse treatment, no legal problem arises when a mentally competent adult refuses lifesaving or life-support treat-

## FROM THE HEART

Here's a picture of nursing ethics straight from the heart. Nurses like you sent in these letters with their responses to nursing ethics surveys. Two of these nurses graphically describe the conflicts they felt when the care ordered for terminally ill patients clashed with their personal nursing ethics.

"Before taking my present position as office nurse for an internist, I worked in a coronary care–intensive care unit for 4 years. I became thoroughly convinced that people should be allowed to die with dignity. To have to resuscitate an 80- or 90-year-old patient when he was tired of living and requesting to die, is cruel. Or to keep a patient on life-sustaining equipment even with a flat EEG, is cruel for the family as well as the patient. A class I recently took on bioethics helped me look closer at my feelings and face some of the ethical questions that we often try to run away from."

"I believe my values have not changed in 25 years of nursing, but that my experience and maturity have helped me to reaffirm them....the dignity of the patient in terminal illness must be maintained. And the patient and his family continue to need education in these matters.

"There are many things worse than death. I would never hesitate to give a respiration-depressing drug to a terminal patient in pain. Yet, I would never intentionally give an overdose.

"The definition of what constitutes life should not be a matter for the courts. Termination of life-support systems should follow consultation between family, physician, and spiritual advisor."

"I was recently involved in a situation that put me in the middle of a family's request and the doctor's order. The patient was a man in his seventies with a past history of severe cardiac disease, CVA [cerebrovascular accident], and now terminal cancer and a recent respiratory arrest, leaving him in our intensive care unit on a respirator and unresponsive. During my shift, the patient arrested again, and our resuscitation efforts were successful once more. His wife and son then came to visit, and when I told his wife about her husband's most recent condition, the wife asked why he was being 'tortured' this way, since she and her son had both expressed their desire to let him die in peace without further 'heroics' after the first time he had been coded. She said the attending physician was aware of her wishes, however we had no legal no-code order at that time. The physician had been notified of the patient's second respiratory arrest and was now on his way to the hospital. I explained the situation to the wife and son, and told them we would all speak with the doctor when he arrived and get the order not to resuscitate. Unfortunately, the patient then had a cardiac arrest before the doctor arrived and one of the other nurses began CPR [cardiopulmonary resuscitation]. While we worked on the patient, his son came into the room and very calmly, but adamantly, told us, "No! No more—stop and let him die." The son then left the room, leaving us standing there quite stunned. The resident in charge of the code then told us to continue CPR. I immediately refused as did the other two nurses present, telling the resident of the earlier conversation I had with the wife and son. I suggested to the resident that if he wanted CPR resumed, that he should do it, but he also just stood there, unsure of what to do. At that time, the intern and respiratory therapist resumed CPR, until the attending physician arrived about 5 to 10 minutes later. After he asked about the surrounding circumstances, he finally decided to stop the CPR, and our patient died.

"We discussed the whole experience with our nursing supervisor. She agreed it was a 'sticky' situation, but said since we did not have a no-code order, we could not take an order from a family member, as when the son came into the room and told us to stop our efforts—we should have continued CPR. This just left all of us upset and confused. It's a shame that our society is so 'sue-happy' that we have to become so legally aware during a time like this, even when a family's wishes were being so clearly expressed but we had to wait for the physician to 'give the word'."

ments (see *Withdrawing Life Support: Who Decides?*, page 450).

But what if the patient later becomes incompetent? For example, suppose a competent patient refuses dialysis. Eventually, because of increasing uremia, he becomes obtunded and unable to make decisions. If he then develops pneumonia and needs ventilatory support, should the doctor prescribe it?

Each situation would have to be judged on its own merits. Generally, however, courts have ruled that—when no reasonable chance of recovery exists—extraordinary medical care may be withheld from terminally ill and incompetent patients who have previously, "clearly and convincingly,"

## YOUR ROLE IN WITHHOLDING OR WITHDRAWING LIFE SUPPORT

Suppose the terminally ill patient you're caring for refuses life-support treatment. You've been trained to provide, not withhold, health care. What's your role now?

Your frequent contact with the patient puts you in an opportune position to support his decision. This includes letting the patient express his feelings about his situation and assisting him in getting answers to questions about his prognosis, treatments, side effects, and so on.

If the patient is unconscious and the family participates in making the decision to withhold life-support measures, they'll need your help. Family members will probably experience ambivalent feelings. In part, these feelings stem from confusion over prognosis. Family members may be torn between a belief that "where there's life, there's hope" and a desire to end the loved one's suffering. They'll also feel grief, which may be disrupted by the slowness of the dying process and by confusion over the meaning of slight changes in the patient's condition. Some family members feel guilt; many feel anger.

With family dynamics disrupted as different members deal with their grief at a different pace, the family will need you to help prepare them for the crisis and to assist them through it. Encourage them to express their feelings. Reassure them concerning their participation in making the decision. Answer all their questions about alternatives. Help them cope by encouraging them to use supportive resources. If members experience spiritual distress, you may refer them to the chaplain, if appropriate. In some hospitals, life support can be withdrawn over a period of hours, instead of abruptly. This method can help the family cope because it facilitates a peaceful, more natural dying process.

Whenever you're caring for the terminally ill patient on life support, you should know your state law regarding the definition of death and the binding nature of living wills. For more information on both subjects, see Entries 17 and 30. Also, keep accurate and complete documentation of events surrounding life-support termination and the patient's death. The legal importance of your records can't be overestimated.

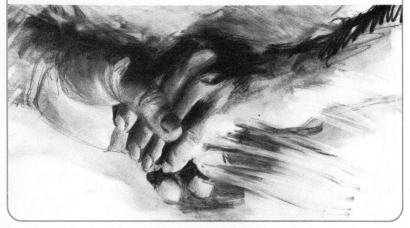

expressed opposition to the use of extraordinary life-support measures. Thus, a living will—a prior directive—would "clearly and convincingly" express his wishes, and should be followed.

## The rights of incompetent patients

The question of a patient's right to refuse treatment is more complicated, of course, if the patient is incompetent.

Generally, however, the courts have relied on substitutive judgment when they decide this question for incompetent adults. That is, they try to decide what the patient would have decided if he'd been legally competent. The courts attempt to balance such diverse factors as discomfort and pain, possible side effects of treatment, and prospective benefits.

Only rarely, out of a conviction that treatment would permit the patient to live a useful life, do the courts overrule the patient's decision or wishes. Sometimes, if the patient's death would leave his children orphaned, the court might use this as a basis to overrule his decision.

## Four court cases

Among court cases involving incompetent patients, four deserve mention here:
- *In re Quinlan* (1976)
- *Superintendent of Belchertown State School v. Saikewicz* (1977)
- *Eichner v. Dillon* (1980)
- *In re Storar* (1981).

In both the Quinlan (New Jersey) and Saikewicz (Massachusetts) cases, the courts emphasized that a patient's right to refuse treatment is not forfeited by incompetence. In the Quinlan case, the court allowed treatment to be withdrawn; in the Saikewicz case, the court allowed treatment to be withheld. Both rulings were based on what the patient would presumably have decided if he'd been able to make the decision personally (substitutive judgment).

The New Jersey court gave Ms. Quin-

lan's "guardian and family" the right to withdraw Ms. Quinlan's life support in the face of conflicting prognoses. Her parents were thus granted the authority to make a decision on her behalf. The guardian can exercise this authority if the family and the doctor concur that "no reasonable possibility" exists that the patient will return to a "cognitive, sapient state," and if a hospital ethics committee agrees.

In the Saikewicz case, the Massachusetts court allowed withholding of cancer chemotherapy from a developmentally disabled man because prolonging his life for a few months wasn't in his best interest. The Saikewicz case involved substitutive judgment to withhold treatment for a patient who could never have made a competent decision

---

*"The courts rarely over-rule the patient's decision regarding life support."*

---

himself. The court upheld the decision to withhold treatment because of the likelihood of adverse side effects, the small chance of remission, and the certainty that treatment would cause the patient further suffering.

In the Eichner case, the New York State appeals court accepted a patient's earlier wishes as sufficient reason not to maintain his life by "extraordinary means." The patient, a priest, had discussed Karen Quinlan's situation with other priests and indicated that if he were ever in the same situation, he would want the respirator disconnected.

These three cases seem to show the role of substitutive judgment clearly. The *In re Storar* case, however, muddies the water. In this case, the New York State appeals court ruled that Storar's transfusions should be continued despite a prognosis of only 6 months to live. Because Storar had never been competent and could never have made his own decision, the court said it had no way of knowing what the patient would have wanted. Although some doctors and attorneys disagree with the decision, further clarification must await another court challenge.

In reviewing these four decisions, several points clearly emerge. First, the courts are most concerned with protecting the patient's right of self-determination. Second, the courts are ready to leave medical decisions, specifically diagnoses and prognoses, in the doctors' hands. And third, when making decisions on behalf of incompetent patients, the courts look closely at the patients' previous wishes, medical prognoses, potential suffering, and quality of continued life.

## Deciding on what action to take

As a nurse who cares for terminally ill patients, you don't have the luxury of waiting until all the ethical and legal arguments are settled. You will often be forced to implement a medical regimen, whether you agree with it or not. To handle this difficult situation, remember these guidelines.

You can contribute to the medical decision-making process in several ways. You can observe and report a patient's physical and emotional status. And you can support your patient's decisions and make sure his doctor and other members of the health-care team hear about them.

In addition, you can volunteer for hospital committees charged with developing policies on life support, resuscitation, no-code, and critical care unit admissions. (See Entry 74.) Be sure all new policies both spell out criteria to be applied in specific situations and require written documentation of any clinical decisions and discussions with patients and families.

If you work with patients receiving extended life support, someday someone (most likely a doctor) will order you to "pull the plug" or to stop further treatment. When this happens, protect yourself—and the patient—by observing these precautions:

• Ask your hospital's legal department about the legality of the decision to discontinue treatment.

• Insist that the order be put in writing, with the doctor's signature, before you carry it out. (See Entry 74.)

• Check the patient's medical record to make sure it either clearly states that the patient is brain dead or indicates why treatment is being discontinued. For example, the record might show that a court decision was obtained. Or it might elaborate on the patient's prognosis and summarize discussions with the patient and family regarding continued treatment.

• Review hospital documentation policies to verify that the record is complete.

• Make sure the person making the decision to discontinue treatment is authorized to do so. In some hospitals, the attending doctor may write the order; in others, a doctor's department head may need to concur in the order. If an organ will be removed for transplantation, the doctors involved with either the transplantation or the organ retrieval program cannot make the decision.

• Keep your nurses' notes current. Make sure they supply a complete record of continuing care and indicate exactly when you reduced or terminated each treatment. If brain death is the basis for withdrawing treatment, the pronouncement of death should precede the discontinuation of life support.

### A final word

Apart from all legalities, your job is to make sure the patient's last hours are as comfortable as possible. And pay special attention to his family's needs; even though they've agreed to the patient's death, this is a difficult time for them. In short, be a nurse in the fullest sense of the word—a professional who's caring and compassionate.

# 71 Patients who want to die

Who should decide whether to give or withhold lifesaving treatment? In the two situations that follow, the patients have made decisions about how their lives should end. How would you respond?

Mrs. Keeley, an 85-year-old widow, has lived at the Shady Valley Nursing Home for nearly 4 years. You've always considered her a bright, cheerful person—one who loves to mix with the other residents.

But she's also a practical person. "When my time comes," she's often told you and other nurses, "I want you to let me go naturally. After all, I've had a full life, my children are all busy raising large families of their own, and my money won't last forever. Besides, my husband Jack is waiting for me to join him in heaven."

This morning, while making your rounds, you find Mrs. Keeley slumped over in her bed. You speak to her, but she doesn't answer. When you check her pulse, you find it weak and irregular.

The question: What do you do now?

Mr. Perillo, a carpenter in his early fifties, has spent the past 4 days on your surgical unit, where you're working the night shift. His problem is lung cancer, which is causing severe pain and a frightening shortness of breath. Even worse, his doctor told him earlier today that the cancer will no longer respond to medical therapy.

At about 3 a.m., Mr. Perillo complains of pain, so you bring him an as-needed medication. While you sit with him, he tells you his health insurance benefits are about to run out. He mentions that he and his wife have drifted apart during the past several years. Despite this, she's agreed to continue working to support the family, which includes two teenage children.

"Look," he suddenly tells you, "I want to die. It'll spare me a lot of pain, free my wife, and provide insurance money so my kids can go to college. Please, help me get some pills so I can end it all right away."

The question: What do you do now?

These two stories are fictional. Still, they represent situations you may face if you work with dying patients.

At any given time, a million Americans are living with a terminal prognosis. And each year, 2 million Americans die—80% of them in hospitals or other institutions where nurses have direct-line responsibility. Obviously, the more you know about the ethical and legal dimensions of caring for the dying, the better you'll be able to handle situations such as the ones just described.

## The ethics of withholding care

Given America's cultural and religious diversity, you would expect viewpoints about elective death to vary widely. For some Americans, the thought of withholding life support is abhorrent. This view probably comes from our society's preoccupation with youth and health and a perception of death as something apart from life—a stark tragedy to be avoided at all costs.

For other Americans, letting a patient die a natural death is not only a

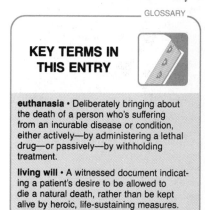

GLOSSARY

**KEY TERMS IN THIS ENTRY**

**euthanasia** • Deliberately bringing about the death of a person who's suffering from an incurable disease or condition, either actively—by administering a lethal drug—or passively—by withholding treatment.

**living will** • A witnessed document indicating a patient's desire to be allowed to die a natural death, rather than be kept alive by heroic, life-sustaining measures.

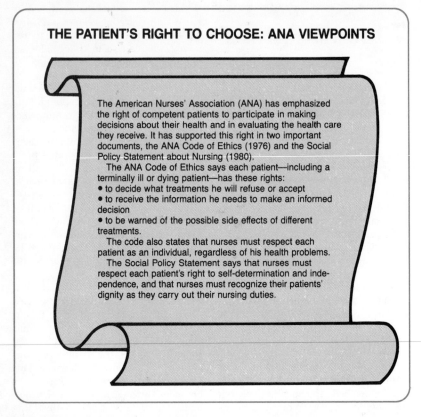

## THE PATIENT'S RIGHT TO CHOOSE: ANA VIEWPOINTS

The American Nurses' Association (ANA) has emphasized the right of competent patients to participate in making decisions about their health and in evaluating the health care they receive. It has supported this right in two important documents, the ANA Code of Ethics (1976) and the Social Policy Statement about Nursing (1980).

The ANA Code of Ethics says each patient—including a terminally ill or dying patient—has these rights:
- to decide what treatments he will refuse or accept
- to receive the information he needs to make an informed decision
- to be warned of the possible side effects of different treatments.

The code also states that nurses must respect each patient as an individual, regardless of his health problems.

The Social Policy Statement says that nurses must respect each patient's right to self-determination and independence, and that nurses must recognize their patients' dignity as they carry out their nursing duties.

mark of clear thinking but also of love and concern for a suffering patient.

This group views mercy as a moral obligation, and compassion as the motivating force behind any decision to let a patient die. Accordingly, death isn't the worst thing that can befall an individual. Thus, acts of omission (not instituting life-support measures) as well as acts of commission (withdrawing already instituted life-support measures) are moral when the result and the intent are in the patient's best interest.

In regard to a patient like Mrs. Keeley—who told you many times to let her die a natural death—this group would urge you not to try to prolong her life. They would tell you that your patient's integrity as a human being demands that she be given the right to choose, and that protecting her choice is more important than continuing her biological functions.

Most religious groups agree that health professionals aren't obligated to preserve life in all terminal cases. The religious position is also based on the proposition that human life is more than biologic function—it must also evidence certain qualities of self-awareness and cognition to merit the name "human life." Thus today's religious thinkers agree with their ancient counterparts who asserted that the essence of human character lies in a person's rational faculties.

## Applying general principles
But theory sometimes falls apart in practice. Even those Americans who support the general principle that a patient has a right to choose a natural death may feel differently when the

general principle is applied to a specific patient, especially someone they know.

Mrs. Keeley's children, for example, may suddenly reverse their previous support for their mother's right to die in the emotionally charged hours when you have to implement her decision to "do nothing." Because of guilt, fear, anger, or an overwhelming feeling of loss, they may insist on continuing life support regardless of her wishes.

Your dilemma may also be complicated by pressure from doctors and other nurses who urge the use of new or experimental techniques that may help others in the future.

And, finally, you may face the stress of your own contradictory impulses. You may recognize all patients' rights to be spared heroic yet futile procedures. Yet you may feel that actually withholding those procedures from a particular patient conflicts with your professional (and, usually, legal) commitment to do everything possible.

## Look for guidelines
Before you find yourself in a situation where you're forced to make crucial decisions between life and death and ordinary and extraordinary measures, try to clarify your professional and legal obligations.

Read your institution's policy on withholding care. If your hospital doesn't have one, volunteer to develop one.

Read your state or provincial nurse practice act, and examine the standards and codes of ethics of professional societies (see *The Patient's Right To Choose: ANA Viewpoints*).

Find out which laws your state has passed protecting patients' right to die natural deaths. The most common laws protecting this right are called right-to-die laws or living-will laws (see Entry 30). But your state may have other laws relating to death and the care of the dying, such as laws covering brain death, resuscitation, defibrillation, and medication administration.

And, finally, keep up with nursing

## HOSPICE CARE: A GROWING ALTERNATIVE

Hospice care shifts the emphasis of care from the traditional goal of lifesaving at all costs to that of palliative care or assistance with dying. Using a multidisciplinary team, a hospice tries to provide the highest quality care for the remaining life of the terminally ill patient.

By concentrating on pain and symptom control and psychosocial and spiritual support, the hospice staff practices euthanasia in its most literal sense—it aims to provide an easy, painless death.

According to Cicely Saunders, founder of the modern hospice movement, active listening, support, and adequate pain and symptom control decrease patients' yearning for a quick death. With adequate support during the dying process, they'll want to be able to experience all the "good" living time they have left. This assertion, however, has only anecdotal, not statistical, support.

For some patients and their families, hospice care represents a natural, humane, dignified, ethical, and legally uncomplicated approach to death.

For nurses, hospice care theoretically resolves the legal dilemmas about the validity of informed consent, the appropriateness of calling a "no code," and the possible liability for being involved in involuntary euthanasia. In the last decade, the movement has grown rapidly and has been virtually unchallenged in the courts.

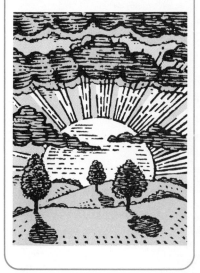

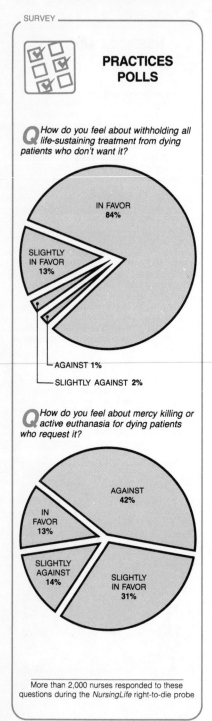

**PRACTICES POLLS**

**Q** *How do you feel about withholding all life-sustaining treatment from dying patients who don't want it?*

IN FAVOR
84%

SLIGHTLY IN FAVOR
13%

AGAINST 1%

SLIGHTLY AGAINST 2%

**Q** *How do you feel about mercy killing or active euthanasia for dying patients who request it?*

AGAINST
42%

IN FAVOR
13%

SLIGHTLY AGAINST
14%

SLIGHTLY IN FAVOR
31%

More than 2,000 nurses responded to these questions during the *NursingLife* right-to-die probe

literature that tells you how current court decisions reflect and shape the ethics of letting a patient die.

## Court decisions on the right to die

The courts have generally upheld the right of competent patients to make life-or-death medical choices. In this way, courts have supported the ethical view that doctors and nurses are consultants who provide expert advice. But patients are the final arbiters of their own lives.

True, the courts sometimes overrule a patient's right. For example, they may empower doctors to give lifesaving treatment to minors even though the minors' legal guardians seek to withhold treatment. And the courts may empower doctors to give lifesaving treatment to competent adults if failure to give such care could leave orphaned children.

But these exceptions are rare. The decision of *In re Osborne* (1972) is more typical of the courts' attitude toward patients' right to die. This case involved a Jehovah's Witness who refused blood transfusions on religious grounds. Citing the First Amendment, the court supported his right to refuse lifesaving treatment even though he had a young wife and two dependent children.

In the case *In re Quinlan* (1976), the court established the right of patients or their proxies to authorize the withdrawal of life-support mechanisms. And in *Superintendent of Belchertown State School v. Saikewicz* (1977), the court supported the right of incompetent patients to refuse life-prolonging measures, such as chemotherapy.

## Implementing your decision

If you can ethically support the decision to let a patient like Mrs. Keeley die, continue to provide all normal nursing support and comfort. Pay special attention to the patient's hygiene, grooming, and mouth care. Also, continue to talk to her and explain what's happening—even if she's comatose.

In short, show the same care and respect you'd show if her recovery were certain.

If you can't accept the decision to let a patient die, explain your position to your supervisor and ask to be relieved of your assignment.

### Letting someone die versus helping someone die
The ethics involved with a patient like Mr. Perillo—who asks you to give him a fatal overdose of pills—are very different. Although social and legal prohibitions against suicide have been modified, the ancient Western religious injunction against suicide continues to exert a powerful legal and ethical influence. Even those who agree with the idea of letting a disease run its course make a moral distinction between this inaction against death and the direct action of causing death.

One ethical basis for this distinction comes from the biblical injunction "You shall not kill" (Exodus 20:13). Its adherents insist that all killing is wrong, that the body must be respected, and that the sanctity of life, not the quality of life, is the paramount principle.

Clearly, you can't act alone to help a patient like Mr. Perillo die. But that doesn't mean you can't help him at all. When you find yourself in such a situation, try to determine whether the patient is acting out of a firm conviction or expressing a temporary depression. If he seems sincerely committed, ask his permission to contact his doctor to try to find ways to support his wishes.

Depending on your state laws, charting his comments, or the existence of a living will, may lay the groundwork for withholding life-support measures later in his care.

### A final word
For you, as a nurse, an ethical and compassionate response to a patient who wants to die involves listening, accepting, and trying to help him fulfill his wish. You needn't do more—but you should never do less.

# 72 Organ donation and transplantation

Jack Bowen, a 20-year-old university student, was driving home for Christmas vacation. Suddenly, his car swerved off the road and crashed head-on into a tree. A passing motorist found Jack unconscious with his head against the steering wheel.

An hour later, Jack was brought into the emergency department of the nearest hospital. He had no spontaneous respirations and no reflex response to painful stimuli. His pupils were nonreactive with no doll's eye movement. After being stabilized on a respirator, Jack was transferred to the intensive care unit.

By the time his parents arrived the next morning, Jack had had two flat EEGs, 24 hours apart. Each showed no brain wave activity. Jack's doctor told the parents that these and other tests met the generally accepted medical criteria for death and the state's legal definition of brain death. He offered his sympathy, answered a few questions, and left.

Jack's nurse stayed with the parents after the doctor left. She listened to their expressions of pain and confusion and tried to comfort and support them. The nurse also got more information for them when they asked about donating

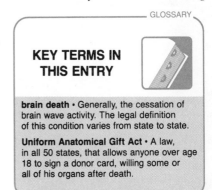

GLOSSARY

### KEY TERMS IN THIS ENTRY

**brain death** • Generally, the cessation of brain wave activity. The legal definition of this condition varies from state to state.

**Uniform Anatomical Gift Act** • A law, in all 50 states, that allows anyone over age 18 to sign a donor card, willing some or all of his organs after death.

# ANSWERING YOUR PATIENT'S QUESTIONS ABOUT ORGAN DONATION

Your dying patient may want to discuss organ donation with you. So that you can help him reach a decision, the National Kidney Foundation has prepared answers to some of the questions you'll probably be asked.

**Q** *Is there a need for organ donors?*

**A** Yes. Thousands of lives every year are lost because donors of kidneys and other organs are so scarce.

**Q** *How can I become a donor?*

**A** Sign a donor card in the presence of two witnesses who also sign. You have several donor options: You can donate any organ or part that is needed; you can restrict the donation to the organs or parts you specify; or you can donate your entire body for anatomical study.

**Q** *Is there an age requirement for donors?*

**A** Yes. Anyone older than age 18 may become a donor. A person age 18 or younger must have his parents' permission.

**Q** *Do I have to register with an agency?*

**A** No. Your signed, witnessed donor card is all that's needed.

**Q** *Do I have to mention the organ donation in my will?*

**A** No. You may mention it in your will if you wish, but your donor card is a kind of pocket will and is all you need. Obviously this makes the card important. Tell your family and your doctor of your wishes to ensure their cooperation.

**Q** *Can I change my mind later?*

**A** Yes. Simply tear up the card. Nothing else is necessary.

**Q** *Can I be sure my gift will be used?*

**A** You can be sure it will be used if possible. Sometimes, of course, an organ can't be used because no compatible recipient can be found or because the organ isn't healthy.

**Q** *When will my gift be used?*

**A** The organ will probably be removed within an hour after death. According to the Uniform Anatomical Gift Act (the model law that governs organ donation issues in each state), the doctor in attendance is responsible for determining that life has ceased and that the donor's wishes may be carried out. The act specifies, however, that the doctor attending the dying person not participate in either the removal or the transplantation. That's the job of the hospital and the transplant team.

**Q** *Does organ donation affect funeral and burial arrangements?*

**A** No. Removal of organs or tissues won't interfere with customary funeral or burial arrangements. These remain the responsibility of relatives or persons in charge of the estate. If you want to will your body to a medical center for anatomical study, you must make arrangements with the medical center.

Adapted with permission from The National Kidney Foundation, Inc.

some of Jack's organs. As the mother said, "At least it'll make some sense out of this senseless situation."

The next day, Jack was pronounced dead and taken to the operating room, where the organs to be donated were removed. His eyes went to a man who'd been blind for 5 years. And his kidneys

went to two people: a mother with two children and a young college student like Jack.

Jack's case is hardly unusual. For example, some 5,000 kidney transplants are performed each year in the United States. In addition, doctors performed 309 heart, 268 liver, 37 lung, and 49 pancreas transplants in a recent sample year.

You may already have cared for a transplant donor or recipient. If you haven't, you probably will. At that point, you'll find yourself facing a number of important medical, ethical, and legal issues.

## Medical and ethical issues

Medically speaking, the number of transplants is increasing because of three main developments:
* improved surgical techniques
* more success with medications to suppress immunologic response to transplanted organs
* improved ability to type tissues correctly.

In addition, today's technology allows organs to be preserved for a longer time—and, if necessary, to be flown to recipients all over the world. And organs are welcomed in more and more nations, as both the idea of transplantation and the acceptance of brain-death criteria gain increasing approval.

Ethically, the decision to donate or accept an organ usually rests with the answer to the key question: Dare I make a decision that involves taking organs from one person's body to save or improve the quality of another's life? The answer usually depends on a person's social, cultural, and religious values.

In general, Western society has supported the idea of saving or improving another's life by giving of oneself. But Western society has also considered body mutilation, either before or after death, taboo.

Today, this attitude is slowly changing. One reason is growing public awareness of successful organ transplants. Another is the pro-transplant stand being taken by the major religions.

The Roman Catholic Church, for example, generally views organ transplantation as permissible, provided the organ recipient will benefit and the donor (if not already brain dead) will survive without being deprived of some vital function. Other Christian churches also support organ transplantation. Although they don't consider anyone obliged to donate an organ, they support donation as a gift of love freely given.

Traditional Jewish ethics have forbidden body mutilation, except to save a life. Orthodox Judaism still adheres to this view; but Conservative and Reform Judaism have broken with this view and impose no restrictions on organ transplantation.

Despite such changing views, many people still have a strong aversion to mutilation, even after death. Some, for example, can't bring themselves to allow a loved one's body to be autopsied. And others can't tolerate the thought of

*"Western society has supported the idea of saving or improving another's life by giving of oneself."*

their own or a family member's body being surgically invaded to obtain a donated organ.

Although mutilation is the basic issue to be resolved, for many people, organ transplants raise other ethical questions, such as, How should society allocate its resources? If an infant and an elderly person both need corneas, for example, or a professor and a prisoner both need a kidney, who should get the organ? And who should decide?

And how should society allocate its limited financial resources? Is an experimental liver transplant for one patient *worth* hundreds of thousands of dollars in public funds? Or should these be spent to meet the needs of a greater number of people?

As a nurse, you may find yourself torn by such conflict when you're counseling patients or families about organ donation or when you're caring for a

## UNIFORM DONOR CARD

Here's a facsimile of a uniform donor card:

### Uniform Donor Card

x _____

*Print or type name of donor*

In the hope that I may help others, I hereby make this anatomical gift, if medically acceptable, to take effect upon my death. The words and marks below indicate my desires.

I give: (a) _____ any needed organs or parts

(b) _____ only the following organs or parts

_____

*Specify the organ(s) or part(s)*

for the purposes of transplantation, therapy, medical research or education;

(c) _____ my body for anatomical study if needed.

Limitations or special wishes, if any: _____

**FRONT**

Signed by the donor and the following two witnesses in the presence of each other:

_____

Signature of donor            Date of birth
                                of donor

_____

Date signed        City and State

_____

Witness                         Witness

This is a legal document under the Uniform Anatomical Gift Act or similar laws. For further information consult your physician or local National Kidney Foundation Office.

**BACK**

Reprinted with permission from the National Kidney Foundation, Inc.

cadaveric organ donor.

Resolving such conflicts requires a willingness to examine your beliefs and identify their sources. Only then will you be able to feel comfortable with providing care.

### Legal issues

Whatever your ethical beliefs, you should be aware of certain legal responsibilities in organ donation and transplant situations.

First, for a donation to be made, the donor's consent is necessary. Getting consent from an adult who wants to donate a kidney is routine, for example—removing one kidney doesn't decrease life expectancy, and the transplant success rate is considerable.

If the donor can't consent, either because he's mentally incompetent or a minor, the courts allow parents or guardians to consent as long as the donor and recipient are related. In *Strunk v. Strunk* (1969), a Kentucky court authorized a transplant from a developmentally disabled 27-year-old to his brother. And in *Masdev v. Harrison* (1957) and *Hart et al v. Brown et al* (1972), Massachusetts and Connecticut courts ruled that parents could allow transplants between minor identical twins.

For cadaveric organ donation, all 50 states have adopted the Uniform Anatomical Gift Act, which provides two ways to donate organs:

• In Canada and the United States, any person 18 or older may indicate his desire to become an organ donor by signing a uniform donor card (or similar document) in the presence of two witnesses. In many states this intent is recorded on the back of a driver's license. Legally, this decision is binding on the person's family after his death. As a practical matter, however, most hospitals will comply with the family's wishes. (See *Uniform Donor Card*.)

• A family member may authorize donation of a decedent's organs by signing an appropriate document. If death occurs within 24 hours of admission to a hospital or results from an accident, homicide, or other unnatural cause, a medical examiner must also consent to the organ donation.

Of course, for any cadaveric donation to occur, death must be legally established first. By 1980, 28 states and several provinces had recognized brain death as a valid definition of death. But even in states and provinces without brain-death laws, medical practice—and court decisions—have upheld the brain-death concept (see Entry 17).

### Your role

Given these medical, ethical, and legal considerations, what's your role as a nurse assigned to care for a prospective organ donor or recipient?

As in any other medical or surgical procedure, getting consent for organ transplants and donations is a medical responsibility. But you can help by answering questions, or by referring patients and their families to someone who can.

With a prospective donor, your first job is to help the patient or his family decide whether to donate an organ. Tell them that this is a question they'll need to answer, then give them objective information (or find someone who can) so that the patient or his family can make an informed decision.

When your patient is a prospective recipient, outline the advantages and disadvantages of transplant procedures as objectively as possible. Then let the patient (or, if necessary, his family) decide whether or not to consent.

### A final word

What if you're opposed to the idea of donations and transplantation? If you don't know why you feel this way, try to identify the reasons. Until you understand your feelings better, ask to be excused from caring for prospective donors or recipients.

If you're opposed to the procedure for a specific donor or recipient, share your concerns with the medical team. If you still feel uncomfortable, share your concerns with the hospital administration.

# 73 Abortion

Mention the word "abortion" to a group of nurses, doctors, or other health-care workers, and the debate begins. Some are for it, some against it, and some aren't sure.

As an individual, you have a right to your opinion about abortion. But as a nurse, you must try not to let your personal opinion interfere with your care of patients exercising their legal right to abortions. To meet that duty, you need to be familiar with abortion's current legal status.

## KEY TERMS IN THIS ENTRY

**illegal (criminal) abortion** • Induced termination of a pregnancy under certain circumstances, or at a gestational time, prohibited by law. In Canada, an abortion not approved by a hospital therapeutic abortion committee. Many illegal abortions are performed under medically unsafe conditions.

**legal abortion** • Induced termination of pregnancy by a doctor before the fetus has developed sufficiently to live outside the uterus. The procedure is performed under medically safe conditions prescribed by law.

**pro-choice** • The philosophy that a woman has the right to choose either to continue or to terminate her pregnancy.

**pro-life** • The philosophy that the unborn fetus has the right to develop to term and to be born.

**therapeutic abortion** • Induced termination of pregnancy to preserve the health, safety, or life of the woman.

## Changing laws on abortion

Abortion's been practiced since the dawn of recorded history. In the United States, however, before the 1960s state laws severely limited or outlawed abortions. Women faced with unwanted pregnancies were caught between the laws against abortion and society's intolerance of out-of-wedlock pregnancies and illegitimate births.

In the 1960s, some states passed less restrictive abortion laws. But in *Roe v. Wade* (1973), the U.S. Supreme Court took the question out of the states' hands. The Court ruled that abortion was a right derived from the constitutional right to privacy. Although the Constitution nowhere specifically declares such a right, the Court found it in the framers' intent and in the Fourteenth Amendment, which, the Court said, precludes government intrusion into the personal matter of "whether to

beget and bear a child." According to the Court, a woman and her doctor could jointly decide whether to abort a fetus during the first two trimesters. Thus, the decision-making power was taken away from state legislators and given to those directly involved in the question. (In Canada, abortion is legal only with the approval of a hospital's committee on therapeutic abortion.)

The ruling didn't shut the states out entirely, however. It said that a state's interest began when the fetus became viable. That, of course, prompted increased debate on when life begins.

## When does life begin?

A biologist might say life begins at conception. A theologian might back up the moment into eternity, or he might move it ahead to "when the woman feels life" (quickening). But for many centuries, the courts had their own reference point: life, most suggested, began at birth. For example, only persons had rights under common law, and the unborn weren't considered "persons." Neither were the stillborn. Thus, a birth attendant, by reporting either "life" (even a few fleeting breaths) or "no life," had the power to secure or cut off an infant's rights. But gradually, both statutory and common law began to view life as beginning before birth. Among other things, this allowed compensation for prenatal injuries.

In questions of abortion, the emphasis has shifted from "birth" to "viability." The revised (1979) fifth edition of *Black's Law Dictionary* defines abortion as: "the intentional expulsion or removal of an unborn child from the womb other than for the principal purpose of producing a live birth or removing a dead fetus." While this definition suggests that abortion is unlawful, modern common law accepts the definition but considers the conduct lawful. This shift demonstrates the law's capacity to catch up with the issues and the times.

In 1976, the Supreme Court upheld viability as the earliest point at which a state could interfere with a woman's right to have an abortion. Thus, in *Planned Parenthood of Central Missouri v. Danforth* (1976), the Court ruled unconstitutional a Missouri law that required health-care workers to protect fetal life *before* viability, under threat of civil and criminal penalties.

The state can place some restrictions on the abortion itself, however. In the *first trimester,* the state can require that the doctor be duly licensed (*Roe v. Wade,* 1973) and that reasonable records be kept (*Planned Parenthood of Central Missouri v. Danforth,* 1976), but not that the abortion take place in a hospital accredited by the Joint Commission on Accreditation of Hospitals (*Doe v. Bolton,* 1973). (Nearly 80% of legal abortions now take place outside hospitals, a decided increase from 50% in 1973.)

In the *second trimester,* the state may impose more stringent regulations to protect the pregnant woman's health and safety. But because the state has no overriding interest in the nonviable fetus, it can't prohibit the use of saline procedure or require the protection of fetal life (*Planned Parenthood of Central Missouri v. Danforth,* 1976).

In the *third trimester,* the state's interest in the viable fetus becomes sufficient to prohibit abortion unless the doctor believes that continuing to carry the fetus poses a danger to the pregnant mother's health.

### Who pays for an abortion?

Although the courts have upheld women's right to have abortions, they've been less willing to say that the state must pay for it. In some instances, therefore, a woman's inability to pay for an abortion effectively cancels her right of choice. (In Canada, provincial health plans cover the cost of abortions done in a hospital for health reasons.) Even so, an estimated 1.2 million legal and illegal abortions were performed in the United States in 1980. According to some estimates, 15% of U.S. women of childbearing age (15 to 44) have had

at least one abortion.

Compared to other countries, the U.S. abortion rate is near the middle. Canada and western European countries have lower rates. Eastern European countries, the Soviet Union, and Japan have higher rates.

Until 1976, abortions were covered under federal Medicaid programs. But in that year, Congress accepted the Hyde Amendment to the Labor–Health, Education, and Welfare Appropriations Act, effectively removing abortion from federal Medicaid coverage.

In *Harris v. McRae* (1980), the U.S. Supreme Court upheld the constitutionality of the original Hyde Amendment and its later revisions. As a result, state Medicaid programs may subsidize childbirth but exclude all abor-

---

*"For years, the courts have suggested that life began at birth."*

---

tions, even those deemed "medically necessary." However, some state courts (California, New Jersey, and Massachusetts) have held that the *state* constitution requires Medicaid funding for medically necessary abortions if the state also pays the costs of childbirth.

### The continuing controversy

Despite the laws and court decisions regulating abortion, the ethical controversy continues. Two organized groups are particularly prominent: the National Right to Life Committee (NRLC) and the National Abortion Rights Action League (NARAL).

The NRLC, a pro-life group, focuses on fetal rights and seeks to restrict or eliminate maternal choice. The group favors a constitutional amendment that would grant the fetus rights at the time of conception. Such an amendment would void the *Roe v. Wade* right-to-privacy ruling.

In contrast, NARAL, a pro-choice group, places maternal rights first and favors abortion as an alternative to unwanted pregnancies. The group contends that women should be free to choose when (and when not) to have a baby, and that abortion is safe.

## Your role

You have a personal right to side with either argument, of course. But that right normally shouldn't interfere with your professional duty.

Some states have laws giving nurses a "conscience" right to refuse to participate in abortions because of moral or ethical reasons. In states without such laws, you could be subject to an employer's disciplinary action for refusing to participate in an abortion. However, as a practical matter, most institutions can and do adjust staffing patterns and schedules to accommodate objections, when possible.

You may provide abortion counseling, though getting the patient's informed consent, as you know, is the doctor's province. Many patients are uncertain about the procedures and risks involved in abortion—and about possible alternatives. As a counselor, you can help patients consider available options, resolve their conflicts, and make their decisions.

One caution, though. If *you* have conflicts about abortion, discuss them with a competent supervisor or counselor—not with the patient. If you can't resolve the conflicts, you may need to transfer to another unit.

## First- and second-trimester care

Technical procedures during a first-trimester abortion are relatively simple, not unlike those used for dilation and curettage. Follow prescribed protocol before and during the operation. Postoperatively, watch for excessive bleeding and check vital signs, urine flow, and signs and symptoms of possible complications.

The patient's emotional needs, however, may be the major complications you face. For example, a freckle-faced, adopted 16-year-old was admitted to a hospital for a first-trimester aspiration. Although her parents had approved the abortion, they were angry that she needed one. The patient tearfully told the nurses about her parents' accusations. "You're just like your real mother when she had you," they'd said. The implication obviously was, "You're no good, either." To help improve her self-image, her nurses spent extra time listening attentively to her feelings. They tried to show her, "You're good." When she was discharged, she said, "You know, I expected this to be a horrible day, but you made it bearable. Thanks for being so good to me."

A second-trimester abortion poses technical difficulties, so you'll need to give more support. When the exact expulsion time can't be predicted (as in the saline solution procedure), monitor the patient's contractions and coach her. Delivering a fetus unattended can be very frightening.

Your own role in dealing with an aborted fetus can also be frightening and upsetting, especially if the fetus shows any signs of life. In this situation, follow prescribed procedures or standing orders.

Following expulsion of the fetus, give care similar to immediate postpartum care, watching vital signs, cleanliness, and bleeding.

The patient who undergoes a second-trimester abortion may also need more emotional support. Most of these patients have experienced more conflict, more barriers, and more hassles. And some, particularly those undergoing the abortion of a wanted pregnancy (after amniocentesis, for example), may feel an extra-acute sense of loss.

## A final word

You can alter a patient's perception of abortion by kindness and consideration. A quality nurse-patient relationship will also improve the patient's self-image and promote a quick recovery.

In addition, such a relationship will help the patient respect her reproductive potential—and to make responsible choices that will eliminate the need for another abortion.

---

# 74 No-code and slow-code: The legalities and ethics

As a nurse, you've undoubtedly struggled from time to time with conflict between your ethical concerns for patients and the certainty of what the law requires of you. This conflict can be acute when you're the first to arrive at the bedside of a terminally ill patient in cardiac or respiratory arrest. His life depends on whether or not you call a code and initiate resuscitation efforts.

This entry discusses the legal status of no-code and so-called slow-code orders and provides guidelines for managing the difficult ethical conflicts that can arise.

## Understanding no-code orders
When a patient's terminally ill, and his imminent death is expected, his doctor and family (and sometimes the patient, too) will often agree that a no-code order is appropriate to end his suffering. The doctor writes it, and the staff carries it out when the patient goes into cardiac or respiratory arrest. This is a legal order, and you'll incur no liability when you don't attempt to resuscitate such a patient and he subsequently dies. But it must be a written order. *Any unwritten or undocumented no-code order is a so-called slow-code order—an illegal order.* So if the doctor gives you a verbal no-code order as he's rushing off to attend another patient, or gives you such an order over the telephone, or instructs you not to write down his verbal no-code order, remember—only a *written* no-code order

is legally defensible. *You must document the verbal order in your nurses' notes and insist that the doctor sign off on it—and you must refuse a no-code order he gives over the telephone.* (For more information on verbal orders, see Entry 87.)

All this sounds pretty serious, doesn't it? Well, it is. Why? Because if a patient you didn't try to resuscitate dies, and no written no-code order exists, you can be charged with *murder or manslaughter.* This isn't the typical nursing malpractice situation, which usually involves a patient who's still alive, though injured. This patient's injuries, and the damages a court may exact from a nurse-defendant who's found liable, obviously can't compare in severity with the situation of a dead slow-coded patient and a nurse charged with

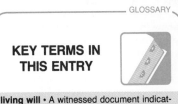

### KEY TERMS IN THIS ENTRY

**living will** • A witnessed document indicating a patient's desire to be allowed to die a natural death, rather than be kept alive by heroic, life-sustaining measures.

**no-code order** • A note, written in the patient record and signed by a doctor, instructing staff not to attempt to resuscitate a terminally ill patient if he suffers cardiac or respiratory failure.

**nurse practice act** • A law enacted by a state's legislature outlining the legal scope of nursing practice within that state.

**slow-code order** • A verbal or implicit order from a doctor instructing staff to refrain from resuscitating a terminally ill patient after apparent death, until a point is reached when CPR is unlikely to be successful. *An illegal order.*

**standards of care** • In a malpractice lawsuit, those acts performed or omitted that an ordinary, prudent person in the defendant's position would have done or not done; a measure by which the defendant's alleged wrongful conduct is compared.

**verbal order** • An order given directly and in person by a doctor to a nurse.

murder. With so profound a risk of liability, you need to be secure in your knowledge of legally correct nursing practice in no-code situations.

But even a written no-code order can pose problems for you. Suppose you think a doctor's order may be premature, because your nursing assessment and nursing diagnosis indicate the patient's death may not be imminent. If you've any doubt about the timing of a doctor's written no-code order, you have a legal and professional obligation to question the order. This is because you have the duty, as your patient's advocate, to exercise independent professional judgment in caring for him. (See Entry 1.)

In this situation, you can delay carrying out the order until the doctor confirms or corrects it to your satisfaction. Here's how to proceed:
• Before you speak with the patient's doctor, document your nursing assessment and nursing diagnosis, which caused you to question the no-code order, in the patient's chart.
• Next, discuss your concerns with the doctor. Ask him to clarify his reasons for no-coding the patient. If his explanation removes your doubts, you'll probably decide to withdraw your objection and carry out the no-code order. If his explanation isn't satisfactory, or if he refuses to discuss the matter with you, request an administrative opinion on how you should proceed. Begin with your head nurse, but be prepared to go through your institution's entire chain of command if necessary. (Of course, if your institution has a written policy for how to assess no-code orders, you should follow it.) You may also want to talk with the medical chief of staff.

Until you're satisfied that the no-code order is appropriate, you can delay carrying it out. This means you'll call a code, and attempt resuscitation, if the patient goes into cardiac or respiratory arrest.
• Document your request for clarification of the no-code order, and the doctor's satisfactory or unsatisfactory explanation (or refusal to give one), on the patient's chart.

Of course, you know that challenging a doctor's order can be very unpleasant. (For more information, see Entry 87.) But it couldn't be more unpleasant than the consequences—a patient's premature death and a possible lawsuit—if you're right about the timing of the order but carry it out anyway.

The ethical issues involved in no-code orders center on the dying patient's rights to care, comfort, dignity, and self-determination. (See *From the Heart*, pages 452 and 453.) The nursing staff in an ICU or CCU must often accept no-code orders for patients they've become close to. In this situation, you know you must act professionally and not let your emotions overpower your concern for giving proper care.

But keeping your emotions in check during a personally painful no-code situation isn't easy. What can you do? Try to accept a patient's imminent death, and to work through your feelings, *before* the crisis occurs. One way to do this is by consciously recalling the grief you felt when someone you loved died. This is a painful process, but preparing yourself this way will help you make unclouded nursing decisions when the no-coded patient goes into cardiac or respiratory arrest. If you *don't* work out some of your feelings about a patient's death beforehand, you (and other staff members) may become caught up in unrealistic rescue fantasies that impede clear-headed responses to the no-code order. To best serve the patient's interests, you must put your personal feelings aside.

You can also prepare yourself for no-coded patients' deaths by regularly assessing your reactions to death and dying, and by keeping up with studies in this area.

Sometimes, because of your attachment to a patient, you may feel angry at his doctor, his family, or both for their decision to issue a no-code order. Remember, this decision is a very painful one for everyone involved, not just for you. Don't make the situation worse by standing in judgment of the patient's family or by publicly criticizing their decision.

### Slow-code order? Refuse it, document it

*Any unwritten, documented but unsigned, or unstated but "understood" no-code order is an illegal slow-code order.* If you carry out such an order, and the patient dies because you didn't make an effort to resuscitate him, you can be liable for wrongful death (and for practicing medicine without a license).

Strictly speaking, the existence of such a serious and clear-cut legal risk should mean that so-called slow-codes are never agreed to, or carried out, by health-team members. But, as you probably know, slow-codes *do* happen. Maybe you've even been involved.

If so, why?

● Maybe you weren't aware of how serious the legal consequences could be for you.

● Maybe you lacked the confidence to speak up and ask the doctor to put the slow-code order in writing as a no-code order.

● Maybe you thought that documenting the order in your nurses' notes, without the doctor's countersignature, was sufficient to make the order valid.

● Maybe you and the rest of the health team, including the doctor, had a strong personal attachment to a terminally ill patient that made writing a no-code order emotionally difficult. So no one discussed or wrote it, but everyone silently agreed to it.

Only one way exists to avoid a slow-code order's dire legal consequences: *Every no-coded patient must have a written order.* Unless the doctor has written a no-code order or signed off on documentation of his verbal order, always initiate resuscitation efforts for a terminally ill patient in cardiac or respiratory arrest.

Never forget that your primary legal and professional responsibility to every

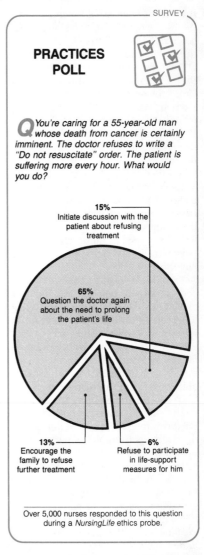

**PRACTICES POLL**

**Q** *You're caring for a 55-year-old man whose death from cancer is certainly imminent. The doctor refuses to write a "Do not resuscitate" order. The patient is suffering more every hour. What would you do?*

**15%**
Initiate discussion with the patient about refusing treatment

**65%**
Question the doctor again about the need to prolong the patient's life

**13%**
Encourage the family to refuse further treatment

**6%**
Refuse to participate in life-support measures for him

Over 5,000 nurses responded to this question during a *NursingLife* ethics probe.

patient, including terminally ill patients, is to give care that meets applicable standards—care that a reasonably prudent nurse with equivalent education, training, and experience (see Entry 2) would give in the same circumstances. *Preservation of life* is the overriding duty of nursing and medical staff; you can never relinquish this duty *except* when a doctor writes a no-code order for your patient.

Remember, too, that if a lawsuit results from your involvement in a patient's death because of slow-coding, you'll have no written evidence that the doctor gave the verbal no-code order. (Without evidence, juries usually find that a claimed event did not occur.) Don't forget that doctors commonly have an edge when lawsuits come to trial: until nurses attain a fully professional image, most juries will give a doctor's testimony more weight than a nurse's.

Another way to provide evidence that a doctor gave a verbal, unsigned no-code order is to keep a personal journal in which you document unusual events, including slow-codes, that occur on the unit. Of course, if you've refused to take part in the illegal order, you won't need any other defense.

The ethical considerations of a slow-code situation pale beside the legal ones. Consider this: If you fail to meet a personal ethical requirement on the job, you may have trouble facing yourself in the mirror for awhile. But if you fail to meet a legal requirement, you may have trouble that won't go away, and you'll wind up facing a jury.

Of course, you feel pity and grief for a terminally ill patient whose suffering must continue for lack of a no-code order. In this situation, the patient's best helped by your efforts to *get* a written order—not by ambivalence and equivocation on the part of the health team. In effect, a staff that permits an illegal slow-code response to end a patient's life is inviting a jury to decide whether the failure to call a code was reasonable under the circumstances.

## What if a patient wants a no-code order, but his doctor and family refuse?

This is a truly difficult dilemma for you—and for the doctor, who may want to no-code the patient but, to avoid any legal repercussions, yields to the family's pressure. At stake here is every competent adult's right to participate in the formulation of his treatment plan, to choose among alternative treatment modalities, and to *refuse treatment.* (See Entries 11 and 13.) If a terminally ill patient has expressed his wish not to be coded, and you call a code when he goes into cardiac or respiratory arrest, you're violating his right to refuse treatment. But if you *don't* call a code (in the absence of a written no-code order), you're practicing medicine without a license, and you're liable for his death if he dies.

In a double-bind situation like this, one way to proceed is as follows:

● If a terminally ill patient tells you he doesn't want to be resuscitated in the event of a crisis, document his statement (in his own words) and chart his apparent degree of awareness and orientation.

● If the doctor knows of the patient's wish and still refuses to write a no-code order, document this in your notes. The doctor has the same conflict with the patient's right to refuse treatment that you have, and he may be liable if he doesn't comply with the patient's request.

Without a written no-code order, should you attempt resuscitation on a patient who's said he doesn't want it? In the final analysis, the answer's "yes." Your best course, though, is to try to get the doctor to write the no-code order *before* a crisis occurs. This may prove difficult in the face of a family's denial of the patient's imminent death, or a doctor's concern about a possible lawsuit. But it's your duty to your patient, if your nursing assessment and nursing diagnosis corroborate the patient's belief that his death will occur soon. (Of course, if his status is such that recovery still seems possible, defer asking for the no-code order—and resuscitate if needed.)

● If your terminally ill patient has prepared a living will, make sure his doctor has seen it. It may or may not be legally binding in your state (see Entry 30). The doctor, perhaps in conjunction with a hospital administrator, will decide what action to take concerning it.

## A final word

No doubt about it—no-code/slow-code situations are tough for nurses. They're painful ethically, and they're fraught with legal peril in which the unsigned verbal no-code order (the so-called slow-code) figures prominently.

If a doctor gives you a slow-code order, you'll need courage and self-confidence to insist that he countersign your documentation of the order. You'll need these qualities if he *doesn't* sign, too. Why? Because you'll have to resuscitate the patient as needed, in spite of the doctor's order and, possibly, in spite of your ethical feelings about the situation.

If your institution doesn't have a written policy for assessing no-code orders, work to get one. (The American Heart Association's guidelines can help you get started.) Ask your head nurse and your nursing colleagues to help you put a proposal together and get administrative approval of it. Then, when a doctor gives you a questionable no-code order, that policy will lend weight to your request that he follow legally correct no-code procedures.

# 75 When a colleague is incompetent

The American Nurses' Association (ANA) Code for Nurses says you have a professional responsibility to "safeguard the client and the public when health care and safety are affected by the incompetent, unethical, or illegal practice of any person."

The International Council of Nurses Code of Nursing Ethics, adopted by the Canadian Nurses Association, has a similar provision: "[Nurses should take] appropriate action to safeguard the individual when his care is endangered by a co-worker or any other person." But how do you know when a

colleague's behavior should be reported? Or how to go about it?

## When should you report a colleague?

Before reporting a colleague or other health-care professional for incompetent, unethical, or illegal conduct, assess the situation carefully. Make sure you have a solid case by asking yourself questions such as these:

• Is the conduct truly a matter of incompetence, poor ethics, or illegality, or is it simply conduct with which you disagree?

• Would the conduct be acceptable if the outcome had been different? If so, are you judging the results rather than the conduct?

• Has the conduct harmed a patient, or does this possibility exist?

You may not know the answers, especially in situations where the conduct is mediocre but not necessarily incompetent. In these situations, you'll have to weigh the consequences of waiting or taking action. Obviously, the more likely patient injury seems, the more pressure you'll feel to take action.

When you're reasonably sure of your ground, what next? The ANA code suggests that you first approach your colleague directly. Share your concern that her conduct is hurting patient care.

The exchange may have one of sev-

## STEPS TO FOLLOW WHEN YOU REPORT UNSAFE PRACTICES

Consider this scenario: The night medication nurse on your unit keeps an accurate narcotics count, but you continually see evidence of poor pain control on her shift. You're suspicious, but you know she's one of the most conscientious workers on your understaffed unit. She's also the sole supporter of two young children. What should you do?

Blowing the whistle is never easy. But because you're committed to patient health and safety, it's a responsibility you can't shirk. To give information about a co-worker's unethical or incompetent conduct, follow these guidelines:

Go through channels. Follow your institution's procedures for dealing with complaints of unethical or improper conduct. If the person you're reporting to is part of the problem, go to that person's supervisor.

 Be clear. Describe in writing the questionable or dangerous conduct and its consequences.

Be accurate. Describe the facts of the situation that you know to be true. Describe why you're not sure of certain things (for example, because a medical record is locked in the hospital administrator's office).

Be consistent. Get the story right the first time, and stick with it.

Be discreet. Don't gossip about the situation with co-workers, and don't contribute to rumors about it.

Be candid. If you try to hide aspects of the situation, your credibility will be damaged.

Get support. Get the support of co-workers you know and trust. Encourage them to contribute written statements corroborating your report.

Be persistent. If the situation is a sensitive one, you may be pressured to forget it. Remember that the issue is an important one: you owe it to your profession and your patients to pursue it.

eral outcomes. The colleague may convince you that what she's doing is indeed acceptable. Or you may convince her she's wrong; she may agree to change her ways. These outcomes don't present any problem. But what do you do if she agrees she's wrong and asks you to cover up?

### When a colleague asks you to cover up

You may be tempted to say yes when a colleague asks you to cover up her mis-takes, incompetence, or unethical conduct.

Maybe she's a close friend who you feel needs a little more time to cope with the alcohol problem or whatever problem you've uncovered. Even if she isn't a friend, maybe you've been taught not to sit in judgment of others, or you just don't like to tattle. Besides, maybe you'll be the one making the mistake next time, and you'll want your colleagues' support. Or maybe you simply feel your life has enough stress, and the

# GUIDANCE WHEN DEALING WITH COLLEAGUES

### Danger to patients: The alcoholic nurse

*I work with a 40-year-old nurse who had a good employment record until a few weeks ago.*

*Since then, she's made many medication errors—including giving the wrong preoperative medication to a patient. She's come in late several times, and she's often absent from the floor. I've also smelled alcohol on her breath. Do you have any suggestions on how to handle this?—RN, Mich.*

Sounds like your colleague may be suffering from some kind of stress and using alcohol to cope with it. Unchecked, her use of alcohol could turn into a more serious problem than the stress.

Since your colleague's problems are endangering her patients, talk to her or tell her supervisor what you've observed. The supervisor should sit down with her, tell her the behavior problems that have interfered with her work, and ask her what's causing the problems.

If the nurse admits she's abusing alcohol, the supervisor must first make absolutely clear that reporting for duty under the influence of alcohol will not be tolerated. Then the supervisor should help her identify some alternate coping mechanisms and, if possible, some solutions to her stress.

In the meantime, if the nurse's behavior continues to endanger her patients, the supervisor must take the steps necessary to protect them—either by limiting the nurse's contact with patients or by relieving her of her duties until she's learned to cope effectively with her stress.

Either way, once you've talked to the supervisor, you can best help your colleague by keeping her problem confidential.

### Reporting an abusive colleague

*I saw a nurse in my pediatric unit slap and shake a 2-year-old recently when he refused to take his medication.*

*I was horrified that she might be abusing children. So far, no one else has said or done anything about her behavior.*

*What's worse, I've only been working here a couple of months, and I don't want to rock the boat. I know my colleague is generally a good nurse. She's been on this unit 15 years.*

*What's my responsibility in this situation? Where can I turn for help?—RN, Ohio*

First, tell your supervisor. Isolated or not, the incident could be grounds for legal charges from the child's parents.

If you continue to suspect that your colleague is abusing children, insist that your supervisor talk to her. If she refuses, talk with your director of nursing.

Why do you have to get involved? The safety and well-being of your young patients is the first priority, of course. But consider this, too: At least one court decided that health-care professionals who didn't report suspected child abuse were liable for further injuries the child sustained.

### Protection for reporting negligence

*When a nurse asks what to do about poor patient care, attorneys and ethicists advise her to compile records, then talk with her supervisor. Doesn't the nurse run the risk of being fired or having to resign? Or is there some legal protection for nurses who report poor practices?—RN, N.Y.*

Some states do offer protection to encourage nurses and other health-care professionals to report poor practices. Two new additions to New York's Public Health Law grant immunity from civil problems that interfere with nursing practice. In exchange, however, the laws make reports of patient abuse and professional misconduct mandatory for doctors in residential health-care facilities. Failure to report such actions is unprofessional conduct.

Other states have mandated peer accountability in the rules and regulations that accompany their nurse practice acts. Check with your state nurses associations for the latest news on your legal responsibilities and protection in such situations.

---

These letters were taken from the files of *Nursing* and *NursingLife* magazines.

# TAKING HOSPITAL SUPPLIES:
# WHERE DO YOU DRAW THE LINE?

Attitudes and norms about taking hospital supplies for personal use vary considerably from place to place. That's what a recent *NursingLife* magazine ethics probe discovered.

What's considered theft by staff persons in one hospital might be a fringe benefit in another. Taking ends of gauze rolls that would be thrown out anyway, for example, wouldn't be considered wrong in many places. As one nurse respondent wrote, "We look on it as conserving and reusing items that would've ended up in a wastebasket."

Despite a certain amount of accepted practice, however, hospital theft is an increasingly serious problem that certainly contributes to escalating health-care costs. A U.S. Department of Commerce report, *Crime in the Service Industry*, estimated typical losses for hospitals at about $1,000 per bed per year.

When asked whether *other* nurses take supplies for personal use, 12% of those who responded to the probe said yes, commonly, and 21% said most nurses do sometimes. That's *one third* reporting a rather prevalent condition. Close to half said a few do sometimes, and the rest said they'd heard of it but had no firsthand knowledge.

Still, the incidence of stealing seems lower today than in 1974. *Nursing74*, in a similar poll, found that about 20%—8% more nurses than in the recent survey—thought stealing was common.

Yet how much of the stealing does anyone see? For each hospital employee who's caught stealing, there are probably 10 or more who aren't, estimated Steve M. Rhodes, LPN, RCST, in a 1981 article for *Hospital Topics* magazine. As central service director at Lutheran Hospital in Fort Wayne, Indiana, he's seen various methods for sneaking supplies out—such as stuffing linens and towels into knitting sacks, or taping instruments inside empty cartons.

Taking supplies like these raises the cost of health care, but stealing medications is potentially more serious. Although aspirin and antacids top the list, 3% of the probe respondents said they had stolen narcotics, and 18% had stolen other prescription drugs. Over a third said that medications other than aspirin and antacids were at least occasionally stolen from the hospital. The statistics on nurses stealing such medications for their own use, when compared with statistics from *Nursing74* magazine's poll, show some decrease over the years:

|                        | 1974 | 1982 |
| ---------------------- | ---- | ---- |
| It's very common ....  | 10%  | 7%   |
| It occurs occasionally | 40%  | 28%  |
| It seldom occurs ....  | 40%  | 47%  |
| It never occurs ......  | 10%  | 18%  |

Many respondents felt justified in stealing a medication they needed to keep on working. As one nurse supervisor wrote, "Usually it's for headache, nausea, diarrhea, or sometimes asthma or sinus problems. We're so short-staffed that it's almost impossible to let nurses go home. We often work when we're less than well because we know there's nobody to replace us."

Such a situation in itself may make nurses want to take drugs. Psychologist John W. Jones has correlated nurses' theft of drugs with their degree of burnout. As reported in the November 1981 issue of *Nursing Management* magazine, burned-out employees tend to steal more hospital supplies and drugs than those who *don't* suffer from frustration, interpersonal tension, work pressures, and anger toward patients, co-workers, and supervisors. And sometimes burned-out employees steal, not because they really want the items but because they want to commit an aggressive act against their employer.

A Canadian nurse who responded to the probe wrote that she'd taken narcotics and other drugs to cope with burnout and depression. She confessed, "I took Valium, Dalmane, chloral hydrate, and Librium to help me to sleep and to cope with an uncaring and demanding administration. I worked in a place where we were encouraged to 'tell' on our fellow employees; where hostility between nurse and nurse's aide was actively promoted... where mistakes we admitted won us a day's suspension from duty without pay, even for a first offense."

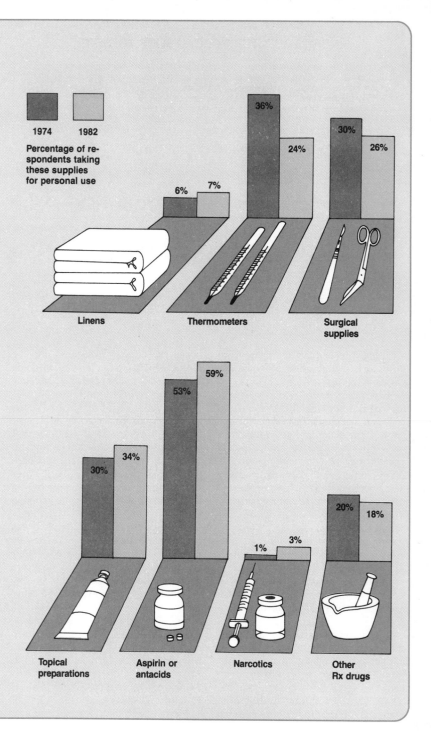

1974   1982

Percentage of respondents taking these supplies for personal use

Linens

6%   7%

Thermometers

36%   24%

Surgical supplies

30%   26%

Topical preparations

30%   34%

Aspirin or antacids

53%   59%

Narcotics

1%   3%

Other Rx drugs

20%   18%

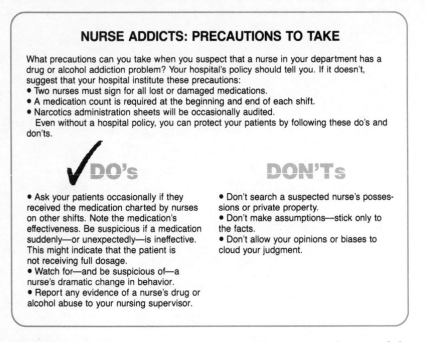

## NURSE ADDICTS: PRECAUTIONS TO TAKE

What precautions can you take when you suspect that a nurse in your department has a drug or alcohol addiction problem? Your hospital's policy should tell you. If it doesn't, suggest that your hospital institute these precautions:
- Two nurses must sign for all lost or damaged medications.
- A medication count is required at the beginning and end of each shift.
- Narcotics administration sheets will be occasionally audited.

Even without a hospital policy, you can protect your patients by following these do's and don'ts.

### ✓DO's

- Ask your patients occasionally if they received the medication charted by nurses on other shifts. Note the medication's effectiveness. Be suspicious if a medication suddenly—or unexpectedly—is ineffective. This might indicate that the patient is not receiving full dosage.
- Watch for—and be suspicious of—a nurse's dramatic change in behavior.
- Report any evidence of a nurse's drug or alcohol abuse to your nursing supervisor.

### DON'Ts

- Don't search a suspected nurse's possessions or private property.
- Don't make assumptions—stick only to the facts.
- Don't allow your opinions or biases to cloud your judgment.

---

last thing you need is more stress from the notoriety that often accompanies whistle blowing.

Before you give in to these very human considerations, think about the likely consequences if you *do* cover up:

- In some states and provinces, failing to report a colleague's unacceptable conduct may be considered unprofessional conduct and grounds for disciplinary action by the licensing agency.
- The cover-up might harm patients, bringing legal as well as moral and ethical consequences.
- You might lose your job.
- You might be named in a malpractice lawsuit if you were aware of your colleague's negligence.
- You might be subject to criminal penalties if the cover-up involves narcotics.
- The cover-up might harm the person you're trying to help. If your colleague has a drug problem, for example, she may delay getting treatment.
- If discovered and publicized, cover-ups damage the relationship between the nursing profession and the public. A public that knows nurses hide each other's incompetence is unlikely to trust or respect nurses.

Then what should you do when a colleague asks you to cover up her incompetent or unethical conduct or if she simply refuses to change and, in effect, tells you to get lost? If this happens, tell her you can't agree to cover up or remain silent. If her patients are endangered, take appropriate action to protect them. Then, follow your employer's established procedures for reporting incompetent, unethical, or illegal conduct. (By the way, if your employer doesn't have a clear statement of such procedures, urge that one be developed now—before you need to use it.)

You may want to draw on help from unbiased sources, such as clergymen or ombudsmen. They may be able to provide valuable guidance—and minimize your risk of reprisal. (See *Steps To Follow When You Report Unsafe Practices,* page 474.)

If your employer fails to act, your next

step is to report the conduct to the appropriate state or provincial licensing agency. Reports to such agencies may be protected from reprisal by statutory law or administrative rule. If not, consider sending an anonymous complaint. To learn about current requirements and protections, contact your state or provincial board of nursing.

## A final word

Reporting a colleague is difficult—personally and professionally. But one of the marks of any profession's maturity is its members' willingness to police themselves. Through your willingness to share in that often unpleasant task, you'll help nursing maintain its integrity and justify the public's trust.

## Selected References

American Nurses' Association. *Code For Nurses With Interpretive Statements.* Kansas City, Mo.: American Nurses' Association, 1976.

American Nurses' Association. *Nursing: A Social Policy Statement.* Kansas City, Mo.: American Nurses' Association, 1980.

American Nurses' Association. *Standards of Nursing Practice.* Kansas City, Mo.: American Nurses' Association, 1973.

Annas, George J., et al. *The Rights of Doctors, Nurses and Allied Health Professionals.* Cambridge, Mass.: Ballinger Publishing Co., 1981.

Aroskar, M.A. "Anatomy of an Ethical Dilemma: the Theory...the Practice," *American Journal of Nursing* 80:658-63, April 1980.

Binkin, N., et al. "Illegal Abortion Deaths in the United States: Why Are They Still Occurring?" *Family Planning Perspectives* 14:163-67, May/June 1982.

Cazalas, Mary W. *Nursing and the Law,* 3rd ed. Rockville, Md.: Aspen Systems Corp., 1979.

Creighton, Helen. *Law Every Nurse Should Know,* 4th ed. Philadelpia: W.B. Saunders Co., 1981.

Creighton, Helen. "A Nurse's Freedom of Speech," *Supervisor Nurse* 5:45-48, April 1974.

Curtin, Leah, and Flaherty, M. Josephine. *Nursing Ethics: Theories and Pragmatics.* Bowie, Md.: Robert J. Brady Co., 1981.

Davis, Anne J., and Aroskar, Mila A. *Ethical Dilemmas in Nursing Practice.* East Norwalk, Conn.: Appleton-Century-Crofts, 1979.

Davis, P.S. "Medico-Legal Considerations and the Quality of Life," *Topics in Clinical Nursing* 3:79-85, October 1981.

Fletcher, J. "Ethics and Euthanasia," *American Journal of Nursing* 73:670-675, April 1973.

Hemelt, M., and Mackert, M. *Dynamics of Law, Nursing and Health Care,* 2nd ed. Reston, Va.: Reston Publishing Co., 1982.

Hiscoe, S. "The Awesome Decision," *American Journal of Nursing* 73:291-93, February 1973.

Kalish, Richard A. *Death, Grief and Caring Relationships.* Monterey, Calif.: Brooks/Cole Publishing Co., 1981.

Kollar, Nathan. "Terminal Suicide: Priority of Life? Priority of Death?" in *Death Education and Counseling: Priorities Today and Tomorrow.* Edited by Pacholeki, Richard A., and Copp, Charles A. Arlington, Va.: Forum for Death Education and Counseling, 1982.

McCloskey, Joanne C., et al. *Current Issues in Nursing.* Boston: Blackwell Scientific Publications, 1981.

Olson, Janice. "To Treat or to Allow to Die: An Ethical Dilemma in Gerontological Nursing," *Journal of Gerontological Nursing* 7:141, March 1981.

Rothman, Daniel A., and Rothman, Nancy L. *The Professional Nurse and the Law.* Boston: Little, Brown & Co., 1977.

Saunders, Cicely. "The Care of the Dying Patient and His Family," in *Ethics in Medicine: Historical Perspectives and Contemporary Concerns.* Edited by Reiser, Stanley J., and Dyck, Arthur J. Cambridge, Mass.: MIT Press, 1977.

Thompson, Joyce B., and Thompson, Henry O. *Ethics in Nursing.* New York: Macmillan Publishing Co., 1981.

Veatch, Robert M. *Case Studies in Medical Ethics.* Cambridge, Mass.: Harvard University Press, 1977.

Walker, A. *Cerebral Death,* 2nd ed. Baltimore: Urban & Schwarzenberg, 1981.

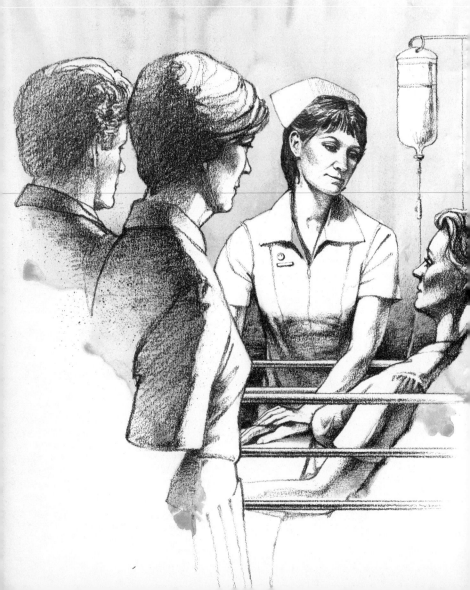

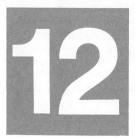

# Relating with Patients and Their Families

## Introduction

By any standard—legal, professional, or ethical—meeting the emotional needs of patients and their families is one of the most important tasks you perform as a nurse. Your therapeutic relationships with patients and their families can increase their willingness to participate actively in the patient's care plan. And close communication, as you know, can help prevent dangerous medical errors.

This chapter provides you with guidelines and techniques for communicating effectively with patients and their families. You'll learn how to assess the emotional needs of young and elderly patients and their relatives, as well as patients who present special nursing problems. You'll discover ways to handle patients' complaints and methods for intervening skillfully in the family crises that often accompany illness. And you'll find out how to recognize your personal biases concerning certain patients—biases that can reduce your effectiveness as a nurse unless you take preventive action.

### In this chapter
Entry 76, "Communicating effectively with patients," describes how nurses and patients communicate with each other through their actions as well as their words. This entry also explains several techniques you can use to gain

patients' trust and open yourself to giving and receiving clear communications.

Entry 77, "Providing emotional support," describes how, by observing the interactions of patients and family members, you can decide on techniques for helping them work through illness-related emotional difficulties. You'll also learn to be aware of the kinds of patient problems you can't, and shouldn't, try to handle alone. This entry shows you how to use other resources, inside and outside the hospital, to help patients and their family members when *your* help isn't enough.

No matter where you work in the hospital, you sometimes have to listen to complaints from patients and family members. Entry 78, "How to deal with patients who complain," shows you how to avoid reacting defensively to complaints and describes how you can evaluate complaints to determine patients' and their families' need for emotional support.

Of all patients, children often react most strongly to the stress of hospitalization. Entry 79, "Communicating with pediatric patients," gives you helpful techniques for dealing with children whose illnesses trigger depressed, manipulative, or aggressive behavior.

Caring for geriatric patients is *not*

the same as caring for children—although too many nurses treat both groups of patients the same way. Entry 80, "Communicating with geriatric patients," sums up the stereotypes that people commonly associate with old age and discusses helpful attitudes and techniques you can use for giving individual care to geriatric patients.

No nurse can avoid having to care for problem patients—the patients who challenge our concepts of ourselves as professionals and as human beings. Entry 81, "Patients who challenge you," explains why alcoholics, drug abusers, and the suicide-prone (among others) are so often successful at manipulating and frustrating nurses. This entry also describes how to control your initial reactions to these challenging patients so you can give them the emotional support they need in addition to your skilled nursing care.

When a medical crisis occurs, the patient and his family may cope with it poorly or not at all. Entry 82, "Families in crisis," describes the problems family members may confront as they attempt to deal with a crisis. This entry also details, in a case study, the steps you can take to help a family recognize crises and cope with them successfully.

With your guidance and support, family members can greatly improve a patient's willingness and ability to respond to treatment. Entry 83, "Helping a patient's family participate in his care," presents a case study of how one nurse helped a patient's family make their own emotional adjustments to a crisis so they could then participate effectively in the patient's care.

Of course, you're familiar with situations where family members' concern for a patient—along with their awareness of his rights—can complicate your nursing care. This chapter's final entry, "Why some families are difficult" (Entry 84), helps you manage these situations more confidently and avoid the stressful confrontations that can otherwise develop between nurses and patients' families.

### A final word

Meeting the emotional needs of your patient and his family takes skills that you can't acquire simply by reading about them. But reading this chapter is a good starting point. Try out the tips and techniques included in the following pages. Some of them will work for you. With practice, you'll probably find that you're more relaxed with patients and their families—and more confident about the quality of your nursing care.

# 76 Communicating effectively with patients

The patient who says he's feeling fine, as he lies in bed stiff as a board, is probably saying one thing and feeling another. His health depends on your knowing the difference. This entry explains many of the techniques you can use to establish effective and useful communication with your patient.

## Do you discourage patients from communicating?

"Of course not!", you'll surely answer. But maybe some things you're not aware you're doing *are* discouraging patients from communicating with you. How? By encouraging patients to be meek and compliant. Every day, patients are told (in actions if not in words) that they shouldn't bother busy nurses about minor discomforts or with long conversations. Don't think this doesn't happen in your hospital. How many times have you seen a staff member nod mechanically as a patient describes in minute detail the onset and progression of his illness? When a patient who "rides" his call bell must wait a long time before the nurse responds, while the patient who makes few calls gets immediate attention, isn't the first patient being punished for his behavior and the second patient being rewarded?

Naturally, you won't always have time to have an extended conversation with a talkative patient or to answer a demanding patient's repeated calls immediately. But once a patient learns that being "good" means taking up as little of your time as possible, establishing meaningful communication becomes much more difficult.

## Creating the right communication environment

Take these three steps to create the right environment for effective communication:

• Watch for patients' nonverbal cues, and incorporate nonverbal cues into *your* communication with patients.
• Listen carefully to every patient.
• Be aware of your personal biases, and don't let them affect your performance as a nurse.

Most patients will say and do several things to "test you"—to find out how receptive you are to their real or imagined needs. By creating the right communication environment, you can begin to pass this test before even one word is exchanged.

To understand the importance of creating the right environment, consider your familiar work surroundings from the point of view of a new patient. Placed in a small hospital room, usually with a stranger, he's probably frightened and anxious. Few of us would want to divulge our feelings immediately in this situation.

Once the patient has had time to settle in, what can you do to set the stage for effective communication? First, eliminate unnecessary interruptions by leaving word with the ward clerk that you should be disturbed only in an emergency. Minimize external noises and other distractions by closing the door and drawing the curtain around the patient's bed.

To begin your conversation, tell the patient you're interested in how he's feeling and in hearing anything else he has to say. No matter how busy you are, be sure you look and act as if you

have no other concerns but his. You must be conscious of the nonverbal cues you and your patient exchange. These cues include gestures, facial expressions, posture, and voice tone and quality.

Obviously, you want to send a patient nonverbal cues that encourage him to communicate. Looking at your patient in a relaxed and steady way, without staring, will tell him that you're interested and concerned. So will standing or sitting in a comfortable position—without shifting from one leg to the other, glancing at your watch, or backing toward the door.

Consider the nonverbal cues your patient is sending. A blank look may mean he hasn't understood what you've told him. When he says, "I'm just not getting any better," does he meet your eyes with a steady, determined look? Or does he shrug his shoulders, avoid looking at you, begin to cry? The same words, accompanied by different nonverbal actions, reflect very different feelings. You must watch the patient to detect those different feelings.

Less subtle nonverbal cues also can help you understand a patient's condition. For example, does your male patient comb his hair and shave? Is your female patient wearing any makeup, and are her nails trimmed? Observations like these can tell you quite a bit about the patient's current self-image.

Other cues to watch for include blanched skin, body tremors, voice changes, sweating, increased muscle tension, and increased heart or respiratory rate. These physiologic changes may indicate how your patient is feeling more accurately than what he says.

As you talk with the patient, reinforce the rapport you've established with him by moving closer. If the patient seems startled or draws away, he probably needs more time to become comfortable with the situation. Touching the patient as he talks, when appropriate, can also convey warmth and empathy. But if he seems uncomfortable with your attempt to touch his hand or shoulder, accept his feelings

---

*"Listening carefully to the patient means accepting his right to feel the way he feels at that moment."*

---

and don't force physical contact. If you do, you'll undermine your efforts to communicate. Remember that patients can easily distinguish a warm hand from a stiff and unsure one, so don't use this technique unless you're comfortable with it.

### Listening carefully

Most of us become nurses because we want to help people. Often this means giving them advice. So when you think you understand a patient's problem, you may want to plunge in with suggestions or words of encouragement. Resist this temptation, at least for awhile. Say nothing—just listen. By doing this, and by interpreting nonverbal cues, you'll be able to understand not only what he says but also *why* he's saying it. For example, suppose a terminally ill cancer patient asks you, "Do you think there's any hope for

me?" He might really be asking, "Have you given up on me?", "Has my doctor given up on me?", "Has my family given up on me?", or "Am I dying?" Whatever his specific concerns, one thing is certain: The patient does not want a "yes" or "no" answer. Instead, he wants to discuss his feelings about the situation, and you can learn specifically what he's concerned about by listening.

Active listening will also help you pick up a barely audible phrase, or a trail of words at the end of a patient's comment, that may give you additional significant clues to his feelings. Here's another tip: don't feel you have to be talking if the patient isn't. Silent periods allow both of you to think about what the other person has said and give you time to organize your thoughts.

Listening carefully to a patient's choice of words can help you adjust your vocabulary to the patient's level of understanding. For example, if the patient says "pee" and you insist on using the words "urinate" or "void," the patient may not grasp your meaning. Having to constantly explain yourself will make both of you feel foolish. On the other hand, you may be led to believe that a patient who uses complicated medical terms is knowledgeable when he really isn't. In both situations, you must determine the patient's level of understanding so that you communicate clearly with him.

Listening to your patient also means accepting his right to feel the way he feels at that moment. This is easy to forget. One student nurse, for example, was caring for a patient about to undergo a breast biopsy and, probably, radical mastectomy. The nurse attempted to calm the patient by gently probing her feelings about the surgery. The tearful patient said, "No woman wants to lose her breast." The young nurse could have replied, "I can understand why you're upset. Would you like to tell me more about it?" Instead, she said, "Oh, well, maybe they won't have to do it." No patient in this situation wants to be told she has no reason

## ENCOURAGING YOUR PATIENT TO TALK

Information about your patient's feelings and needs can significantly enhance the quality of care you provide. The chart below contrasts effective communication techniques with ineffective ones. The *effective communication techniques* encourage the patient to continue talking so you can learn as much about him as possible. The *ineffective communication techniques* cut off communication and can raise a wall of misunderstanding between you and your patient.

### EFFECTIVE COMMUNICATION TECHNIQUES

| Patient's statement | Nurse's response | Why is this response appropriate? |
| --- | --- | --- |
| "I just haven't felt comfortable since I went on this new treatment schedule." | "How are you handling your new treatment routine?" | *Open-ended questions* allow the patient to clarify and elaborate on his thoughts and feelings. |
| "I've been depressed ever since I returned from vacation." | "Tell me, just how do you feel when you're depressed?" | *Closed questions* direct the patient toward providing specific information. |
| "Right after New Year's Day, I went in for tests. At that time they found the cause of my abdominal pain immediately. I followed my medication very carefully, but I had to go back to the hospital again last month because the gastritis had started up again." | "So, this is your third visit this year. You were admitted in January and again in May, each time for gastritis." | *Restatement* (summarizing) clarifies meaning for your understanding as well as the patient's. |
| "My folks have gone out of their way recently to care for me and I'm grateful to them. But I find myself thinking back to just a month ago when I was completely on my own." | "It must be hard to be dependent on your parents after being independent for so long." | *Communicating support* (empathy) encourages the patient to continue and reflects your concern. |
| "I don't know.... My family is so upset by my illness that I guess I've tried to ignore other treatment possibilities." | "You say your family has been so upset by your illness that you haven't explored alternative treatments." | *Reflecting* (echoing) allows the patient to evaluate his thoughts and feelings through your restatement of them. |
| "I guess what it comes down to is that I felt too guilty about being a burden." | | *Silence* allows the patient to collect his thoughts and reflect on the conversation. |

### INEFFECTIVE COMMUNICATION TECHNIQUES

| Patient's statement | Nurse's response | Why is this response inappropriate? |
| --- | --- | --- |
| "I think I'm doing all right today." | "What time does your doctor usually come in?" | *Changing the topic* makes the patient feel you don't care or aren't listening. |

*(continued)*

## ENCOURAGING YOUR PATIENT TO TALK *(continued)*

### INEFFECTIVE COMMUNICATION TECHNIQUES

| Patient's statement | Nurse's response | Why is this response inappropriate? |
|---|---|---|
| "I'm afraid the test results will be bad news." | "Maybe they won't be bad at all." | *Giving false assurances* misleads the patient and doesn't help him cope with the possibilities of his illness. |
| "You know, the thing I've been..." | "Would you like to sit up?" | *Interrupting* forces the patient to reinitiate the conversation. |
| "I haven't felt this way for days." | "I know what you're saying." | *Failing to clarify what's being talked about* can cause confusion for the nurse and the patient. |
| "I'm not sure I'm doing the right thing, asking my sister to come here." | "Well, you know what they say, 'nothing ventured, nothing gained.'" | *Making trite comments* trivializes the patient's feelings. |
| "What do you think I should do about telling my children?" | "Tell them the truth. They're old enough to handle it." | *Giving advice* places the patient in a dependent role, in effect absolving him of the consequences of his decision because he didn't make it himself. |
| "I don't think this hospital is very clean." | "It's as clean as any hospital you'll find." | *Being defensive* interferes with getting to the root of problems and feelings. |

to be upset. Not surprisingly, the patient kept her further feelings on the subject to herself.

Of course, communicating with your patient usually involves more than just listening. If you want to know how a patient feels, ask him. Once he responds, verbally and nonverbally, you can determine if you need to ask additional questions. For example, a patient may respond to your "How are you today?" with "Okay, I guess." By adding that "I guess," the patient is hinting that something is on his mind, and he's inviting you to probe further. And finally, if you've been sensitive to your patient's cues, you'll know when to *stop* asking questions as well. (See *Encouraging your patient to talk,* page 485.)

### Know your own limits
All of us have strong feelings and even biases on certain issues. These feelings and biases can affect our ability to communicate with patients. Being aware of your own feelings and biases can help you recognize, anticipate, and avoid problems.

Suppose, for example, that you're strongly opposed to abortion for any but life-threatening reasons. If you'll occasionally be caring for patients getting abortions, you must decide how you're going to deal with your feelings. Tell the charge nurse how you feel and either ask for counseling or request that you not be assigned to care for patients getting abortions. If you opt for counseling, it may or may not change your mind on the issue. But as a professional, you're obliged to separate your feelings about abortion from the patient's need for care. (See Entry 71.)

### A final word
Everything you say and do communicates something to your patient, just as everything your patient says or does

# WHAT ABOUT TIPPING?

*In 6 years of nursing, I've been offered anywhere from $1 to $50 in tips. Some of the patients I hardly knew; others, I knocked myself out for. Some were rich, some poor; some I loved, others I dreaded. But in no case have I ever accepted the tip. This has caused such bad feelings: I'm embarrassed, the patients and their families are embarrassed—some deeply hurt. I've honestly come to wonder if it might not be the generous gesture on my part just to accept the money with thanks. How do you handle this?—RN, Wyo.*

A person commonly offers a gratuity, or tip, to a person who fulfills his *requests* or *demands*. A nurse, however, through her unique professional training, assesses and meets a patient's *needs*. This distinction dictates your correct professional stance: accepting only your salary in return for your nursing services.

Unfortunately, you can't count on patients' knowing—or observing—*your* professional standards. You must consider any patient's offer of a tip as carefully as you plan his care. Your patient's manner may offer a clue to his motivation for tipping. Is he offering you a tip because he believes one is expected of him? If you think so, tell him he just gave you the *best* tip—the only

tip you can accept—by getting well again. But what about the elderly pensioner who gratefully slips a quarter in your hand as she's leaving? Clearly, this gesture means a great deal to that patient, and you have no real choice but to accept. When you must choose between ethical priorities, the patient's dignity and well-being always supersede your personal feelings about professional conduct.

The simplest solution is for everyone in a unit to agree on what to do with any tips that can't be gracefully refused. Some hospitals have "floor funds" in which all tips are pooled to buy textbooks or equipment or coffee-break treats for that unit. Others have a "sunshine" fund to supply toys for children or shaving kits for the needy.

In your question you made no mention of personal gifts, which can also be considered a form of tipping. This suggests that you've already recognized the important difference. Money is a universal form of exchange that can be as correctly offered to a maitre d' as to a paperboy. But a personal gift, which someone has given special thought and effort to selecting, is an intimate interaction between two people. To decline such a gift can only appear as a rejection of the giver. You should accept it graciously.

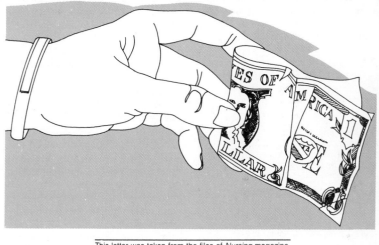

This letter was taken from the files of *Nursing* magazine.

should tell you something. Knowing how to read these verbal and nonverbal cues will help you build a sense of trust between you and your patient and greatly increase your effectiveness as a nurse.

# 77 Providing emotional support

For years, nurses were expected to function as technicians and concern themselves only with caring for a patient's body. Today, nurses are assuming more responsibility than ever for treating the *whole* patient, as an individual and as a member of a family, by providing emotional as well as physical care.

Although you have many techniques to assess the emotional needs of a patient and his family and to help them work through problems, giving emotional care is rarely easy. Doctors, traditionally more concerned with a patient's physical needs, may resist your efforts to offer advice or to arrange consultation on emotional care. Sometimes patients may resist your attempts to

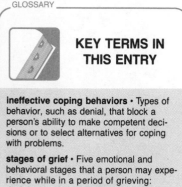

## KEY TERMS IN THIS ENTRY

**ineffective coping behaviors** • Types of behavior, such as denial, that block a person's ability to make competent decisions or to select alternatives for coping with problems.

**stages of grief** • Five emotional and behavioral stages that a person may experience while in a period of grieving: denial or avoidance, anger, depression, rationalization, and acceptance.

provide guidance and support. Still other patients, because of what they see on television, may have unrealistically high expectations of your capacity to carry emotional burdens. And here's another consideration for giving effective emotional care: you must be aware of the kinds of problems you cannot and should not handle alone. You need to know how to use resources inside and outside the hospital that can help the patient. This entry will help you learn how to deal with all these challenges.

## How to assess the emotional climate

The pain and anguish a patient and his family feel may or may not be proportional to the seriousness of the patient's medical problem. So your first task is to determine how much emotional support, if any, the patient and family require.

Without being obvious, you can observe the patient and family members during your routine activities and find answers to these questions: How much emotional support passes between the patient and family members? Do they seem to communicate openly and to respect each other's feelings and opinions? When family decisions must be made about treating the patient, who makes them? Several patterns of behavior you identify may indicate the family's need for emotional support. For example, such behavior as denial, emotional distancing, or ineffective problem solving indicate that the patient or family is coping ineffectively. Denial occurs, for example, when a family member refuses to accept the reality of the patient's condition. Emotional distancing occurs when the patient avoids discussing his feelings about his condition and instead dwells on "safe" topics. Ineffective problem solving occurs when a family member can't make a decision when faced with several alternatives. In all these situations, your intervention can help.

Patients and family members who exhibit these patterns of behavior may

## HANDLING YOUR OWN EMOTIONAL NEEDS

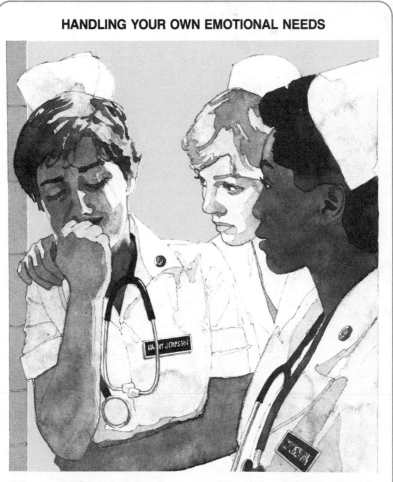

Patients generally think nurses have been "through it all" and expect them to be able to handle just about any situation that arises. You may even expect this of yourself. Of course, this is unrealistic. No nurse can *always* maintain that level of professionalism.

When you deal with a burn patient or a terminally ill child, for example, you may find yourself unable to cope with your feelings or to assess the patient's condition objectively. Learn to recognize when your own behavior signals that you need emotional support. For example, if you are often ill, or have chronic difficulty dealing with your family problems, these may be signs that you're overstressed.

When you feel unable to manage a particular patient, ask another nurse to take over. But then *you* must take action: before the same situation arises again, examine your feelings and fears. If necessary, get help to deal with them. You can do this in several ways. In many hospitals, chaplains are available to help staff members cope with patients' illnesses and deaths. Or you may wish to join (or to establish) a support group where nurses can discuss common problems. Another way to deal with your fears and concerns is an inservice workshop your hospital's nursing-education department can offer. Here you can review conversations you've had with patients and family members during stressful periods and consider how to improve future interactions.

not always be willing or able to recognize their need for your help. The patient who says, "I'm dying of cancer and you can't do anything about it," may at that moment be trying to cope with his own legitimate feelings of grief. The family member who resists your assistance may fear becoming too dependent on an outsider for help. Your success in overcoming this resistance depends on how skillfully you intervene. You can do this by actively listening to what the patient or family member is saying, following the tips presented in Entry 78.

Once the patient or family member is willing to accept your help, you can better assist him at each stage of the grieving process by recognizing which stage he's in and by continuing to use active listening techniques to help him work through his feelings. According to Patricia Sue Sharer, the stages of grief include denial or avoidance, anger, depression, rationalization, and acceptance. The patient or family member demonstrates denial or avoidance when he refuses to discuss the importance of a problem or only acknowledges nonthreatening situations. He demonstrates anger when he expresses his feelings in an explosive or volatile manner. He demonstrates depression when he experiences overwhelming episodes of loneliness and hopelessness. He demonstrates rationalization

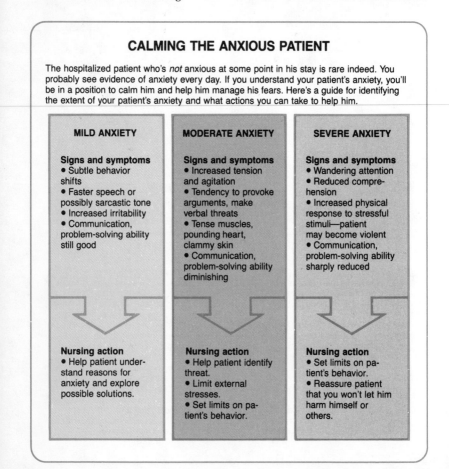

## CALMING THE ANXIOUS PATIENT

The hospitalized patient who's *not* anxious at some point in his stay is rare indeed. You probably see evidence of anxiety every day. If you understand your patient's anxiety, you'll be in a position to calm him and help him manage his fears. Here's a guide for identifying the extent of your patient's anxiety and what actions you can take to help him.

| MILD ANXIETY | MODERATE ANXIETY | SEVERE ANXIETY |
|---|---|---|
| **Signs and symptoms** <br> • Subtle behavior shifts <br> • Faster speech or possibly sarcastic tone <br> • Increased irritability <br> • Communication, problem-solving ability still good | **Signs and symptoms** <br> • Increased tension and agitation <br> • Tendency to provoke arguments, make verbal threats <br> • Tense muscles, pounding heart, clammy skin <br> • Communication, problem-solving ability diminishing | **Signs and symptoms** <br> • Wandering attention <br> • Reduced comprehension <br> • Increased physical response to stressful stimuli—patient may become violent <br> • Communication, problem-solving ability sharply reduced |
| **Nursing action** <br> • Help patient understand reasons for anxiety and explore possible solutions. | **Nursing action** <br> • Help patient identify threat. <br> • Limit external stresses. <br> • Set limits on patient's behavior. | **Nursing action** <br> • Set limits on patient's behavior. <br> • Reassure patient that you won't let him harm himself or others. |

and acceptance when he's able to discuss the problem and come to terms with it.

Sometimes, helping the patient or family member through these stages is more than one person can handle or more than your time will allow. That's when you should turn to your colleagues, in and out of the hospital, for assistance.

### Using resources within the hospital

Often nurses, doctors, and social service personnel care for the same patients without knowing entirely what the other professionals are doing. As a result, the patient receives fragmented care. To prevent or remedy this, you and the other health-care professionals involved should consider holding informal conferences, regularly or as necessary, to exchange opinions, solve problems, and coordinate care.

Ideally, you and the hospital doctors should always be considering therapeutic alternatives to current treatment in order to satisfy the patient's physical and emotional needs. In that consideration, remember that other staff members within the hospital—from mental health consultants to music therapists—are available to you. Don't hesitate to use their expertise, especially when you start to feel that a particular patient is becoming too difficult for you to handle, either professionally or emotionally.

### Using resources outside the hospital

If you aren't already familiar with services outside the hospital that can help you provide patient care, you'll discover that you have a wide range to choose from. These services include independent health-care providers, community agencies, and self-help groups. They can assist the patient or his family with such problems as coping with grief, overcoming a drug or alcohol dependency, even managing the home. To find out what's available to your pa-

tient, contact your hospital's social services department or your hospital's community health nurse. You'll find the community health nurse to be a valuable link between you and your patient and the community. She may even assume the coordinating responsibilities involved in matching your patient with the appropriate community service.

But before you call in or refer your patient to such a service, you have a professional obligation to understand

---

*"You can assist the patient in grief by using active listening techniques to help him work through his feelings."*

---

your patient's needs, the service's admission criteria (if any), and the service's objectives and methods. Referring a patient to a service that's inappropriate for him will not benefit any of the parties involved. To ensure that the referral is appropriate, consult with the patient's doctor. To make the referral, you'll probably have to get the doctor's written permission as well. His permission is needed to satisfy hospital protocol, to assure the outside service that the professionals caring for the patient are in agreement, and to meet Medicare and insurance company requirements for third-party reimbursements.

### A final word

As nurses assume more authority for planning and managing patient care, they also assume more responsibility for meeting the emotional needs of patients and their families. This means treating each patient and family member as a person with feelings and values that you understand, acknowledge, and respect.

# 78 How to deal with patients who complain

The patient who deals with the stress of hospitalization by constant complaining strains the tolerance of the entire nursing staff—and probably affects the care he receives. We're all familiar with what can happen to the constant complainer: he gets the substitute or part-time nurse; his call light is answered last; his questions and complaints receive terse and incomplete responses; he's avoided; he's given tranquilizers to help "manage" him; his behavior's harshly recounted in reports so as not to leave an unbiased nurse on the unit. If any of this happens on your unit, it's a clue that you need to deal more constructively with patients' complaining behavior.

You can't change some patients' complaining behavior. Maybe you don't have time to make an intensive effort, or maybe complaining is ingrained in your patient's personality. Often, however, you *can* encourage a positive attitude and lessen negative behavior by reading clues the patient gives you and then practicing specific interventions.

GLOSSARY

### KEY TERMS IN THIS ENTRY

**behavior modification techniques** • Techniques used for eradicating or reducing negative behaviors, or for reinforcing positive behaviors, by adjusting the amount of attention and approval a person receives or by manipulating certain aspects of the person's environment.

**stress** • Any emotional, physical, social, economic, or other change that produces physical or mental tension and may contribute to the onset of illness; also, the tension itself.

## What you need to know

What are some possible causes of complaining behavior? First and foremost—but often overlooked—is the fact that the patient may truly have something to complain about. "Nurse, my food is never hot." "Nurse, the physical therapist is always late coming for me." Do the complaints have a basis in fact? It's your job to find out.

Complaining also may indicate that the patient is having trouble dealing with deeper feelings, feelings acted out as complaining behavior. Here are some examples:
• *Anger and resentment.* "If the doctors and you nurses did your job better, I could have been out of here by now."
• *Fear and anxiety.* "It's not right that we're lined up in those drafty halls waiting for X-ray. What if I get taken in for the wrong test?"
• *Distancing behavior.* "Nurse, it's very important that you set the blinds so the light doesn't shine in my eyes. I also expect not to be disturbed until dinner."
• *Regression.* "Why can't anyone get anything right around here? I declare, I'll die just trying to correct things."

## What you need to do

If the complaints are legitimate, correct their causes if you can—no matter how many complaints the patient has. If you can't correct them, explain courteously to the patient why you can't. A simple explanation may be all that's needed.

When complaining indicates deeper feelings, such as anger or fear, or when it's a by-product of distancing or regression, you need to identify the feeling and to help the patient deal with it.

Begin by scrutinizing your own response to the patient. A complaint made in an angry tone will probably generate an angry feeling, if not an angry response, in you. An anxious or depressed patient can make you feel the same way. If the patient mimics a demanding, complaining child, you may find yourself reproaching the patient in

## PLANNING CARE FOR THE COMPLAINING PATIENT

When you, the nurse manager, make a care plan for a patient who complains a lot, keep these guidelines in mind:
• Assign a staff member with good communication skills.
• Limit the number of staff providing care, to minimize the chance of faulty communication. In this situation, primary care is best.
• Expand the patient's care plan to include ways of improving the patient's communication. Discuss these with the entire staff.

• Adopt the attitude that you can change complaining behavior, rather than that you just have to live with it.
• Consider using behavior modification techniques. (Whether you decide to do so may depend on the availability of an appropriate consultant.)
• Respect the patient's individuality. Using pat formulas or faulty and incomplete interpretations of his behavior is demeaning to him and unworthy of you as a professional nurse.

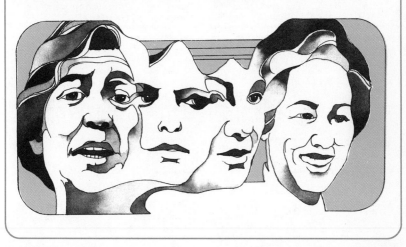

a parentlike way.

After you've identified the feelings involved, help your patient identify the feelings, too. By helping him understand his feelings and concerns, you'll lessen your patient's stress—and his complaining behavior.

How can you respond to complaining behavior? Try these approaches to encourage the patient to deal more effectively with what may be underlying his complaint:
• *Anger and resentment.* "Mr. Smith, being in a hospital and being sick are aggravating and disruptive for most people. I'll do anything I can to make this experience less difficult for you. You can help by sharing your concerns with me."
• *Fear and anxiety.* "Mrs. Jones, I know that hospitals, with all the dif-

ferent routines and staff, can be confusing. If I can explain anything to you or if you have any questions, please let's talk about them. Maybe that will make your stay here less confusing."
• *Distancing behavior.* "Hospitals usually don't allow as much privacy as people like. Perhaps we can work out some ways to prevent so many intrusions. Are there any particular interruptions that you find especially aggravating?"
• *Regression.* "If you can be more specific about what's bothering you, I think we'll work better together. Your complaining is making it difficult to care for you. Since I'm going to be the nurse most responsible for your care, I'd like to spend 10 minutes each day just talking with you. This will be your time to let me know what you need."

Be sure to perform these key steps

## IDENTIFYING DEFENSE MECHANISMS

Why does your patient use defense mechanisms? To protect himself from anxiety by changing, concealing, or falsifying the threat he believes a stressful event poses. As you know, defense mechanisms aren't always harmful. But they can interfere with a patient's daily functioning. That's why you need to understand them and be able to identify them. This chart defines and describes some of the defense mechanisms patients commonly use.

| DEFENSE MECHANISM | DEFINITION | BEHAVIOR TRAITS | REASONS FOR USE |
|---|---|---|---|
| **Denial** | Refusing to recognize some aspect of reality | Denying known facts or reality | Protects patient from painful reality |
| **Rationalization** | Justifying behavior by using a plausible excuse | Intensely defending position | Maintains patient's self-respect and wards off guilt feelings |
| **Displacement** | Shifting feelings and attitudes about a person from that person to another | Developing compulsive habits or phobia toward object of displaced feeling; exhibiting excessive emotions | Allows patient to express repressed feelings |
| **Conversion** | Translating psychological problems into physical complaints | Claiming physical problems that have no clinical cause | Helps patient avoid the anxiety-producing situation because he's "ill"; gives patient legitimate reason for seeking help and support or takes the focus away from the psychological problems |
| **Regression** | Returning to a previous, immature way of behaving | Abandoning adult role and embracing child or infant role | Permits patient to avoid anxiety of real situation |
| **Projection** | Transferring unwanted thoughts and tendencies to others | Distorting personal world view; minimizing own guilt by making others feel guilty; blaming others for own problems | Provides an outlet for patient's repressed thoughts and tendencies |

when you approach the patient:
- Begin the discussion in an open, non-judgmental way.
- Set an adult, but caring, tone.
- Acknowledge that being in a hospital can cause stress.
- Encourage the patient to talk about whatever is bothering him: Let him select what he wants to share.
- Accept his feelings—no matter what they are—and don't attribute a negative value to them.
- Share your observations on what you think his feelings and concerns are. This allows the patient to affirm or correct your perception.
- Dignify the patient by inviting him to share in problem solving. This will help reinstate in him a sense of independence and competence.

You may find behavior modification techniques effective for eliminating negative behaviors or for reinforcing desirable ones. Even without training in such techniques, you can use positive reinforcement in your everyday interactions by giving your patient attention and approval, by showing him respect and caring, by providing comfort, and by relieving his pain. All these are powerful rewards.

No matter how distressing the patient's behavior may be, as long as you do not act defensively or match his anger or anxiety with your own, you can communicate constructively with him and promote further understanding. To borrow from the language of transactional analysis, a patient is often responding out of his petulant "child." If you can respond with "adult" rather than with "child" or "parent" behavior, you'll be more likely to encourage productive communication with him.

### A final word
Sometimes, of course, a patient who complains persistently must be confronted directly about his behavior. But you'll usually be able to avoid communication problems, or at least deal with them effectively, when you've gained your patients' respect and trust.

# 79 Communicating with pediatric patients

A child's hospitalization presents a crisis for the child, of course, but also for his family. As a nurse, you know you're in a unique position to help them cope. How? By anticipating the child's emotional needs as well as his physical needs. You can assess a child's developmental level and establish a thorough nursing history during the admission interview. By doing this, you'll be better able to help him and his parents throughout his hospital stay. You'll provide better nursing care, too.

First, you need to find out what hospitalization means to the child. For example, a child may view his hospitalization as a form of punishment. Even if his mother stays with him in the hospital, separation from his father, siblings, or extended family and familiar surroundings may be confusing and upsetting. Changes from his daily routine and loss of his ability or opportunity to care for himself can be

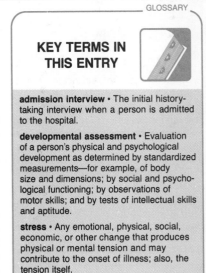

GLOSSARY

**KEY TERMS IN THIS ENTRY**

**admission interview** • The initial history-taking interview when a person is admitted to the hospital.

**developmental assessment** • Evaluation of a person's physical and psychological development as determined by standardized measurements—for example, of body size and dimensions; by social and psychological functioning; by observations of motor skills; and by tests of intellectual skills and aptitude.

**stress** • Any emotional, physical, social, economic, or other change that produces physical or mental tension and may contribute to the onset of illness; also, the tension itself.

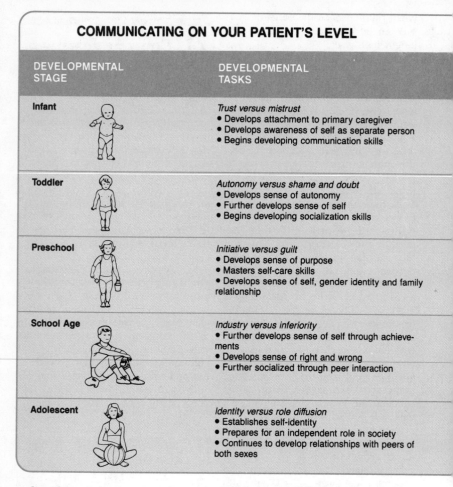

## COMMUNICATING ON YOUR PATIENT'S LEVEL

| DEVELOPMENTAL STAGE | DEVELOPMENTAL TASKS |
|---|---|
| **Infant** | *Trust versus mistrust*<br>• Develops attachment to primary caregiver<br>• Develops awareness of self as separate person<br>• Begins developing communication skills |
| **Toddler** | *Autonomy versus shame and doubt*<br>• Develops sense of autonomy<br>• Further develops sense of self<br>• Begins developing socialization skills |
| **Preschool** | *Initiative versus guilt*<br>• Develops sense of purpose<br>• Masters self-care skills<br>• Develops sense of self, gender identity and family relationship |
| **School Age** | *Industry versus inferiority*<br>• Further develops sense of self through achievements<br>• Develops sense of right and wrong<br>• Further socialized through peer interaction |
| **Adolescent** | *Identity versus role diffusion*<br>• Establishes self-identity<br>• Prepares for an independent role in society<br>• Continues to develop relationships with peers of both sexes |

as disturbing as the treatments he must endure.

A child's age, developmental level, and past experience play a big part in influencing the meaning that any situation has for him. The key to recognizing hospitalization's meaning to a child of any age is being able to communicate with him. This involves taking a detailed nursing history and using it to understand the child's fears and concerns, and to learn about his usual daily routine. Then you can fashion a care plan that takes these into account and facilitates effective communication with the child throughout his hospital stay.

## Taking a child's history: what you need to know

Carry out the admission interview in a quiet, unhurried setting. Include the child during the initial portion of the interview; tell his parents they can talk privately with you later.

*Display a friendly, reassuring manner.* Tell the child and his parents that the information they share with you will help you develop a care plan that will include easing the stress of hospitalization.

Use the interview to *determine the child's behavioral pattern*, as well as his response to stress. What does he know about his illness? What does he

| MAJOR FEARS | TIPS FOR SUCCESSFUL COMMUNICATION |
|---|---|
| • Separation from parents<br>• Pain | • Allow mother or primary caretaker to be involved in care.<br>• Allow him to see your face when talking; use facial and vocal expression.<br>• Use nonverbal soothing communication, such as rocking and stroking. |
| • Separation from parents<br>• Bodily injury and pain<br>• Loss of control | • Allow some independence; provide safe environment so he can use acquired skills.<br>• Use terms he's familiar with for body parts and functions.<br>• Continue familiar routines as much as possible. |
| • Separation from parents<br>• Bodily injury and pain<br>• Loss of control | • Encourage parents to bring photos, toys, or security objects from home.<br>• Encourage interaction with other children on unit.<br>• Acknowledge and deal with fears; provide information in clear, easy-to-understand terms.<br>• Set limits for behavior. |
| • Separation from parents and peers<br>• Bodily injury and pain<br>• Loss of control | • Encourage contact with friends as well as family.<br>• Allow privacy, place him with children of same sex.<br>• Provide information about illness and treatment prior to any event to let him get used to the situation.<br>• Tell jokes and play games.<br>• Provide limits, positive reinforcement for accomplishments. |
| • Separation, especially from peer group<br>• Bodily injury<br>• Loss of control | • Provide privacy, information about routines and therapies.<br>• Explain limits; allow privileges not allowed younger children on unit.<br>• Let him express fears; do not be drawn into his anger with family, doctors, or other nurses. |

think hospitalization will be like?

*Note the parents' anxiety level.* Parental anxiety will affect the child and may frighten him. Here's an example:

Billy, age 5, was admitted for possible leukemia. His parents naturally were upset. The father was impatient, angry, and abrupt when he spoke. He paced up and down and often became hostile during the interview. The mother acted nervous and edgy. She appeared to have been crying and seemed to be about to cry frequently during the interview. Billy sat on his mother's lap throughout the interview, stroking her arm, squeezing her hand, and staring at his father. He seemed bewildered and frightened.

You can prevent unnecessary anxiety for a child like Billy and his parents by providing information and support. This can be the most important thing you accomplish during the admission interview. If the parents seem to be very anxious, share this information with the medical and nursing staff.

*Include a family history.* Ask about recent events, such as the birth of another child, travel, divorce, separation, or the death of a family member, friend, or pet. If you learn that a child's parents are divorced or separated, ask the parent who has custody about whether—and how often—the other parent will visit the child. Ask the child about this, too—what does he expect will happen? Remember that a child whose parents are divorced or separated may have some behavior problems including withdrawal, aggression, and manipulative behavior.

*Find out about the child's usual habits,* his daily living activities.

*Develop a baseline of the child's verbal and motor ability.* How self-reliant is the child at home? This information is particularly helpful if your patient is a small child or preschooler. Children who dress and feed themselves at home need opportunities to do so when they're hospitalized. Often they're very proud of these accomplishments and will become angry or depressed if they can't continue to demonstrate them. A

---

*"Knowing the normal behavior for a child's age group helps you recognize when his behavior is abnormal."*

---

child who's toilet trained also needs the opportunity and encouragement to maintain this developmental level.

*Obtain information about the child's sleeping habits.* Bedtime can be traumatic when a child must sleep away from home. But if you know that a child age 10 months who wakes up late at night is used to having his back rubbed, you can do this and comfort him.

Does the child usually sleep in a bed or a crib? Does he have set routines at bedtime? Does he sleep with a special doll or blanket? Find out if he's a light sleeper, if he sleeps alone in his room at home, and if he naps during the day. If he's a light sleeper, you can try to place him in a room away from active areas on the unit. If he usually sleeps alone, be sure to explain that he'll probably have a roommate. (If this is

a problem after the child is placed in his room, create a private cubicle for him by drawing the curtains around his bed.) If he reads, watches TV, or listens to the radio at bedtime, try to arrange to continue this routine in the hospital.

Be sure to *assess the child's language skills* and to identify any special words the child uses for his body parts or functions, for his parents, or for a security object (for example, a blanket or a toy). When you know these special words, you can communicate more effectively with him. When you don't, you may be unable to comfort him. Imagine a 2-year-old calling for "Bobby": you may think he wants his brother, when what he's asking for is a bottle.

Finally, *assess the child's developmental level,* particularly whether he's mastered the tasks of each stage of childhood he's passed through. (See *Communicating on Your Patient's Level,* pages 496 and 497.) Include in your notes specific abilities the child has that were reported, or that you observed, during the admission interview.

## Making your care plan

Once you know the behaviors and activities that constitute a child's life at home, you can structure a care plan tailored to his developmental level and designed so he can use newly acquired behavior in his daily hospital activities. This way, he'll feel more in control of his environment, and less frightened and anxious, during his hospital stay. For example:

• Try not to limit a very young walker's mobility.

• Don't put a toilet-trained child in diapers.

• Don't start an intravenous line in a preschool or school-age child's dominant hand.

• Help school-age children to call their friends at home. Ensure privacy.

• As much as possible, let your pediatric patients participate in decisions about their care. (See *How to Achieve Pediatric Nursing Goals.*)

## Signs and symptoms of some common behavior problems

You'll find your thorough nursing history and developmental assessment very helpful when problems arise with pediatric patients. Knowing a child's normal behavior lets you recognize when his behavior is *abnormal*. Regression, aggression, rejection, manipulation, and depression are some common abnormal behaviors that can cause problems in caring for pediatric patients.

*Regression* is common in children experiencing stress. Normally, a child works hard to achieve and maintain new developmental levels. But when he's in a stressful situation, continued development becomes difficult. In order to reduce his stress, the child may regress to a simpler, less difficult level he has previously mastered. Unfortunately, he may also display troublesome behavior.

You'll usually have no trouble recognizing *aggression* or *rejection*. Recognizing them early and dealing with them promptly, before they become behavior patterns, are essential.

A child suffering from *depression* may lie quietly in his bed, tolerate procedures without crying, or even sleep for long periods during the day. Sometimes he is thought of as an ideal patient, and his depression isn't recognized. A depressed child who's using *manipulation* to get what he wants can be even harder to recognize, because his personality changes may be subtle and subject to misinterpretation.

## HOW TO ACHIEVE PEDIATRIC NURSING GOALS

| NURSING GOALS | INTERVENTIONS |
|---|---|
| Help the child feel loved and cared for as an individual. | • Use the child's name or nickname when talking to him.<br>• Don't show disapproval of the child.<br>• Encourage the parents to remain with the child and to demonstrate their affection for him. |
| Establish a trusting relationship with the child. | • Provide primary care as often as possible.<br>• Be honest with the child, using explanations he can understand; involve the parents in care.<br>• Have consistent expectations; set reasonable and fair limits on his behavior; reward positive behavior. |
| Allow the child to have some control over his situation. | • Use terms familiar to the child; explain procedures and treatments, and allow him to handle equipment; whenever possible, allow him to make choices about the timing of care.<br>• Continue routines the child is accustomed to; provide the child with opportunities for self-care.<br>• Allow the child time for play, uninterrupted by treatments and care. |
| Provide opportunities for the child to display feelings of fear, anger, or frustration. | • Accept the child's feelings, absolve him of any guilty feelings.<br>• Provide an atmosphere that allows him to express himself; use play as an anxiety-reducing technique; provide toys and hospital equipment for him to act out his fears. |
| Allow the child to regress during periods of illness. | • Help the parents recognize regressive behavior as a reaction to stress.<br>• Help the child with any dependency manifested during regression. |

# THE HOSPITALIZED CHILD: HELPING HIM COPE WITH HIS FEARS

How would you manage a child, age 6, suffering from a head injury and possible internal injuries, who's been admitted to your unit for observation and testing?

Here's one important consideration: because he's unprepared for hospitalization, he may cope poorly with the stress of a new environment and even suffer some long-term emotional effects.

Fortunately, most children who are treated with kindness and respect cope with the stress of hospitalization remarkably well. And your sensitive nursing care can make the difference.

Although a child who enters your unit with little or no emotional preparation may need extra attention and support, you'll use the same basic techniques to care for him that you use to help *all* your patients cope with the stress of hospitalization. Follow these guidelines:

• *Provide one-to-one nursing care,* if possible. You or another nurse, a nurse's aide, or any other staff member can serve as the child's special friend throughout his hospital stay. In addition to playing with him, this staff member should be available for support during any stressful treatment procedure, especially if the parents aren't present.

• *Assess the child's understanding of his illness and treatment* by asking him why he thinks he's in the hospital. Use his re-

sponses to plan patient teaching and to assess his need for emotional support.

• *Plan teaching sessions* for times when the child is rested and alert. Don't prolong them beyond the child's attention span.

• *Foster the child's trust* with consistent behavior and honest communication. Tell him that you'll warn him before you do anything that'll hurt; then, keep your promise. This way, he won't feel he must be on guard all the time.

• *Prepare him for treatments,* including surgery, by describing the events and sensations he'll experience. But avoid being *too* specific, because he may become upset if events don't happen exactly as you predicted. To prepare the child to cope with any unexpected event, ask him to remember anything that happens to him that's different from what he expected. Then you can discuss it with him later.

*Important:* Tell him about painful or unpleasant aspects of his treatment last. Otherwise, he may become too anxious to listen to the rest of your explanation.

• *Choose your words carefully,* especially if your patient is a preschooler. Remember, a child this age thinks in literal terms and in terms of his own experience. For example, if you tell him that he'll be "put to sleep" for surgery, he may think of the old family dog who never returned from the veterinarian. Likewise, if you tell him that surgery

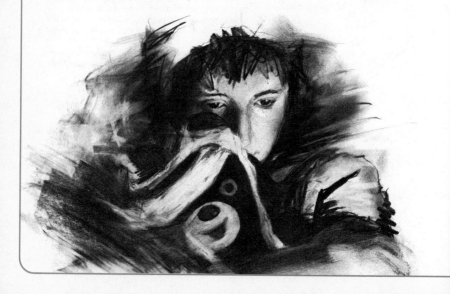

will occur when he's asleep, he may be reluctant to fall asleep at night, fearing that something awful will happen if he does. Emphasize that anesthesia is a *special* sleep he'll experience only when the doctor gives him a special medicine, and that the doctor will wake him up when the surgery is over.

• *Question the child* about his understanding of treatments and procedures. Suppose he asks you, for example, "How does the doctor take out my tonsils?" Reply by saying, "How do *you* think he does it?" Listen carefully to his explanation: in addition to revealing the extent of his understanding, it can help you understand his unique fears and fantasies.

• *Use group-teaching techniques,* when possible. In addition to saving you time, group teaching provides peer-group support for each child.

• *Perform all painful or upsetting procedures in the treatment room*—not the child's hospital room. Let this room be a safe haven for him.

• *Give him a sense of control* by offering realistic choices. For example, you can't allow him to choose whether or not to have an injection. But you *can* ask him if he'd like another minute to get ready.

• *Ask another child to help you prepare a newcomer* for an unpleasant procedure. For example, if the new patient is afraid of an injection, a more experienced child may be able to reassure him that it's not so bad.

• *Build playtime into your daily routine.* This encourages the child to associate you with comfort and fun, not just pain. And it gives you a chance to learn more about him.

• *Use play therapy* to explain procedures to the child and to help him work through his emotions. For example, before you change his dressings, you might bandage the head of his teddy bear or other toy, to show him what you're going to do.

Play provides clues to how well the child is adjusting to his illness and treatment. Play also helps him work through his feelings. For example, violent play suggests anger or fear; drawings that distort body parts suggest a poor self-image and fear of mutilation. If the child seems unusually disturbed, consult with a child psychologist or specially trained social worker.

• *Tell the child that no one will be mad if he cries.* Remain supportive of the child regardless of how he behaves.

In general, a manipulative child uses the fact that he's ill to ensure constant attention. He does this by crying when he's left alone, ignoring his parents when they visit, or complaining continually about how he feels.

## How to manage problem behaviors

A child who demonstrates aggressive, protesting behavior is usually a challenge for the unit. He may be verbally or physically abusive to his nurses or to other children on the unit. Unfortunately, often the nurses' response is to avoid the child—which only intensifies his behavior. Remember, an aggressive child needs to know that others are in control and that he can rely on the people taking care of him to set the behavior limits he needs.

Don't allow a child's abusive behavior to continue unabated, even if you feel the child has reason to be angry. Point out that this type of behavior is unacceptable, but be sure the child understands that you disapprove only of his behavior, not of *him.* Always remain calm, and avoid taking any aggressive action yourself. You may have to restrain a child who's out of control, but you should never respond angrily.

Whenever possible, leave a child who's having a temper tantrum alone with one nurse until the tantrum is over. Once the child has calmed down, talk with him about a system that will reward and reinforce appropriate behavior. Your part in this system will be to ignore or appropriately subdue aggressive outbursts. Discuss this idea at a level the child can understand. Here are some examples of reward systems for pediatric patients:

• You might offer extra TV time, or a half hour later bedtime, to a school-age child for each day he gets through without fighting with other children in the playroom.

• Offer a preschooler who's having a tantrum, because another child is playing with a toy he wants, a chance to play with the toy later if he'll first play quietly with other toys for a specified period of time. (An automatic timer can be useful for this purpose. Keep the time span short for young children.)

Allowing yourself to openly pity a sick child invites manipulative behavior. A child who recognizes that certain behaviors will get him attention will naturally repeat them. You'll commonly see this in a child who's been hospitalized repeatedly or for a long time. He notices that other children with more acute health problems get more attention, so he looks for ways to attract the staff's attention to *his* problems. Along with obvious attention-getting behaviors like crying or sulking, the child may use so-called withholding behaviors: refusing to eat, to take medicines, or to talk. The staff's usual reaction is to focus on the withholding behavior. The coaxing, cajoling, and even bribing that often result serve the child's primary purpose: he becomes the center of attention.

The remedy for manipulative behavior is generally the same as for aggressive or abusive behavior. Early recognition of the problem and a willingness to set limits for the child are very important. Talk with him at a level he can understand. Acknowledge his need for attention, and assure him that cooperative behavior will get him more attention than manipulative behavior will. Once you've established this mutual understanding, implement a plan of care that supports this philosophy. Communicate the plan to all the nursing and medical staff as well as to the child's parents, and stick to it even if it's a drastic change from earlier ways of dealing with the child.

For example, you can tell a child who refuses to eat that his behavior isn't acceptable and won't get him extra attention, now or in the future. Then offer meals only at the designated time, and have one person (either a nurse or a parent) stay with the child throughout the meal, *without coaxing or forcing him to eat*. When mealtime is over, remove the food and offer no more until the next mealtime. The child will begin to associate his withholding behavior with social isolation—the opposite of what he wants—and with hunger. As you continue to give attention to the child as a reward for acceptable behavior, he'll become less dependent on manipulative behavioral patterns.

A child in danger of becoming depressed because of his illness and hospitalization will first begin to withdraw from social interaction. If you're alert to this possibility, you'll be able to recognize depression's early signs and to intervene appropriately. The child's withdrawal is a sign of despair. He may have misconceptions about his hospitalization so that, for example, he feels that the separation from his family is a punishment, or that his need for isolation means his disease is fatal. After all, such a child may reason, he's been confined to bed (you know this doesn't mean he's seriously ill, but *he* doesn't), and his parents visit infrequently (because they live a long way from the hospital). But he may not communicate these fears to you. In fact, his quiet, docile behavior may not be consistent with your expectation that he'll cry to display sadness. This is why recognizing the signs of depression can be difficult. But because early intervention to relieve depression can be so

---

## "Play sessions can help to reveal a child's state of mind."

---

important to a child's comfort during a stay in the hospital, you need to evaluate the concerns and fears of any child who begins to withdraw from others.

Of course, if his illness *is* serious or fatal, you must help him and his family manage their very real fears and concerns. And what if his parents *are* rejecting him, or you suspect he's been abused? In a situation like this, you must intervene to help the child. Consult your institution's social work department, and perhaps even a family therapist, to help the parent and child build a stronger relationship and to help ensure the child's safety after discharge (see Entry 27). During the child's hospitalization, you'll need to find other ways to provide the security he's lacking. For example, with parental permission, you might arrange the visit of a relative, neighbor, or teacher the child cares for and has a loving relationship with. A volunteer foster grandparent may be able to spend time with an infant or young child. Teenage volunteers can provide consistent, dependable companionship for school-age children during busy visiting times, to help combat loneliness and the feeling of rejection.

**Supportive actions you can take**
Play sessions can help to reveal a child's state of mind. When you offer a child opportunities to act out his fears and to clarify his misconceptions, you can help him relieve his tensions and understand the reasons for his hospitalization. Encourage his parents to establish a consistent visiting pattern, even if these visits have to be infrequent. Other ways of helping him feel connected to his family include phone calls and cards from them, photographs to display in his room, and even audio tapes he can make and exchange with his family. For example, his parents can tape a family mealtime where everyone at the table tells the child what each did that day. Talking about things that will happen once he's home again will help the child realize that his hospitalization is not permanent. (See *The Hospitalized Child: Helping Him Cope With His Fears,* pages 500 and 501.)

**A final word**
A hospitalized child has many needs. As a nurse, you're often in the best position to meet his needs. But unless you can communicate effectively with the child, identifying his needs may be impossible. Effective communication with children means you must give them clear messages they can understand, and you must understand the sometimes disguised or obscured messages they give you. Your nursing history and your powers of observation will help you recognize a young patient's developmental level, his usual coping behavior, and what the hospitalization means to him. If you're able to tailor your care to his specific needs, you'll soon find you're able to reduce his stress. You may even find that other staff members consult you to help ensure quality care for all children on the unit.

# 80 Communicating with geriatric patients

You're probably aware that between the years 1980 and 2030, the number of persons in the United States who live past age 75 will increase by about 150% (see Entry 8). This means that many elderly people will live to be extremely old, and that gerontologic nursing concepts will be increasingly important in nursing practice. At the core of gerontologic nursing is the principle that elderly people can continue as full participants in their own health care provided they receive sensitive, knowledgeable teaching and kindly, consistent encouragement in self-care.

**How society stereotypes the elderly**
Elderly people are too often viewed as throwaway commodities that have far outgrown their usefulness. Many people believe that all the elderly are ill and infirm, cluttering hospitals and nursing homes with their uninteresting chronic illnesses. They're grouped together, in many people's minds, as nonconsumers who are mentally unfit to voice opinions and make decisions.

## KEY TERMS IN THIS ENTRY

**gerontologic nursing** • A type of nursing care, in which a nurse may specialize, that provides specifically for the physical, intellectual, and emotional needs of the elderly.

**reality orientation techniques** • Nursing techniques for keeping patients oriented to time, place, and person.

**stereotyping** • Using subjective judgment to view people with certain characteristics in common as a group, conforming to a standardized mental image.

Have you noticed how often the media portray elderly people as senile, dependent, unfashionable, and unattractive? Human-interest news stories tend to focus more on the abnormal activities of a few elderly people than on the numerous achievements of the vast majority of elderly persons. Even what's considered normal behavior for a younger person (such as having sex, holding a job, being creative, getting married) is often considered abnormal if an elderly person does it. Interestingly, many elderly people believe these myths themselves.

### A look at nurses' attitudes

Chances are you've occasionally shared in society's stereotyping of the elderly—especially if you've worked mainly with acutely ill, severely chronically ill, or terminally ill adults. Here's a statistic that may surprise you: Only about 6% of the elderly population are institutionalized at any given time. Most of the other 94% lead full lives and make their own decisions about their daily activities. (See *How to Avoid "Stereotype Backlash" with Geriatric Patients.*)

No one's unconcerned about aging and death. Elderly patients remind us all of our mortality. This discomfort could be a reason why (until recently) gerontologic nursing was an unpopular career choice.

If you're a nurse who's cared for many very ill elderly patients, but who hasn't been trained in gerontologic nursing, you may erroneously believe that elderly people can't learn new things or care for themselves. Maybe some of your nursing colleagues feel this way, too. Do some of them treat elderly patients as babies or children? Do some nurses you know consult elderly patients' relatives and friends to discuss the patients' hospitalization and obtain decisions about the patients' care? This attitude stems from the belief that elderly people no longer control their own lives. For most, this simply isn't true. Elderly people are commonly lucid and rational, quite capable of making their own decisions. (They also have the same legal rights as all other citizens—such as the right to consent to treatment or refuse it. See Entries 8, 11, 12, and 14 to 18.)

Or maybe you've been frustrated, in caring for elderly patients, by a lack of understanding of the aging process. Elderly patients *do* require special nursing care. An elderly patient who can't comply with a treatment regimen or cooperate with your nursing efforts may not be recalcitrant or senile—he may just be demonstrating the effects of old age.

Patient teaching offers a prime example of how stereotyped views can have a negative effect on older patients' care. Believing that an elderly patient won't be able to understand, a nurse may explain his home care to a family member or friend. The patient may learn about his care almost by accident instead of from his nurse. He may have practical problems, too: in written self-care instructions, the print is often too small for aging eyes to read easily.

Most often, however, the elderly patient's need for teaching is simply ignored, and the patient has to use his own ingenuity at home to compensate. Then, when he must return to the hospital, a nurse is likely to remark, "He

# HOW TO AVOID "STEREOTYPE BACKLASH" WITH GERIATRIC PATIENTS

You're familiar with the stereotyped portrait of the geriatric patient: mentally numb, senile, child-like. You also know how inaccurate and unfair that portrait is. You know that geriatric patients are as different from each other as patients in any other age group, and that each geriatric patient has individual needs—which deserve your individual attention. But even with your enlightened attitude, you need to watch out for a kind of "stereotype backlash" that can cause problems for you in caring for geriatric patients. These patients are typically aware that they're stereotyped— and sensitive about it. This means that unless you're extra careful, a geriatric patient may take offense because of a remark or gesture you make with no intent to insult him. Here's a list of reminders about what *not* to do when you're caring for a geriatric patient:

• Don't use baby-talk. A geriatric patient is an adult, no matter how many disabilities he has, and you shouldn't treat him like a child.

• Don't think of, or describe, a geriatric patient as senile. Look for ways to enhance his memory processes.

• Don't call a geriatric patient by his first name unless he gives you permission to use it.

• Don't perform a procedure on a geriatric patient without first explaining to him what you're going to do. Make sure you get his permission to perform the procedure. Encourage him to participate in his care.

• Don't distance yourself from the geriatric patient. Touch him (unless he objects), because touch gives a sense of belonging and self-worth. But don't patronize him by mechanically patting him on the shoulder or arm.

• Don't say, "Everything's going to be all right," when that's not true. The geriatric patient may have to cope with chronic illness, severe disability, or permanent frailty. Don't set him up for coping with extra disappointment, too.

• Don't speak for the geriatric patient when he's able to speak for himself and make his own decisions.

• Don't use judgmental language, such as, "Don't you know you should ...," "You have to ...," or "Why can't you ...?" Instead, use language that enhances your geriatric patient's self-esteem.

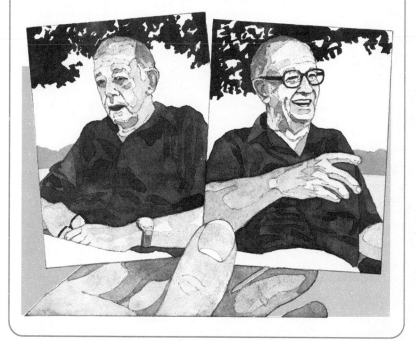

wouldn't follow our instructions at home. No wonder he's back in the hospital!"

## Nursing the elderly: understanding is the key

The primary rule in communicating with an elderly patient calls for you, as a nurse, to be warm, empathic, and nurturing. Don't behave in an authoritarian manner, and don't treat him as your parent (or child). If you relate to your elderly patient on a person-to-person level, adult to adult, age and gender will be of little importance. What *is* vital to your relationship? Genuine caring and feeling for your elderly patient.

Explore your elderly patient's value system so you can understand his background and the way he makes decisions. Be prepared to find that his values, reflective of an earlier time, sometimes clash with yours. This can lead to conflicts in the way you develop and use your nursing care plan. For example, suppose your elderly patient has always dressed in a suit and tie when in public. He'll feel uncomfortable if you insist that he wear only a hospital gown when he's in the hospital corridors and elevators. Or an elderly patient who's been married for 40 or 50 years may be offended by the staff's glib talk about divorce.

Remember, Abraham Maslow's *hierarchy of needs* is as valid for older adults as it is for people of other ages. Your elderly patient still has the same needs for shelter and safety, belonging, self-esteem, and self-actualization. In fact, when he's unable to have these basic needs met, illness (especially depression) may result. He has extra difficulty keeping his needs met, however, because of the changes—external as well as internal—that aging brings. For example, social losses (job, friends, neighbors, and family) lessen feelings of belonging. If he's frequently chided because he can't think, move, eat, or react as fast as a 20-year-old, he may lose self-esteem. If he can't feel satisfied

with his experiences and interactions with others, he won't feel actualized—his goals of living won't be achieved.

An elderly person's mood may be the result of influences you have no experience with yet. For example, toward the end of life, elderly people go through a process Robert Butler terms a *life review*, in which they psychologically review their lives as they remember them, critiquing the good and the bad aspects. Erik Erikson underscores the life review's importance; elderly persons need to integrate their successes and failures into an acceptance of life as it

---

## *"Be prepared to find that an elderly patient's values may clash with yours."*

---

was. Unless your older patient does this successfully, despair will mark the rest of his life.

When you're communicating with elderly patients, keep these aspects of memory theory and learning theory in mind:

● Don't give too much information too rapidly: instead, wait until your elderly patient finishes processing earlier verbal or visual stimuli. If you present new stimuli too quickly, he'll miss part of it. Ask for feedback as you go along.

● If you want your patient to remember what you tell him, write the information down, or tie it in conversationally with something he already knows. Otherwise, he may forget the information quickly.

Age-related sensory changes also may affect communication:

● Age-related changes in the ear (presbycusis) decrease elderly persons' ability to hear high-frequency speech, especially consonants. Your patient may not be able to hear something spoken at a normal loudness level, or the sound may be distorted so he misses hearing exactly what's being said.

• Yellowing of the eyes' lenses may distort color, especially in the blue-green range, so that your elderly patient doesn't see colors the same way you do.

• These changes in his sensory perceptions may make your elderly patient anxious or confused. Ask for feedback often as you talk with him—and take time to clarify your message if you think he didn't understand something.

## Communication pointers

When you make the effort to acknowledge that your elderly patient is an adult, you'll find that your conversations with him, as well as his behavior, will usually remain on an adult level. Don't talk baby talk. Elderly patients have adult developmental needs. They are definitely *not* children—who have a different set of developmental tasks.

Always call your elderly patient by his formal name—"Mr. Smith," for example—and don't offend him by using his first name or such familiarities as "Gramps." Avoid using terms like "senior citizen" or "oldster," too. Many elderly people dislike these terms. Of course, if your elderly patient gives you permission to use his first name or a pet name (and many do), feel free to do so.

When giving information, speak in a normal tone of voice, using a medium to low pitch. You don't need to shout. (In fact, hearing-impaired persons usually lose the ability to hear loud, high-frequency sounds.) Always face your patient, so he can *watch* what you're saying. (You probably know that multiple stimuli, both verbal and visual, aid information retention.) Wear bright lipstick or lip gloss so your elderly patient can follow your lip movements readily. If you're a male nurse working with the elderly, avoid wearing a heavy mustache and beard.

If your elderly patient has poor vision, always identify yourself by touching him on the arm and saying who you are. When you give him written instructions, use nonglare paper, and write or print the information in large

black or red letters, using a broad felt-tip pen. Read the information to the patient, and ask for feedback to ensure that he understands. Do you know that many elderly people have problems reading elite or pica type, as well as light print? Yet hospital menus and discharge instructions are often lightly duplicated from small print. Many health-teaching pamphlets are also inappropriate for older adults. Why? Because they're printed on high-gloss paper with small print in low-contrast ink. If you can't obtain commercially printed materials that are easy to read, develop your own.

Don't forget patience and tact! If your older patient's talk is becoming too tangential or too descriptive, gently take his hand and say, "I'd like to hear more about . . . , but I believe we'd better get back to our subject," or "Mr. Smith, when I come back to change your dressings, you can tell me the rest of the story about Uncle Harry." This way, he knows you're interested in him but that you must keep to a work schedule. Never admonish your patient with, "That's not important. Now answer my question," or "I'm interested in you, Mr. Smith, not your Uncle Harry." By using your periodic visits with your patient to continue your conversation with him, you can eventually hear all the stories he wants to tell you. At the same time, you'll be facilitating one of his important developmental tasks—his life review.

*Touch* is a major means of communicating with your elderly patient. But don't pat him on the shoulder, because he may think you're being condescending. Instead, clasp his hand while you talk. If you've come to know him well, you can embrace him around the shoulders and give him a big hug, unless he asks you not to.

Speak directly to your elderly patient when you're discussing his care. In order to maintain his self-worth and sense of belonging, he needs to retain his identity. Never "talk through" your older patient as if he wasn't there

("Mrs. Jones, I'm going to start an I.V. on your father.").

Let your elderly patient speak for himself and be in control of his own life as much as possible. This is his right. For example, if Mr. White states that he doesn't want his 2 p.m. tranquilizer because it makes him feel weak and stuporous, and he wants to be alert to enjoy his daughter's forthcoming visit, remember he has the right to refuse the medication. Using pressuring statements such as, "You *have* to take the tranquilizer, Mr. White, because the doctor *ordered* it for you" are totally inappropriate and thoughtless.

You can be an effective advocate for your elderly patient by helping him to assert his right to be included in decision-making about his health. Try to protect him from the depersonalizing rounds made by attending and academic doctors and nurses, with their student entourages. Too often, professors poke, prod, uncover, and talk about an elderly patient, and make plans for his management, without ever once acknowledging the presence of a human being in the bed.

Keep in mind that you can psychologically abuse an elderly patient without recognizing it. Here's an example:

Mr. Carter was scheduled for a chest X-ray. His nurse admonished him for eating too slowly, taking his bath too slowly, and even transferring to his wheelchair too slowly. "Hurry up, Mr. Carter. We can't wait all day for you. You aren't the only patient, you know." By being so impersonal with him, she lowered his self-esteem and isolated him from an appropriate social interaction: chatting with her as she performed these tasks, at *his* pace. She forgot that elderly persons are slow because the time they need to react increases with age.

Remember that performing several activities too close together will quickly deplete your elderly patient's energy.

When he's feeling anxious, or when he's under the influence of mood-altering drugs, or when he's very ill, an elderly patient may be unable to speak in complete sentences. This doesn't mean he doesn't have something important to communicate. As Lilian Weymouth describes in a sensitive article, an elderly woman with a hip fracture could only say, "Bananas in the window." That was a clue to what she was trying to tell the nurses about her fear that she wouldn't be able to return home. The nurses labeled her confused. But a sensitive graduate student slowly helped the patient tell her story: she was afraid the social workers would consider her an unfit housekeeper, and not let her return home, when they found rotting bananas on her kitchen window ledge—where she'd put them to ripen just before she fell and was hospitalized.

Sometimes a patient isn't spoken to at all. Here's an example:

In one nursing home, two graduate nursing students observed that the staff said absolutely nothing to Miss Webber, a very elderly and ill patient who followed all activities with her eyes. She was bathed, fed, gotten out of bed into a wheelchair, and given medication without one word said to her. The staff talked only among themselves. The two graduate nursing students asked to care for Miss Webber. They began caring for her using reality orientation techniques and touch to communicate. They asked her permission to give her each bit of care, and they carefully informed her of what they were going to do. They brought her bright ribbons for her hair and flowers for her table.

Miss Webber made no verbal response to the students for almost a week. Then, just as the students were becoming discouraged, she uttered one word, "Yes." From then on, she began to talk with the students and to participate actively in her own care. Later, she told them that because the staff had seemed to have no use for her, she just hadn't bothered to be responsive. She'd hoped she would just die. She was glad that someone finally recognized her as a person.

## A final word

If you remember that elderly people are adults who have a wealth of worldly experience, who are individuals with the same legal and human rights we all can claim, and who can be interesting people and challenging patients, you'll have no difficulty relating to them.

If you remember that the elderly are subject to certain age-related changes in both their information-processing capabilities (input, storage, and output) and their sensory perceptions, you can adapt your methods of communicating with them and achieve therapeutic interaction.

If you remember that elderly people continue to have basic human needs throughout their lives, and that they also continue to have developmental tasks to accomplish, you can relate more closely and professionally with them. You'll feel gratified when your elderly patient brags about the kindness and competence of "my nurse."

A final word about elderly persons' rights: recognizing that their numbers are increasing, they're no longer content to be treated as second-class citizens. Instead, they're demanding high-quality health care, especially nursing care, and they're also demanding that their nurses be knowledgeable in gerontologic theory and practice. As a result, this is becoming a dynamic, exciting nursing specialty. More and more colleges of nursing are adding gerontologic nursing to their courses of study. Nursing students are increasingly given clinical assignments in nursing homes. More often now than in the past, nurses are assigned to care for acutely ill elderly patients as *people* with special needs, not as human organisms hooked to high-technology equipment.

As all these trends continue, you can expect elderly patients to assert their rights with increasing confidence— and nurses to respond to these patients' needs with equal confidence in the quality of their nursing care.

# 81 Patients who challenge you

The patient who challenges you most, the one who's most frustrating to care for, may well become your favorite patient if you accept some simple assumptions about yourself. First, accept yourself as a good nurse, one who's competent, caring, and knowledgeable. Second, accept your inability to be all things to all people. (Perfection was never meant to be a part of the basic nursing curriculum.) Third, look closely, but kindly, at yourself: in your work, when do you most often feel discouraged, frustrated, or angry? Finally, look within yourself for ways that you can change your responses to patients' challenging behaviors.

Categorizing patients into packages with convenient labels has been an unfortunate part of nursing practice. It's easier to say that old Mr. George is a problem patient who will never change than it is to look at the many variables in Mr. George's life that are eliciting troublesome behaviors. Frail Mrs. Edgar is less painful for you to think about if you tell yourself that she's better off

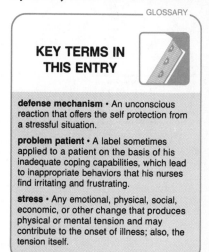

GLOSSARY

**KEY TERMS IN THIS ENTRY**

**defense mechanism** • An unconscious reaction that offers the self protection from a stressful situation.

**problem patient** • A label sometimes applied to a patient on the basis of his inadequate coping capabilities, which lead to inappropriate behaviors that his nurses find irritating and frustrating.

**stress** • Any emotional, physical, social, economic, or other change that produces physical or mental tension and may contribute to the onset of illness; also, the tension itself.

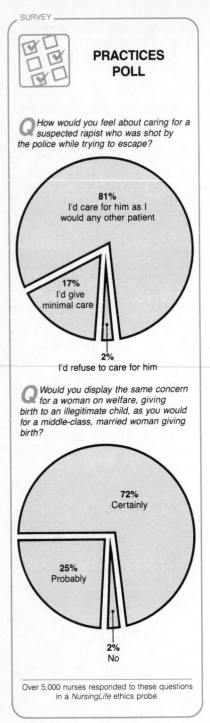

# PRACTICES POLL

**Q** *How would you feel about caring for a suspected rapist who was shot by the police while trying to escape?*

**81%**
I'd care for him as I would any other patient

**17%**
I'd give minimal care

**2%**
I'd refuse to care for him

**Q** *Would you display the same concern for a woman on welfare, giving birth to an illegitimate child, as you would for a middle-class, married woman giving birth?*

**72%**
Certainly

**25%**
Probably

**2%**
No

Over 5,000 nurses responded to these questions in a *NursingLife* ethics probe.

---

left alone, because she's tired, than if you allow yourself to think about her fear of being alone during the process of dying.

The type of patient who challenges one nurse may present less of a problem to another. So no types of patients who are universally thought of as difficult can be identified. The patients discussed below represent some of the common behaviors that staff nurses find challenging. (Discussion of patients like these frequently dominates staff patient-care conferences.)

## Recognizing challenging patients

*The noncompliant patient* balks each time you try to give him care. Your simplest requests are met with stubborn resistance despite your use of good patient teaching. When a patient refuses fluids, prevents you from making a neat hospital bed, or resists your attempts to encourage ambulation, maintaining your usual high quality of nursing care becomes difficult. (See *What Types of Patients Make You Uncomfortable?*)

*The aggressive patient* almost always presents a challenge to the nursing staff. (See *Identifying Defense Mechanisms,* page 494.) Everyone wants to be liked by others—even you, as a nurse. The aggressive patient's illness and hospitalization make him feel trapped, so he strikes out at those around him. He challenges your ability to keep from striking back at what you may view as an attack on your self-image as a likeable person.

*The clinging patient,* regressing to an immature state in response to the stress of hospitalization, may invoke contempt in nurses who particularly value strength of character. You may find this type of patient troublesome if your ethnic background, early childhood teachings, or philosophical point of view disagree with this type of behavior. This is the patient nurses often refer to as demanding—taking more time than they have to give.

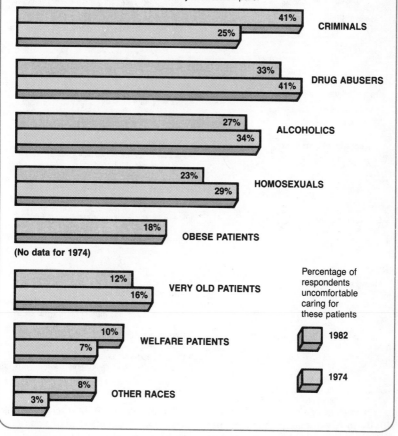

## WHAT TYPES OF PATIENTS MAKE YOU UNCOMFORTABLE?

Do you feel uncomfortable caring for certain types of patients? Most of the more than 5,000 nurses who responded to a *Nursing74* survey and the *NursingLife* 1982 Ethics Probe don't. But a sizable minority admitted that some types of patients made them uncomfortable. Here's how the 1974 and 1982 survey results compare.

CRIMINALS — 41% / 25%

DRUG ABUSERS — 33% / 41%

ALCOHOLICS — 27% / 34%

HOMOSEXUALS — 23% / 29%

OBESE PATIENTS — 18%
(No data for 1974)

VERY OLD PATIENTS — 12% / 16%

WELFARE PATIENTS — 10% / 7%

OTHER RACES — 8% / 3%

Percentage of respondents uncomfortable caring for these patients

1982

1974

*The suicidal patient* on a unit raises questions that trouble all his caregivers: Does anyone have a right to end his own life? How hard should you work to save him if he doesn't want to live anyway? Do you really have the power and the means to stop him if he chooses to end his life? Do you know enough to assess the behavioral clues that indicate how strong his suicidal tendencies are?

*The dying patient,* well on the road to his exit from life, brings you face to face with your own mortality. More than any other patient, he forces you to be involved. You're committed to caring for him so that his death dignifies both him and his family.

*The alcoholic patient* has no typical set of personality characteristics. He may be noncompliant, aggressive, clinging—or cooperative. Your own values about the use and abuse of alcohol will play a part in your response to this patient. Because an alcoholic is so often stigmatized, he may deny hav-

## MANAGING DIFFICULT PATIENTS

| TYPE OF PATIENT | CLUES TO IDENTIFYING BEHAVIOR |
|---|---|
| **Noncompliant patient** | • Refuses to participate in care<br>• Refuses to comply with rules and regulations |
| **Aggressive patient** | • Uses negative, abusive language<br>• Has a defiant attitude |
| **Crying, clinging patient** | • Constantly demands attention<br>• Has bouts of uncontrollable crying |
| **Suicidal patient** | • Makes self-deprecating statements<br>• Suggests plans to harm himself<br>• Lacks interest in what's going on around him |
| **Dying patient** | • Displaces anger, denies illness<br>• Withdraws from others<br>• Has a compulsion to talk about death and dying<br>• (Medical diagnosis may confirm what clues suggest) |
| **Alcoholic or drug-abusing patient** | • Denies addiction<br>• Uses manipulative techniques to secure contraband<br>• Undergoes withdrawal<br>• (Medical diagnosis may confirm what clues suggest) |

ing the disease of alcoholism. Your sensitivity to his dilemma may help him reveal information about his drinking patterns so that the health team can prepare a complete treatment plan.

*The drug abuser,* like the alcoholic, fears rejection, yet he may be demanding or manipulative. Why? Sometimes he acts this way because he's afraid his higher tolerance for pain-relieving drugs means his pain will continue. This is true for ex-addicts, too. For both groups of patients, anxiety about getting adequate pain relief medication at regular intervals leads to demanding or manipulative behavior.

The patient with an *alternative lifestyle* may challenge you if you're accustomed to a patient population representing the mainstream of middle-class American values. These patients require special understanding. Otherwise, for example, a nurse may not understand a partner's need to be involved in a homosexual patient's care. Or staff may be rude and abrupt with the father of an unwed mother's child. Or a patient whose religious beliefs contradict lifesaving treatment may feel alienated in the hospital environment.

*The patient with threatening professional credentials* may challenge you in

Difficult patients present a special challenge to your abilities to deal with others. The information in this chart will help you meet that challenge as effectively as possible.

| POSSIBLE CAUSES OF THE BEHAVIOR | NURSE'S INSTINCTIVE REACTION TO THE BEHAVIOR | NURSE'S MOST HELPFUL REACTION TO THE BEHAVIOR |
|---|---|---|
| • Fears pain, disability<br>• Lacks understanding of the reasons for compliance | • To force compliance | • To reward the patient when he cooperates<br>• To stimulate him to ask questions about his care<br>• To fully explain the benefits of treatment |
| • Feels threatened<br>• Lacks self-confidence | • To strike back | • To encourage him to express his anger<br>• To include him in planning care<br>• To stay calm and listen objectively |
| • Wants help<br>• Fears treatments' consequences | • To be impatient with his inability to cope | • To assure him that she understands his fear<br>• To provide him with specific information to ease his fear<br>• To make time to stay with him and offer to talk |
| • Despairs about illness or personal problems<br>• Seems overwhelmed by sense of worthlessness or guilt | • To be anxious about her ability to help him pull through | • To encourage him to express his hopelessness<br>• To offer constant, frequent exchanges |
| • Appears unable to adapt to fatal illness | • To deny death<br>• To be uncomfortable in the patient's presence | • To agree to talk with him about dying<br>• To provide comfort and companionship |
| • Needs alcohol or drugs<br>• Fears rejection | • To be judgmental about his dependency<br>• To mistrust what he says | • To understand him as a person with disease<br>• To set up a constant, consistent treatment regimen to break the addiction |

a way that leads to mutual avoidance. For example, a doctor who's ill with terminal cancer has the same emotional needs as any other patient. But his greater medical knowledge, and perhaps his hostility, may intimidate you and cause you to spend minimal time with him. And a hospitalized minister or counselor, with intellectual expertise in theories of loss and grief, still needs you to be attuned to his unmet psychological needs.

## Controlling your reactions to challenging patients

Why do challenging patients cause your level of anxiety to rise? Possibly because they threaten your self-confidence as a nurse. Will you be able to handle the problems they present? That depends on many factors, including these:
• *Progress in the nurse-patient relationship.* Newly admitted patients are generally highly anxious, spilling out erratic behaviors to staff involved in their care. Being hospitalized is traumatic due to fear of treatment procedures, uncertainty about the illness's outcome, lack of privacy, worries left behind at home or on the job, and financial burdens, along with a whole host of issues peculiar to each patient's

## DEALING WITH THE MANIPULATIVE PATIENT

No one has to tell you how resourceful the manipulative patient can be when he wants to cause trouble. The manipulative patient has a seemingly limitless variety of behaviors to make your job harder. But you know you can't give in to his scheming, or he'll take

| | Set limits | Tell him your expectations | Ask for clarification | Allow choices | Encourage constructive expression of feelings | Stay with him | |
|---|---|---|---|---|---|---|---|
| **Plays one staff member against another** | ● | ● | | | | | |
| **Insists on bargaining** | ● | ● | ● | ● | | | |
| **Makes demands** | ● | ● | | ● | ● | | |
| **Uses intimidation** | ● | | ● | ● | ● | ● | |
| **Makes derogatory remarks** | ● | | ● | | ● | ● | |
| **Exploits others' weaknesses** | ● | ● | | | ● | | |
| **Uses flattery** | ● | ● | ● | | | | |
| **Urges other patients to oppose care** | ● | ● | | | ● | | |
| **Uses socially unacceptable behavior** | ● | ● | | | ● | | |
| **Views self as deserving or special** | ● | ● | | | | | |
| **Questions excessively** | ● | ● | ● | ● | ● | ● | |
| **Violates rules and procedures** | ● | ● | | ● | ● | ● | |
| **Hides things** | ● | ● | | | ● | | |
| **Uses self-pity** | ● | ● | | | ● | | |
| **Acts helpless** | ● | ● | | ● | | | |
| **Changes the subject constantly** | | | | | ● | ● | |
| **Dawdles and causes delays** | ● | ● | | | ● | ● | |
| **Exploits others' generosity or sense of responsibility** | ● | ● | | | | | |

advantage of you and others. You must take appropriate nursing action to discourage manipulative behavior. This chart lists the most common patient manipulative behaviors and your most effective responses to them (A dot [•] indicates those actions that most effectively discourage each manipulative behavior.)

| | Listen carefully | Create a predictable environment | Focus on the current task or discussion | Comply with his reasonable requests | Give constructive responses | Hold a conference with staff | Devise plan of action with staff | Educate him about his behavior |
|---|---|---|---|---|---|---|---|---|
| | | • | • | | | • | • | |
| | | | • | • | • | • | • | • |
| | • | | • | • | | | | • |
| | | | • | | | | | |
| | • | | • | | | | | • |
| | | | • | | • | | | |
| | | | • | | | | | • |
| | | | • | • | • | • | • | • |
| | | | • | | • | | | • |
| | | | • | • | | | | • |
| | • | | • | | | | | |
| | • | • | • | • | • | • | • | • |
| | | • | | | | | | • |
| | | • | | • | • | | | • |
| | | • | • | | | | | • |
| | • | | • | | • | | | • |
| | • | • | • | | | | • | |
| | | • | • | • | | • | • | |

situation. Little wonder, then, that your initial encounter with a patient may be less than ideal. But a well-timed and appropriate intervention now may make a crucial difference throughout your patient's hospitalization.

• *Your expectations about how "good" patients behave.* If your preconceived expectations about "good" patients' behavior aren't met, your anxiety may increase. Some nurses are blessed with a wide repertoire of life experiences, so they have less difficulty responding to potentially threatening situations. Other nurses must develop greater tolerance for a variety of patient behaviors.

• *The emotional armor that you bring to work.* Are you experiencing stress in your personal life? If so, you're more vulnerable to real or imagined attacks on your sense of self-worth. This will strain the objectivity you need for handling challenging patients. Remember, feeling upset about something personal is okay, but acting on that feeling isn't, if the patient suffers.

• *Your sense of security on the job.* What's your relationship to your supervisor? How much do unfair labor practices where you work threaten you? Are you aware of a gap in your knowledge of psychological principles of patient care? If you feel satisfied and secure on the job, you're more likely to tap into the listening skills you naturally use when you're feeling relaxed.

## A case in point: Joseph Brown

Joseph Brown, who's been admitted for emergency abdominal surgery 3 months after the death of his wife, has character attributes his nurses have defined as "cantankerous", "stubborn", and "impossible."

His admission notes include observations about his high level of anxiety complicated by grief. He's been continuously uncooperative about rules concerning smoking in his room, and his notoriety as a problem patient has spread. About the time you begin to care for him, he becomes even more anxious, using abusive language and belittling the hospital staff. Having lost his spouse, his physical strength, and his ability to control his own life—all within the space of a few months—this formerly independent man begins to use defense mechanisms that evoke further rejection from the staff.

He denies the seriousness of his illness and refuses to follow directives in his treatment plan that would promote healing. He rationalizes his troublesome behavior by citing apparently plausible reasons that aren't actually the basis for his actions. He displaces his anger about absent family members onto the staff. He projects his own thoughts onto others, too. Finally, he regresses to a state in which he's more withdrawn—and appears more cooperative. But you realize that, because his psychosocial needs haven't been met adequately during his hospitalization, the course of his illness has changed for the worse.

To your dismay, you note that most of the nurses caring for Mr. Brown react with defense mechanisms of their own. They treat him like a deterrent to the accomplishment of their assigned tasks. They're angry at Mr. Brown because his doctors admonish *them* for some of his problems, and because his family members blame the hospital for his deteriorating condition. Originally motivated by a sense of confidence, these nurses are becoming frustrated and discouraged, and they're using rationalizations of their own. They say, "We can't do much if he refuses to cooperate," "Everybody has a right to make decisions about his life," and "Maybe he belongs on the psych unit."

As a thoughtful and caring nurse, you're naturally concerned that Mr. Brown's condition, and his care, have seriously deteriorated.

## Understanding challenging patients

Patients like Mr. Brown have the same human needs as anyone else. They also have the same right to quality care.

# THE VIOLENT PATIENT: HOW TO PREVENT HIS OUTBURSTS

When a patient becomes violent, it's a frightening situation. But by just watching for a few clues, you can predict violence and even prevent it from occurring. Here's a list of guidelines to help you do this.

 Don't discount any feeling that your patient is growing hostile or showing inappropriate anger. Act on these intuitions, and document them even if your patient has not behaved in an overtly dangerous way. Share your feelings and concerns with the staff and your nursing administration.

 Review a potentially violent patient's history for indications of alcoholism, drug addiction, reaction to a medication change, or a metabolic or emotional disturbance. Then, if you think medication would help prevent a violent outburst, request an appropriate medication p.r.n.

 Don't undervalue information that a patient's family or staff members give you about your patient's potential for violence. If you think he'll be different with you, or that *you* can handle it where others couldn't, think again. You could be setting yourself up for trouble. If you listen to others' information about a patient's previous violence, about what's apt to provoke him and how he behaves when provoked, you may avoid a frightening and possibly harmful incident.

 Don't continue treatment if a patient is obviously growing more and more agitated. Discontinue touching him and moving toward him, too—he may misinterpret these actions and react with physical aggression. Instead, tell the patient that he appears to be angry or agitated. In a few calmly expressed words, ask him if he's felt this way before. If he has, ask him how he ordinarily handles such feelings and what others have done to help him. You want him to know that *his* feelings and point of view are being respected, so he'll feel less victimized and powerless. But be careful to observe his responses closely during this brief discussion. If his agitation continues or increases, find an excuse to leave his room, and then take appropriate action to get him calmed down or controlled.

 Don't isolate yourself with a patient who has a history of violence or any potential to be violent. When he's assigned to your unit, put him in a room near the nurses' station—not at the end of a long, relatively unprotected corridor. When you're with the patient, keep the door open—and never turn your back on him. Have a nurse, or, if possible, a security officer or male aide within immediate call.

 Don't disturb this patient (even for treatment, or to take vital signs) any more than necessary. Arrange opportunities for physical activity, if you think it will help siphon off his excess energies. Arrange for time out of his room, if this seems appropriate—and if he agrees to it.

 If you're a nurse manager, don't assign a timid or inexperienced nurse to care for a potentially violent patient. Instead, assign a mature, easygoing, experienced nurse. (In this kind of powder-keg situation, only one anxious person should be present in the room—the patient.) And don't overlook the significance of gender. Consider assigning a male staff nurse to a female patient who's potentially violent, and a female nurse to a male patient. Observers have learned that a female patient may be inclined to react negatively to another woman but positively to a male staff member. This gender crossing also works for the male patient, who may hesitate to strike or injure a female nurse.

True, you can't always control their behavior, but you *are* in charge of your own. The outcome of your care may not be as successful as you'd like. But you need to feel sure you've done everything possible, in terms of selecting treatment approaches and using available resources, to give optimal patient care. (See *Managing Difficult Patients,* pages 512 and 513.)

Spend some time reflecting about particular patients who've been troublesome for you. Be specific. What kind of person do you most dislike finding in your patient assignments? Is it a person of a certain age, or from a particular ethnic group? Or a patient with a particular diagnosis? Or is it someone who reminds you of a person you used to know—and didn't like?

Examine your feelings often. Get in the habit of reflecting on how your patients make you feel. Do this in the early stages of your relationships with patients, so that problem behaviors don't have a chance to escalate. At the same time, be aware of your resources for support. Use colleagues for feedback and reassurance. Accept the fact that you may need someone with special skills to help you sort out your feelings. Take advantage of inservice opportunities where you can learn more about human behavior.

Keep your own level of well-being high by regularly practicing healthy self-care habits. Become familiar with stress-reducing techniques that work for you. (See Entry 68.) Above all, leave your job behind, emotionally as well as physically, when you go home.

Undoubtedly, demands at work will sometimes be high. Remember to reward yourself when you've done a good job; only by nurturing yourself will you be able to continue working in nursing year after year.

Here are some basic steps to follow when you're assigned to a patient with particularly challenging behavior:

• Keep in mind that you are not, *you cannot be,* responsible for your patient's behavior.

• Set up a series of approaches toward gaining his confidence. Start by simply initiating frequent interactions. Sit down by his bed, call him by name, and use some general opening remark to begin a conversation.

• Let him know how often you can spend time with him.

• Your intuitive sense is a tool in the art of nursing: use it. Touch, humor, and other interactive techniques will help, too.

If you find you're unable to provide complete care to a particular patient, discuss the situation with members of your team and with your supervisor. Participate in problem-solving sessions where you can work out a consistent approach. You may decide together that a particular nurse gets along with Mr. George, while another does well with Mrs. Edgar, or you may settle for a rotating assignment schedule. After open discussion of the problems involved in providing care to challenging patients, you'll have a stronger sense of staff support—and greater confidence in the quality of your nursing care, even under difficult conditions.

### A final word

Every patient's emotional response to his illness has a significant effect on its course. Because every illness has an emotional component, you must care for the whole person, even when his behavior impedes your efforts.

People have always reacted to the stress of illness with behaviors that challenged their caregivers. They always will. Accept this challenge. It's part of the excitement and the satisfaction of being a nurse.

# 82 Families in crisis

As a nurse, you frequently have to deal with families in crisis—parents of critically ill newborns, families of severely burned patients and accident victims,

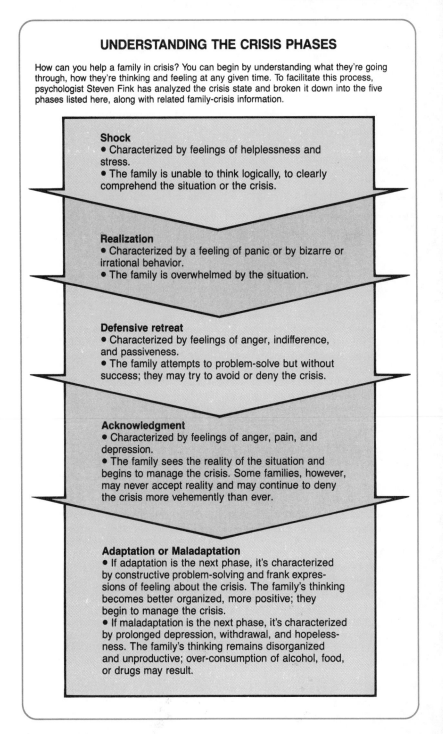

# UNDERSTANDING THE CRISIS PHASES

How can you help a family in crisis? You can begin by understanding what they're going through, how they're thinking and feeling at any given time. To facilitate this process, psychologist Steven Fink has analyzed the crisis state and broken it down into the five phases listed here, along with related family-crisis information.

**Shock**
● Characterized by feelings of helplessness and stress.
● The family is unable to think logically, to clearly comprehend the situation or the crisis.

**Realization**
● Characterized by a feeling of panic or by bizarre or irrational behavior.
● The family is overwhelmed by the situation.

**Defensive retreat**
● Characterized by feelings of anger, indifference, and passiveness.
● The family attempts to problem-solve but without success; they may try to avoid or deny the crisis.

**Acknowledgment**
● Characterized by feelings of anger, pain, and depression.
● The family sees the reality of the situation and begins to manage the crisis. Some families, however, may never accept reality and may continue to deny the crisis more vehemently than ever.

**Adaptation or Maladaptation**
● If adaptation is the next phase, it's characterized by constructive problem-solving and frank expressions of feeling about the crisis. The family's thinking becomes better organized, more positive; they begin to manage the crisis.
● If maladaptation is the next phase, it's characterized by prolonged depression, withdrawal, and hopelessness. The family's thinking remains disorganized and unproductive; over-consumption of alcohol, food, or drugs may result.

GLOSSARY

## KEY TERMS IN THIS ENTRY

**coping strategy** • The plan of action a person develops to adapt to temporary stress-producing situations.

**crisis** • An emotionally significant event, an extreme change of status, or an uncertain or crucial time or situation where the outcome will decisively affect a person's future life.

**nuclear family** • A family unit consisting of the biologic parents and their children.

**support group** • People whom a person confides in and draws on for support, either as individuals or in a group setting.

friends and loved ones of alcoholics and pregnant teenagers, and children and adults caught between illness and the emotional turmoil of divorce or job loss.

When a crisis occurs, family members may cope with it well, poorly, or not at all. Your ability to intervene during critical stages of a family crisis can make a vital difference in how that family functions, now and for years to come.

This entry probes a case study illustrating the problems family members may confront as they attempt to deal with a crisis. Also discussed are the steps you can take, as a nurse, to strengthen a family's ability to recognize crises and to cope with them.

### What is a crisis?

A crisis occurs when any stressful or hazardous event causes a family's normal routine to break down. Typically, people are unable to handle crisis situations for three reasons:
• Family members don't completely understand what has happened.
• They've never developed strategies for coping with a crisis.
• They lack support from friends, relatives, and social service professionals.

Crises may be situational or matu-rational. A sudden death, an accident, or an unplanned pregnancy is a *situational crisis* because it occurs unexpectedly and can overwhelm individuals' and their families' ability to cope. Even an event that may seem relatively unimportant, such as forgetting a loved one's birthday, can become a situational crisis for someone.

In contrast, *maturational crises* occur when people arrive at—and can't cope with—transition points in their physical, social, or emotional growth. Here are some examples:
• a woman who enters menopause
• a teenager who reaches puberty
• a father who's beginning to confront his fears of growing old.

Often these people have no role models to follow, and their attempts to develop new roles bring resistance from friends, co-workers, and family members.

Keep in mind that parents and children (the so-called nuclear family) are usually not the only persons a family crisis affects. Defined in the broadest sense, "family" includes neighbors, co-workers, friends, and relatives who play significant roles in the family's life.

### Early intervention with a family in crisis

Skillful nursing intervention early in a crisis situation can do a great deal to relieve a family's stress. (See *Comforting the Family*, page 523.) So you must be alert to crisis signs and symptoms in the patients and families you encounter. For example, a nurse working in the intensive care unit may realize that the parents of a child injured in an automobile accident are entering a crisis state. Or an emergency department nurse may note that a rape victim is experiencing feelings of guilt, embarrassment, and loss of self-worth. Another nurse may be involved with a family who has just learned that one family member is abusing drugs. For all patients and their families, feelings of dismay and anger may signal impending crises.

As you're probably aware, no two family crises are alike. But certain stages are common to all crisis situations, and you can use them to gauge how far a family has progressed in recognizing their crisis situation and dealing with it. These stages include *shock (or impact), realization, defen-*

---

## CARING FOR THE FAMILY IN CRISIS, USING THE NURSING PROCESS

Do you know you can use the nursing process to provide support and comfort to the family of a critically ill patient? If your institution doesn't already have a care plan for families in crisis, you can use the one provided here.

### 1 Assessment
- Who are the significant family members?
- Are their needs emotional or informational?
- What is the family's present emotional state?
- What are the outside stresses?
- Are the family members in crisis, depressed, grieving, overwhelmed with guilt?

### 2 Planning
- Set up a time for listening to the family, and note it in your nursing care plan.
- Explore family and outside resources.
- Explore resources within the hospital setting.
- Set up a time for a private (if possible) and comfortable visit for patient and family, and note this in your care plan.
- Talk with the patient's doctor. Find out the best time for the family to contact him, and what he's told the family. Share information about the family and their needs.

### 3 Interventions
- Allow for reliving of the critical incident and general expression of feelings.
- Introduce the family to staff, describe staff functions, and reassure them about staff competence and commitment.
- Encourage (and provide for) a comfortable and private family visit with the patient.
- Make appropriate referrals for psychological support and treatment if the family's needs are greater than you can handle.

### 4 Evaluation
- Make a specific evaluation visit with the family.
- Has their emotional state changed—have their needs changed?
- Have they followed through on referrals?
- Is the family receiving enough support to solve their problems?

*sive retreat, acknowledgment,* and *adaptation* or *maladaptation.* (See *Understanding the Crisis Phases,* page 519.)

Here's a case study that illustrates how you, as a nurse, might intervene with a family in crisis.

Mr. and Mrs. Jeffrey Martinson have one child, a daughter age 16, who they've recently discovered is 3 months pregnant. The daughter says she wants to bear and raise her child, and the parents have accompanied her to the hospital for tests. This is when you first meet the family.

(Obviously, few people in this situation will pour out their hearts to a stranger. Before family members can begin to trust you and talk with you openly, your words and actions must assure them of two things: first, they have every right to feel what they're feeling at that moment, and second, that you're willing to accept the family members at any point in their attempts to manage their situation.)

As you talk with the Martinsons, you can see that their first reaction to their daughter's unplanned pregnancy is to feel helpless and panicky. The family clearly doesn't want to talk about the pregnancy, but you know you need to press the issue. They seem anxious when you mention the pregnancy, and you acknowledge this by saying, "None of you seems very comfortable talking about what's happening."

Mrs. Martinson responds, "It's so hard to talk about it. We didn't want this to happen to our daughter." You show sympathy by saying, "You're struggling with a difficult situation. It sounds as if you're wondering why this happened to you." This approach opens the Martinsons up to a candid conversation.

The Martinsons' situation is relatively straightforward, but you know you can improve your understanding by finding out if similar problems have occurred in the past. You ask: Have family members argued about the daughter's dating habits or sexual activity? Has she been pregnant before?

---

ADVICE

## FACING UP TO DEATH

*One of my patients, a 34-year-old father of two, has cancer of the liver. He's lost 30 lb (14 kg), and he looks terrible. Since he knows he probably won't go home again, he wants his sons, ages 7 and 9, to visit him in the hospital. I'm afraid his appearance will frighten the boys. His wife shares my concern. Any advice?*—RN, Fla.

Letting the boys see their father may help them understand what's happening and perhaps adjust to his imminent death. To make their visit as comfortable as possible, help the whole family prepare.

First, encourage the man to discuss with you how he feels about dying. The more comfortable he is talking about it with you, the easier time he'll have talking about it with his sons. Suggest that he wear his own clothes for the visit, rather than a hospital gown, if he's up to it. The boys may feel more at ease if they see him in, say, a familiar shirt that he frequently wore around the house.

Talk to his wife, too. Encourage her to discuss her fears with her husband so the atmosphere will be as relaxed as possible when the boys visit. Discuss how she might prepare the boys by describing how their father looks before they visit, so they won't be shocked. (She might even want to take a picture to them.) And explain to her the importance of reassuring the boys that *she's* healthy and will be there to take care of them.

---

This letter was taken from the files of *NursingLife* magazine.

## COMFORTING THE FAMILY

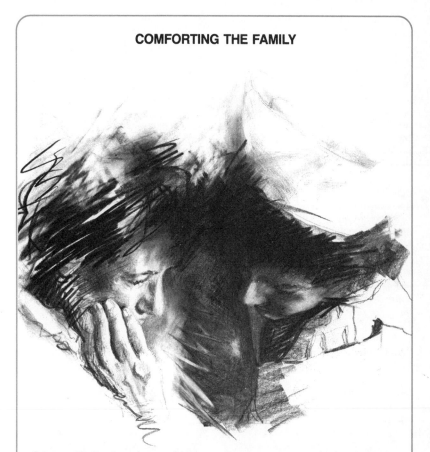

Put yourself in the place of your patient's mother, Mrs. Ciani. Her son John, age 22—until today strong, athletic, and healthy—has just suffered a cerebral aneurysm. She comforts herself with all of the familiar clichés—"He has so much to live for," and "A cerebral aneurysm won't topple John." She feels so helpless, so vulnerable, so dependent on the machines. She watches your face, searching for the smallest sign of hope. But she sees no sign. You and your colleagues remain detached, as though you see someone like John die every day.

How would *you* feel if you were Mrs. Ciani? Or if the patient in the hospital bed were your mother, father, brother, sister, or child? Most likely, you'd want a word of encouragement, an arm around your shoulder, and a sympathetic ear.

Supporting your patient's family during a crisis is one of your vital responsibilities. Performing your nursing duties effectively doesn't mean you must be detached and objective. Here are some things to remember when dealing with grieving family members:

• Listen to the family's fears and anxieties, encourage discussing them, and be sure to answer any questions the family may have.

• Family members are likely to be awed by complicated medical procedures and equipment, so go out of your way to explain to them what's going on.

• Maintain eye contact when you're talking with family members; when appropriate, touch them on the arm or the shoulder.

• Involve them in caring for their family member (when appropriate) by teaching them procedures they can perform.

What are the keys to dealing with your patient's family? Understanding, compassion, kindness. Don't be reluctant to spread them around.

As you gather background information from family members, you also begin to assess their coping strategies and the support systems they've developed over the years. Suppose you find that the Martinsons have few sources of emotional support outside their home, and that they value their independence. This information will help you in later planning. (See *Caring for the Family in Crisis, Using the Nursing Process*, page 521.)

Suppose you also discover that communication within the Martinson family is minimal. The parents and their daughter freely admit that they never discuss their feelings with each other. Mr. Martinson makes most of the family's decisions, and although all three say that this coping strategy has caused problems in the past, no one has attempted to alter it. You recognize that this, too, will become important later.

Although the Martinsons' present crisis doesn't appear to be so serious that suicide is a possibility, you listen to the family for clues to determine if any member is a suicide risk. You assess their degree of hope or despair, and you ask how they've handled severe family stress in the past. Have they made any plans to handle the present crisis—their daughter's pregnancy? Has any family member's behavior changed as a result of this crisis?

### Helping the family cope
Most family crisis situations won't require your involvement for more than short periods of time. However, before you're finished, a family in crisis should have both short- and long-term goals that you've developed and agreed on with each family member. Creating these goals together will give the family a feeling of control over the crisis.

For example, suppose that all three members of the Martinson family have agreed that the daughter will bear and raise her child. One short-term goal of this plan can be helping the family to choose a single-parent support group for the daughter. A longer-term goal

can be helping the family to expand its support system. Once family members agree this goal is important, you can offer to call a local social service agency and make an appointment for them.

Establishing long-term goals will help the family put this crisis in perspective, too. As you work with the Martinsons, you can help them realize that their long-established strategy for coping—not communicating openly at all—will not help any of them deal with this crisis or future ones.

Keep in mind that in any family crisis, certain family members may dig in their heels at any time and refuse to cooperate further with you. If you feel that they need continued help, you have a professional and ethical responsibility as a nurse to refer the family to social service personnel inside or outside your hospital.

In most family crises where you intervene, your actions will be enough to make family members realize the necessity of dealing directly with you and with each other. As the family's crisis is being resolved, identify the behaviors that the family used successfully in managing the crisis, and reinforce those behaviors by your approval. Provide them with ideas for coping more effectively in the future, too. As you bring your intervention to a close, emphasize how the family has grown stronger because of what its members have learned about coping with crises.

### A final word
Understanding how a crisis develops and can overwhelm its victims is essential to your work with patients and their families. Sometimes helping them to strengthen their crisis-coping strategies and meet their short- and long-term emotional needs may demand more of your time and skills than any other part of your job. But you'll find that successfully intervening in family crisis situations is an important nursing function—one that can do much to satisfy some of *your* personal and professional needs.

# 83 Helping a patient's family participate in his care

You may know that, before nursing became a widely recognized profession, relatives would often accompany a family member to the hospital. There they assisted in preparing the patient's food and caring for his basic hygiene needs. This practice continues in a number of countries.

This entry presents a case study of how you, as a nurse, can include relatives in a patient's plan of care. Properly directed, family members can greatly improve a patient's willingness and ability to respond to treatment, in the hospital and at home. But no matter how eager they are to participate, a patient's relatives will often need your help to begin. Why? Because they need to make their own emotional adjustments to the situation before they can work effectively with the patient.

Many families, you'll find, will go to considerable lengths to care for a stricken relative or to be near him. Family members are often willing to use an extra room in the home to shelter an aging relative. Parents commonly uproot themselves from small towns to be closer to medical centers in large metropolitan areas where their children are receiving treatment.

These people and others like them are resources you can draw on to enhance patient care. The key is learning how to assess the family's strengths and needs, then directing their efforts to care for the patient.

## Introducing Mr. Giraldo, his family, and his nurse

Ideally, family members should become involved in a patient's care as soon as possible after a crisis occurs. As an illustration of how a nurse can achieve this goal, consider this fictional example: Mr. Joseph Giraldo, age 42, hospitalized with an acute myocardial infarction.

When Mr. Giraldo was admitted, the nurse in charge, Ellen Stallman, RN, began to carefully assess not only the patient but his family as well. She noted which family members accompanied Mr. Giraldo to the hospital and what kinds of questions they asked the staff. She observed how the family members talked with the patient and with each other, and she noted whom they turned to, among themselves, for guidance and emotional support.

As the family members talked, Ellen could begin to see how they reacted to Mr. Giraldo's illness and discussed problems among themselves. She listened for clues about the family's economic condition, and she watched for gestures and actions that might stem from the family's ethnic or religious background. All of this information, Ellen knew, would help her develop a care plan that effectively involved Mr. Giraldo's family.

## Understanding types of families

Obviously, no two families react to the illness of a loved one in the same way. But in general, families can be categorized as either disengaged or close-knit.

Of the two, *the disengaged family* is more difficult to involve in active caring

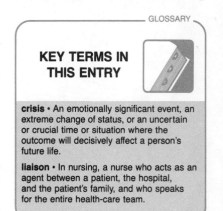

GLOSSARY

## KEY TERMS IN THIS ENTRY

**crisis** • An emotionally significant event, an extreme change of status, or an uncertain or crucial time or situation where the outcome will decisively affect a person's future life.

**liaison** • In nursing, a nurse who acts as an agent between a patient, the hospital, and the patient's family, and who speaks for the entire health-care team.

## STRENGTHENING FAMILY TIES

Once your patient's discharged, his family will provide much of his long-term health needs. That means you'll be meeting your patient's needs if you help strengthen his family ties. How? By accommodating his family as much as possible in the hospital and by helping to improve patient-family communication. Here are some guidelines to follow, when appropriate:

### Accommodating the family
• Manipulate visiting hours and telephone rules to make patient-family contact more convenient.
• Allow family members to sleep in the patient's room, or in hospital-sponsored housing.
• Use police and hospital security guards, when necessary, to protect your patient and his family from a hostile relative, such as an abusive spouse.
• Arrange for professional consultation and therapy, such as nurse counselors or social service or psychiatric help.

### Improving communication
• Encourage your patient and his family to discuss his illness, its consequences, and his needs for recovery at home.
• Encourage your patient and his family to share their feelings.
• Remind your patient and his family of their mutual (and sometimes divergent) needs.

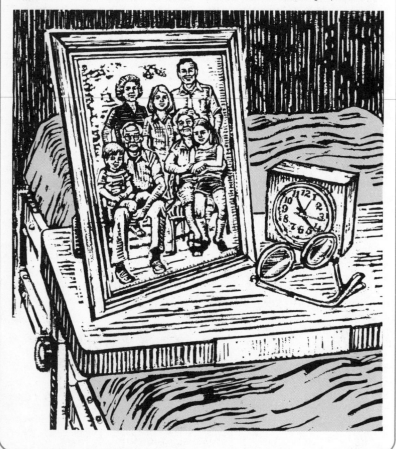

for a patient. Why? Because when the boundaries between family members are mostly rigid, a change in one member's health will have little effect on most of the other members. So they may show little apparent interest in their stricken relative.

However, family members who seem disengaged are often willing to become involved; they may just be uncomfortable around sick people or in the hospital setting. They may feel unimportant or in the way. Only by carefully observing and assessing family members can you discover which ones care enough about the patient to help him in a meaningful way.

In a *close-knit family*, the members tend to react quickly and emotionally when a loved one becomes ill.

In either type of family, members may want to participate in caring for the patient. This means that you or someone else on the hospital staff must assume the role of principal liaison with the family. Essentially, the person who acts as liaison becomes the spokesperson for the entire health-care treatment team. (See *Strengthening Family Ties*.)

### Helping family members explore their own needs

As liaison for Mr. Giraldo and his family, Ellen Stallman quickly discovered that Mr. Giraldo's wife was the principal family decision maker. She also seemed extremely close to her husband, who listened carefully to everything she said. Ellen realized that if she directed Mrs. Giraldo properly, the woman could become an important ally in planning Mr. Giraldo's care so it included his family.

In the first few days after her husband's admission, Mrs. Giraldo arranged for their two children, ages 6 and 10, to be cared for after school. She insisted on waiting silently in the hospital corridor for a verdict from the doctors. Staff members found that she responded best to specific and direct questions.

Mrs. Giraldo seemed unable to talk about her feelings with anyone on the hospital staff. But Ellen realized this reaction was common under the circumstances. Over the next several days, as Mrs. Giraldo's initial feelings of shock subsided, Ellen decided to approach Mrs. Giraldo and ask her to participate in her husband's care.

As they talked, Ellen discovered that Mrs. Giraldo had several problems of her own to deal with before she'd be able to help her husband. So they could

> *"Family members who seem disengaged often want to become involved."*

talk together privately, Ellen led Mrs. Giraldo to a conference room. When they were alone, Ellen encouraged Mrs. Giraldo to express her fears and concerns for her husband, her children, and herself. As Mrs. Giraldo talked, Ellen sat quietly, nodding and listening. Occasionally she uttered broad, accepting statements such as "And then?" and "Please go on." Ellen offered reassurance, too, by acknowledging Mrs. Giraldo's feelings with comments such as, "You seem particularly worried about . . . " and "That must have been frightening for you."

During their conversation, Ellen found out that Mrs. Giraldo had several concerns. She was having a difficult time disciplining her children and answering their questions about their father. In particular, her 10-year-old daughter had quickly assumed many of her mother's roles, reorganizing items in the kitchen cabinets for no reason and attempting to discipline her younger brother in ways that increased the stress everyone felt at home.

Finally, Mrs. Giraldo acknowledged a deeply distressing concern: she told Ellen she felt largely responsible for her husband's heart attack. A week before her husband was admitted, Mrs. Giraldo revealed, he'd started a major remodeling project in their kitchen. But the work progressed slowly over the next few days. Exasperated, Mrs. Giraldo had confronted him about his tendency to put things off. As a result, he'd worked late for the next several nights to convince her that he'd finish the task. Then came the heart attack. Tearfully, Mrs. Giraldo blamed her "nagging" for causing it.

Ellen also learned that Mrs. Giraldo felt unable to plan for her husband's and her family's future. She seemed confused about plans for her husband's rehabilitation, especially concerning sexual practices and exercise programs. She spoke of unresolved issues from her own childhood.

## Bringing the family into the picture

Now that she understood Mrs. Giraldo's state of mind, Ellen worked to convince the woman that helping herself was the best way she could help her husband and children. As a start, Ellen gave Mrs. Giraldo general information about her husband's condition. She emphasized the fact that heart attacks occur for many reasons, so Mrs. Giraldo shouldn't blame herself for what had happened to her husband.

To help resolve Mrs. Giraldo's practical concerns, Ellen arranged for her to attend cardiac rehabilitation classes in the hospital's outpatient department. Ellen also referred Mrs. Giraldo to a local mental health center for counseling on emotional issues.

Ellen was also careful to include other family members and friends in Mr. Giraldo's care. She established specific times for Mr. Giraldo's children to visit; when she observed that seeing his children in the evening seemed to tire Mr. Giraldo, Ellen suggested to him that they visit in the late afternoon. One regular evening visitor was Mr. Giraldo's pastor. Thoughtfully, Ellen made sure that Mr. Giraldo wasn't given his evening care until the pastor had gone.

From the beginning, Mr. Giraldo's mother had tended to overreact to her son's situation. She catered excessively to what she felt were his needs; for example, she appeared in the hospital at all hours to visit him and started bringing him food that wasn't allowed on his diet.

When this activity started, Ellen set up a conference with Mr. Giraldo's mother. When they met, Ellen first stated that she appreciated the older woman's concern for her son. Then Ellen helped her set up a regular schedule for visiting him. As a result of this conference, Mr. Giraldo's mother also decided to help babysit with the children so Mrs. Giraldo could have some relief from her exhausting schedule.

Typically, some elements in a family-assisted care plan must be changed or discontinued because they're not working effectively. Fortunately, most of Ellen's interventions worked as planned. The entire family adhered to their planned visiting schedules. Mrs. Giraldo visited the mental health center for regular counseling and began looking forward to her husband's return home. In fact, with the help of Ellen's counseling, Mrs. Giraldo grew confident enough to become her husband's principal emotional support. She encouraged her husband to follow his treatment carefully, allowed him to make appropriate decisions about household matters, and prudently avoided expressing her concerns about the family's finances.

Within a few weeks of his admission, Mr. Giraldo appeared much less worried about his family and was participating eagerly in his treatment program.

## A final word

In this case study, the nurse worked carefully and directly with family members interested in helping the patient. Perhaps most important, the nurse's intervention enabled the patient's family to provide, within the hospital setting, many familiar and comforting features of the patient's home environment.

Ideally, whatever benefits a patient's family members derive from their hospital experience will strengthen the family unit and make the patient's re-entry to home life easier.

# 84 Why some families are difficult

As you know, hospitalization is a stressful event for the patient *and* for his family. For nursing staff, "patient care" increasingly means meeting the family's needs as well as the patient's. But when family members aren't coping or communicating well, the nursing staff may tend to regard the whole family as difficult, and avoid them. This, of course, is the exact opposite of meeting their needs. When a family isn't communicating its needs very well, that's just when they need your help the most.

Knowing how to intervene can help minimize the disruption that illness introduces into family life. For example, when a family member has a terminal illness, the family experiences significant changes. Family members can become emotionally unstable as they attempt to adjust to role changes, loss of security, and disrupted family goals. They may experience underlying feelings of mistrust, guilt, anger, and fear as they respond to the family member's illness. To successfully help such a family, you need to have a working knowledge of family types and an understanding of the reasons why family members may feel the ways they do. With this knowledge, you begin to see not so much a "difficult" family as a family under enormous stress. The difficult part comes in helping the family cope effectively with that stress. (See Entry 82.)

**What you need to know**
Sociologists have identified several family types, among them the single parent family, the nuclear family, the extended family, and the non-blood-related family. The *single parent family* consists of a father or mother and a child or children sharing a household. The *nuclear family* consists of a father, mother, and child or children sharing a household. An *extended family* includes family members, such as grandparents, in addition to the nuclear family. The *non-blood-related family* consists of individuals who share a household, share mutual goals, and fulfill some of the emotional and physical needs of "family members." Because specific family needs vary depending on the family type, knowing the family type enhances your ability to meet those needs. Why? Because by understanding family dynamics, you'll know who's appropriate to include in family care.

Once you identify the family type, you need to understand what the family is going through, what emotions they may be experiencing that make the ordeal of hospitalization so difficult for them. Here are the most common emotions families experience when a member is hospitalized:

● *Mistrust.* Family members who exhibit signs of mistrust may be influ-

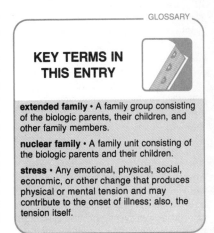

GLOSSARY

**KEY TERMS IN THIS ENTRY**

**extended family** • A family group consisting of the biologic parents, their children, and other family members.

**nuclear family** • A family unit consisting of the biologic parents and their children.

**stress** • Any emotional, physical, social, economic, or other change that produces physical or mental tension and may contribute to the onset of illness; also, the tension itself.

## HOW TO TELL IF RELATIVES ARE UPSETTING YOUR PATIENT

How can you tell when your patient's relatives upset him? Look for certain behaviors—which may or may not be clearly due to his feelings about his relatives—that may be telltale signs. Here's what to look for:

**Behaviors probably due to feelings about relatives**
• Your patient refuses to see his relatives, or asks that no one be allowed to visit.
• Your patient argues with his relatives.
• Your patient exhibits anger toward his relatives—or the relatives exhibit anger toward him.

**Behaviors possibly due to feelings about relatives**
• Your patient usually sleeps during relatives' visits.
• Your patient doesn't interact with his relatives.
• Your patient refuses to be discharged.
• Your patient exhibits physiologic changes such as rapid heart rate, agitation, perspiration, or flushed skin.
• Your patient experiences a return of signs and symptoms such as chest pain, wheezing, or shortness of breath.

enced by previous unpleasant experiences with hospitalization. They may also be mistrustful if they don't understand what's happening to their family member or if they don't understand the roles of the many professionals involved in the family member's care.

• *Guilt.* Family members may feel guilty if they think something they did or didn't do was responsible for the hospitalization. Families may also blame themselves if the patient's illness has been genetically transmitted.

• *Anger.* Family members frequently become angry when they have unrealistic expectations of medical care. They may express anger if they believe the family member is not receiving the kind of care that they expected or that he's not responding as quickly as they expected. This anger increases with the frustration the family may feel over their inability to hasten the patient's recovery or to change his prognosis.

• *Fear.* Family members may fear loneliness, death, a change in the patient's body image, a change in the family's economic status, or simply the unknown. A family's fear of the unknown may arise when they haven't been fully

informed about (or don't fully understand) the family member's condition or treatment regimen. Fear of loneliness occurs when family members are particularly dependent on one another. Family members who fear death will become withdrawn and depressed. When family members must adapt to changes in the body image they have of the patient, they're forced to make major, often painful adjustments. The family that fears a change in their economic status—faced with the possibility that they'll have to sacrifice any financial security they'd built up over the years—will exhibit increased anxiety and a sense of powerlessness. The patient's illness may also force a realignment of family roles, such as when the homemaker must seek employment to support the family.

### How you can help
Families experiencing these emotions and fears will often create difficult situations that challenge your ability to deal with them. To give such a family effective support and minimize their stress, follow these guidelines:

• *Be empathetic.* Remember that illness diminishes feelings of worth. Encourage the family to express their concerns, and respect what they say even if those feelings seem superficial or passing. This will help minimize any guilty feelings they have—and build up their trust in you.

• *Teach the family.* Supply the family with information about the patient's condition, diagnosis, therapy, and medications. Also teach them about the purpose of any apparatus (tubes, catheters, I.V.s, respirators) that's included in the patient's care. Finally, explain unit policies, and give the family a tour of the unit. This will contribute to their trust in you as someone they can turn to.

• *Involve the family.* When appropriate, try to involve the family in feeding and bathing the patient, and in reading to him. This will comfort the family and diminish their stress.

• *Honor your commitments.* Follow through with any commitments that you make to the family. If, for example, you've agreed to extend visiting hours for the family, you must follow through with that agreement. This will assure the family that they can trust you.

• *Remember to use your hospital's resources to increase your effectiveness in helping families cope with stress.*

Nurse consultants can help you manage specific family problems, such as marital conflicts or acting-out behaviors. Also, ask your inservice training department to conduct a class on helping families cope with such adversities as illness, death, or emotional disturbances.

• *Recognize that not all families will be responsive to nursing interventions.* In fact, some may reject your attempts to intervene. If they do reject your efforts, don't take this personally. It may reflect their inability to confront the illness. Persistence and tact on your part may eventually bring results, but if the family continues to cope ineffectively and to resist your help, consider bringing in a nursing consultant to help manage the problem.

## A final word

Knowing how to intervene with a difficult family benefits you, the family, and especially the patient. When you help resolve a difficult situation, you gain satisfaction from a job well done. The family that's coping with their stress more effectively is happier for it. And the patient gets the support from you and his family that he needs to facilitate his recovery.

## Selected References

Alford, D.M. "Tips for Teaching Older Adults," *NursingLife* 2(5):60-63, September/October 1982.

Butler, Robert. "The Life Review: An Interpretation of Reminiscence in the Aged," *Psychiatry* 26(1):65-76, 1963.

Erikson, Erik H. *Childhood and Society.* New York: W.W. Norton & Co., 1964.

Gunter, Laurie M., and Estes, Carmen A. *Education for Gerontic Nursing.* New York: Springer Publishing Co., 1979.

Knowles, R.D. "Preventing Anger," *American Journal of Nursing* 82:118, January 1982.

Leifer, Glora. *Principles and Techniques in Pediatric Nursing,* 3th ed. Philadelphia: W.B. Saunders Co., 1977.

Maslow, Abraham H., ed. *Motivation and Personality,* 2nd ed. New York: Harper & Row Publishers, 1970.

Molter, N.C. "Needs of Relatives of Critically Ill Patients: a Descriptive Study," *Heart and Lung: Journal of Critical Care* 8:332-9, March/April 1979.

Paterson, Josephine G., and Zderad, Loretta T. *Humanistic Nursing.* New York: John Wiley & Sons, 1976.

Weymouth, Lilian. "The Nursing Care of the So-Called Confused Patient," *Nursing Clinics of North America* 3(4):709-715, December 1968.

Wong, Donna L., and Whaley, Lucille F. *Clinical Handbook of Pediatric Nursing.* St. Louis: C.V. Mosby Co., 1981.

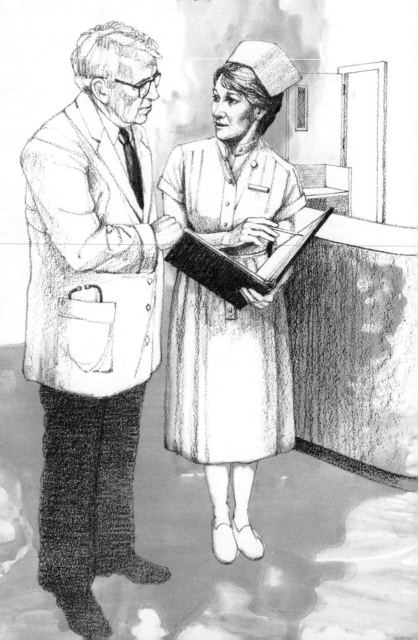

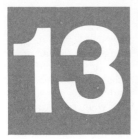

# 13 Understanding and Working with Doctors

## Introduction

Patients are usually admitted to the hospital into the doctor's care—he's the one who prescribes drug therapy and medical treatment. But you're the one who usually administers the drugs and monitors the effects of the prescribed treatments. You're also the one who has the opportunity to assess the patient over time and to recognize his signs and symptoms, as well as his fears and anxieties. How you use this information to ensure the best patient care depends on your communication skills.

How well you communicate with the doctor, how well you present information concerning the patient's health status, and how well you present your ideas for improving his care—all may influence how the doctor reacts. With the patient's well-being as your ultimate goal, communicating effectively and working productively with the patient's doctor is imperative.

The doctor-nurse relationship has been strongly influenced by the fact that the majority of doctors are men and the majority of nurses are women. Historically, the roles and prestige assigned to each professional group have reflected the groups' sex-determined roles in society. In the same way, communications between doctors and nurses have reflected the general communication patterns of men and women.

As the role of women has changed in society, so has the role of nurses in the doctor-nurse relationship. This change began in the 1940s, when society recognized the importance of advanced education for women in general, and for nurses in particular. And since the late 1960s, the increasing willingness of nurses to speak up about hospital problems has upset the traditional dominance of doctors in health-care decision making.

These changes in nurses' roles have had far-reaching effects, not only on nurse-doctor interactions but also on patient care and on doctor-patient relationships. For one thing, nurses are aggressively identifying patient problems. This patient-advocate role, however, need not make you and the doctor adversaries. In fact, an antagonistic relationship will undermine, not promote, quality patient care. If the patient is to benefit, you and the doctor need to respect each other as professionals and as people.

How can you begin building such a nurse-doctor relationship—one based on mutual respect? This chapter will tell you how. First, you must understand the difference between interdependent and dependent nursing functions (Entry 85, "Dependent nursing functions: Who's dependent on whom?"). The scope of your practice, as defined by your state's nurse practice

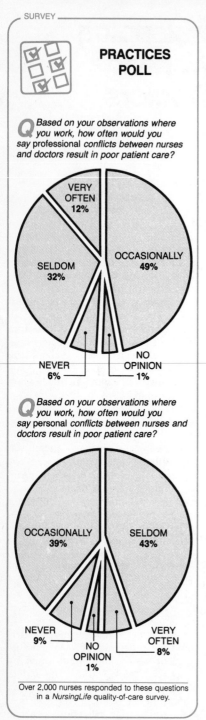

SURVEY

**PRACTICES POLL**

**Q** *Based on your observations where you work, how often would you say* professional *conflicts between nurses and doctors result in poor patient care?*

VERY OFTEN
12%

OCCASIONALLY
49%

SELDOM
32%

NEVER
6%

NO OPINION
1%

**Q** *Based on your observations where you work, how often would you say* personal *conflicts between nurses and doctors result in poor patient care?*

OCCASIONALLY
39%

SELDOM
43%

NEVER
9%

NO OPINION
1%

VERY OFTEN
8%

Over 2,000 nurses responded to these questions in a *NursingLife* quality-of-care survey.

act, includes certain functions that you can perform only with a doctor's orders. On the other hand, often the doctor can't knowledgeably give an order without your input or data collection, making your relationship interdependent. Understanding this interdependence helps clarify your respective roles in providing health care. You'll find that clarifying these roles is the first step toward effective communication.

To fully understand your role in relation to the doctor's, you also must understand his relationship with the patient (Entry 86, "Understanding the doctor-patient relationship"). What's involved in the fiduciary doctor-patient relationship? When are you violating this fiduciary relationship, and when are you protecting the patient's rights? Entry 86 gives you the answers.

A discussion of patients' rights naturally leads to the sensitive topic of challenging doctors' orders (Entry 87, "How and when to challenge a doctor's order"). When should you challenge a doctor's order? How can you do it without marring your professional working relationship? What if the doctor confirms the order and you refuse to carry it out? Should you carry it out even though you disagree with it? The way you deal with these situations has a profound effect on your relationship with doctors.

What if you follow all the rules, but the doctor is just impossible to work with (Entry 88, "Dealing with problem doctors")? Then you need to adopt some special strategies—to protect yourself, the patient, the institution you work for, and sometimes even the doctor.

This chapter also deals with the situation of a nurse who's employed by a doctor in an office setting (Entry 89, "Office nursing: The doctor as employer"). At times, office nurses find themselves functioning as jacks-of-all-trades. How you fare in such a situation depends on the understanding you develop with the doctor you work for.

Your ability to get others to listen to your ideas and accept them is a vital factor in your relationships with doctors (Entry 90, "Abandoning the handmaiden image"). Often the satisfaction you get from your work is directly related to your ability to influence others. To influence doctors, you must be prepared to abandon the handmaiden role for a more collegial relationship. Such a move has its risks, but after all, that's what building effective working relationships is all about—taking risks. If you take those risks and win—developing productive nurse-doctor relationships—you'll help bring about important changes in the quality of your professional life and in the quality of your care.

# 85 Dependent nursing functions: Who's dependent on whom?

You know, of course, that nurses are dependent on doctors for direction in performing some nursing functions. Many nurses lament this dependence and relate it to the traditional "handmaiden image" of nurses. But what really matters most is that, most of the time, doctors and nurses are *dependent on each other* and share accountability for patient care. This entry:

• describes and discusses dependent nursing functions

• examines the interdependence among health professionals and considers the difficult situations that can result when a disagreement occurs

• discusses how health-care professionals' interdependent ways of caring for patients affect their interventions' outcome

• recommends some methods for improving nurses' working relationships with other health-care professionals—particularly doctors—to promote a positive view of dependent nursing functions.

A nurse performs dependent functions on the basis of someone else's assessment and judgment and under circumstances where someone else—generally the doctor—is mainly accountable. Generally speaking, a dependent function can't be performed without another professional's written order. Examples of dependent nursing functions include pharmacologic and surgical treatments, blood and blood-product administration, tube insertion, and prosthesis-fitting.

Where drug administration is concerned, you know about the usual dose, route, interactions and reactions, and expected efficacy of a prescribed drug. Even so, you must have the doctor's order for the drug before you can put this knowledge into effect. Once he gives the order, you assess whether the patient is ready for the drug, teach him about it, and of course, administer it.

Dependent functions are, to some extent, inevitable. But they're not just "necessary evils." In fact, the opposite is true: these functions contribute importantly to patients' health and wellbeing. If nurses didn't perform dependent functions, other health-care professionals couldn't implement their practice—just as, without other health-care professionals, nurses couldn't im-

GLOSSARY

## KEY TERMS IN THIS ENTRY

**change agent** • A nurse or other health-care professional who works to bring about beneficial change for co-workers or patients.

**dependent nursing function** • A function the nurse performs, with another professional's written order, on the basis of that professional's assessment and judgment, for which that professional is accountable.

**nurse practice act** • A law enacted by a state's legislature outlining the legal scope of nursing practice within that state.

# UNDERSTANDING NURSING FUNCTIONS

When you work with a doctor, you may function dependently, interdependently, or independently. A number of factors determine, at any given time, which function is most appropriate for you: the type of patient you're caring for, his particular situation, your level of education, the professional standard of care that should be met for that patient, and the requirements of your state nurse practice act.

| FUNCTION | RESPONSIBILITIES |
|---|---|
| **Dependent** | |
| The nurse depends on another health-care professional for patient assessment and decision making and has no control over, and limited accountability for, treatment outcome. | • carries out established policies, procedures, and care plans<br>• obtains patient data, but not for use in nursing assessment<br>• implements the medical treatment plans for patients<br>• carries out medical orders after evaluating them and determining that they're safe and therapeutic for the patient<br>• reports her observations of medical treatment |
| **Interdependent** | |
| The nurse contributes to patient assessment and decision making and controls the nursing aspects of patients' treatment. | • continually questions the assumptions that patient care is based on<br>• communicates patient data to the entire health-care team<br>• determines the relationship of nursing diagnosis to each patient's total health-care plan<br>• communicates and validates care plans with the other nurses and professionals involved; specifies protocols for emergency situations<br>• communicates, consults on, and validates care-plan outcomes with other involved nurses and professionals<br>• represents nursing on committees and decision-making groups at interdisciplinary conferences, and during grand rounds |
| **Independent** | |
| The nurse has control over patient assessment and is accountable and responsible for treatment outcomes. | • continually questions the assumptions that patient care is based on<br>• systematically and continually collects and records data about patients' health status<br>• derives nursing diagnoses about the health status of patients, families, and patient groups; compares data to norms; identifies patients' capabilities and limitations<br>• formulates and implements a plan of care based on nursing diagnosis, including measurement criteria and time frames<br>• determines progress or lack of progress toward improved health status for patients' families and patient groups; reorganizes care plans, as appropriate<br>• creates an environment conducive to the maintenance or restoration of patients', families', and patient-groups' health |

plement *their* practice. Who, then, really "depends" on whom? The answer is that no health-care provider is completely dependent or independent in practicing his profession. Each must seek not only to control his own practice but also to function interdependently for the sake of improving, maintaining, or restoring patients' health. Only by functioning interdependently can all health-care professionals achieve their practice goals.

## Sources of conflict in dependent nursing functions

Medication orders—or, for that matter, any doctor's orders—are often a source of conflict between the two professions. The doctor orders the drug, and the nurse is usually the person who administers it. Sometimes errors are made in ordering drugs or administering them. What should you do when you're functioning in a dependent role and you believe a medication order is in error? Or when an error has occurred in administration?

Consider the following hypothetical example:

Billy Glenn, age 3, is hospitalized for treatment of acute lead poisoning. He's had two series of EDTA injections, with good urine lead output but little decrease in serum lead level. X-rays of the long bones reveal widespread lead deposits.

Nurse Diane Wilson usually follows an approved medical protocol for lead-poisoning treatment when no doctor is readily available. The protocol for Billy's situation calls for a third series of EDTA injections. She has informed Billy's mother about the planned treatment, assuming medical backup. But Dr. Wetzel, who is conducting pediatric rounds today, countermands the planned treatment, prescribes D-penicillamine—an oral chelation medication—and recommends that Billy be discharged. Diane objects to the orders. She outlines the rationale for the usual protocol to Dr. Wetzel—in a condescending manner. Dr. Wetzel doesn't show

appreciation for either her unasked-for information or her attitude.

Diane also tells the doctor that Billy's home is in poor condition, with obvious and accessible sources of lead, and that Billy's mother has three other preschool children. She adds that she questions the mother's ability to follow the complex directions for administering the drug. Dr. Wetzel persists in his original judgment.

What are Diane's alternatives? She can:

• *Examine her approach to the doctor.* Diane should be sure to use her communication skills in presenting her objections and her ideas. This may seem a trivial point, but it isn't; you get much further with good communication skills than without them. Diane could probably get a better response from Dr. Wetzel with an opening statement such as, "I'd really like to see Billy off those shots, too, Dr. Wetzel, and I'd like to see him back home, but I know this family. Could we possibly …" The issue here isn't Diane's authority; it's appropriate treatment for Billy.

• *Suggest that the doctor talk with the family.* He could explain the change in treatment and the rationale for that change. Talking with Billy's mother would let Dr. Wetzel assess her ability to follow the directions. It would also give him the opportunity to reacquaint himself with Billy as a person, rather than as a series of laboratory and X-ray values.

• *Follow the order as given,* knowing full well that little probability exists that Billy's mother will follow up on the treatment Billy needs. But perhaps Diane can arrange for a clinic assistant, a community health nurse, or a visiting nurse to visit frequently enough during the medication regimen to ensure that the drug is administered properly. Ethically, this alternative is questionable because, in Diane's judgment, Billy is likely to receive inadequate treatment.

• *Follow the protocol, regardless of the consequences.* Obviously, this approach violates Diane's legally defined scope of nursing practice (see Entry 1). Here's another consideration: refusing to follow a doctor's valid order and substituting another treatment procedure could be interpreted as practicing medicine without a license.

• *Use a combination of the alternatives described.* Diane could follow the doctor's order but formally register her objections to it with the doctor and her supervisor. She should fully document the incident as well as the outcome of the treatment. Diane would be at least personal risk if she did this. Legally and ethically, this alternative is sound.

---

*"The issue here isn't whether dependent functions are appropriate or fair. They're a fact of modern health care."*

---

### Some theoretical underpinnings to interdependent care

Nurses, doctors, nutritionists, social workers—all health-care personnel—share the same ultimate goal: improving the patient's mental and physical health. And all depend on each other to meet this goal. How they contribute to this goal depends on their professional roles in health-care delivery.

In Billy's case, the health-care team wants to cure the effects of lead intoxication and eliminate the possibility of future intoxication. Here's what the goals for the professionals involved might be:

• *Doctor's goal:* to reduce serum blood lead levels to less than 30 mg/100 ml

• *Nurse's goal:* to help restore a normal 3-year-old's growth and development level within the context of the family's life-style

• *Nutritionist's goal:* to provide iron-rich foods to raise the patient's hemoglobin level above 11 mg/dl

• *Social worker's goal:* to provide ad-

equate social support so that lead-poisoning treatment will continue and be completed.

### Treatment

To attain these goals, each profession develops its own treatments (or processes). The doctor treats the patient's blood level with drugs. The nurse treats the patient's family's physical and mental responses to lead poisoning by nurturing the child, giving his mother emotional support, and helping her provide a safe (lead-free) environment for her children. The nutritionist treats the family's dietary deficiencies by recommending foods that are high in iron, that children like, and that the mother can buy and prepare. The social worker treats the mother's need for financial and social assistance by securing the necessary child care, home repairs, and food.

### Setting

The setting (or structure) in which the health-care professionals carry out the treatments can make the difference between success and failure of treatment. For instance, professionals working together without formal opportunities to discuss case-management issues are working in a setting that lacks an effective communication system. The result: mixed messages between professionals (and transmitted to the patient), duplication of effort, and a potential breakdown in treatment. A good setting provides policies and procedures for interprofessional practice, adequate interdisciplinary staffing, and feedback mechanisms for input from patients, staff, and outside experts. In such a setting, each professional can collaborate with and depend on the others.

### A final word

The issue here isn't whether dependent functions are appropriate or fair. They're a fact of modern health care. But, as health-sciences knowledge bases grow, opportunities for interdependence will probably grow as well.

How will greater interdependence affect you, as a nurse? First, because interdependence requires increased responsibility and accountability, every nurse must practice at her absolute best, basing her practice decisions upon tested nursing science and theory. Second, the setting for interdependent practice must accommodate nursing's increased accountability and responsibility. This means that functions that don't fall within the updated definition of nursing should be delegated to health-care assistants. And finally, by being freed of some of the old nursing functions, nurses will be able to provide a higher level of patient care.

---

# 86 Understanding the doctor-patient relationship

The doctor-patient relationship is changing in very positive ways. And you, as a nurse, deserve some of the credit for these changes. Why? Because you serve as a liaison between doctor and patient, acting as the doctor's agent and the patient's advocate. As you know, a willingness to communicate is the foundation of any relationship. You've done all you could to facilitate communication between doctors and patients. You need to remember, though, that this role places you in a position where, to be effective, you must understand their relationship. This way you'll know when you're enhancing it and when you're interfering with it.

## What you need to know
Historically, a patient's relationship with his doctor was a purely dependent one. Doctors talked *to* patients, not *with* patients. The patient blindly put his life

in the doctor's hands—rarely asking questions, never participating in decision making.

Today, the doctor-patient relationship is like a partnership between the professional delivering care and the consumer receiving it. More and more, doctors understand the value of involving patients in their own care. And the typical patient is no longer satisfied with a "no questions asked" relationship. If he's faced with undergoing an invasive procedure, for example, he'll first want to discuss the expected outcomes, possible side effects, and possible alternatives. The result: a healthy dialogue between patient and doctor.

## Your legal concerns as a staff nurse
Legally, the doctor and patient have a fiduciary relationship. The doctor is the fiduciary to the patient, who relies on the doctor's advice and judgment. Even when the patient participates fully in his treatment plan, he's still not on an equal footing with his doctor.

What does this mean to you, as a nurse? Well, you know you should never deliberately violate this fiduciary relationship. But you're right in the middle of it; how can you tell when you're improperly interfering with it and when you're enhancing it? Here are some examples to help you.

You enhance the doctor-patient re-

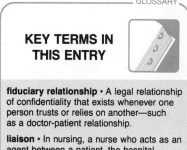

GLOSSARY

## KEY TERMS IN THIS ENTRY

**fiduciary relationship** • A legal relationship of confidentiality that exists whenever one person trusts or relies on another—such as a doctor-patient relationship.

**liaison** • In nursing, a nurse who acts as an agent between a patient, the hospital, and the patient's family, and who speaks for the entire health-care team.

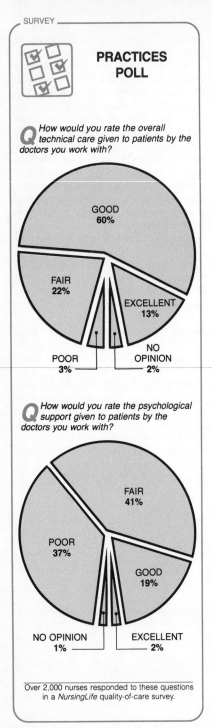

SURVEY

**PRACTICES POLL**

**Q** *How would you rate the overall technical care given to patients by the doctors you work with?*

GOOD
60%

FAIR
22%

EXCELLENT
13%

POOR
3%

NO OPINION
2%

**Q** *How would you rate the psychological support given to patients by the doctors you work with?*

FAIR
41%

POOR
37%

GOOD
19%

NO OPINION
1%

EXCELLENT
2%

Over 2,000 nurses responded to these questions in a *NursingLife* quality-of-care survey.

lationship by helping coordinate health care. Before a patient has surgery, for example, you can allay his fears by explaining routine procedures and answering questions that you, as a nurse, may properly answer (see Entry 5). Don't discuss alternative treatments with the patient unless the doctor's already discussed those alternatives with him.

Consider the following hypothetical situation.

Lisa Berryman, RN, enters Alice Taylor's room to obtain procedural consent for an intravenous pyelogram (IVP). Lisa can tell that Alice, who's hypertensive, is afraid. Alice asks Lisa what kind of test the doctor's ordered. Lisa sits down to explain the preparations and the procedures that will take place in the X-ray department. She also explains that the dye they'll use may cause a hot flash or a salty taste. She does *not* tell the patient what the doctor is looking for (pheochromocytoma). Instead, she suggests that Alice ask her doctor why he's ordered the test and what he expects to find. This action is within the scope of her nurse's license.

Here's a case that, although the board of nursing's decision against the nurse was eventually overturned, nevertheless illustrates why you should never contradict what a doctor has told his patient or give a patient any medical advice. This kind of interference can lead to the suspension of your license. Consider the case of *Tuma v. Board of Nursing* (1979). Ms. Tuma, a clinical nursing instructor, counseled a terminally ill female leukemia patient about treatments other than the chemotherapy the patient was undergoing. And she told the patient that she would help make the arrangements if the patient decided on one of the alternative treatments. Over the next few hours, the patient did consider changing her treatment regimen; in fact, because of her change of attitude, her doctor discontinued his order for chemotherapy but reinstated it about an hour later. Two weeks later, the patient died.

Shortly thereafter, hospital personnel filed complaints with the state board of nursing.

Acting on the staff's complaints about Ms. Tuma, the board found her guilty of violating the section of the nurse practice act that prohibits "unprofessional conduct" because she improperly interfered with the doctor-patient relationship. On appeal, the Idaho Supreme Court did not agree with the board, stating that the section of the nurse practice act that Ms. Tuma was accused of violating was too vague. So the court did eventually rule that Ms. Tuma was not guilty of violating her state's nurse practice act; it never decided whether Ms. Tuma's actions violated the patient-doctor relationship. The chance that Ms. Tuma would have her license suspended for this reason, however, was high—too high for you or any other nurse to risk. So, if you want to enhance, not hinder, the doctor-patient relationship, you need to become familiar with the licensing laws and regulations of your state.

You may find yourself in situations where your professional responsibilities force you to actively intervene in the doctor-patient relationship. *Darling v. Charleston Community Memorial Hospital* (1965) is an example. A young man, age 18, was admitted to a hospital emergency room with a broken leg. A doctor applied traction and a plaster cast; a heat cradle was placed over the cast to quicken the drying. Over the next few hours, the patient had a great deal of pain, and his toes swelled and changed colors. When the cast was loosened, "blood and other seepage were observed by the nurses and others...", and an overpowering odor filled the room.

The nurses never reported the patient's condition or questioned the doctor's treatment. No one called the supervisor or the medical director. No one suggested to the parents that they might want to have the patient examined by another doctor or transferred to another hospital. Ultimately, the patient's leg had to be amputated. An Illinois court found fault not only with the doctor but also with the nurses and the hospital. The court ruled that the nurses had a duty to speak up and report the improper treatment of the patient to their supervisors. The *Darling* decision was upheld by the Illinois Appellate Court and Illinois Supreme Court.

## A final word

The doctor-patient relationship is changing, from one-sided dependency to a provider-consumer partnership. Legally, however, the relationship remains a fiduciary one; the patient relies on and needs to trust his doctor. As a nurse, you can promote beneficial doctor-patient communication that enhances their relationship. But be careful—make sure your actions as liaison don't cause you to exceed the legal scope of nursing practice.

# 87 How and when to challenge a doctor's order

Dr. Smith's order reads, "digoxin 50 mg given now." You call Dr. Smith to clarify the order, expecting him to say he meant 0.5 mg of digoxin. But to your amazement, he states that he does want *50 mg* of digoxin given *now*. Would you challenge this order, or give the medication as prescribed?

Following doctors' orders is a large part of your practice. However, nursing practice also requires that you evaluate every order for its safety and appropriateness. The doctor is no longer the captain of the ship, and you, as an independent professional, are held accountable for every order you carry out.

Evaluating every order will lead you either to challenge some of them for the patient's protection or to question who

## KEY TERMS IN THIS ENTRY

**"the handmaiden image"** • A term that reflects the outdated view of nurses as doctors' servants.

**liability** • Legal responsibility for *failure to act*, so causing harm to another person, or for *actions* that fail to meet standards of care, so causing harm to another person.

**scope of practice** • In nursing, the professional nursing activities defined under state or provincial law in each state's (or Canadian province's) nurse practice act.

should carry out some of them. But the real challenge you face as the nurse is deciding *when* to say no to a doctor and then *how* to say it in an effective way.

## The problem with saying no

Saying no to anyone is one of the most difficult things we ever have to do. The word "no" is a red flag signaling disagreement, and disagreement causes stress. We feel that by saying no, we're rejecting the other person. We feel guilty for hurting his feelings.

Women, in particular, typically have been socialized to make other people happy. And if other people aren't happy, women have been made to feel responsible. Although women have come a long way in recognizing their own needs and in learning to take responsibility for their feelings, some of the guilt about saying no still lingers.

For a female nurse, saying no to a doctor is especially difficult. As both a nurse and a woman, you have to deal not only with your socialization as a woman but also with the intimidating effects of the doctor's perceived power and influence. The response that you probably anticipate most is not rejection, but anger. You've probably gotten such responses as, "How dare you question my order?" or "Are you questioning my judgment and experience?"

So, more than feeling guilty about saying no to a doctor, you probably feel scared. But even though you may find that saying no to a doctor is extremely difficult, you have a professional right and a responsibility—when it's appropriate—to do just that.

*Who may benefit from your decision to say no?* The patient? The doctor? The hospital? The nurse? Nursing itself? Answer: All of the above.

## Benefits for the patient

Patients rightfully expect that the care they receive will be appropriate and necessary. By assuming responsibility for your own actions, saying no when you feel you should, you provide a double-check to ensure high-quality patient care.

As you know, giving high-quality care includes avoiding such dangerous practices as giving the wrong drug or the wrong dose of a drug. It also means that doctors' orders must be executed only by qualified personnel. For example, suppose a doctor orders you to reprogram a pacemaker. You feel that the procedure is outside your scope of practice. You and the patient will benefit if you say no and suggest that the most qualified professional—in this instance, the doctor—perform the procedure.

The patient also benefits when you challenge *unnecessary* orders. He doesn't need the unnecessary risk. And care is expensive enough without adding the cost of unnecessary procedures, tests, or drugs.

## Benefits for the doctor

The doctor benefits, too, when you question an order. Why? Because your action may protect his patient from harm—and him from liability for malpractice. The doctor also gains a better understanding of your role in the health-care process. Every time you explain your reasons for questioning a care plan, you reinforce his perception of you as an accountable health-care professional.

# WHEN YOU DISAGREE WITH A DOCTOR'S ORDER

### Doing what he tells you not to do

*For the past several weeks, our intensive care unit (ICU) has been caring for a patient who's had massive intracranial bleeding. He's relatively unresponsive and has little or no rehabilitation potential.*

*Besides his other problems, he has copious pulmonary secretions that require suctioning every 30 to 45 minutes. A neurosurgeon filling in for the patient's regular doctor (who was on vacation) took one look at the patient and wrote an order to suction the patient no more than once every 4 hours.*

*I feel that carrying out such an order would be negligent on my part, especially in the ICU—where, by definition, we provide intensive care. What do you think?—RN, Tex.*

You're right. Determining when and when not to suction is a nursing assessment based on throat and breath sounds, respiratory rate, and significant signs.

Also, from a physiologic viewpoint, an order for suctioning every 4 hours (or even every 3 or 2 hours) is a poor one, because secretions may not peak within any specific time frame.

Discuss your concerns with the doctor immediately, but continue to suction the patient as necessary.

If the doctor disagrees with you, let him know, as a professional courtesy, that you intend to pursue the matter through channels with an incident report.

### Not doing what he tells you to do

*A member of our medical staff insists on ordering heparin given intramuscularly (I.M.), despite protests from our pharmacists and other hospital personnel.*

*I administered it once, as he ordered, but I regretted doing it. When I returned after my weekend off, I could see large hematomas on the patient's buttocks, resulting from the injections.*

*I'd like to refuse to give heparin I.M. the next time—but my action won't be taken lightly in the small community hospital where I work.*

*Before I take my stand, I'd like to know: Is there a therapeutic reason for administering heparin by the I.M. route?—RN, Mich.*

The fourth edition of the American Medical Association *Drug Evaluations* says this about heparin: "The intramuscular route should not be used because of the likelihood of producing tissue irritation, local bleeding, or hematoma; in addition, absorption is unpredictable after intramuscular administration."

When you returned and noted the hematomas, you should have filed an incident report: "Hematomas noted on same sites as I.M. heparin injections"—and included the hematoma's measurements as well as the patient's complaints about pain.

But that experience is past. Before it happens again, decide that the next time a doctor asks you to administer heparin I.M., you'll tell him you're uncomfortable about doing it—and why. Speaking up this way is both your right and your responsibility. Of course, you should first ask if he has a special reason for choosing the I.M. route, or if he has new information on the subject that you're not yet familiar with. If he offers neither a medical reason nor new information, call in your pharmacist. He's the expert in this matter.

When you've done your groundwork, you can feel comfortable telling the doctor you'll administer the drug by any recommended route. But if the doctor insists on I.M., give him the option of administering the heparin himself. (And, of course, document fully as you go.) If you're knowledgeable and confident, and if you handle the matter discreetly (so the doctor isn't publicly put on the defensive), he probably won't insist that you carry out the order.

What should you do, however, if he still insists on ordering the heparin to be given I.M.? Present your documentation to your supervisor. Emphasize that your objections are based on your understanding of the nurse's role and function in the situation. Your supervisor will probably back you up, but if she doesn't, keep going up the administrative ladder until you get results. Finally, when things calm down, work to get a procedure for heparin injection added to your nursing procedure manual.

---

These letters were taken from the files of *Nursing* magazine.

## Benefits for the hospital

You might think that the hospital would frown on a nurse's refusal to follow a medical order. But the hospital's first responsibility is to the patient, and it will support all efforts to protect patients from harm or injury.

Remember, the hospital is responsible for all the actions of its employees. This responsibility is termed "vicarious liability." It means that if an employer has hired you to further its interests (patient care), the employer is held liable for your actions. As a nurse employed by a hospital, therefore, you're representing the hospital, as well as yourself, when you question a medical order. The hospital has a vested interest in your ability to evaluate—and your willingness to challenge—services you're instructed to deliver to patients.

---

### GETTING A DOCTOR TO SAY "YES"

Saying "no" to a doctor's order is hard enough. But suppose you have an idea that you'd like to suggest to the doctor? How do you convince him to say "yes"?

Obviously, this is a delicate situation. Doctors can be very sensitive, even defensive, when nurses challenge their original care plans and suggest changes. The last thing you want to do is become defensive yourself, so you need to proceed cautiously and tactfully.

First, offer your suggestions from a *nursing* perspective, and, if possible, explain to the doctor how the care regimen you're suggesting has worked for you or other nurses. Then, give examples of other patients you've cared for, using a similar regimen. This way, the doctor needn't feel threatened, because you're basing your suggestion on your nursing knowledge, and you're backing up your suggestion with concrete examples.

Of course, you'll want to phrase your suggestion in such a way that the doctor knows you trust his judgment. Saying something like, "In a similar case, we did such and such, and it worked quite well; I believe it will work in this case, too," opens the door for discussion between you and the doctor. On the other hand, if you say, "If I were you, I'd do such and such," you may get the door to discussion slammed in your face.

The following examples illustrate the best approach:

Suppose you're caring for Mr. Yeats, who's been hospitalized for 3 weeks with a head injury. Mr. Yeats is losing weight and becoming progressively weaker, and you're getting concerned about his nutritional status. But the doctor has never mentioned this aspect of his care. You might say, "Dr. Brooks, I have a nursing problem I'd like to discuss with you. I've noticed that Mr. Yeats has been losing weight and that his strength is diminishing. It's also becoming more difficult to get him out of bed. I think this is related to his nutritional status. If it is, what can I do to help?"

This way, you've made your point, but you've left decision making up to the doctor. He'll probably agree that Mr. Yeats' nutritional status needs improving and add this to the care plan.

Here's another example:

Suppose you've noticed that Mrs. Webb's response to an antiemetic hasn't been effective. You've just attended a workshop on the use of these medications and have some information about a new antiemetic. How do you tell the doctor about it without implying that you're more up to date on these medications than he is?

Once again, your best approach is to discuss the patient's problem with the doctor, telling him of your nursing observations. Then explain that you've just attended a workshop on the subject. State your own tentative conclusions, make your recommendation, and ask him how he views the situation. Then watch what happens. Chances are, the doctor will do one of three things: take your advice and act on it, share his views with you, or do some research of his own and come up with the same information you presented to him.

Of course, many care plans still legally require a doctor's order, but you, the doctor, and the patient benefit when you offer your ideas and unique skills. Getting a doctor to say "yes" takes planning and tact on your part, but with the right approach, you'll both be glad you spoke up.

### Benefits for you

When you refuse to carry out a questionable medical order, you benefit by protecting your own practice. The doctor is responsible, on the basis of his skill and education, for ordering the therapy; you're responsible, on the basis of your skill and education, for implementing the order. Therefore, both of you have to answer for any consequences of an action. Challenging an order at the time it's given is better than having to justify your actions later. Keep in mind that having to say "The doctor ordered it" is humiliating. Your license is on the line, so your future depends on your ability to challenge medical orders appropriately.

### Benefits for nursing

Nursing benefits as a profession every time you make clear distinctions be-

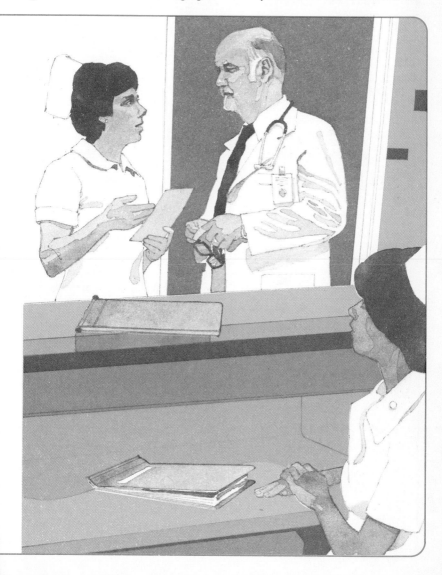

tween responsibilities you can and can't assume. Nurses need to have a good understanding of what they contribute to patient care *and* confidence in their ability to evaluate the effects of *total* care—not just of their own contribution. Improving the status of the nursing profession depends on nurses who are assertive, who know how to set limits, and who are responsible for their own actions.

### Suggested strategies for action

*How* you challenge a doctor's order will determine how effective you are in ensuring safe patient care. What can be done to make challenging easier? Entry 90, "Abandoning the handmaiden im-age," gives some helpful communication techniques to use when saying no to a doctor. Here are some practical suggestions for formulating the most effective strategy when you challenge a doctor's order.

*When you need to say no.* Ask yourself what you would do in the following situations:

• The doctor orders occupational therapy for a psychiatric patient who was admitted to the hospital a week ago with a diagnosis of attempted suicide. You feel that the patient is still suicidal, and you're concerned about exposing him to the occupational therapy room's equipment and supplies.

• You're caring for a patient who's supposed to receive Nephramine, which is made with 70% dextrose. The doctor orders that the solution be run at a rate of 150 cc/hr, but you feel that's too fast.

• It's 3 a.m., and your patient's chest tube doesn't appear to be functioning. You call the doctor on the phone and tell him the situation. He asks you to irrigate the chest tube with normal saline solution while he stays on the line. You feel that this procedure is neither within your scope of practice nor appropriate for the situation.

In each of these situations, you must challenge the doctor—either because a procedure or drug is inappropriate or because you feel that you're not the most qualified professional to perform the procedure. Here are the steps you should take:

*Talk it over.* The first step in questioning any doctor's order is to clarify the order with the doctor. Many times the doctor has forgotten the order or is unaware of the mistake. If either of these is true, the issue is easily resolved. If the doctor insists that the order be carried out as prescribed, you'll have to tell him why, in your nursing judgment, you cannot carry it out. Before taking such a position, however, you should know exactly what your state's nurse practice act permits and prohibits a nurse to do. (Entry 1 contains a discussion of nurse practice acts.)

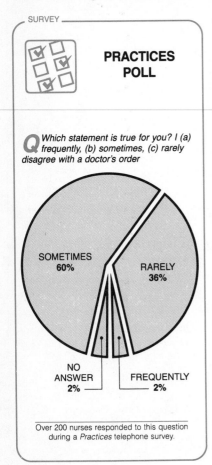

SURVEY

**PRACTICES POLL**

**Q** *Which statement is true for you? I (a) frequently, (b) sometimes, (c) rarely disagree with a doctor's order*

SOMETIMES
**60%**

RARELY
**36%**

NO ANSWER
**2%**

FREQUENTLY
**2%**

Over 200 nurses responded to this question during a *Practices* telephone survey.

Ask the doctor about his rationale for giving the order. His explanation may be very reasonable. Knowing his rationale will help you make an informed decision.

*Document the incident.* If the issue remains unresolved, you must document, for the record, the steps you've taken. Include in your documentation a description of the incident and the

---

"*Nurses need to have confidence in their ability to evaluate the effects of the health care that their patients receive.*"

---

names of any witnesses. (Chapter 5 provides information on nursing documentation that will help you record the incident correctly.)

*Report the incident to your supervisor.* If possible, let your supervisor know about a problem you think may occur. The most urgent time to talk to your supervisor is *during* an incident. She may have some suggestions for handling the doctor. Many times a doctor will respond when someone from nursing administration talks to him. But don't neglect to talk to your supervisor after the incident has been resolved. You never know when a doctor will agree with you at the time but complain to your supervisor later. By telling your supervisor immediately after you resolve the problem, you'll give her time to prepare for any challenges by getting the facts.

*Follow the chain of command.* Most medical staffs have a chain of command or a committee to deal with patient-care issues. Your supervisor, once involved, should initiate the process. If your supervisor won't proceed, then you should do so, documenting it carefully. Continue up the chain of command until the issue is resolved—

either in your favor or in the doctor's.

Following the chain of command takes a lot of time. And you may be in situations that don't allow you that time. The quickest solution to your problem is to allow the doctor to administer the drug or perform the procedure personally. By doing so, he assumes sole accountability for any consequences of the action.

These suggestions for challenging a doctor's order will help you do it in a logical and professional manner. Your institution's system for handling disagreements should provide you with the kind of support you need. If it doesn't, get legal advice from an attorney, preferably one experienced in employees' rights. Knowing that you've protected a patient is itself satisfying. But having the support of your colleagues will mean you don't have to take on this kind of challenge alone.

### A final word
Nursing practice and medical practice are constantly changing and evolving. One trend is the health-care system's increasing respect for nurses' professional judgment. In this context, challenging a doctor's order can be as proper and necessary as carrying one out.

---

# 88 Dealing with problem doctors

Problem doctors? Chances are this phrase rings a bell with you. Maybe some of the following four situations remind you of incidents in your own nursing career:

A patient's admitted to your floor for surgery. The surgery schedule indicates that the attending doctor is the patient's surgeon. You know that this doctor's surgical privileges in your hospital are limited—and don't include the scheduled procedure. *What can you do?*

## KEY TERMS IN THIS ENTRY

**hospital quality assurance program** • A program developed by a hospital committee that monitors the quality of the hospital's diagnostic, therapeutic, prognostic, and other health-care activities.

**liability** • Legal responsibility for *failure to act*, so causing harm to another person, or for *actions* that fail to meet standards of care, so causing harm to another person.

**standards of care** • In a malpractice lawsuit, those acts performed or omitted that an ordinary, prudent person in the defendant's position would have done or not done; a measure by which the defendant's alleged wrongful conduct is compared.

A patient's in a body cast. You observe that he isn't doing well. You document the problem in the clinical record, then you phone the doctor's office and leave a message. The doctor doesn't respond to your phone call. When he does come to the unit, he reads the record but takes no action. *What can you do?*

The clinical record notes that your patient is allergic to penicillin. The attending doctor prescribes penicillin, and doesn't want to discuss the matter with you. *What can you do?*

On the day he's had disc-removal surgery, you find that the patient can't move his legs and complains of numbness, pain, and weakness. After unsuccessfully trying to reach the surgeon, you document the patient's signs and symptoms in the clinical record. You also document that your attempts to contact the surgeon haven't been successful. *What else can you do?*

Nurses frequently ask how they should act in situations like these. What's the key to simultaneously acting in the patient's best interests *and* following the doctor's orders? You know, of course, that the doctor has primary responsibility for the patient's total medical regimen. And you know that nurses aren't permitted to alter that regimen or to take nursing actions that conflict with it. But sometimes—!

Although situations like the ones described don't occur frequently, most nurses occasionally encounter a doctor who may be stretching the limits of his ability. This can happen if the doctor becomes too busy to keep up with recent medical developments, if he drinks heavily, or if he takes medication that affects his performance. Such a doctor needs assistance. And his patients need protection.

## Understanding interprofessional responsibilities

Only the medical community can set standards for the doctor's professional practice. As a nurse, however, you share a responsibility with the doctor—to protect the public. You must ensure that patients receive care that's consistent with their needs and with prevailing medical and nursing standards.

The Arizona Supreme Court emphasized the importance of this responsibility by saying, "If the medical staff was negligent in the exercise of its duties of supervising its members or in failing to recommend action by the hospital's governing body, then the hospital would be negligent." (*Tucson Medical Center v. Misevch*, 1976.) The same court implied that the hospital has a duty to the patient to ensure that only professionally competent persons are on its staff. You and your fellow nurses, as part of the hospital staff, share this responsibility and are required to assist the hospital administration whenever and however possible. Some state laws, such as those of the state of Washington, require that any incident of professional medical misconduct, in any health-care setting, be reported.

Although nursing doesn't set standards for any other professional discipline, or determine the adequacy of

## WHEN THE PROBLEM ISN'T INCOMPETENCE

Thankfully, incompetent doctors are the exception, not the rule, so you probably won't meet too many of them in your career. What you *will* meet, though, are doctors like these, who can make your life miserable:

● the foul-mouthed doctor, who uses obscenities freely

● the commanding-officer doctor, who orders everyone around

● the Don Juan doctor who can't keep his hands to himself.

From your own experience, you can probably add to this list of doctors we can all do without.

Let's face it, work is hard enough without these kinds of problems. But you can't keep ducking these doctors if they work on your units, and you can't just "grin and bear it" forever without feeling resentful. Then what *can* you do? Here are a few suggestions:

● Tell your supervisor about the doctor's behavior and about specific incidents, especially incidents involving patients.

● Confront the doctor. Tell him you find his behavior offensive, and say that if *you*

feel this way, chances are some of the patients do, too. In fact, the doctor's behavior may get him in legal hot water, if an offended patient decides to sue.

● If the doctor is overly commanding, try establishing standard procedures for certain situations where he tends to get overbearing. This way, at least in these situations, the doctor has less reason to issue arbitrary commands.

● Document all the incidents that involve that doctor, and your actions. This way, if hospital administrators investigate any situations, they have written records to refer to that will help them determine the extent of the doctor's involvement.

If a problem persists in spite of your efforts, move up to the next rung of authority. Talk with someone above the department heads, such as a hospital administrator. (First, tell your supervisor of your plans to talk with the administrator.) Remember, you're acting for the benefit of your patients as well as yourself. So keep at it until someone gives the matter attention. And remember, document all your actions.

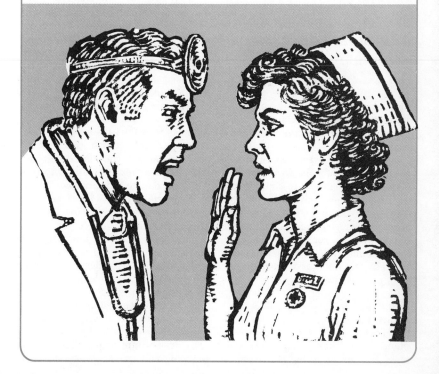

the performance of practitioners in other disciplines, nurses do have a legal obligation to report inadequate or unresponsive care rendered by an attending doctor. If you fail to carry out this duty, you expose yourself and your institution to liability. And nurses also have an ethical obligation to patients. The American Nurses' Association code for nurses states, "The nurse acts to safeguard the client and the public when health care and safety are affected by incompetent, unethical, or illegal practice of any person."

These obligations require observing, questioning, and reporting known instances of doctors' inadequate responses to patients' needs. Reporting such instances contributes to the medical staff's peer review process—a process through which the medical staff

*"If you fail to carry out your duty to report a doctor's misconduct, you expose yourself and your institution to liability."*

monitors itself. Reporting also provides input for medical staff decisions related to granting or limiting a doctor's privileges.

So you can't afford to remain uninvolved. Sympathy for the doctor, or fear of him, won't help you in court if you fail to take proper action. And it certainly won't contribute to good patient care. Whether you dread involvement in hospital politics or perhaps don't feel like taking the time to document these incidents, your duty to report a doctor's misconduct is clear.

### Who decides that a doctor's incompetent?
Dictionaries commonly define incompetence as inefficiency, inadequacy, and lack of ability in the performance

of functions. *Black's Law Dictionary,* 5th edition, defines incompetence as "lack of ability, legal qualification, or fitness to discharge the required duty." So, the term *incompetent doctor* generally means that the doctor is consistently unable to practice medicine with reasonable skill and safety to patients.

Of course, determining a doctor's liability for inadequate patient care is a matter for the courts. Poor results alone are not enough to assign liability; the expert testimony of other doctors is usually needed to show that the poor results stemmed from the doctor's failure to meet a required standard of care.

But when you're taking care of patients, you don't have a court to help you if you're concerned about a doctor's competence. You *do* have a kind of "expert testimony," though—consultation with other doctors and nurses—that either will clarify a doctor's order or action or will confirm the existence of a problem you've observed.

Of equally pressing concern is the doctor, surgeon, or anesthesiologist who appears to be under the influence of alcohol or other drugs, who regularly doesn't attend to his patients' needs, or who orders medication or treatment that clearly contradicts normal practices. A doctor like this places all of his patients in potential jeopardy.

### Actions you can take
When you find yourself in any of the above situations, you have several responsibilities. You're required to protect your patient from undue risk, to share information with those who have responsibility for monitoring the doctor's performance, and to assist the medical staff in trying to change the doctor's performance if necessary. After talking with two colleagues, if you're convinced that a problem exists, then what do you do?

If the patient's health or safety requires immediate attention—particularly at night or on weekends—inform your immediate supervisor. She'll probably call the health-services supervisor or the person in your institution who has authority to take immediate action, such as the head of medical services on the unit.

The health-services supervisor or head of medical services may take one or more of the following actions: notifying and consulting with the medical director, specialty staff, peer review committee, or the medical committee;

ADVICE

## PROPER CHANNELS FOR REPORTING IMPROPER CONDUCT

*One of our in-house anesthesiologists has been behaving in a totally unprofessional way and we're beginning to fear for our patients' lives.*

*Here's a sampling of this doctor's behavior:*

*He leaves the delivery room in the middle of deliveries and cesarean sections, swears at nurses and patients, and resuscitates newborns very vigorously. He doesn't check the $O_2$ or $NO_2$ tank levels and doesn't check the equipment to make sure it's working properly.*

*And as if these things weren't bad enough, one day he gave a patient the wrong anesthesia. If another doctor hadn't intervened, the patient might have died.*

*For the past 3 months, we've documented each of these incidents and sent the reports to the director of nursing. Our charge nurse has also reported the problem to the director. And now I call the nursing supervisor whenever a new incident occurs.*

*We nurses have lost all faith in "proper channels." So far, absolutely nothing has been done about this doctor. Do we have to wait until a patient dies before someone takes us seriously?—RN, Pa.*

This is definitely a problem that calls for alerting two department heads— the doctor's and yours—using a double-barreled approach: talk to the department heads and send a thoroughly documented report through the proper channels.

If, after a week or two, you've had no word and no action, then it's time to move up to the next level of authority: take the matter up with those who are over the department heads who've failed to act. (Professional courtesy requires that you let your department head, and the doctor's,

know that you're taking the matter further.)

If you have to, you can go a step further—to the hospital's board of directors. If you can't get *any* response within the hospital, you can even go to an outside authority. Call your state's Office of Complaints in the Bureau of Professional and Occupational Affairs. Request an official complaint form and fill it out. (If you wish, you can request that your name be withheld.) You'll be notified by mail about the action this state agency decides to take.

No obstetric or gynecologic procedure should be started when the dangerous situation you describe exists. For example, if the proper equipment checks haven't been made, as you report, the surgeon and the charge nurse should be told. They have to know that a dangerous situation exists in the delivery room. Until that situation is remedied, the procedure should not begin.

Be prepared: a confrontation is inevitable. Be sure the patient is not present when it happens, or at least not aware of what's going on.

If you conduct yourself knowledgeably and with conviction, both the nursing and the medical staffs will recognize that you and your co-workers mean business when it comes to safe and effective patient care.

There's another danger here: If you work right along with this anesthesiologist, knowing that he's set up a dangerous situation for the patient, you could be legally liable.

Before the matter is settled, there may be a lot of sound and fury. But when calm is restored, the entire health team will have avoided serious trouble—and you'll probably have earned new respect from your colleagues.

This letter was taken from the files of *Nursing* magazine.

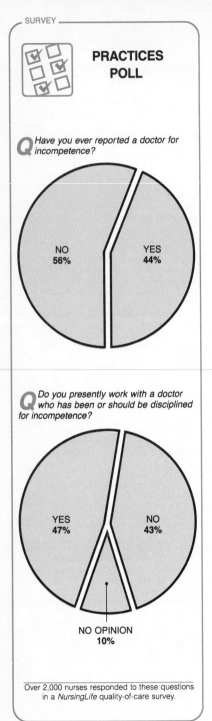

## PRACTICES POLL

**Q** *Have you ever reported a doctor for incompetence?*

NO
56%

YES
44%

**Q** *Do you presently work with a doctor who has been or should be disciplined for incompetence?*

YES
47%

NO
43%

NO OPINION
10%

Over 2,000 nurses responded to these questions in a *NursingLife* quality-of-care survey.

or consulting with someone from outside the institution—for example, from a neighboring medical center—who has the knowledge and expertise to determine the appropriateness of the doctor's order or action. That person may speak with the attending doctor and share his expertise to help resolve the problem.

After your observation has been validated and you've taken the immediate action necessary to protect the patient, how do you bring about a permanent solution? How do you ensure that the problem behavior won't happen again? First, discuss the matter with your supervisor. Depending on your institution's protocol, she'll either pursue the matter up the nursing chain of command or turn it over to the person responsible for quality assurance, who'll pursue it himself.

If your institution has no provision for such actions or your supervisor ignores your request for action, you may have to approach the medical director, administrator, or member of the governing body yourself for additional assistance. (As a courtesy, you should tell each person you speak with that you plan to go to yet a higher authority.) You should know, however, that such action is not without risk. Prior to or concurrent with taking any steps beyond the nursing supervisory level, you may be wise to consult an attorney to minimize exposing yourself to unnecessary legal risks and to increase your awareness of any risks inherent in the situation. You also may want to consult your state nurses' association, state board of nursing, or some other professional group you belong to. These bodies may have their own counsel who can provide you with additional advice and assistance.

If your institution has no protocol for dealing with such matters, you should work with the person in charge of your institution's quality assurance program to see that one is developed. Most hospitals will support you in this effort, because a hospital's governing body is ultimately responsible for any privileges it grants to a doctor, making it responsible, in turn, for a doctor's in-hospital performance. Hospitals that don't take action to correct inadequacies expose themselves to liability.

Finally, *if you've done everything you can within the hospital and nothing happens*, you may have to go outside the hospital—to the county medical society, to the state medical society, or to the state agency responsible for the discipline of medical practitioners.

### The importance of documentation

Whenever you pursue matters such as those discussed here, remember to document all your observations and all your actions. Do this on a quality-assurance report or on some other kind

---

*"By knowing how to take appropriate action when action is needed, you can minimize personal frustrations and feelings of helplessness."*

---

of incident report—one that's signed by you, the charge nurse, and any supervisor you've consulted. The summary should include the date, the time, the patient's case number, a description of the facts, and signatures of any observers. The original report goes to the person in charge of quality assurance in your institution, and copies go to the medical director and to the medical review or medical audit committee. Also, keep copies of all your documentation for your own files.

Even if the problem is resolved early on, you should still document what happened. Your careful documentation may take on crucial importance if the problem recurs.

### Facing up to the challenge

As you know, your discretion about such a situation is required at all times. Don't get angry, hostile, or irritated. Your goal should be to assist, not to antagonize, the doctor or other professional needing help. Don't ever confront the doctor in front of others. Also, avoid criticizing the doctor's professional skills. Your attitude should be one of quiet confidence, based upon nursing standards of practice.

Taking action against problem doctors is never easy. Knowing that you have a professional duty to do so doesn't lessen the burden. You may be ostracized, even threatened, but you mustn't back down. You've made a commitment to standards that you now must defend. If the worst happens—if you're fired or forced to resign—consult an attorney. The law is on your side in this matter, and you stand a good chance of vindication in a court.

### A final word

You help to improve patient care when you know the proper way to handle a serious situation with a problem doctor. By confronting the situation, you contribute to patient safety and community welfare, and you also minimize the risk of liability—the doctor's, the hospital's, and your own. In addition, by knowing how to take appropriate action when action is needed, you can minimize personal frustrations and feelings of helplessness. And finally, you may be helping the doctor to get the assistance he needs.

---

# 89 Office nursing: The doctor as employer

Most nurses have little professional experience with doctors' offices. Nursing students spend little or no time training in them. And only about 1 in 20 nurses ends up working in one. In fact, many nurses don't even know a nurse who works in a doctor's office. So whom do you turn to for answers if you're considering office nursing? This entry will give you the guidance you need.

## Personal and professional qualifications

What does a doctor look for when he's hiring an office nurse? He'll sometimes want a nurse who's been trained in his specialty. This isn't always true, however. If he expects the nurse to perform mostly basic nursing tasks, he'll probably want a nurse with varied—not specialty—experience.

More important than previous experience, however, are the nurse's personal qualities and abilities. Because of the pressures of office nursing, she'll need to be highly organized, able to keep track of several situations at once, able to set priorities for taking action, and flexible enough to do tasks she wouldn't normally do, when necessary.

Some doctors don't want to hire registered nurses for jobs that require doing many basic nursing tasks, yet they require staff with more nursing knowledge than a medical assistant would have. Thus, they frequently hire LPNs/LVNs to fill their office-nursing positions.

## Duties and responsibilities

What does an office nurse usually do? Some state nurse practice acts have addressed this question. According to the Minnesota Nurse Practice Act, for example, an office nurse should "Provide a nursing assessment of actual or potential health needs.... Provide nursing care supportive...of life by functions such as...health teaching, health counseling,...and referral to other health resources. Perform delegated medical functions."

Surveys of practicing office nurses also help to define office nursing. In a recent survey conducted by Solberg and Johnson, office nurses listed the following tasks as those which they perform most frequently: giving injections, handling telephone consultations, placing patients in examining rooms, giving patients health-care instruction, taking health histories, and collecting specimens. Both Kergin and Winter reported similar findings for Canadian office nurses. According to these surveys, less than one third of nurse time was spent on direct patient care. This will probably be true for some time to come. As doctors strive to decrease costs by keeping patients out of the hospital, office nurses will probably perform more and more health monitoring and health-care teaching.

As an office nurse, you may be called on to perform tasks totally new to you, particularly if your background is in hospital nursing. One of the new tasks may be telephone management of patients' medical problems. A nurse can save a doctor hours every week by effectively handling routine telephone consultations.

Another aspect of office nursing that may be new to you is laboratory work, including specimen collection and interpretation of cultures and slides. However, because you learned the theoretical base for these procedures in school, acquiring these new skills should not be difficult. You may need to learn about taking EKGs and X-rays, which also are procedures that you

## DEVELOPING YOUR OWN OFFICE-NURSE JOB DESCRIPTION

Compared to a hospital job, an office job can be very unstructured—you might not even have a written job description. If this is your situation, write your own job description. Start by jotting down what the doctor lists as your nursing duties; then, after you've been on the job a few more months, add any other duties you regularly perform. Present your list to the doctor for his approval.

A typical job description might include the following:

- Prepare patient for doctor's visit by taking history, discussing problem, and taking appropriate vital signs
- complete patient visit by giving immunizations, discussing medications, and ordering laboratory tests and other diagnostic tests as indicated; provide health-risk information and help plan life-style changes as needed, including scheduling follow-up support visits
- assess patient's understanding of care plan and ability to carry it out
- arrange for consultations and referrals to community agencies as indicated, including scheduling outside diagnostic procedures and preparing patient appropriately
- handle patient phone calls, give patients advice concerning self-care, and determine if and when a patient requires the doctor's attention; give out medication refills and test results according to office protocol
- gather and organize patient-education materials—pamphlets, posters, newsletters, reference books—and develop specific materials which the patient can use to practice a procedure
- order supplies and stock examination rooms
- supervise nonprofessional staff, direct patient flow, and handle patient problems
- assist doctor with procedures as needed

should be able to pick up easily.

Most certainly, you'll also be responsible for teaching patients, for community resource referrals, and for counseling. You may need to assist in office procedures, such as inserting intrauterine devices, setting up equipment, preparing patients, instructing patients after procedures, and resterilizing equipment.

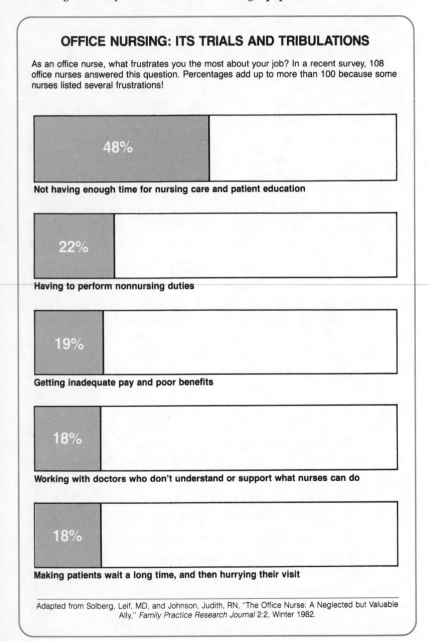

## OFFICE NURSING: ITS TRIALS AND TRIBULATIONS

As an office nurse, what frustrates you the most about your job? In a recent survey, 108 office nurses answered this question. Percentages add up to more than 100 because some nurses listed several frustrations!

**48%**

Not having enough time for nursing care and patient education

**22%**

Having to perform nonnursing duties

**19%**

Getting inadequate pay and poor benefits

**18%**

Working with doctors who don't understand or support what nurses can do

**18%**

Making patients wait a long time, and then hurrying their visit

Adapted from Solberg, Leif, MD, and Johnson, Judith, RN, "The Office Nurse: A Neglected but Valuable Ally," *Family Practice Research Journal* 2:2, Winter 1982.

Nonmedical tasks—such as receptionist duties, bookkeeping, office management, and research—may also be part of your duties.

Finally, you may be expected to do tasks that are neither medical nor office-related—ones that you may feel take advantage of you, such as making coffee or running errands. But if there's a spirit of cooperation in the office, with everyone taking turns, such tasks shouldn't be a problem.

## Benefits of office nursing

Know what benefits are really important to you before you discuss the possibility of joining a doctor's office staff.

• *Hours.* In the Solberg and Johnson study, 50% of the office nurses responding indicated that their primary reason for choosing office nursing was better hours. Working hours for office nurses are probably better than those for hospital nurses, but these hours may not be perfect. Many doctors have office hours in the evenings and on Saturday mornings. Also, your day may not end at the stroke of five. If the patients' problems are more complex than you anticipated, treatment will probably take longer than the time scheduled. Moreover, if the doctor starts his day late—a common complaint among office nurses—he'll probably end it late. In some practices, nurses are expected to teach classes held in the evening. Before you accept a position, you and your employer should agree on what time commitments he expects. If you're salaried rather than paid by the hour, ask about extra compensation.

Another advantage to office practice is that you get holidays off on the day of the holiday. Of course, this means you have no opportunity to log overtime or save up days, as you might be able to do while working in the hospital. You also may not have as many days off as staff nurses do. In addition, ask about time off for vacations and sickness and about leave of absence without pay. Ask about time off for conferences as well: about half of the nurses

surveyed by Solberg and Johnson receive time off and reimbursement for attending conferences.

• *Salary.* Though office nursing hours may be better, you should expect a lower salary and fewer benefits than you'd get for hospital nursing. According to the Solberg and Johnson survey cited earlier, the average salary of an office nurse is about 80% of that of a hospital nurse with comparable experience. In addition, most practices don't pay professional dues or give uniform allowances, but you lose nothing by asking about them. Larger offices may offer their employees profit sharing, year-end bonuses, and pension plans, but none of these benefits is common.

• *Insurance.* One benefit of office nursing that *is* common is free health care in the office; most doctors offer life and health insurance as well.

Professional liability insurance is a different matter. Doctors don't usually

---

*"Working hours for office nurses are probably better than those for hospital nurses, but these hours may not be perfect."*

---

offer it. A doctor's practice will have some "umbrella" coverage, but you should have an individual policy, even if you have to pay for it yourself. This kind of insurance is necessary wherever you work. These policies are relatively inexpensive—about $50 a year for $200,000 liability for each incident. And, of course, the insurance is tax deductible (see Entries 41 and 42).

• *Expanded role.* Professional liability insurance becomes even more important if you take advantage of another of office nursing's benefits: becoming a nurse practitioner. As an office nurse, you may have opportunities to develop

## WORKING IN A DOCTOR'S OFFICE: RESPONSIBILITIES OF ASSOCIATED HEALTH-CARE PROFESSIONALS

| TITLE | EDUCATION | LICENSING/CERTIFICATION |
|---|---|---|
| Medical assistant (MA) | 6 to 12 months, including an office internship | Not licensed; certified nationally by American Association of Medical Assistants (AAMA) |
| Physician's assistant (PA) | 18 months to 5 years | Not licensed; certified nationally by the National Commission on Certification for Physician Assistants; certified in state of practice by state board of medical education and licensure |
| Nurse practitioner (NP) | Nursing degree prerequisite, then 3 months to 2 years additional study | Licensed as RN; usually certified by national specialty organization (some specialties currently do not require certification) |

the special skills of a nurse practitioner through on-the-job training or formal classwork. Depending on your setting, the skills needed, and the doctor's willingness to delegate responsibility, you may develop an expanded role that will enhance your professional standing and improve your patients' care (see Entry 6).

• *Patient teaching.* Here's another work-related benefit: You may find that ambulatory patients are more receptive to health-care information than very sick hospital patients. In an office setting, you'll have the chance to see the patient and become acquainted with him and his family over time. You'll also have a chance to influence health-related behavior. The patient and family may come to regard you as a health-care expert who knows their special needs.

### Getting an office nursing job

Probably the most common way doc-tors find nurses for their offices is by recruiting them in hospitals. If you know of a doctor you'd like to work with, let him know that you're interested. Even if he has no current job openings, he may remember your interest in the future.

If you work in a hospital with a residency program, you're in a position to know the plans of many young doctors who are about to open practices. This is a decided advantage, because you and the doctors already know each other and have a sense of how well you may work together.

Doctors may even use employment agencies to recruit nurses. In such instances, you may have to interview with the agency and then be screened by an office manager before you even get to see the doctor. If you go this route, be sure you know who pays the agency's fee, which can be sizable—15% of your first year's salary, for example. Usually, you'll have to pay it. In some instances,

## RESPONSIBILITIES

- Takes vital signs
- Assists with procedures
- Gives injections
- Collects blood and urine samples
- Performs diagnostic tests, such as electrocardiograms (EKGs)
- Performs laboratory tests, such as complete blood counts
- May also perform nonmedical tasks, such as bookkeeping

- Performs all the responsibilities of a medical assistant
- Performs treatments, such as suturing or applying casts, following preestablished protocols
- Performs physical examinations
- Makes medical diagnoses
- May share on-call duty with doctor

- Performs all of the responsibilities of a registered nurse
- Performs physical examinations
- Makes medical diagnoses
- May share on-call duty with doctor

the employer pays the fee or will split it with you after you've been on the job for a certain length of time.

Some doctors advertise for office nurses. If you respond to such an ad, send along your résumé and get ready for an interview. To help you evaluate a job offer, make a list of questions to ask during the interview (see Entry 59).

Unless the doctor's office where you'll be working is large, you probably won't be given a formal contract to sign. Your employment agreement will be oral. You'll most likely be on probation for your first 3 to 6 months, during which time you may not receive any benefits— such as sick days or health insurance. Usually, you'll get a performance review at the end of the probationary period—or halfway through it—to give you feedback on your performance. You can expect the probationary period and the performance review to be less structured in the office setting than in the hospital setting.

A job description is very important. If the doctor doesn't provide one, jot down what the doctor lists as your duties. You can be sure that he doesn't know them all, though, unless he has a very small practice. He may take tasks such as ordering supplies or restocking rooms for granted. So you may have to write your own job description. (See *Developing Your Own Office-Nurse Job Description,* page 555.)

### A final word

Economics will determine the nurse's future in the doctor's office. The question is: Can someone else besides an RN (medical assistant, LPN/LVN) do the job for less? The answer is yes *if* the job stays the same. But if the nurse's role is expanded to include medical-related tasks, she may become indispensable to a doctor's practice.

Nursing in general is becoming more technical, but the nurse's basic roles as counselor, teacher, and "wellness manager" are also assuming greater importance. No setting offers the nurse more opportunity to develop and refine these roles than office nursing.

# 90 Abandoning the handmaiden image

Nursing was formalized as a profession during the Victorian era—a time of rigidly defined roles for women. The role assigned to the Victorian woman was that of an inferior, submissive creature who was inherently gentle, affectionate, and nurturing. She was physically weaker than men, to whom she looked for guidance and protection and who were, for her, a source of power.

Although the nursing profession has made great strides since then, many nurses are still unwittingly trapped by the Victorian image. Likewise, members of other health professions often expect handmaiden behavior from the nurse. A nurse who deliberately or unknowingly chooses to assume the handmaiden role limits her effectiveness as a professional and compromises her self-respect. For example:

Rita Henry, RN, was seething. "If Dr. Steed really is one of the hospital's finest doctors," she said, "then why isn't he attending to his patients?" She'd paged Dr. Steed three times in the past hour; he hadn't responded. One of his postoperative patients had developed a fever. And Dr. Steed hadn't left a medication order.

As Rita Henry waited by the phone, other nurses nervously joked about her impending confrontation with Dr. Steed. He had an explosive temper and was demeaning to nurses who tried to match fire with fire.

"I hope we're not scraping you off the ceiling in 5 minutes," one staff member warned. "Just remember, Dr. Steed thinks all nurses are handmaidens!"

But Rita was tired of being careful, self-effacing, and apologetic every time she had to approach Dr. Steed and some of the other doctors. Today, she knew she had no reason to apologize: the patient needed medication that couldn't be given without Dr. Steed's order. And the sooner he gave it, the better. Still, an apprehensiveness crept over her as she waited for his call.

Like most nurses, Rita had been socialized—in school and on the job—to the idea that being self-effacing was the best way to avoid conflict with doctors. To be the ideal nurse was to be cool, efficient, and conciliatory. Experience had taught Rita to be passive and indirect with doctors. "Just remember," one veteran nurse said, "the idea is to let him think it was his idea to see the patient. That's what the smart nurse does!"

## Role conflict: "ideal" vs. "real"

As you probably know, "ideal nurse" behavior results in almost trouble-free relationships. Why? Because if both you and the doctor see your role as that

## SQUELCHING THOSE STEREOTYPES

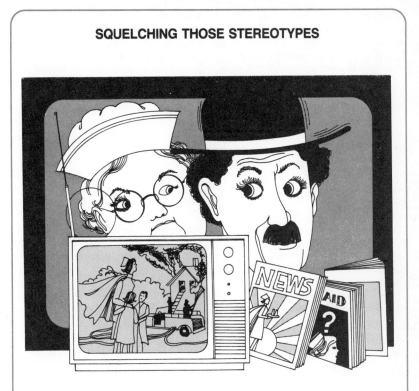

Nursing has come a long way in the last 100 years, but you wouldn't know it from the image the public still has of nurses. The women's movement notwithstanding, nurses are still plagued by stereotypes. As a group, nurses are perhaps the most maligned and misunderstood professionals.

The media, in particular, foster the handmaiden image—and other, worse, images. Nurses have been stereotyped on TV and in movies and magazines as temperature-takers, bedpan-carriers, doctor-chasers, airheads, and sexpots. Or, for a change of pace, they've been portrayed as motherly, self-sacrificing souls whose job (*not* profession) is "a good one for a woman."

What can you do to improve nursing's image in the media? Well, some nurses' groups have already organized media-watch committees. These groups include the American Nurses' Association, the National League for Nursing, the American Academy of Nursing, the American Association of Critical Care Nurses, and some local and district organizations. You can contact these groups for more information, or you can form your own media-watch group. Your group can write letters of protest (or praise) to television and movie producers, magazine editors, and advertisers. You can also send editorials to your local newspapers and picket theaters that show offensive movies. And you can work to promote a positive image of nursing by asking media representatives to attend nursing conferences, by offering your services as a consultant to local radio or television shows that cover health-related topics, or by contacting your local paper and asking if you might write a regular health column.

You're probably thinking this sounds like a lot of work. Of course, it is. You're also probably thinking, "Why should anyone from the media listen to me?" But they *will* listen, maybe not to one voice, but to many. After all, the women's movement may not have been around for long, but it's now a voice to be reckoned with. To effect change, nurses need a strong voice, too.

of a helpmate less important and less powerful than the doctor, he'll simply dictate orders, and you'll follow them. When you *must* question orders or treatment plans, you'll do so delicately. When he loses his temper, you'll understand and ask yourself what you could have done to ease his load. You'll never show anger toward him. If you did, he and other nurses would label you a malcontent or even question your rationality. By following this behavior, you do indeed make the doctor the leader, and yourself his dedicated helpmate.

Most doctor-nurse relationships take this form to one degree or another, but it certainly isn't the only form—or the best. For example, you'll also have minimal communication problems when you and a doctor view each other as professional colleagues. As in the "ideal nurse" relationship, you share the same

---

> *"Communication problems have to be solved by persistent individual efforts in real-world situations."*

---

viewpoints—but the nature of a problem determines who should lead. If the problem is nursing-related, your expertise will prevail; if medical, his will prevail.

Disagreements in such a relationship will usually occur over issues, not personalities, and neither of you will be afraid to ask the other for clarification. Since openness and negotiation are natural components of such a relationship, compromise is probable.

### When sparks fly
Problems develop in nurse-doctor relationships when the nurse and doctor have different views of their roles. Although conflict is the usual outcome of such differing viewpoints, it can set the stage for interpersonal and individual growth. Nurse Rita Henry and Dr. Steed are examples. As the nurse's confidence in her own professional capabilities grew, she decided she'd no longer apologize for being "only a nurse." Gradually, she was beginning to see herself as equal to other professionals, including doctors. Unfortunately, Dr. Steed had continued to think of her as a handmaiden.

Imagine yourself in Rita's place, standing by the phone, when Dr. Steed finally walks onto the unit. You're angry that he hasn't answered the page, but you put that behind you. You call to him as he walks by, but he doesn't stop. His behavior humiliates you because you know the other nurses on the unit are watching. Still you persist. Keeping your voice even, you call to him again. He stops, turns, and approaches you. "You called me?" he asks.

"Yes, doctor," you reply firmly. You look right at him—with confidence, not hostility—as you continue. "I need to talk to you about Mrs. Jones—." Before you can finish, he interrupts, remarking condescendingly, "Oh, you do?"

At this point you might be tempted to answer with some sarcasm of your own. This isn't the first time he's derided your professionalism, and you've been holding back your anger for months.

Still, if you're smart, you'll keep on holding back. An angry retort *would* momentarily relieve your frustration, but it would also elicit another negative remark from the doctor—and only compound the problem.

What you want to do is to foster a collegial relationship. You know that in such a relationship, disagreements center around issues, not personalities, so you focus on the issue at hand and reply evenly, "Mrs. Jones has an elevated temperature, 102.6°." You go on to explain her condition.

He listens, at first impassively and then intently. What you've said has surprised him. He wants to see Mrs. Jones.

You accompany him to her room. After examining her, he writes new medication orders on her chart. Before leaving the unit, he asks you to notify him immediately if her condition changes. You assure him you will.

The minute the elevator doors close, the rest of the staff expresses amazement that Dr. Steed has come and gone without a scene, and you sigh with relief. You have a right to be pleased with the exchange: you recognized that your task was not to become Dr. Steed's friend, not to change his personality, not to change his attitude toward nurses. Your task was to inform him of the patient's condition, and you did so. Although you didn't try to "manage" Dr. Steed, your successful *self*-management did bring about a minor change in *his* behavior. He never did live up to his bad reputation. Why? Because *you* didn't live up to his image of you as the fearful handmaiden.

### Self-respect works

You may think such a small personal exchange doesn't matter. ("The rest of the doctors in the world will still demean nurses anyway.") Many nurses have these feelings, and they choose to fight the handmaiden role in much larger forums. They work with inter-disciplinary committees and try to change hospital policies. Such formalized groups of nurses and doctors may prove helpful in a general way by clarifying roles and functions. But they're only remotely helpful in day-to-day situations like the one Rita Henry faced. After all, communication problems are grass-roots problems; they have to be solved by persistent individual efforts in real-world situations.

Imagine, for example, how a committee would have handled Ms. Henry's situation. Suppose she'd called the supervisor and had written out an incident report, claiming Dr. Steed's unanswered page was symbolic of his contempt for nurses. Then what? Her complaint might eventually have been reviewed by the Ad Hoc Committee on

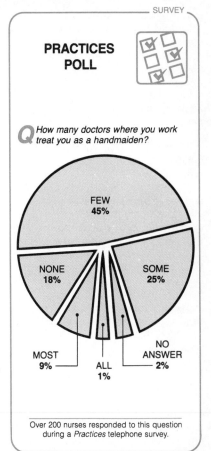

SURVEY

## PRACTICES POLL

**Q** *How many doctors where you work treat you as a handmaiden?*

FEW 45%

NONE 18%

SOME 25%

MOST 9%

ALL 1%

NO ANSWER 2%

Over 200 nurses responded to this question during a *Practices* telephone survey.

Nurse-Doctor Friction. She might eventually have received their conclusion that Dr. Steed should have answered his page. In the meantime, their relationship would have deteriorated. Instead, she focused on the issue at hand and approached the doctor individually. The result: A needed medication order and a small step toward an effective working relationship.

### Step-by-step guide to abandoning the handmaiden image

If you agree that relationships have to be hammered out, one-on-one, you'll find the following guidelines helpful for restructuring your relationships with doctors and improving the quality of your communication.

• *Establish your position.* The way you represent nursing to a doctor is the way he'll perceive it. If you cower when he gives an order, he'll continue to see you—and the nursing profession—as subordinate. When you're giving patient care and a doctor walks into the patient's room and asks you to get a chart from the desk, try answering, "I can't stop what I'm doing right now, but the chart is in the rack. Please help yourself."

This message carries several important implications for the doctor. First, it lets him know that patient care takes priority. Second, it demonstrates that you're independent of doctor control and able to refuse requests. Third, it gives him permission to get the chart from territory he may perceive as yours.

• *Respect yourself.* Expecting courtesy and equity in interpersonal exchanges almost guarantees them. Even in the heyday of handmaiden relationships, certain nurses in every organization commanded respect from doctors, who wouldn't have considered approaching them in less than a professional manner.

What was those nurses' secret? Their high regard for their profession and themselves gave them more than self-confidence—it gave them a presence that demanded respect. The handmaiden has to deny both her professionalism and her feelings. When a person does this to herself, it's easy for others to treat her similarly.

• *Know your rights.* Read your job description and be familiar with the rights inherent in your role. By knowing your rights, you can elicit support from others when you're in conflict with a doctor. If a doctor persists in demanding that you do something outside the realm of your duties, delay acting until you can consult with your supervisor or a knowledgeable peer. Most important, don't be intimidated into acting until you fully understand your options.

• *Evaluate requests and directives be-fore responding.* Some nurses treat every issue raised and every request made by a doctor as if it deserved an immediate response. They respond automatically to the doctor's presence before he even makes a request. How many times has a nurse given up a chart to a doctor before completing her notes—even before the doctor asked for it? This happens because some nurses assume a doctor's time is more valuable than their own.

The solution is to evaluate the urgency of each request. If you believe the doctor's needs deserve prompt attention, proceed immediately; but evaluation will show that doctors, like the rest of us, *can* usually wait for what they need. If your task seems more urgent than the doctor's request, let him know you'll handle his request as soon as possible and get back to him.

• *Relax and be yourself.* This is probably the simplest and yet the most important guideline for improving the quality of your professional relationships. Many nurses become extremely anxious when dealing with some doctors, and their anxiety is like negative energy that disrupts the balance of power in the relationship, giving the doctor the upper hand.

If you're anxiety-prone with doctors, explore some relaxation techniques like deep breathing or muscle relaxation. Treat yourself to a personal growth experience like assertiveness training that will help you to use specific communication techniques in difficult interpersonal situations.

Finally, be yourself, not that stereotyped image of the ideal nurse that you've been trying to live up to since graduating from nursing school. The ideal nurse is a myth in the minds of nurses and doctors alike. The modern nurse is one who lives up to her nursing potential, regardless of circumstances, situations, or people. The more self-accepting you are, the freer you'll be to recognize your worth and to communicate with anyone, even a Dr. Steed, as just another health-team member.

## A final word

Relinquishing the handmaiden role may feel alien at first. It may even create new skirmishes for you with doctors and other health professionals. But think of the benefits you'll receive. Remember that a self-assured nurse who can question an order or request and comfortably say "no" is preserving her-self—personally, professionally, and legally. Furthermore, her behavior will encourage other health-care professionals to demonstrate self-respect and professional confidence. A handmaiden can never be a colleague. In contrast, collegial relationships benefit everyone, including, and most important, the patient.

## Selected References

American Nurses' Association. *Nursing: A Social Policy Statement.* Kansas City, Mo.: American Nurses' Association, 1980.

American Nurses' Association. "A Statement on the Scope of Maternal and Child Health Nursing Practice," *Texas Nursing* 54:11, September 1980.

Christman, L., and Kirkman, R.E. "Nurse-Physician Communications in the Hospital," *Nursing Digest* 6:64-70, Summer 1978.

Donnelly, G.F. "RN's Assertiveness Workbook: How to Soothe a Savage Surgeon (Without Making A Doormat of Yourself or Blowing a Fuse)," Part 1. *RN* 41:45-47, November 1978.

Feinstein, Alvan R. *Clinical Judgment.* Melbourne, Fla.: Robert E. Krieger Publishing Co., 1974.

Friedman, F.B. "The 'Joy' of Telling a Physician He's Wrong," *RN* 45:34-37, April 1982.

Halas, Celia, and Matteson, Roberta. *"I've Done So Well—Why Do I Feel So Bad?" (Conflicts in the Female Experience and What Women Can Do About Them).* New York: Macmillan Publishing Co., 1978.

Hardy, Margaret E., and Conway, Mary, eds. *Role Theory: Perspectives for Health Professionals.* East Norwalk, Conn.: Appleton-Century-Crofts, 1978.

Huttmann, Barbara. *The Patient's Advocate: the Complete Handbook of Patients' Rights—How to Get Them and How to Use Them to Save Your Time, Your Money, and Your Life.* New York: Viking Press, 1981.

Kergin, D.J., et al. *A Study of Nurse Activities in Primary Care Settings.* Hamilton, Ontario: McMasters University School of Nursing, 1972.

Maas, M., and Jacox, A.K. *Guidelines for Nurse Action and Patient Welfare.* East Norwalk, Conn.: Appleton-Century-Crofts, 1977.

Mechanic, D., and Aiken, L. "A Co-Operative Agenda for Medicine and Nursing," *New England Journal of Medicine* 307(12):747-51, 1982.

Moses, E., and Roth, A. "Nursepower: What Do Statistics Reveal About the Nation's Nurses?" *American Journal of Nursing* 79:1745-56, October 1979.

National League for Nursing. "Nursing's Role in Patients' Rights," *Nursing Outlook* 25:725, November 1977.

"Opinion Exchange: Is It Better to Know the Worst?" *RN* 45(3):49, March 1982.

Regan, William A. "How to Cover Yourself When the MD's Wrong," *RN* 44:79-80, June 1981.

Sheard, T. "The Structure of Conflict in Nurse-Physician Relations," *Supervisor Nurse* 11:14-15, August 1980.

Solberg, L.I., and Johnson, J.M. *Physician and Nurse: A Manual for Collaboration.* Minneapolis: University of Minnesota Press, 1981.

Winter, S.J., and Last, J.M. "Registered Nurses in Office Practice...Canada," *Canadian Nurse* 70:18-20, November 1974.

# Working with Other Professionals

## Introduction

No one works in a vacuum. Each of us, regardless of profession or occupation, interacts with others in some way. Today, this is especially true for nurses. Because of the increased specialization among health-care personnel in general, and among nurses in particular, you communicate frequently with other professionals and nonprofessionals who contribute to patient care. You provide them with vital information about the patient and obtain equally vital patient information from them. If problems arise during the patient's care, you collaborate with them to arrive at solutions. Because the quality of the care your patient receives depends to a great extent on how you interact with other health personnel, your ability to work cooperatively with them is as important a challenge as any that you face in nursing. Consider the following scenario.

Mrs. Camilla Jones, age 43, is admitted to your medical-surgical unit for diagnostic studies to determine the nature of her illness. As she arrives on the unit, she complains of weakness that appears to be of muscular origin. Her doctor orders X-rays, blood work, and a special diet to prepare Mrs. Jones for gastric studies.

Within minutes you've contacted numerous health-care professionals within the hospital who will contribute their special skills to Mrs. Jones' care: the radiologist and his technicians, the pathologist and his assistants, the therapeutic dietitian and his aides, the gastroenterologist, and the physical therapist. In addition, you've assessed the patient's immediate needs for direct nursing care. The situation sounds chaotic, but it isn't—you've successfully coordinated all the independent efforts, including your own nursing assessment and intervention, that will culminate in a diagnosis and treatment plan for Mrs. Jones.

This scenario clearly indicates that you're an interdependent health-care professional who must maintain a close and cooperative working relationship with other health professionals. Unfortunately, conflict can disrupt the harmony of that working relationship. When it does, you need to act quickly to restore harmony and to ensure your patients' and your own physical and emotional well-being.

### You've come a long way

Nurses weren't always recognized as significant contributors to patient care. Before the 1960s, nurses weren't permitted to provide a good deal of patient care without doctors' orders. But several events occurred that changed the health-care community's view of nurses.

# HOW DO YOU COME ACROSS?

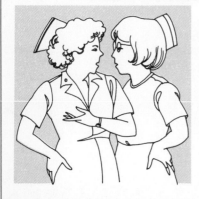

Imagine you're a head nurse in a medical-surgical unit. One of the nurses you supervise hasn't been doing her share of the work lately. The other nurses blame you, and you're getting angry. You've talked with the nurse, but she doesn't seem to understand. Think about how you interact with her. Which of the following behavior types do you use when you deal with her: assertive, aggressive, or passive? Perhaps a change in how you behave toward her will improve communications between you.

| TYPE | CHARACTERISTICS | EXAMPLE | OUTCOME |
|---|---|---|---|
| **Assertive** | • Express your wants, needs, feelings<br>• Stand up for your rights without violating another person's<br>• Do not insult, put down, or attribute motivation to other person<br>• Maintain an "I'm okay, you're okay" attitude<br>• Try to understand other person<br>• Try to get information<br>• Do not apologize for self | • "I'm disappointed that you're not doing your share of the work on the unit, and I'm not comfortable with the position you've put me in. I'd like to talk with you about your performance. I want to understand why you're not completing your work. Then we can come up with a plan you can follow to correct the situation." | • Other person will know how her behavior is affecting you.<br>• Other person understands consequences of her behavior.<br>• Other person will explain her point of view, needs, objectives.<br>• Problem solving is possible.<br>• Mutual good feelings are established and maintained. |
| **Aggressive** | • Attack, insult, put down other person<br>• Patronize<br>• Show contempt<br>• Attribute motivation<br>• Maintain a "you're not okay" attitude | • "You obviously don't care at all about me or the unit. You're one of those people who'll take a free ride whenever they get the chance." | • Other person feels hurt, defensive or fearful.<br>• Other person attacks or withdraws.<br>• Mutual problem solving is impossible. |
| **Passive** | • Don't stand up for your rights<br>• Put yourself down<br>• Apologize inappropriately<br>• Take blame but don't believe it<br>• Maintain an "I'm not okay" attitude | • "I don't understand why you're not finished with your work. I probably wasn't clear about your responsibilities. Maybe I should have been more available to answer your questions." | • Other person feels guilty or loses respect for you.<br>• Other person feels manipulated.<br>• Open communications and problem solving are extremely unlikely. |

Adapted with permission from Pamela Cuming, *The Power Handbook*, CBI Publishing Co., Inc., 1981.

To begin with, in the 1960s an acute doctor shortage occurred. To alleviate problems caused by the shortage, the role of nurse practitioner was developed. (See Entry 6.) This nurse specialist was educated to assess patients' physical and emotional needs—independent functions previously reserved for doctors.

At the same time, the nursing profession was promoting nursing research to define elements of care specific to nursing. The research resulted in the formulation of a number of nursing theories that, for the first time in the history of nursing, were recognized as the basis of nursing practice.

Influenced by the expanded role of the nurse practitioner and supported by a firmly laid foundation in nursing theory, nurses began to think and act independently and with increasing confidence. As their confidence grew, they contributed increasingly to the patient-care decision-making process. Today, nurses who were once considered totally dependent practitioners are recognized as interdependent professionals—willing and able to initiate appropriate nursing interventions and to collaborate with other professionals on an equal footing (see Entry 110).

## Interacting effectively

Because your professional philosophy and approach to nursing care, as well as your personal values and attitudes, may differ from those of other professionals, your views are likely to come in conflict with colleagues' from time to time. To help you deal with this side of nursing practice, this chapter will give you advice on how to work effectively with other professionals and how to successfully resolve any conflicts that may arise.

Effective communication is the basis of all productive relationships. Entry 91, "Communicating effectively," tells you how to communicate your patient-care goals to other professionals. You'll learn how to listen attentively and how to respond clearly and concisely. You'll also learn about the importance of nonverbal communication.

When conflicts do occur, you need to know how to deal with them quickly and effectively. Entry 92, "Conflict on the unit—what causes it?", discusses different types of conflict and why they occur, and suggests various techniques for dealing with them. It also tells you how to safeguard yourself from the negative effects of conflict.

For advice on smoothing feathers ruffled by professional clashes, read Entry 93, "Defusing personal conflict." It tells you how to deal with the usual causes of personal conflicts—differing feelings, ideas, or beliefs.

Entry 94, "Working with nonnursing personnel," discusses how your patients, and the hospital staff in general, can benefit from a sound working relationship between nursing and nonnursing personnel. It also explores the common causes of these conflicts and the best ways to resolve them.

As you become more aware of your interaction with other health-care professionals, you'll gain insight into your attitudes about yourself, your profession, and your colleagues—and your working relationships will improve.

# 91 Communicating effectively

Everyone knows how to communicate—on one level or another. The problem is, not everyone communicates effectively. Because you're a health-care professional working with others to care for patients, your ability to communicate effectively is crucial.

## Planning your communication

The first step in communicating effectively is to know exactly what you want to communicate. If, for example, you're trying to tell a nurse's aide what you expect of her, make sure your expectation is clear in your own mind. This will make planning your communication easier.

Planning how to communicate your message (encoding it) consists of assessing and dealing with your feelings about the message and choosing the words you'll use. First, think about your feelings regarding the message you want to communicate. For example, if you have experience teaching diabetic patients, you'll probably feel comfortable doing so. But if you're teaching a diabetic patient for the first time, you'll probably be anxious or uncertain.

After you've identified your feelings, determine whether they'll affect your communication. If you think they will but don't do anything about it, your message may be unclear or misinterpreted. Instead, try to change the situation before communicating your message. If you're anxious or uncertain, build your confidence by role playing. If you're frustrated or angry, consider talking with the person another time.

Next, consider your choice of words. You want to tailor them to your listener. Begin by considering his mood. If he's anxious or angry, you should use sim-ple words and sentences, speak slowly and clearly, and repeat your message several times.

Also, consider the person's physical state. If you're like most nurses, you probably do this with a patient who's in pain. But you may not do it when dealing with a co-worker who, for example, has a headache. Remember, physical discomfort will affect the way a person listens.

In addition, when weighing your choice of words, think about your listener's ethnic and geographic background. Depending on the culture he's part of and what part of the country (or the world) he comes from, different words and phrases may mean different things.

### Getting your message across

How well you communicate your message will depend on these factors:
- timing
- location
- verbal and nonverbal signals
- active listening.

- *Timing.* Timing influences how effectively you transmit your message. You'll find no better rule than common sense to guide you in determining when you should try to communicate with another person. Your timing will depend on that person's schedule and mood and on the nature of your message. If your goal, however, is to correct a colleague's inappropriate actions, you should talk with that colleague as soon as possible.

- *Location.* Privacy always makes open and honest communication easier. But, as you know, privacy is a scarce commodity in a hospital. Try to choose a place where noise and distractions won't disrupt your conversation. If, for example, you're going to broach a difficult subject with your charge nurse, invite her to a conference room or to the cafeteria.

- *Verbal and nonverbal signals.* Make sure you use appropriate verbal and nonverbal signals when communicating your message. Your tone of voice

GLOSSARY

## KEY TERMS IN THIS ENTRY

**communication barriers** • Any factors—such as noise, language differences, or emotional preoccupations—that interfere with messages transmitted from one person to another.

**decoding** • Deciphering and understanding another person's verbal or nonverbal message.

**encoding** • Preparing a verbal message—identifying the content of the message, including emotional content, and planning how to articulate it—before transmitting that message to another person.

**transmission** • Verbal or nonverbal communication with another person.

## YOU CAN IMPROVE YOUR COMMUNICATION SKILLS

Communication is an important key to working successfully with other people. You're probably not aware of your communication habits and aren't sure whether you're a good communicator. Here are some ways to analyze—and improve—your communication skills:

For 1 day, keep a chart recording every conversation you have. Ask yourself if you've primarily been a listener or a talker. Make a note of which role you *should* have taken in each conversation. This practice will make you conscious of your proper role in future conversations.

Before an interview or meeting, write down what you expect to come out of it. Afterward, decide if your expectations were accurate or realistic. What did or didn't you do to fulfill them? Did others seem to have different expectations? What could you have done to resolve the differences?

After the next meeting you attend, jot down what you think the major points were. Ask three people who attended the meeting to tell you what they thought the major points were. If you get differing responses, try to understand what caused those differences.

Start a discussion with someone. Try to win the other person over to your point of view. If you succeed in winning her over to your side, ask her what you did or said that was convincing.

should always be consistent with your intent. If you're not punishing the person, don't use a punishing tone. Communicate the same message nonverbally that you're communicating verbally. For example, when you ask, "Do you have any questions?", don't immediately look away and pick up papers on your desk. This nonverbal signal says, "Don't ask any questions; I'm too busy."

Use assertive techniques, such as the "I" statement, to help communicate your message. Try speaking to your charge nurse, for example, in this manner: "I was upset when I didn't get the day off that I requested. Can you tell me why I didn't get it?" Remember, assertiveness, based on respect for yourself and for the other person, differs from aggressiveness. A give-and-take attitude demonstrates a willingness to compromise and problem-solve (see Entry 69).

Finally, maintain good eye contact when talking to another person. To facilitate this, sit if she's sitting, stand if she's standing. Also, use touch when appropriate.

• *Active listening.* You can further aid communication by using active listening techniques (see Entry 76). Work to develop your ability to listen and to assess whether the other person received your message. Many communications experts feel that active listening is the most crucial factor in communicating effectively.

## AVOIDING OR OVERCOMING BARRIERS TO COMMUNICATION

To succeed in your relationships with your co-workers, you need effective communication skills. During your life, you've probably learned some lessons that have actually *discouraged* communication. As a child, for example, you may have been punished for "talking back." As an adult now, you may be conditioned to shut off your feelings when you talk to someone, building barriers to communication. At work, this can result

| BARRIERS TO COMMUNICATION | HOW THEY RESULT IN MISCOMMUNICATION |
|---|---|
| Being fearful | If you're not honest about your feelings, (because they may reveal what you perceive as inadequacies), you may lie about your feelings to project the proper image. |
| Not listening | The person who wants to tell you something will not get through to you if you're thinking about something else while she's talking. |
| Being defensive | Instead of listening, you may be thinking of ways you can enhance your image, escape punishment, dominate, or win. |
| Suppressing feelings | Refusing to recognize your own feelings during a conversation prevents you from taking proper action in the situation. |
| Not giving feedback | Refusing to communicate your reaction to what someone is saying to you increases the chances of misunderstanding. |
| Giving advice | Telling someone what you think she should do makes her defensive, reduces her self-esteem. |
| Being excessively repetitive | Repetition lulls the person into not listening because she's heard it before. |
| Being distracted | Being concerned with other things prevents you from listening effectively, making you miss or misunderstand the other person's message. |
| Using inappropriate language | Using words unfamiliar or offensive to the other person prevents her from understanding (sometimes from accepting) your message. |

in frequent misunderstandings, poor morale, and low productivity. Here are some common barriers to communication and some tips for avoiding or overcoming them.

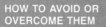

### HOW TO AVOID OR OVERCOME THEM

Think of someone you're afraid to be honest with and say to her, "I have trouble telling you what I really feel and think about this matter." She'll probably be just as relieved as you are to talk about it.

Use active listening: concentrate on the speaker's words and restate them to be sure you heard them correctly. This clarifies communication and shows the speaker that you understand her feelings.

Recognize the kind of behavior that makes you defensive. When someone displays that behavior, tell her you're uncomfortable with her message as you're hearing it

Learn to analyze your feelings during a conversation, and then to communicate them, such as, "I'm feeling annoyed... happy...afraid."

Offer feedback in a supportive way. Also, provide feedback as soon as possible after the conversation, so both of you can remember details. Confine your feedback to your own feelings: don't try telling her how she feels.

Practice active listening; give the person your time, not your advice or opinions.

Listen to yourself. Say what you want to say once, as clearly as possible, and ask for a specific response.

Concentrate on using active listening techniques. If you can't concentrate, interrupt to deal with the distraction.

Choose your words carefully and thoughtfully, being aware of the situation you're in and the person you're talking to.

## Understanding the message

A person's values, preconceptions, and assumptions usually will influence the way he understands (decodes) a message. Similarly, when you receive a message, your own values, preconceptions, and assumptions will influence what you hear.

For instance, a colleague's conflicting values may affect her ability to understand your reservations about caring for an alcoholic patient. Or your assumption that you understand your colleague may make you interrupt or stop listening to her. How often have you thought or said, "Oh, sure, I know what you mean," only to find out later that you didn't?

To understand a message correctly, you should do two things. First, clarify the message by asking questions. This can be time-consuming, but if you have any doubts about the message, do it. Second, resist the natural inclination to let your values, preconceptions, and assumptions overinfluence the way you interpret the message.

## Evaluating and improving

How can you evaluate the effectiveness of your communication? Here's a list of questions that should help:
• What is the nonverbal response of the person you're talking to? Does she seem restless or look away?
• Do people frequently interrupt you, finish your sentences, or ask questions that seem off track?
• Do people *seem* to understand you—until their actions prove that they don't? If you answered yes to any of these questions, you may not be communicating as effectively as you should.

To make your communication more effective, first identify any obvious communication barriers (see *Avoiding or Overcoming Barriers to Communication*) and then practice the appropriate communication skills (see Entry 76). Here are some ways you can practice them:
• Write down what you want to say, so you can analyze whether your message

is accurately stated.
- Use a tape recorder, so you can hear how you communicate your message.
- Use a mirror, so you can see the non-verbal messages you send.
- Role-play with a colleague, so you can practice your message and evaluate how it comes across.
- Attend a communication workshop that uses some of these techniques.

### A final word

As you can see, communicating effectively isn't simple. It requires skill and practice. Fortunately, as a nurse, you already possess most of the skills you need. You know how to set goals and formulate plans to achieve them. And you're already a trained listener and observer. So your keys to more effective communication are practice and ongoing evaluation of your success as a communicator. Remember, the more you exercise these skills, the more effectively you'll communicate.

# 92 Conflict in the unit—what causes it?

As a nurse, you work in a fast-paced and demanding environment that allows little or no margin for error. You're expected to function at peak efficiency at all times and to work cooperatively with all the people you come in contact with—patients and health-care personnel—each with his own attitudes and philosophies about health care. Together with the pressures inherent in nursing, these elements make your unit a potential hotbed for conflict.

If conflicts materialize, they can affect your physical and emotional well-being. You may find yourself going to work each day with a knot in your stomach, wishing to escape once you've arrived, suffering from frequent headaches, and seriously doubting that you made the right career choice. If the conflicts continue, they may even adversely affect the quality of your nursing care.

Conflicts are inevitable, and resolving them isn't always easy. But with the right kind of knowledge and skills, you can learn to cope with any conflicts that arise. To resolve long-standing problems on your unit and to handle future conflicts quickly and effectively, learn what causes conflicts and acquire techniques for managing them effectively. Equipped with this knowledge and what you already know about problem solving, you'll be able to turn potential losses from conflicts into real gains for yourself, your patients, and your unit.

### Understanding conflict

Are you aware that conflict can be the best medicine for the problems on your unit? It can help solve problems if it's *constructive conflict,* the kind that helps you exchange productive ideas with co-workers and eventually achieve goals for your unit. What you want to avoid is *destructive conflict,* the kind that impedes communication, creates job dissatisfaction, and prevents you from reaching your professional goals. By understanding the nature of conflict, you can help make conflicts constructive when they happen in your unit.

Many factors can cause conflict among staff members on a particular nursing unit. These factors include:
- *differing goals.* For example, if one nurse places her professional advancement ahead of every other concern, she'll be in conflict with other staff members.
- *differing ways to meet a mutual goal.* The goal of all staff is to give high quality care; but if some staff members, for example, think primary nursing is the best way to achieve that goal while others think team nursing is best, then the two groups will be in conflict.
- *differing values.* If one staff member, for example, feels strongly that she can't care for a patient having an abortion but other staff members feel supportive of that patient, they may come in conflict.

# TECHNIQUES FOR RESOLVING CONFLICTS

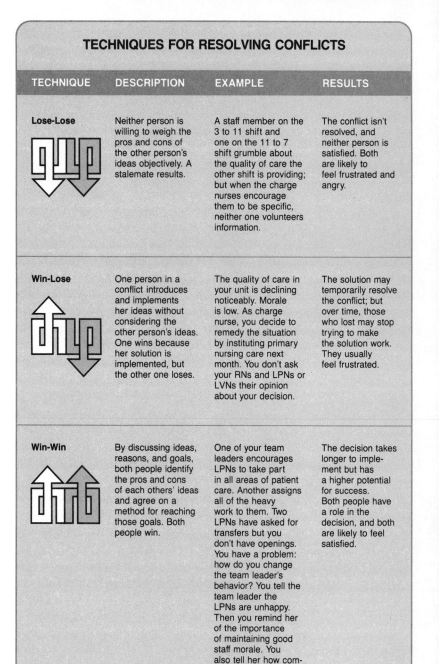

| TECHNIQUE | DESCRIPTION | EXAMPLE | RESULTS |
|---|---|---|---|
| **Lose-Lose** | Neither person is willing to weigh the pros and cons of the other person's ideas objectively. A stalemate results. | A staff member on the 3 to 11 shift and one on the 11 to 7 shift grumble about the quality of care the other shift is providing; but when the charge nurses encourage them to be specific, neither one volunteers information. | The conflict isn't resolved, and neither person is satisfied. Both are likely to feel frustrated and angry. |
| **Win-Lose** | One person in a conflict introduces and implements her ideas without considering the other person's ideas. One wins because her solution is implemented, but the other one loses. | The quality of care in your unit is declining noticeably. Morale is low. As charge nurse, you decide to remedy the situation by instituting primary nursing care next month. You don't ask your RNs and LPNs or LVNs their opinion about your decision. | The solution may temporarily resolve the conflict; but over time, those who lost may stop trying to make the solution work. They usually feel frustrated. |
| **Win-Win** | By discussing ideas, reasons, and goals, both people identify the pros and cons of each others' ideas and agree on a method for reaching those goals. Both people win. | One of your team leaders encourages LPNs to take part in all areas of patient care. Another assigns all of the heavy work to them. Two LPNs have asked for transfers but you don't have openings. You have a problem: how do you change the team leader's behavior? You tell the team leader the LPNs are unhappy. Then you remind her of the importance of maintaining good staff morale. You also tell her how competent you think she is, and you invite her to help resolve the problem. | The decision takes longer to implement but has a higher potential for success. Both people have a role in the decision, and both are likely to feel satisfied. |

• *lack of information.* Some older staff members, for example, may not know how to perform a procedure that the newer nurse graduates were taught in school. Because of this, a conflict may result.

• *personality clash.* If one staff member insists that all staff members include every detail in daily patient reports, while others want to include only the unusual events, they'll come in conflict.

• *overlapping roles.* When staff members on two consecutive shifts are confused about which shift is responsible for gathering admission data on patients who are admitted as shifts are changing, conflict may result.

If one of these conflict situations occurs on your unit, you'll have to act quickly to make sure its outcome's constructive. Confront the persons who're involved in the conflict with your concerns and with your ideas for resolving it. Or tell your head nurse or nursing supervisor what the problem is and what you think should be done about it.

How can you determine whether conflict is being managed constructively on your unit? Look for these indications:

## KEY TERMS IN THIS ENTRY

**conflict management** • Directing and using disagreement creatively so its outcome is constructive, rather than destructive.

**constructive conflict** • A disagreement over such things as goals, methods, or values that stimulates problem solving and is eventually resolved to everyone's satisfaction.

**destructive conflict** • A disagreement over such things as goals, methods, or values that disrupts routine, is counterproductive, and ends in misunderstanding and mutual unhappiness.

• Staff members are generally energetic and enthusiastic, and work well together.
• They openly discuss alternatives and solve problems creatively.
• They state disagreements directly and work through them quickly, without interfering with patient care.

If you don't act quickly and effectively to resolve conflict, it may become destructive. When this happens, indications of poor conflict management will surface quickly. These indications include:
• Staff members are generally irritable and snappish.
• They adopt an "It'll never change" attitude.
• They form cliques.
• They're unwilling to compromise.
• They make few decisions at staff meetings, and not all of the decisions made are implemented.

Destructive conflict can also occur if several conflicting factors surface all at once or in quick succession. When this happens, you must intervene immediately or you'll soon start to notice the signs of too much conflict:
• Staff turnover increases.
• Staff illness and absenteeism increase.
• Staff sentiment is, "We need more meetings to keep up with things, but we don't have the time."
• Staff members compromise and problem-solve but still feel overwhelmed.

Surprisingly enough, nursing units can also suffer from too little conflict. This is often the case on units that have had the same head nurse and a stable nursing staff for several years. The nursing administration places few new expectations on the staff members. They, in turn, become complacent and introduce few new ideas for improving nursing care. On units where conflict is lacking, you'll notice the following:
• Staff members are apathetic.
• Staff members feel that they're in a rut.
• Staff meetings are infrequent, slow-

## TAKING THE REINS

*I'm a new head nurse with three major problems: three staff nurses who have been on the unit for 2 or 3 years.*
*They constantly challenge my authority and undermine my leadership. Last week, for example, I gave one of our aides specific directions on handling an ambulatory patient who refused to get out of bed. Later, I overheard one of the staff nurses saying to the aide, "That's not what I would've told you to do." I'm threatened by their intrusion, but I don't think confronting them is the way to handle the problem.—RN, Ohio*

You're right. A confrontation would force your other staff members to take sides, and you'd probably be the loser. Your first step is to confront your own fears.

Realize that your arrival threatened staff members who are anxious to have everything back to normal. They'd rally behind old leaders in a minute to make things seem normal again—but not because they lack faith in your ability.

Your next step is to infiltrate the "old guard." Ask these informal leaders for their suggestions, and try to use those suggestions. Enlist their individual help on unit projects so that other staff members see that their leaders support you. Hold informal discussions with your staff to air everyone's feelings. The informal leaders will begin to lose their attraction as alternate leaders once you've channeled their leadership into unit goals. When staffers see that you can handle the situation, they'll rally behind you.

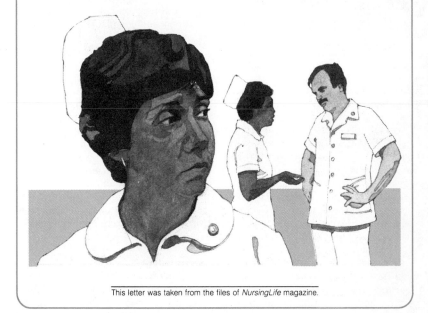

This letter was taken from the files of *NursingLife* magazine.

moving, and unproductive.
● Quality of patient care gradually deteriorates.

### Taking the bull by the horns
Now that you know how to recognize the types of conflict, or lack of it, and its possible causes, what skills do you need to actually remedy a conflict when it arises on your unit? Basically, you'll need problem-solving skills and perseverance.

Suppose, for example, that the staff on your unit's 3 to 11 shift complains regularly and bitterly about what the previous shift did or didn't do. How should you handle this situation? Start by applying your problem-solving skills to determine what caused the current conflict, why it isn't being resolved, and exactly what is blocking its effective resolution. If appropriate, you might consider holding a staff meeting of both shifts to openly discuss the conflict and identify all possible causes. Maybe some of the staff members think the 3 to 11 shift is assuming a disproportionate number of tasks. Maybe one or both of the shifts are understaffed. Or perhaps the conditions of the patients in the unit have become more acute. Write the suggested causes on a black-

---

*"Changing the way your unit resolves conflict will probably take time."*

---

board. Choose the cause most staff members think is the main one and encourage them to problem-solve. Try to get all parties to agree to a solution. (This technique, known as the *win-win technique,* helps each person involved in the conflict feel that she's benefited in some way from the solution.) Then set up a plan to implement the solution. Once the plan's initiated, be sure to hold follow-up meetings to discuss how well it's working. Make modifications, if necessary.

If your first attempt to resolve the conflict fails, don't be discouraged. Through time, every nursing unit has established its own particular way to handle, or not handle, conflict. Changing the way your unit resolves conflicts will probably also take time.

Here are two more examples of effective conflict management. Each demonstrates how you can successfully transform a potentially destructive

conflict into a constructive one.

● *Too much conflict.* You're the new head nurse on a medical-surgical unit and you've immediately implemented a new charting method. At the same time, the administration has introduced a new medication system and a new set of laboratory test forms. Staff members are complaining about the overload of changes on the unit. Absenteeism is up. Several staff members have decided to resign. What can you do? First, identify the problems that you have immediate control over. Then decide whether the changes are all really necessary right now. If they're not, delay implementing a few of them. Then, organize some social functions for the staff to encourage camaraderie and group cohesiveness.

● *Too little conflict.* Staff members on your unit have worked together for 3 years. Everyone knows what her responsibilities are and carries them out routinely and complacently. You notice a lot of inefficiency and duplication of work. What can you do? First, discuss the problems you see with your co-workers and head nurse. They may readily admit that they're in a rut and may welcome a plan to change the situation. Begin by suggesting that small task forces of two or three nurses research new ideas and present them to the department. To get out of your own rut, enroll in courses and keep up with your professional journals. Encourage others to do the same. Give fellow staff members opportunities to grow through active exchange and consideration of new ideas.

### A final word

You don't have to be a head nurse or a nursing administrator to cope with conflict. You and every staff member on your unit can (and should) be prepared to tackle problems whenever necessary. Problems are most effectively resolved when staff members themselves implement the necessary changes.

Managing conflict is risky. Others may criticize you, and you may have to criticize others. But you, your co-workers, and your patients can all benefit when you're willing to take that risk. As health care becomes more complex, conflicts are likely to increase. To ensure continued staff cooperation in your unit, start practicing effective conflict management skills now.

# 93 Defusing personal conflict

Have you ever wondered, "Why didn't nursing school teach us about the problem of personal conflicts with co-workers and patients?" Good question. You don't have to work long as a nurse before you're confronted with personal conflicts. Why are personal conflicts so common in nursing? As a nurse, you're required to interact daily with many people under stressful circumstances. Because everyone has different ideas, beliefs, and feelings, daily interaction and constant stress will naturally lead to some conflict.

You need to know how to deal with personal conflicts on the job—those you anticipate and those you don't. This entry will give you insights into avoiding personal conflicts before they develop—and dealing with those that do.

## Know when you're vulnerable to conflict

Personal conflicts can occur at any time. Usually they occur when you're fatigued, stressed, or involved in a personality clash with a colleague.

When you work overtime, double shifts, or extra days, fatigue makes you less considerate of others' problems and feelings. Even the most trivial issues can set off a conflict. "Why do you always forget to empty the trash?" is the kind of judgmental criticism you might make to a subordinate when you're fatigued.

Stress also diminishes your effectiveness when dealing with others. For example, suppose your medical-surgical unit is full when a recovery room nurse notifies you that a postoperative patient is on the way. Because you're under a lot of stress from the work load, you bark over the phone, "We can't take him now. You'll just have to wait!"

When two personalities clash, personal conflicts are the usual result. For example, a nurse who prefers organization and structure in patient care and a nurse who prefers a less-structured approach make a potentially volatile working combination. Admit it: you probably find some people plain hard to get along with. Your professional challenge is getting along with them anyway.

## Understanding territory's role in conflict

Personal conflict often results when someone challenges another person's territory. *Territory* refers to your unit, your subordinates, your responsibilities, and your authority. For example, if a nurse from another unit criticizes one of your unit's aides, you're likely to become defensive, even if the criticism is justified.

Territory can be a potent force in re-

GLOSSARY

### KEY TERMS IN THIS ENTRY

**constructive conflict** • A disagreement over such things as goals, methods, or values that stimulates problem solving and is eventually resolved to everyone's satisfaction.

**destructive conflict** • A disagreement over such things as goals, methods, or values that disrupts routine, is counterproductive, and ends in misunderstanding and mutual unhappiness.

**territory** • Physical space, aspects of authority, or responsibilities that a person feels belong to him and that he protects.

lationships among professionals. In fact, sometimes your concern for your territory may overshadow your efforts to find a solution. Consider this scenario: The emergency department (ED) transports patients—without a defibrillator—to your coronary care unit. You consider this practice so unwise that you become angry and exchange heated words with the ED nurse. By this action, you create more stress, not less. You should instead focus on the issue and state your view calmly. Then, speak about the subject to your supervisor, who may be in a position to make the changes you believe are necessary.

Personal conflict can even develop between two fellow workers who are also friends. Suppose you work well on your unit with a nurse who's an excellent clinician. She decides to accept a promotion in another unit. Each time she visits your unit, she now makes suggestions about your patient-care procedure, such as, "You know, there's a better way to put on that dressing. On our unit we tape it with silk tape." You feel betrayed and defensive because a respected friend is critical of your work and your unit's performance—in other words, your territory.

### Avoid conflict when you can

Because personal conflict usually makes your job more difficult, you should avoid it when you can. For example, don't get involved in discussing a controversial issue while you're working a double shift. If others ask for your opinion, tell them that you'd prefer to discuss the issue when you're less vulnerable, when your energy level is higher. Besides knowing when you're vulnerable, here are some techniques you can use to avoid conflict:

● *Keep smiling.* A sunny disposition and laughter help relieve stress. Also, not taking yourself too seriously can protect your ego when you're wrong.

● *Use tact.* Say "Would you please?" rather than "You have to." This will make following your instructions easier for others.

● *Be clear.* Make sure that all instructions that you give and receive are as clear as possible. Many personal conflicts stem from a breakdown in communications. Don't hesitate to tell someone the *why* and *how* of an instruction. (See Entry 91.)

● *Use compliments and praise.* A positive word will go a long way in avoiding personal conflict. A sincere compliment motivates someone to continue doing good work.

● *Avoid public disagreements.* Don't embarrass a co-worker in front of patients, doctors, supervisors, or other co-workers. Resolve disagreements in private whenever possible.

### When personal conflict becomes inevitable

Sometimes you can't avoid personal conflict. In these situations, you must at least try to defuse the conflict so that it doesn't interfere with patient care. To do so, use these techniques:

● *Set limits.* Tell the other person that you want to discuss one issue in particular, and keep the discussion on that issue. For example, a nurse with 10 years' experience joins your staff. Your hospital's policy states that antibiotics must be given diluted over 30 minutes. The new nurse repeatedly gives antibiotics by I.V. push. When you ask her why, she says in justification, "I've always given antibiotics by that method." As the head nurse, you realize you can't sidestep this touchy issue. You decide that the new nurse—like all nurses in your hospital—must follow policy. You approach the nurse to inform her of this. But first, you politely tell her that you want to limit the conversation to hospital policy. This will eliminate a source of conflict—the difference between hospital policy and what the nurse is used to doing—and encourage a constructive discussion.

● *Start over.* When you find that you're not getting anywhere in resolving the conflict, say to the other person, "I feel we're both getting angry and I bet if we start over, we'll handle this better."

## HOW TO RESTORE A RELATIONSHIP WHEN THE ARGUMENT IS OVER

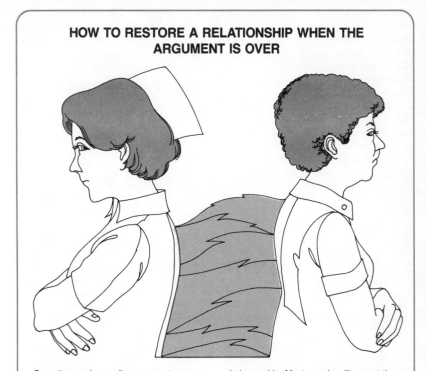

Sometimes, when a disagreement or misunderstanding has caused a rift between you and a co-worker, the rift may persist long afterward. The reason: No one likes to take the risk of suggesting reconciliation only to be rebuffed.

You can master such a situation by establishing positive contact without mentioning the incident that precipitated the rift. First, ask for help. "Do you know how I can do this procedure more efficiently?" By asking for help, you flatter the other person. You tell her you need her and think she's capable. Most people will accept the flattery and forget past problems. Then send a positive comment along the grapevine. Tell somebody else, "She did a great job with the project." Someone might pass the message along, and the gap will narrow.

These techniques are likely to work, especially if the other person has been willing to come around but just didn't know how. If you fail, at least you can feel good about yourself—knowing you made an effort to resolve the conflict.

Adapted with permission from "Head Off a Feud," *Successful Saleswoman* (May 1982), P.O. Box 255708, Sacramento, Calif. 95865.

Or you may want to restate the issue, saying something such as, "I think we've gone off track. Here's the issue as I see it."

• *Take a break.* Sometimes you just need to leave temporarily. When you feel yourself losing control in a conflict with a co-worker, tell her, "I can't talk about this right now. Let's get together after lunch." Arrange a time to resume your discussion. This technique allows you to reconsider all points of a conflict. Taking a break works with patients as well as co-workers. Some patients—for example, those with severe burns—can become extremely angry and lash out at you. You understand the bitterness, but you can't help feeling upset. When this happens, just say, "I'm going to leave the room for 5 minutes. We're both getting frustrated." This way, both of you can regain a reasonable state of mind. Find a corner of the unit you can withdraw to for a couple of minutes. Or just count to 10—taking a break mentally can be as effective as taking one physically.

• *Make the other person think the solution is hers.* A good way to defuse conflict is by guiding the other person to suggest a solution you've already proposed. Early in the conversation, suggest your solution, but don't take credit for it. Then probe the problem by asking questions of the other person. Initially, that person may offer her own solution, but don't be surprised if she introduces a variation on your solution later in the discussion.

### Learning the principles of defusing conflict
No matter how well you plan for conflict, you can't always predict the results of human interactions. But in any conflict, several principles can serve you well in reaching a solution. First, and above all, remember that each person has a right to her own ideas, beliefs, and feelings. Recognizing this right should make you more open to others' solutions.

Next, always try to stay composed, no matter how upset you feel. Angry outbursts only worsen personal conflict. Since the nursing process involves problem solving, you must make sound, unemotional decisions. When you lose your composure, you're less likely to make a logical decision.

Last, keep the problem in perspective. Don't let a disagreement with a colleague push aside the real challenge—how to improve patient care.

### A final word
As your responsibilities grow, you'll increasingly be exposed to stress and conflict. Whenever possible, you must avoid personal conflict and defuse it whenever it develops. Why? Because unless it's defused properly, personal conflict can sour relations among coworkers and reduce the quality of patient care. But once you become adept

at avoiding or defusing conflict, your professional relationships will provide increased opportunity for personal change and growth.

# 94 Working with nonnursing personnel

In the past, a doctor and a few staff nurses provided most or all of any hospitalized patient's care. But health care has grown more complex and specialized. Today, many nonnursing specialists also contribute to a patient's care. These specialists include dietitians, radiology technicians, medical laboratory technicians, physical therapists, occupational therapists, social workers, psychologists, respiratory therapists, and physician's assistants.

Unfortunately, when a number of specialists (as well as doctors and staff nurses) provide care for one patient, that care can become fragmented. As the number of health-care team members rises, achieving effective communication and properly integrated care becomes more difficult.

### Communication: The key to integrated care
You, the staff nurse, generally are responsible for coordinating a patient's care and ensuring effective communication among health-care team members. That's because you're in the unique position of knowing the "whole story," including the patient's medical history, his family history, his work environment, his current health status, and his medical diagnosis and treatment plans. Most nonnursing personnel don't have access to all this information. Instead, they're likely to have only the specific information they need to perform their specialty functions. So, to ensure integrated care, you must share appropriate information with nonnursing personnel and help

promote cooperation among members of the health-care team.

As you know, this is easier said than done. In many hospitals, conflict exists between staff nurses and nonnursing personnel, usually because of role confusion and the misunderstandings that grow out of it. At the root of the problem is poor communication—or even no communication at all.

Here's an example of how such a lack of communication can affect a patient's care.

About 2 hours before Mrs. Annie Law is scheduled for a myelogram, Barbara Peters, RN—the staff nurse caring for Mrs. Law—finds that the patient's extremely anxious about the test. Barbara performs the appropriate nursing tasks: she assesses the reason for Mrs. Law's anxiety, tries to allay it, and documents the problem and her nursing actions. But she doesn't even consider calling the radiologist to alert *him* to Mrs. Law's anxiety. If the radiologist knew about it, he could visit her before the test to further allay her fears. And once Mrs. Law arrived in the radiology department, the staff could make a special effort to explain things to her and reassure her. But because Barbara doesn't call, the radiologist isn't prepared to deal with Mrs. Law. As a result, Mrs. Law doesn't receive the kind of care she should.

## Other benefits of effective communication

Effective communication between nurses and nonnursing personnel not only enhances patient care but also saves time. For example, if you tell other health-care team members which actions you've already taken—including those that weren't effective as well as those that were—they won't waste time duplicating your work. And you'll find that saving other professionals' time is an excellent way to build working relationships.

Promoting effective communication will also help you fulfill your legal responsibilities. Remember, you're le-

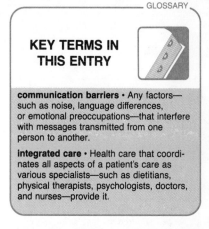

gally responsible for fulfilling your role in properly preparing the patient for any doctor-prescribed procedure. To do this, you must communicate effectively with any nonnursing personnel responsible for carrying out that procedure. Here's an example.

Mrs. Laura Jones has had hip arthroplasty prosthetic surgery. The physical therapy department instructs her twice a day in crutch-walking and conducts her daily exercise program. One night Mrs. Jones begins experiencing unusually sharp and persistent pain in her hip. Arlene Benson, RN, the day staff nurse, notices that range of motion in Mrs. Jones' hip and knee is reduced from the day before. Because an orthopedic doctor can't examine and assess Mrs. Jones' condition right away, Arlene calls the physical therapy department to cancel Mrs. Jones' morning physical therapy regimen. By making this nursing assessment and communicating with the physical therapy department, Arlene protects the patient from unnecessary complications and herself (and those she works with) from potential legal problems.

## What you can do

What can you do to enhance your professional relationships with nonnursing personnel, and thus promote effective communication? Here's some advice.

# ARE YOU TRYING TO CONTROL YOUR PATIENTS' TOTAL CARE?

*I work in an advanced-care unit in an 800-bed teaching hospital. Students from all areas of health care, plus interns and residents, are assigned to our patients. With so many different people providing so many different services, I frequently feel I don't know what's going on with my patients.*

*As a primary nurse, I'm responsible for coordinating my patients' care, yet I feel out of control. Everyone seems to be making decisions about my patients. How can I increase my control?—RN, Ohio*

If you want control of all the health-care disciplines that have input into your patients' care plans, you're asking too much of yourself.

As a primary nurse, you're responsible for coordinating your patients' care— not controlling it.

To ease your frustration in coordinating the contributions of so many health-care providers, hold discussions with those providers who are supervising all the students on your unit. Plan how members of each discipline will handle your patients' care, inform you of their progress, and help you update your nursing-care plans.

Striving for total control of your patients is self-defeating and energy-consuming. By accepting other people's help, you'll feel more satisfied with your work without feeling overwhelmed.

This letter was taken from the files of *NursingLife* magazine.

First, take time to understand the roles of key nonnursing specialists in the hospital where you work. To help gain a good understanding of their roles, find out what kind of education each specialty requires. Share what you learn with your nurse colleagues.

Also, help nonnursing personnel find out more about your role as a staff nurse. Explain your responsibilities for coordinating patient care. If they understand these responsibilities, they'll probably be more willing to cooperate with you.

Get to know key nonnursing personnel. When possible, sit and talk with them at lunch or break. This approach will probably do more to break down communication barriers than any other. By developing personal relationships, you'll enhance your working relationships. Obviously, communication will be smoother if you call the physical therapy department and ask to speak to Mary instead of "the physical therapist."

If you have a conflict with a nonnursing colleague, deal with him directly. Approach him in a professional manner and try to work out your differences. If the two of you can't work out the problem, seek appropriate assistance elsewhere within the hospital, such as from a risk manager. He's there to help solve problems between personnel from different departments.

You can also improve your professional relationships with nonnursing personnel by holding regular multidisciplinary conferences regarding patients you mutually care for. To get the ball rolling, invite one or two nonnursing professionals (such as the occupational therapist and the social worker) to your normal nursing care conference. Hold the meetings regularly and, to avoid inconveniencing anyone, start and end them on time.

Conflicts between nursing and nonnursing personnel may surface during these meetings. Try to solve them within the group. Encourage group members to keep the lines of communication open, no matter how strongly they disagree, for the sake of better patient care. By promoting this approach, you help solve interdisciplinary patient-care problems *and* enhance your own professional status.

## A final word

As health care continues to become more sophisticated and specialized, the need for integrated planning of patient care will grow. More and more, the members of the health-care team will be interdependent. And that will make working effectively with your colleagues—especially nonnursing personnel—one of your top priorities.

## Selected References

Albrecht, Terrance L. "What Job Stress Means for the Staff Nurse," *Nursing Administration Quarterly* 7(1):1-11, Fall 1982.

Ceccio, Joseph F., and Ceccio, Cathy M. *Effective Communication in Nursing: Theory and Practice.* New York: John Wiley & Sons, 1982.

Chaska, Norma. *The Nursing Profession.* New York: McGraw-Hill Book Co., 1977.

Cooper, J. "Conflict: How To Avoid It and What To Do When You Can't," *Nursing79* 9:89-91, January 1979.

Mallory, G.A. "Conflict Can Be Healthy Once You Understand It and Learn How to Manage It," *Nursing81* 11:97-100, June 1981.

Morrison, Ruby S., and Zebelman, Edna. "The Career Concept in Nursing," *Nursing Administration Quarterly* 7(1): 60-68, Fall 1982.

Nuernberger, P. "Freedom from Stress: A Holistic Approach," *NursingLife* 1:61-68, November/December 1981.

Seuntjens, Alice Daly. "Burnout in Nursing—What It Is and How to Prevent It," *Nursing Administration Quarterly* 7(1):12-19, Fall 1982.

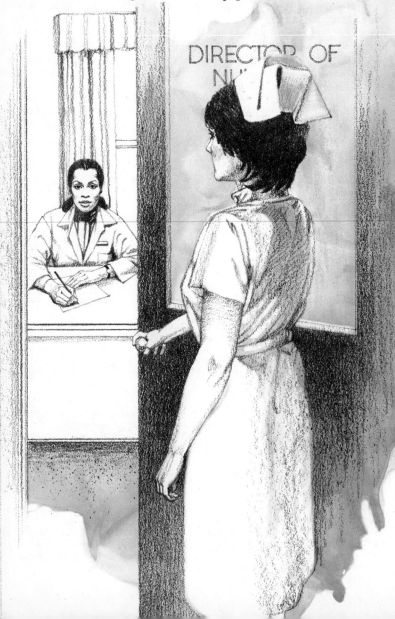

# Dealing with Nursing Management

## Introduction

If you're like most nurses, you probably didn't learn about administrative organization and managerial techniques in nursing school. But now you may wish you had, even if you're not interested in a managerial position. Why? Because knowing these things can help you manage patient care and deal with your supervisors more effectively.

This chapter teaches you what you want—and need—to know about management. The information and advice will help you work more effectively with management, so you can gain a sense of control over your work situation and help bring about change.

### Learning about management

Do you know how your hospital administration is organized? And do you know how much power your nursing service department has? As you'll learn in Entry 95, "Where the real power lies: Looking at the organizational chart," you can begin to get answers to these questions by examining your hospital's organizational chart. This chart tells you how the nursing service department is organized and how it fits into the entire hospital organization. Then you can build on this understanding to determine how much power your department has.

Entry 96, "How (and what) administrators think," discusses the impor-

tance of understanding the administrator's point of view. As a staff nurse, you probably look at most issues from only two perspectives: your patient's and your own. But a director of nursing service must view an issue from many perspectives and consider many points of view. Before you can communicate effectively with her, you need to understand her many concerns.

In Entry 97, "How to relate to supervisors," you'll learn how to establish working and workable relationships with your supervisors. As you'll read, two essential elements for establishing such relationships are an understanding of your role (and your supervisor's) and an ability to communicate effectively. In this entry, you'll discover how to communicate with all supervisors, regardless of their managerial styles. You'll also learn how to disagree with your supervisor without attacking her personally.

Entry 98's entitled "Initiating change." In health-care institutions, change is inevitable. This means you have three options: you can simply let external changes control you, you can resist change, or you can initiate your own changes. This entry gives you a step-by-step guide for making the changes you want.

As you know, your supervisor is responsible for staffing. But when un-

## HOW TO FILE A COMPLAINT

Whenever you have a complaint about your job, bring it to your supervisor's attention, following your institution's grievance procedure. If your institution doesn't have a grievance procedure, follow these guidelines:

• Approach your supervisor and ask to meet privately with her to discuss your complaint. Note the date when you take this step and any subsequent steps.

• If your supervisor puts off your request for a meeting, write up the complaint and submit it to her. Keep a copy for your records.

• Whether you present your complaint verbally or in writing, make sure it's factual (don't include opinion or hearsay), to the point (don't ramble), specific (don't generalize), and fair (don't attack others).

Here are two examples of a complaint—one properly stated and one improperly stated:

| Properly stated complaint | Improperly stated complaint |
|---|---|
| "I've requested two special days off, in October and in June. You've turned down my requests both times. I have not received any explanation why my requests were denied. I'd like to discuss this matter with you." | "Why don't you ever grant my requests for days off? I'm constantly amazed how the rest of the staff always gets what they want. I'd like to know if there's something about me that you don't like. I do my best to please you, but you've obviously chosen to ignore my requests. I demand to know why." |

• Give your supervisor time to respond. Wait several days before approaching her again.

• If your supervisor still fails to respond or doesn't give you a satisfactory answer, tell her you intend to go to a higher authority with your complaint. This will give her one final opportunity to take action.

• If she still takes no action, make an appointment with a higher authority. The higher authority will want to review your complaint and the record you've kept of how you've handled the situation. She may invite your supervisor to come to the meeting with you so the issue is confronted openly.

derstaffing affects the quality of patient care you provide, you must act to improve the situation. How? Entry 99, "Proving you're understaffed (and what to do about it)," supplies the answer. It tells you what information you should gather and whom you should see to remedy understaffing.

Sometimes you have to use sources outside the hospital to solve problems. Entry 100, "Indications for involving outside sources," explains how and when to do this for problems ranging from patient safety to nurses' salaries.

### A final word

As a staff nurse, you're responsible for not only providing direct patient care but also for managing a patient's care. And when your unit has a problem (such as understaffing), good patient care may depend on your ability to understand and deal with management. This chapter shows how you can communicate effectively with your managers to help solve problems. By working together, you and your managers can ensure that patients receive consistent, high-quality care.

# 95 Where the real power lies: Looking at the organizational chart

Many nurses complain of feeling powerless, of being unable to help make changes where they work. They wouldn't feel that way, though, if they understood how their institution was organized and how that organization gives people power. Of course, not all power in an institution is apparent in its organizational structure. But such a strong link exists between power and organization that you must understand their relationship if you want to have any influence where you work.

Here's another consequence of not understanding the power-organization relationship: Because nursing represents the largest department in most health-care institutions, it's become an attractive target for eager executives looking for economies. That means unless you take a direct interest in exercising your nursing department's inherent power, it may be usurped by others who'll then have a big say in such vital issues as staffing.

This entry explains how the organizational structure confers or withholds power, and how you can get more power from your organization.

## Drawing up the organizational chart

To accomplish their objectives, institutions divide necessary work among employees. Job descriptions outline which duties go with each job. As a staff nurse, you're familiar with the duties expected of you. Your job description provides the structure and boundaries you operate within while you're on the job. Such descriptions exist for every person in the institution.

The organizational chart illustrates how each job fits into the institution's structure. You'll find that your institution's organizational chart follows one of three basic structures: centralized, decentralized, or matrix.

## The centralized organization

The primary characteristic of a centralized organization (see *Understanding a Centralized Organization,* page 593) is that all front-line supervisors (head nurses) report to the department head (nursing director), who in turn reports to the administrator. Usually the administrator controls all decision making.

This organization has several advantages, mainly for the smaller hospital. By employing a centralized organization, the smaller hospital can coordinate and control its resources more effectively than with a decentralized or matrix organization. It can also supervise managers more efficiently, allowing it to put less experienced, lower-salaried people in management positions.

The centralized organization also has several disadvantages. Foremost among them: Communication is primarily upward and downward, from superior to subordinate. The organization doesn't

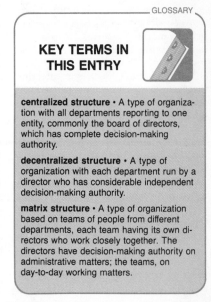

## KEY TERMS IN THIS ENTRY

**centralized structure** • A type of organization with all departments reporting to one entity, commonly the board of directors, which has complete decision-making authority.

**decentralized structure** • A type of organization with each department run by a director who has considerable independent decision-making authority.

**matrix structure** • A type of organization based on teams of people from different departments, each team having its own directors who work closely together. The directors have decision-making authority on administrative matters; the teams, on day-to-day working matters.

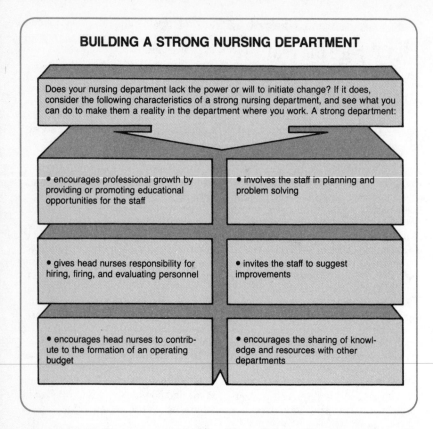

**BUILDING A STRONG NURSING DEPARTMENT**

Does your nursing department lack the power or will to initiate change? If it does, consider the following characteristics of a strong nursing department, and see what you can do to make them a reality in the department where you work. A strong department:

- encourages professional growth by providing or promoting educational opportunities for the staff

- involves the staff in planning and problem solving

- gives head nurses responsibility for hiring, firing, and evaluating personnel

- invites the staff to suggest improvements

- encourages head nurses to contribute to the formation of an operating budget

- encourages the sharing of knowledge and resources with other departments

encourage or facilitate communication between departments, because a few persons maintain control. Head nurses in a centralized organization may possess only a little power to bring about changes or make decisions affecting their staffs. Consequently, the staff nurses in such an organization tend to have even less power.

**The decentralized organization**

A decentralized organization has a horizontal structure that is designed to promote decision-making responsibility at the organization's lower levels (see *Understanding a Decentralized Organization*, page 594). It assumes that qualified managers know best how to maximize the use of resources and to encourage productivity. The organization groups the institution into divisions, each headed by a director.

These division directors report to the vice-president of nursing practice or the assistant administrator for nursing (common titles for the chief nursing administrator). You can usually find the decentralized type of structure in larger hospitals that provide a multitude of services and that attract well-qualified managers.

This structure has many advantages. It provides staff members with greater access to those people—their supervisors—with decision-making power. This accessibility, in turn, allows staff nurses to have greater impact on and more input with decisions involving their work. Theoretically, a decentralized structure is also more flexible and more responsive in solving problems. This organization also allows each department to develop policies and procedures specific to its needs.

The decentralized organization's main disadvantage is its potential for a communication breakdown. Why? Because the organization distributes decision-making authority among division directors whose decisions may conflict. Another disadvantage is that, because the directors have so much power, the organization is only as responsive as the directors choose to be.

### The matrix organization

The third main organizational structure—the matrix—is the most complex (see *Understanding a Matrix Organization,* page 595). Institutions that use a matrix organization are usually large and complex with basically decentralized decision making. The matrix structure's most conventional form involves patient-care teams, made up of members from different departments who work together but who report to different supervisors.

A matrix organization best serves hospitals with objectives that involve

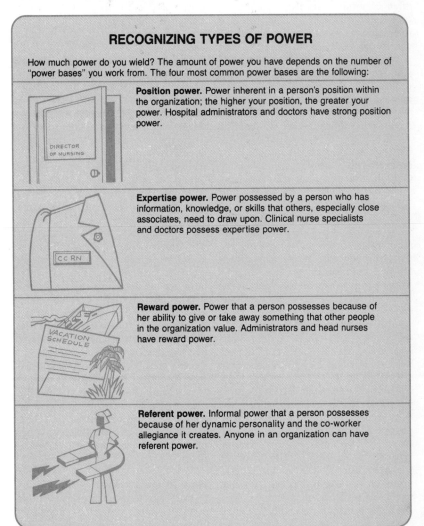

## RECOGNIZING TYPES OF POWER

How much power do you wield? The amount of power you have depends on the number of "power bases" you work from. The four most common power bases are the following:

**Position power.** Power inherent in a person's position within the organization; the higher your position, the greater your power. Hospital administrators and doctors have strong position power.

**Expertise power.** Power possessed by a person who has information, knowledge, or skills that others, especially close associates, need to draw upon. Clinical nurse specialists and doctors possess expertise power.

**Reward power.** Power that a person possesses because of her ability to give or take away something that other people in the organization value. Administrators and head nurses have reward power.

**Referent power.** Informal power that a person possesses because of her dynamic personality and the co-worker allegiance it creates. Anyone in an organization can have referent power.

more than one department. To accomplish such objectives, the hospital usually appoints a coordinator who can go to any department and give whatever directives are necessary to get the job done.

For example, a hospital that wants to begin primary nursing can appoint a coordinator with the power to make the necessary changes. This person crosses nursing department authority lines to work with all the head nurses on education and implementation. Another important advantage of a matrix organization is better communication regarding patient care, because health-care professionals from various disciplines work as a team. But a disadvantage is that the health-care professional is sometimes put in the confusing situation of having to respect his department head's instructions at the expense of health-care teamwork.

## Understanding positions and staff nursing power

Organizational structures are based on line positions and staff positions. A line position includes some form of decision-making responsibility and authority. Examples include the administrator, the chief executive officer, the vice-president, the nursing director, and the head nurse. In a line position, a supervisor directs your work, and you, in turn, direct the work of employees who report to you.

In a staff position, a supervisor directs your work, but no one formally reports to you. Therefore, staff nurses have no *position* power. However, it doesn't mean that staff nurses are powerless (see *Recognizing Types of Power*, page 591). Nurses in staff positions can help achieve institutional objectives through informal means of power. As consultants or advisors, they possess *expertise* power, that is, the power of having a special skill or knowledge that others in the institution rely on. Examples of staff positions include clinical nurse specialist and staff education coordinator.

## Nursing's position on the organizational chart

The way the chief nursing administrator reports to her superiors provides revealing clues to the nursing department's power within the organization. Many of the first U.S. hospitals had strong, centralized organizations, directed by doctors.

Nursing directors, as they were called then, reported directly to the doctors and had little power to initiate change. Most chief nursing administrators still report directly to a chief executive officer—but usually this person is a hospital administrator, not a doctor.

The nursing director can report to her superior by two other, less common, methods. With the first method, she reports to the institution's assistant administrator. This lessens the nursing department's power and authority, because the chief nursing administrator does not deal directly with the hospital administrator.

The second method—called the triad, or collaborative, system—strengthens the nursing department's power. This method calls for a triad at the organization's top—a nursing administrator, a hospital administrator, and a medical staff president—in which each member has an equal voice in policy making.

Whichever system your institution uses, the chief nursing administrator can do several things to maintain and strengthen the nursing department's power. For example, she can:
● insist on reporting directly to the institution's chief executive officer
● maintain regular contact and develop a professional relationship with the institution's board of trustees
● enlarge her referent power by becoming as efficient and effective as possible.

## How to gain power

Nursing's professional growth requires that you commit yourself to expanding nursing's power. What can you do?

## UNDERSTANDING A CENTRALIZED ORGANIZATION

This organizational chart shows a centralized nursing department and its hierarchic relationship to hospital administration. Its structure centralizes decision-making power and authority in the hands of a few people.

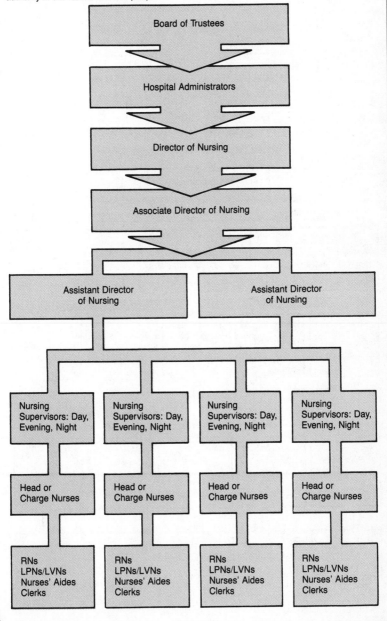

# UNDERSTANDING A DECENTRALIZED ORGANIZATION

This organizational chart shows a decentralized nursing department and its hierarchic relationship to hospital administration. Its structure decentralizes decision-making power and authority and places it in the hands of several assistant directors and division heads.

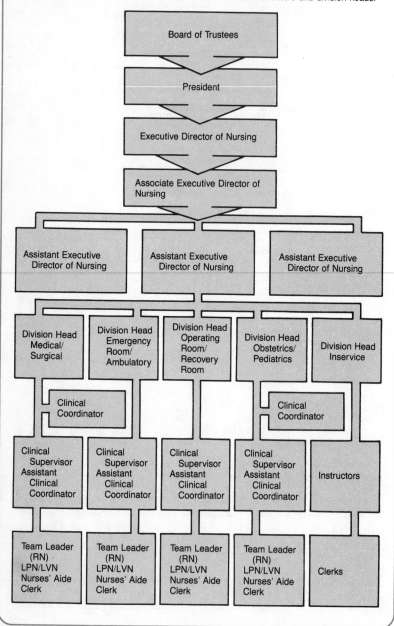

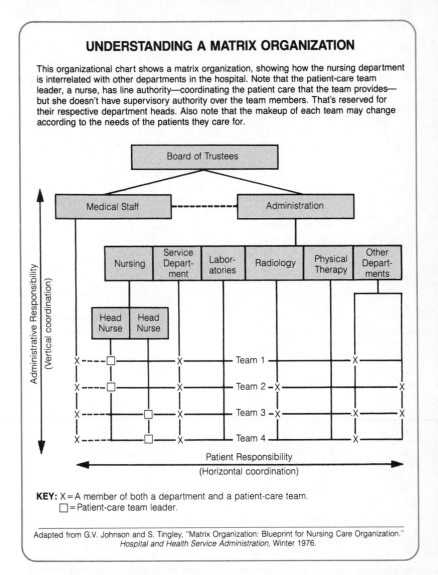

## UNDERSTANDING A MATRIX ORGANIZATION

This organizational chart shows a matrix organization, showing how the nursing department is interrelated with other departments in the hospital. Note that the patient-care team leader, a nurse, has line authority—coordinating the patient care that the team provides— but she doesn't have supervisory authority over the team members. That's reserved for their respective department heads. Also note that the makeup of each team may change according to the needs of the patients they care for.

**KEY:** X = A member of both a department and a patient-care team.
☐ = Patient-care team leader.

Adapted from G.V. Johnson and S. Tingley, "Matrix Organization: Blueprint for Nursing Care Organization." *Hospital and Health Service Administration,* Winter 1976.

Well, one step would be to market your services in a professional manner. That is, demonstrate to patients and doctors that no one can provide better health care for less money than nurses. How? By working efficiently as well as compassionately, using your nursing skills to the best of your ability.

Another step involves developing a network of relationships with individuals and departments outside of nursing. Make an effort to meet the needs of staff members in other departments. For example, suppose the laboratory technician has to draw three stat blood samples on your unit by 1:30 p.m., and he hasn't been to lunch yet. Your cheerful and timely assistance can gain an ally for nursing in the future.

Finally, don't complain about the staff on your unit. Use a positive approach to change things.

## A final word

Knowing how your organization works can help you take the initiative in getting power for nursing. For too long, nurses have considered power the province of other health-care professionals. But now, nurses are beginning to understand that they must seek out power and use it constructively for the benefit of their patients *and* their profession.

# 96 How (and what) administrators think

Part of your responsibility as a nurse is to implement and enforce decisions that nursing administrators make. But what if those decisions seem unreasonable or impractical to you? How do you handle the dilemma of enforcing rules that you yourself disagree with?

You can start by making an effort to learn how administrators view problems and how they arrive at solutions for them. Understanding administrators' reasons for taking certain actions will help you to evaluate the resulting policies with an open mind and to handle policy situations more effectively.

## What makes administrators different?

Generally speaking, administrators are

concerned with the "big picture." They view all of nursing service as a single element within the hospital structure. They continually scan the overall scene, whereas you naturally focus on the day-to-day affairs of your own particular unit—the specific problems and needs that *you* must deal with.

These differing perspectives can cause conflicts. For example, you may feel that your unit's needs would be better met if you used a different nursing care delivery system. So you propose the change to administration. But your administrator balks, declaring your idea unfeasible because of cost and time factors. Unaware that the change you've suggested would require extensive staff training before the new system could be successfully implemented, you feel frustrated and even mad at your administrator. If situations like this happen frequently, you may leave your job or even leave the profession.

You can minimize this type of frustration and disillusionment by understanding the role your administrator plays and the way she makes decisions. Once you achieve this understanding, you'll be in a position to bring about necessary changes, which will improve the quality of your nursing care.

## Understanding your administrator's role

First and foremost, nursing administrators are nurses. Most of them were once practicing clinicians. They've chosen an administrative role because they feel that's how they can best contribute to the profession. You can think of them as professional colleagues whose practice area is administration.

The administrator's primary responsibility is to maintain a conceptual view of all nursing service. She does this by continually monitoring all nursing service units for patterns that indicate developing problems or a need for improvement. Then, based on those patterns, the administrator takes appropriate action. For example, a

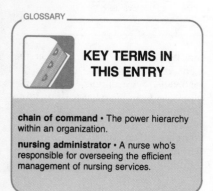

nursing administrator may receive several staffing complaints from various nurses on the same unit who work different shifts. One nurse complains about understaffing, another about the unsafe delivery of nursing care, a third about how the nurses must frequently work overtime. By taking the broad view, the administrator may detect that the unit's basic problem is that it lacks sufficient clerical help. Or she may determine that the problems have been caused by an increase in acutely ill patients. In either instance, she'll develop and implement a plan to remedy the situation. The plan might involve a reorganization of the unit's work load or the employment of additional clerks or staff nurses. Once she implements the new plan, she'll evaluate it periodically to make sure it's remedying the problem her staff helped her identify.

A competent nursing administrator serves as a leader and as a facilitator of change. She's the vital link between you, at the bedside, and the "machinery" of the hospital organization, administration, medical staff, and board of directors. Because she knows your needs and problems, she can communicate them to other administrators and get you the help you need.

### Relating to your administrators

Besides trying to understand the administrator's role and the reasons for various administrative decisions, what else can you do to help establish a productive working relationship with administrators? Consider the following:

• *Get to know your administrators.* They include head nurses and supervisors as well as the chief nursing administrator. You can get to know them by attending staff meetings and by scheduling appointments with them to share your perspectives and ideas about nursing practice. Take the initiative to suggest that administrative personnel other than your charge nurses and supervisors should be invited to your staff meetings. If you're given the job of inviting them, do it in a friendly manner

and explain exactly what you'd like them to contribute. You might ask them to come simply to observe, to discuss the institution's future goals and plans, to explain an administrative decision and the rationale behind it, or to assist staff in negotiating policy or procedural changes. If an administrator agrees to discuss specific issues openly with staff, make sure the meeting stays

---

*"You can minimize frustration by understanding the role your administrator plays and the way she makes decisions."*

---

on a professional level. You can do this by keeping the discussion focused on the issues at hand and by deflecting any accusations leveled at the administrator.

• *Work within the system.* Review the hospital and nursing administration's organizational charts for all staff. Become familiar with the various hospital and nursing committees and functions. Then, when you have a complaint or want to initiate a change, follow the nursing chain of command.

• *Share information with your nursing administrator.* Let your administrator know right away about any problems or concerns that you or the staff have—don't let them linger. By doing so, you help your administrator to prevent or minimize staff anxiety. For example, if a rumor begins to circulate that the hospital has decided not to hire any more LPNs/LVNs, ask your administrator about it. She's the only one who can provide you with accurate information. If the rumor's unfounded, she can squelch it before the staff begins to react. If the rumor's true, she can give you the whole story, which will probably explain the decision.

• *Learn to think like an administrator.* Before you discuss a problem with your administrator, try to identify major issues on your unit; don't just focus on isolated incidents. When you've arrived at a conceptual view of the problem, present the information to your nursing administrator and your co-workers in a logical and objective fashion. Keep in mind the overall impact that the issue may have on all nursing service.

• *Help establish and promote positive attitudes among staff and nursing administrators.* View nursing administrators as professional colleagues. And help your co-workers do the same. Discourage cafeteria gossip about administrative personnel. Don't draw dividing lines by referring to staff members as *we* and administrators as *they.* Support your administration. Try to convey the idea that the nursing staff and administration have the same goal: quality patient care. If staff members are dissatisfied with the way administrators are attempting to reach that goal, encourage them to confront nursing administrators with the issues.

### A final word
Once you understand your nursing administrator's role, you'll be able to assist her in carrying out her responsibilities—which, of course, include helping you to meet your needs. This means you'll increase your own job satisfaction as well.

More and more, health-care institutions are realizing that, to maintain a motivated and productive staff of professional nurses, they must provide a work environment that supports and enhances professional growth. Consequently, more and more nursing administrators are encouraging their staff to participate actively in the decision-making process.

You'll probably find that this type of participative management will become more common as administrators become more aware of its benefits. Now's the time to begin *your* participation in

making decisions that affect your unit—*and* your future.

---

# 97 How to relate to supervisors

As a staff nurse, you may think of your supervisor as your best advocate. If you don't feel that way, your relationship with her may need your attention. To find out if it does, read the following pages. You'll learn the characteristics of a good supervisor-subordinate relationship, how to assess your relationship with your supervisor, and how to improve it.

### Getting started
Your first responsibility in establishing a good supervisor-subordinate relationship is to understand the organizational structure of the institution where you work (see Entry 95). Find out if the nursing service is a centralized, decentralized, or matrix organization. The answer to this question will tell you about the chain of command your supervisor reports to and how many people are between you and the chief nursing administrator.

The next step is to identify your rights and responsibilities as a staff nurse. Find out exactly what your supervisor expects of you. If you have a copy of your job description, study it. If you don't, request a copy.

Then, similarly, try to understand your supervisor's role within the organization. If you didn't request a copy of her job description when you were interviewed for the staff nurse position, request it now. Find out what her rights and responsibilities are.

### What makes a good supervisor-subordinate relationship?
Undoubtedly, your relationship with your supervisor differs from other staff

members' relationships with her. Nevertheless, certain characteristics are common to all good supervisor-subordinate relationships. M. J. O'Brien identifies many of these characteristics in her book *Communications and Relationships in Nursing* (1978). They include:

• *Congeniality.* You and your supervisor don't have to be best friends. In fact, you may not even like each other. However, you should be courteous and kind to one another and acknowledge each other's viewpoints. If your viewpoints differ, don't take it personally. Remember that you're not objecting to her, you're objecting to her ideas.

• *A relaxed manner.* Your relationship with your supervisor should be non-stressful. You should know what your patient-care responsibilities and objectives are and have well-established professional goals. Then you should go about fulfilling those responsibilities and meeting your goals in such a way that your supervisor doesn't have to constantly intervene.

• *Predictability.* You and your supervisor should know what to expect from one another. This will help each of you to establish a relaxed relationship and to build mutual respect, trust, and honesty. Consider the following example: A patient's family complains to your supervisor that you've treated them rudely. You know your supervisor will support you when you both meet with the family, and that she'll talk with you privately about any concerns she has about your behavior. Similarly, she knows that you'll tell her what she needs to know about the situation, positive and negative. Because you and your supervisor have this kind of predictable relationship, the family's complaint won't jeopardize it.

• *Mutual respect.* You and your supervisor should treat each other courteously and professionally, recognizing that each of you is trying to do her job to the best of her abilities. Each of you, of course, expects to be respected on the job—but this respect can quickly

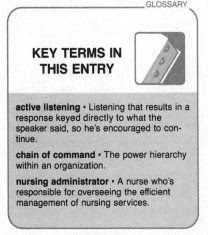

**KEY TERMS IN THIS ENTRY**

**active listening** • Listening that results in a response keyed directly to what the speaker said, so he's encouraged to continue.

**chain of command** • The power hierarchy within an organization.

**nursing administrator** • A nurse who's responsible for overseeing the efficient management of nursing services.

wane if you don't really warrant it. For example, your supervisor undoubtedly respected you when she hired you, based on your educational background and your work experience. And you probably respected *her* automatically, at first. But you can only maintain and enhance that mutual respect by continually working to show each other that you're worthy of it.

• *Trust and honesty.* These may be the two most important characteristics of a supervisor-subordinate relationship. But as with respect, you must work to establish them. As you know, placing your trust in anyone is risky. So proceed slowly, and evaluate your supervisor's trustworthiness carefully. For example, if you confidentially share information with her about yourself or a patient situation, does she keep it confidential, sharing the information only with those who need to know? Or does she reveal it indiscriminately?

Your supervisor will evaluate *your* trustworthiness and honesty the same way. To earn her trust quickly, be sure you discuss job-related problems with her directly. Don't let your feelings about a problem get back to your supervisor secondhand.

• *Openness.* You and your supervisor should freely share information that's important to your professional relationship. To promote this, your super-

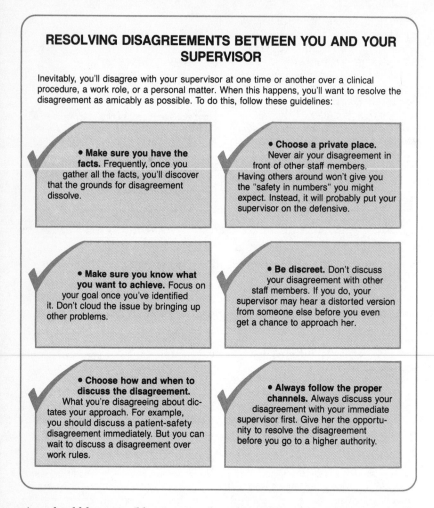

## RESOLVING DISAGREEMENTS BETWEEN YOU AND YOUR SUPERVISOR

Inevitably, you'll disagree with your supervisor at one time or another over a clinical procedure, a work role, or a personal matter. When this happens, you'll want to resolve the disagreement as amicably as possible. To do this, follow these guidelines:

- **Make sure you have the facts.** Frequently, once you gather all the facts, you'll discover that the grounds for disagreement dissolve.

- **Choose a private place.** Never air your disagreement in front of other staff members. Having others around won't give you the "safety in numbers" you might expect. Instead, it will probably put your supervisor on the defensive.

- **Make sure you know what you want to achieve.** Focus on your goal once you've identified it. Don't cloud the issue by bringing up other problems.

- **Be discreet.** Don't discuss your disagreement with other staff members. If you do, your supervisor may hear a distorted version from someone else before you even get a chance to approach her.

- **Choose how and when to discuss the disagreement.** What you're disagreeing about dictates your approach. For example, you should discuss a patient-safety disagreement immediately. But you can wait to discuss a disagreement over work rules.

- **Always follow the proper channels.** Always discuss your disagreement with your immediate supervisor first. Give her the opportunity to resolve the disagreement before you go to a higher authority.

visor should be accessible to you, and you should be willing to approach her with your problems.

- *Tact.* You and your supervisor should be straightforward without being offensive or rude. Express your ideas clearly and concisely, and always maintain a professional manner.

- *Flexibility.* You and your supervisor should be able to respond appropriately to changing conditions by acknowledging each other's viewpoints and problem-solving suggestions.

### Cultivating a good relationship

How do you arrive at a good working relationship with your supervisor? Is relating well to her really something you can learn? In some instances, good relationships just happen naturally; usually, though, you have to work to make a relationship good. You can learn certain skills to facilitate a positive supervisor-subordinate relationship.

Active listening is probably the most important communication skill you need in cultivating a good supervisor-subordinate relationship. Active listening means that you ask your supervisor to repeat her message when you're unsure of what she said, and that you ask

## SUPERVISING EFFECTIVELY BY COMMUNICATING EFFECTIVELY

The key to supervising effectively is communicating effectively. If you're a nurse supervisor, or if you're ever temporarily placed in a supervisory position, keep these communication tips in mind:

● Let staff members know you care about what they have to say by minimizing or eliminating distractions and by listening carefully.

● Encourage staff members to communicate with you, and involve them actively in decisions by asking for their opinions or feelings on matters that affect them.

● Help staff members feel good about their work by acknowledging their efforts and commending them when they deserve it.

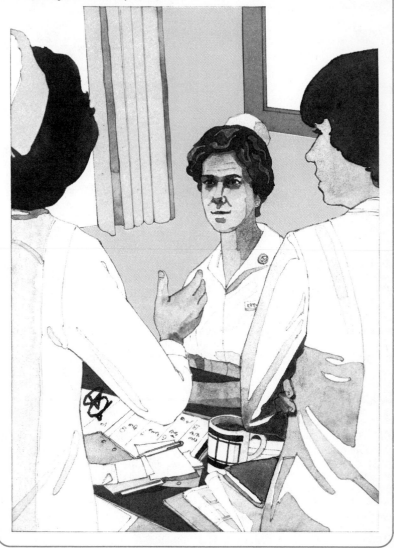

## UNDERSTANDING YOUR SUPERVISOR'S LEADERSHIP STYLE

How well you work with your supervisor depends, in part, on your ability to recognize the primary leadership style she's using—and to understand your reaction to it. Expect her to assume different leadership styles, too, depending on the situation and persons involved. Here's a list of the more common leadership styles and how they may make you feel:

| LEADERSHIP STYLE | SUPERVISOR'S ACTIONS | SUBORDINATE'S REACTIONS |
| --- | --- | --- |
| **Collaborative** (also called democratic, supportive, or participative) | Retains authority and control, but supports subordinate's participation in setting policies and goals | • Derives satisfaction from having some decision-making control<br>• Thinks the supervisor's decisions and tactics are fair because staff participated in making the decisions |
| **Autocratic** (also called authoritative) | Exerts a strong, dogmatic direction and maintains close control over subordinate | • May feel hostile toward the supervisor and criticize decisions because staff were not included in making them |
| **Laissez-faire** (also called free-rein) | Allows subordinate the chance to set goals without direction, giving subordinate maximum decision-making freedom; serves mainly as a resource | • May feel confused because of the lack of direction |

for more specific information when what she's told you seems sketchy. These approaches will minimize misunderstandings.

Once you've received a message from your supervisor—for example, a specific assignment—and interpreted it accurately, acknowledge it and act on it. Your supervisor should do the same with any inquiries or problems you present to her, even if her follow-up response isn't the one you hoped for.

Next, stick to the facts. When discussing situations with your supervisor, avoid assumptions, generalities, and hearsay. For example, if you tell your supervisor that a nurse on your shift is frequently late for work, give her specifics. How many days was this nurse late last month? How late was she?

Finally, be assertive. Use "I" statements to tell your supervisor how you feel, without blaming her or putting her on the spot. "I" statements help prevent your supervisor from becoming defensive and usually lead to constructive conversation. (See Entry 69.)

### Evaluating your relationship with your supervisor

If your relationship with your supervisor needs mending, now's the time to begin. Start by carefully assessing your current relationship and establishing new objectives for improving it. In her book on managing and being managed, Teddy Langford suggests you ask yourself the following questions to evaluate your relationship with your supervisor:

• Am I at ease when I talk with my supervisor?

• Do I state my true opinions when she asks?

• Do I always wait for her to initiate any interaction?

• Do I find myself wanting to get back at her, or not wanting to work in the way she expects?

• Does my interaction with her help me in my work?

Answering these questions honestly will help you discover whether you view your supervisor as a colleague,

---

*"In a positive relationship with your supervisor, you'll gain new respect for your staff nurse role."*

---

who works with you and for you, or as a "parent," who's there to answer your questions and tell you what to do. You'll confirm whether you're comfortable with her and, perhaps, find out why you may be uncomfortable. For example, you may discover that your relationship with your supervisor has been influenced by your experience with a former supervisor, by the way you view your role as a nurse, or by how you think your supervisor expects you to act.

Once you've identified the nature of your relationship, ask yourself if you're satisfied with it. If you're not, why? Then identify those aspects of the relationship that you feel need to be changed. If you're willing to make the effort to change them, talk to your supervisor. Present her with the objectives you'd like to achieve. You and she should decide on deadlines for achieving these objectives and criteria for determining if you've achieved them. For example, you may conclude from your assessment that you need more supervision than your supervisor is currently providing. Tell her this in an assertive, nonthreatening manner. Say, for example, "I need you to make concrete suggestions about my work. Please don't assume that it's OK."

## A final word

Positive relationships usually don't just happen. They require attention and effort. But if you work with your supervisor to identify objectives for improving your relationship, you can expect good results.

In a positive relationship with your supervisor, you'll learn to communicate more effectively, to be more assertive, and to use your energy and nursing knowledge more productively. When problems arise, you'll be able to solve them quickly and effectively because you'll have broken down preexisting communication barriers.

Ultimately, you'll gain new confidence in yourself and new respect for your role as a staff nurse. You may even find new challenge and fulfillment in your job. And if, one day, you're offered a position as a charge nurse, you'll be prepared to handle those responsibilities effectively from the start.

# 98 Initiating change

Change challenges you. No matter what kind of nursing position you have, change is an ever-present force. New technology and procedures—as well as new management ideas—constantly test nursing's status quo. That means you can't avoid change. The effective nurse anticipates change, initiates it, or takes action to direct it.

How profound an impact change has on you depends, in large part, on how you view it. You can become the victim of change or the master of it—you can try to avoid it or try to use it to improve patient care and your profession. This entry tells you how to evaluate your options when change becomes necessary, and how to initiate changes that will help you meet your needs.

## Planning effective change

A bad change—or no change at all—

can cause a crisis, undermine morale, reduce efficiency, and create staff conflict. But properly planned and initiated change can produce the opposite results.

Here's an example of how change that's poorly planned can cause a crisis:

In her new job as director of nursing for a 300-bed community hospital, Janet Green, RN, who recently received an MSN degree, tried to implement several major changes in a very short time. In her first 3 months, she tried to shift the entire nursing staff from a team approach to a primary-nursing approach. Two months later, Janet announced that the nursing department would be reorganized along decentralized lines. As part of this change, Janet indicated that the nursing supervisor position would be eliminated, and that nurses currently in those jobs would be reevaluated and placed in new jobs. Thinking that her staff would welcome the changes as progressive steps in the right direction, Janet neglected to fully involve her management team in either decision, and she didn't ask for any input from other nursing staff. Two weeks after Janet announced the structure change, she received letters of resignation from most of her supervisors and from head nurses and staff as well.

Here's an example of how the lack of change can damage staff morale:

Karen Block, RN, a staff nurse in the delivery unit of a 500-bed urban hospital, angrily told a co-worker, "I can't believe we can't change that dumb rule. This is the 10th single woman we've had in labor this week. These women keep asking for their mother, or sister, or friend to be with them during labor. But we can't let them, because of our fathers-only policy. I've tried for 2 years to get that policy changed." When the co-worker asked why the policy was in effect, Karen said, "I'm told it's to keep the infection rate down and to limit the number of people who'd be in the way in an emergency. But with all the nurses and doctors in and out of the delivery room, one more person wouldn't make that much difference—especially one who'd really support the patient. I think the real issue is the chief of obstetric services—*he* initiated the policy. It'll remain as long as he's here. So much for quality nursing care!" Karen's co-worker sighed in agreement.

Now—here's an example of how change can improve staff morale and efficiency:

Allison Day's first job—as assistant nursing director in a 400-bed hospital—made her responsible for all medical units. Sheila Gray, RN, the charge nurse on a 40-bed medical unit, told Allison that her unit, like many other units, had staffing problems—especially on weekends and evenings. Sheila asked Allison to draw up a unit plan that would allow the staff to develop its own work schedules and to recruit nurses to fill in for staff. Sheila wasn't seeking additional staff; she was asking for a more flexible staffing pattern. All her unit needed was a portion of the hospital's recruitment budget. Allison noted that the plan had appropriate documentation and a method for evaluation. She also considered how efficiently Sheila's unit was run—it had the highest nurse-retention rate among all

# PROBLEM SOLVING THROUGH BRAINSTORMING

Does your unit always seem to be faced with persistent problems that eat away at staff morale or cause staff apathy? If you answer yes, then you're not alone. To surmount such problems, you need to approach problem solving in a logical, creative way.

Invite all staff members affected by the problem to a discussion. Encourage everyone to suggest solutions. If you adopt a nonjudgmental approach, you won't make anyone feel intimidated about offering an idea. If the staff is having problems coming up with ideas, use the categorizing method to stimulate thinking. For example, suppose you want to find out the job-performance problems on your unit. Start by listing all the job-performance categories you can think of—such as salary and benefits, scheduling, work loads, and communication channels. Using categories should help focus staff thinking.

If you think staff members will be afraid to speak out in a group meeting, use the group notebook method instead. How does it work? Put a spiral notebook in a conspicuous place. Write the problem at the top of a clean page—for example, "How can we slow down the increasing staff turnover on the unit?" Then invite the staff to write down any suggestions they have for dealing with the problem. Leave the book out for at least several days. You'll be surprised how staff members' written comments and suggestions will prompt others to offer counter arguments or new ideas, many of them intriguing.

Whichever method you choose—group meeting or group notebook—sift through all of the suggestions on your own, after everyone has had a chance to make one. Select the ideas (even parts of ideas) that seem promising, and try them out.

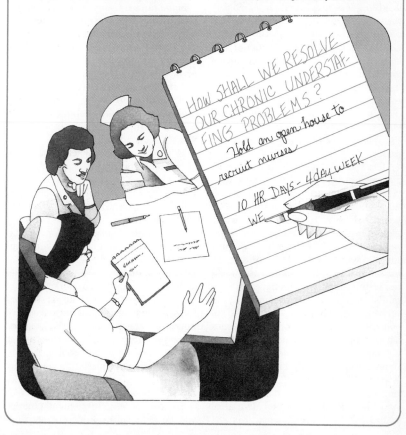

units, and patients there regularly praised the nursing care they received. After meeting with the unit staff, Allison noted that all the nurses had contributed to developing the plan and were committed to it. At the next meeting with the nursing supervisor, Allison presented Sheila's plan and indicated her own support. Within 3 months, the plan was implemented.

## Understanding your options

Change—whether planned or unplanned—is a process that alters behavior. What options do you have regarding that process? Basically, you have three: you can initiate change, you can passively accept change, or you can resist change.

If you're a change initiator, you probably possess these key characteristics: a willingness to take risks; a belief in the value of change; and three kinds of competencies—nursing knowledge, clinical skills, and interpersonal and communication skills. Change initiators tend to be goal-directed and committed to their profession and their institution. Even though change demands a lot of time and energy, as a change initiator you probably welcome the challenge of influencing people and policy.

Here's an example of initiating effective change: Several hospital nurses proposed changing their work schedule from the traditional 8-hour, 5-day workweek to a 10-hour, 4-day workweek. But other nurses, who were mothers, said the change would cause them to worry about their children after school. To satisfy that concern, the nurse-initiators developed a plan to establish a free after-school nursery for nursing-staff children that would be coordinated by the working mothers. Their proposal was accepted.

Some nurses merely accept change—a passive approach that just lets change happen. If this sounds like you or someone you know, stop and think about how "letting things happen" can affect your work. At the very least, this attitude provides no avenue for complaint if you don't like a particular change.

Here's an example of passively accepting change: The administrator at a 350-bed hospital wants to increase the patient census. To do so, she proposes that each unit, regardless of its specialty, will accept any patient, regardless of his illness. The administrator asks each member of the hospital policy committee—representatives from nursing, medicine, dietary, and other departments—to define the problems this change might cause. The nursing director, who represents the nursing staff on the committee, sits back and listens to the others' comments, but doesn't offer any of her own. The result? She must deal with problems she never addressed and winds up complaining about them constantly.

Some nurses choose to resist change, usually for these reasons: They disagree with the change, they have an inaccurate perception of the change, they have a low tolerance for change, or they feel the change threatens their self-interest in some way. Those who feel threatened worry about losing money or job status, about being required to work harder, or about losing valued friendships.

Here's an example where a nurse resists change because she doesn't think it has value: The head nurse in a critical care unit helped shape many of the policies that went into effect when the unit opened 10 years ago. She's respected by her colleagues for her excellent patient care, but she's a change resister. She vigorously tries to maintain the status quo. When two of her staff nurses suggest a policy change based on recent research about site care for a patient receiving total parenteral nutrition, she responds, "We've been providing site care using our technique for years and we've had no major problems. You don't go changing something that works each time a new idea comes along." The idea of change is dropped.

To initiate and implement change, you need to follow a step-by-step approach. The following guide explains 10 practical steps you can take to make change work.

### Step one: Identify the problem correctly

Exactly what's the problem? More change efforts falter at this step than at any other, because nurses fail to understand or fail to carefully define the problem they're tying to solve. For example, after being promoted to head nurse, Lisa Keyes, RN, has become demanding and abrupt—traits she never showed as a staff nurse. What's Lisa's problem? The staff concludes that the

---

*"Nurses who are change initiators tend to be goal-directed and committed to their profession and their institution."*

---

power has gone to her head, and they decide to return her abrupt manner. They don't know that the real problem is that she's frightened about her new responsibilities and doesn't feel equipped to meet them. The staff's negative behavior only compounds the problem.

### Step two: Enlist others who want change

Do others share your desire to bring about change? And are they willing to work for it with you? You'll find that some co-workers want change but aren't willing to contribute to the process. Ideally, you should know from the start how much real support you can count on. Here's an example:

The junior nursing class president called a student meeting to discuss the quality of some of the nursing course lecturers. Most class students attended the meeting, where they planned to hold an open forum with school ad-ministrators to address their concerns. The class president scheduled the forum late in the day so that all program administrators and students could participate. But because most of the students weren't willing to give the time to work for changes, only a handful of students showed up.

You'll be able to help bring about change more easily if you have an effective support group sharing the work. Recruit those who can present your argument for change persuasively—someone who can write, someone who knows her way around the organization and power structure, someone who has influence on the right committees. Once you recruit them, keep them enthusiastic and involved.

### Step three: Gather the facts

Gather data to assist you in identifying the problem's causative or contributing factors as well as its effects on staff, patients, and families. To gather the data you need, ask yourself the following questions:
• What factors have contributed to the development of this problem?
• What are the financial implications of not resolving the problem? (While you may not have all of the financial data you need for this analysis, you can suggest general financial implications of not resolving the problem.)
• What effects has this problem had on staff, on patients, and on patients' families?
• Has this problem raised issues with other departments and disciplines? If so, what are examples of these issues?
• What are the organizational implications of continuing the status quo without resolving this problem?

### Step four: Find a practical solution

Once you accurately diagnose the problem, work with the support group to arrive at a practical solution. How? By brainstorming possible solutions. (See *Problem solving through brainstorming,* page 605.) Compile a list of the

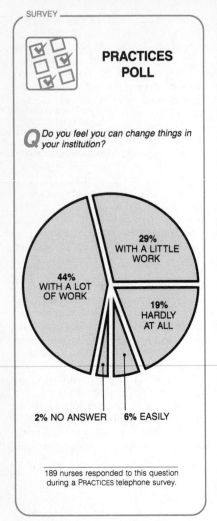

SURVEY

## PRACTICES POLL

**Q** *Do you feel you can change things in your institution?*

29%
WITH A LITTLE
WORK

44%
WITH A LOT
OF WORK

19%
HARDLY
AT ALL

**2% NO ANSWER**     **6% EASILY**

189 nurses responded to this question during a PRACTICES telephone survey.

must know your institution's resources—its power structure and its available materials. Why its power structure? Because you'll never be able to institute lasting change without having access to those who have ultimate responsibility for accepting and implementing new ideas (see Entry 95).

Why must you know your institution's resources? Because those with the power to OK your change will want to know what materials (or personnel) you'll need to implement the change, whether they're available now or have to be purchased (or hired), and the costs involved. You'll be competing for allocations with other individuals and groups, so make careful documentation the cornerstone of your strategy.

### Step six: Plan each step—and choose one course of action

Too many change initiators have good ideas but fail to plan wisely. Develop a course of action to follow, indicating what to do first, second, third, and so on. Then develop alternative plans in case your plan of choice doesn't work. Don't make the mistake of launching several courses of action simultaneously—this causes confusion, wastes energy and resources, and can lead to failure. Also, pursuing several courses at once makes evaluating the effectiveness of any one course very difficult. If your plan of choice doesn't work, try one of your alternative plans.

A practical point to remember: When you choose a solution, start implementing it on a small scale. And remember: You'll stand the best chance of success if you implement it in a unit that's strongly in favor of the change and excited by it.

### Step seven: Choose an effective strategy

Once you've established a plan for change, you need a strategy to implement that plan. Two of the more common strategies are coercion and cooperation. Coercion entails using power or authority to force change. To

suggested solutions that brainstorming yields. Then, examine each solution by asking several questions, such as: What are the risks involved in this solution? Is it feasible in terms of cost, time, resources, and potential obstacles? Will it improve staff morale and productivity, or will it generate resistance? Choose the best solution from among the ones you examine.

### Step five: Define what resources can help you

To succeed in your plan for change, you

use this strategy, you need position power and reward power (see *Recognizing types of power,* page 591). Understandably, this strategy usually breeds resentment and resistance.

Cooperation, the most time-consuming strategy, requires you to use interpersonal skills and open communication techniques. The gains secured by cooperation tend to meet the least resistance and last the longest. You should build into your plan strategies to decrease resistance. For example, include nonnurses—such as doctors—in your support group.

### Step eight: Implement your change
To implement the change, make sure everyone involved clearly understands the new procedures. Spread the word about each bit of success through official channels, such as the institution newsletter, and through the grapevine. Be prepared to iron out any problems that emerge by making adjustments in your plan. Remember, be flexible.

### Step nine: Evaluate the results
Establish evaluation criteria before you initiate the change, as a method for measuring its degree of success. Analyze the change's result by asking the following questions: Was the problem solved? What evidence shows that this happened? Were the best means used to solve the problem?

### Step ten: Make the change stick
Take measures to reinforce and maintain the change. Keep the channels of communication open among co-workers, to minimize any growing resistance to the change. Continue follow-up measures until the change becomes an established part of the system. Remember, unless the change becomes part of everyday routine, you can lose all that you've worked for.

### A final word
To stay abreast of new technologic and managerial developments, nursing must and will change. Don't be reluctant to initiate change when you're convinced that it can yield benefits for patients and staff. But remember, for change to succeed, you must believe in it and be willing to work hard for it.

# 99 Proving you're understaffed (and what to do about it)

Charge nurse Sally Bartley arrived on her unit one morning and learned that two nurses had called in sick. Naturally, she called the nursing office to ask the staffing supervisor to send reinforcements. The supervisor told her that no extra nurses were available. To make matters worse, the supervisor then asked Sally to float one of the nursing assistants from her unit to another floor. Later, when Sally learned that the other unit had fewer patients and more staff on hand than her own unit, she became irate. What's more, the other unit had no absentees and hadn't even requested help!

That evening in the intensive care unit (ICU), five nurses were on duty to care for *only* 15 patients. Though this was the usual evening complement, these nurses felt their unit was and always had been understaffed. They felt they needed at least seven nurses and one nurse's aide to provide proper patient care.

When the staff discussed their concerns with the evening supervisor, she would always point out that some units with 50 patients, more than three times the ICU's census, were covered by only three or four nurses and auxiliary help. Then she'd note that auxiliary staff for the ICU was out of the question because the ICU roster required an all-RN staff on the evening and night shifts.

Do the nurses in these two examples have valid complaints about the balance between the work load and staff

GLOSSARY

## KEY TERMS IN THIS ENTRY

**patient classification systems** • Ways of grouping patients so that the size of the staff needed to care for them can be estimated accurately.

**patient overload/staffing shortage** • The situation that occurs when the number of patients exceeds an institution's medical, nursing, and support-staff resources to care for them properly.

on their respective units? If so, why did the staffing supervisor turn down their requests for help? Would the nurses have been more successful if they had presented their requests differently?

All nurses should consider these questions vitally important, since staff shortages are a chronic concern. If you haven't already experienced problems like Sally Bartley's or the ICU nurses', chances are you will. So read this entry carefully. It will tell you how to prove unit understaffing and get the results you want—for your patients' welfare as well as your own.

## Understanding your administration's approach to staffing

Before you can present accurate and effective proof of understaffing, you should first try to understand your nursing administration's view of staffing in general and the methods it uses to determine what it believes to be adequate staffing. Review your hospital's patient classification systems, budgetary requirements, and staffing alternatives to help you present a more factual and better focused request for your staffing needs. By doing this, you'll be better prepared to counter any arguments administrators may put forth to invalidate your claims.

In the past, hospitals have determined staffing needs for given units based on past experience. Under this system, staffing was based on the occupancy rates of each unit during the previous 6 months or year. The method often wasn't cost-effective because, if the current occupancy rate proved to be less than the previous year's, overstaffing resulted. Or, if occupancy increased over the previous year's rate, understaffing resulted. In addition, this method didn't consider the varying ratio of severely ill patients to moderately ill ones.

To devise new and improved methods for determining staffing needs, hospitals turned to time/motion studies and similar analyses. With these studies, hospitals evaluate a unit's changing needs on a weekly, daily, or even shift-by-shift basis. And the number of patients is no longer the sole indicator of staffing requirements. Instead, patients are classified according to acuteness of illness and the time nurses need to meet each patient's needs. (See Entry 101.)

Hospitals generally use either of two types of patient classification systems to contribute to time/motion studies. With the first type, patient classes are established based on patient-care requirements. Each patient class is assigned a specific number of care hours—the amount of time the nursing staff needs to provide adequate patient care—for each shift or 24-hour period. Equipped with this information, the unit's charge nurse assigns each patient to a class, adds up the number of patients in each class, and multiplies that by the number of greatest patient-care hours assigned to each class. She then adds up the total number of hours for all classes of patients on the unit and divides this overall total by the number of hours in a nurse's normal workday (see *Calculating Nursing-Care Hours*, page 612). The resulting number represents the number of staff or full-time equivalents she needs to provide adequate patient care on the unit. If the hospital has a policy for the use of professional and nonprofessional staff, the nurse will also calculate the correct proportion of RNs to LPNs/LVNs to nursing assistants.

The second type of patient classification system is based on a checklist of particular patient-care requirements and a grading system for each requirement. The charge nurse checks off each patient's care needs, applies predetermined point values to each care need, and adds up the points for each patient. Then, based on patients' point totals, she assigns each patient to a classification that's correlated to the number

---

*"To devise new and improved methods for determining staffing needs, hospitals turned to time/motion studies..."*

---

of nursing-care hours the patient needs. Next, she multiplies the number of patients in each classification by the number of hours assigned to the classification, adds up the total hours for each patient classification, and divides this sum by the number of hours in the workday. The end result is the number of staff required to meet patient-care needs.

Studies have shown both methods to be accurate, although their accuracy, of course, depends on how accurate calculations of the patient-care hours per classification are in the first place. These methods show why the ICU discussed earlier may have more nurses on duty than a gynecologic unit with the same number of patients. The more acute a patient's illness is, the more debilitated a patient is, or the more teaching the patient and his family need, the more nursing care he requires.

## Keeping the budget balanced

Staffing is also influenced by other fac-

tors. Most important: The budget.

The goal of nursing administration is to provide adequate nursing care *efficiently*. Administrators may be unwilling to cut back on admissions during staffing shortages because each filled bed or "patient day" provides the hospital with direct revenue. Administrators also may be unwilling to increase staff during periods of high occupancy because that would increase costs. Most administrators have made understaffing during heavy work periods a policy rather than risk costly overstaffing during lighter work periods.

Administrators have alternatives to understaffing, but they usually prove impractical or costly. For example, when patient loads are excessive, some hospitals request regular staff to work overtime, opt to use per diem staff, or contact supplemental staffing agencies for additional help. From the administrator's viewpoint, however, these are unsatisfactory alternatives because the cost is much more than for routine staffing.

Under extreme circumstances, nursing administrators may choose to cut back on patient services and then to reduce the number of patient-care hours allotted to each patient category. This usually just puts greater pressure on the nurses, who feel they must meet the same number of patient needs in less time.

## What can you do about understaffing?

If you're the charge nurse and you find your unit understaffed, your immediate response is probably the same as Sally Bartley's: to call your staffing supervisor for help. If she says additional help is unavailable, one reaction would be to argue with her about the situation and even threaten to refuse responsibility for an "unsafe" situation.

To avoid adopting this threatening behavior, employ a more effective strategy—a strategy with the long-term goal of minimizing understaffing on your

# CALCULATING NURSING-CARE HOURS

You realize your unit is understaffed, and you want to bring this fact to your administrator's attention. But before you do, you should figure out how many more nurses you need for adequate staffing. To calculate the amount, follow these steps:

### Step 1

Get a copy of your hospital's patient classification system, which categorizes patients by the number of nursing-care hours (NCH) they need each day or each shift. If your hospital doesn't have such a list, here's how to draw one up:

Analyze the care you give your patients. Break down that care into discrete tasks. Determine how much time each task takes to complete. Then, *patient by patient*, take that itemized list and determine how many nursing-care hours each patient needs. Take these totals and divide your patients into classes, as in the following example.

Class I patient needs up to 1 NCH per shift
Class II patient needs between 1 and 2 NCH per shift
Class III patient needs between 2 and 3 NCH per shift

### Step 2

Multiply the number of patients in each classification by the most NCH they need. This figure represents the total NCH your patients require each shift.

| | |
|---|---|
| 25 Class I X 1 hour | = 25 NCH |
| 20 Class II X 2 hours | = 40 NCH |
| 5 Class III X 3 hours | = 15 NCH |
| | 80 NCH |

### Step 3

Now divide the per-shift NCH by 7, the number of NCH hours one full-time nurse provides during a shift, allowing for a meal break. This figure represents the minimal number of nurses your unit needs per shift to meet your patients' needs.

80 NCH ÷ 7 = 11.4 (12 nurses)

unit *before it happens.* Begin by rallying support from your colleagues. Call a meeting with unit staff, your supervisor, and the staffing coordinator. List the attendees and take meeting minutes. At the meeting, review a copy of the hospital's staffing standards and policies. Find out if nurses or their support staff are performing nonnursing responsibilities. Then encourage nurses to air their concerns.

Once you've obtained the basic staffing information you need and identified basic problems, form a committee to develop and present your request for additional staffing. Assign several committee members to obtain information from other hospitals on *their* staffing patterns.

When you're ready to start putting information on paper, remember that management consists predominantly of business people. So you must present your request in their language—numbers. Numbers, especially for business people, put things in black and white. Your task must be to show how your staff's available nursing-care hours fall short of the administration's recommended number to adequately meet patient needs.

Identify patterns in understaffing, too. Does understaffing occur at a certain time of year? On certain shifts? On weekends? If you discover a pattern, try to analyze the reason for it. For example, is staffing allocated unevenly, causing overstaffing on certain days or shifts? Are weekend shifts half-staffed without any supplementation? Does the administration consider staff's vacation days and holidays when they draw up their staffing schedule? Is staff absenteeism a problem?

Once you've discovered a pattern of shorter staffing and learned why it occurs, you must demonstrate the inadequacy of the shorter staffing. Start by listing all nursing tasks and procedures. Indicate the time required to complete each one. Then pinpoint the tasks that are usually left undone, and figure out the number of extra staff

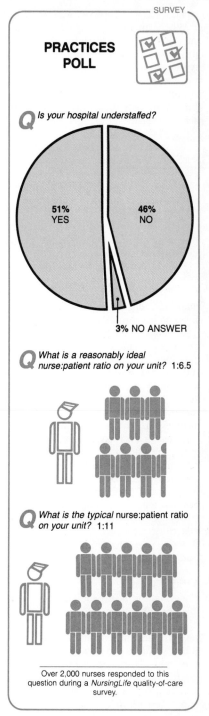

SURVEY

**PRACTICES POLL**

**Q** *Is your hospital understaffed?*

51% YES

46% NO

**3% NO ANSWER**

**Q** *What is a reasonably ideal nurse:patient ratio on your unit?* 1:6.5

**Q** *What is the typical nurse:patient ratio on your unit?* 1:11

Over 2,000 nurses responded to this question during a *NursingLife* quality-of-care survey.

you'd need to complete these tasks.

When you present your request, make sure your timing is right. Don't wait until Saturday afternoon to handle weekend staffing problems. Do it during the week. Likewise, don't discuss summer shortages in May, June, or July. Anticipate the problems, and present your request during the preceding fall and winter months.

Be prepared for counterarguments, such as, "That doesn't have to be done every day," or "That's not necessary on the weekend." Refute these comments with several verifiable anecdotes about patient complaints and incidents, including accidents and errors. You may find that all of these correlate to understaffing periods.

Keep in mind that the auxiliary benefits of solving your unit's staffing problems include easing your own work load and improving working conditions on the unit in general. In the process, you'll stabilize your nursing staff and improve patient care.

Remember, too, that failing to deal with a poor staffing situation, or submitting to the administration's decisions, is legally questionable. By identifying problems and attempting to assure patient-care standards, you'll diminish legal risks on your unit.

If your efforts to get action at the administrative level fail, remember that you have recourse outside the administration. The medical board at your hospital may agree to review your data. If they concur with your conclusion, the board—a powerful ally—can put additional pressure on the administration.

### A final word

Understaffing is a problem that you'll face for some time to come. You must decide how you'll cope with it. Will you be satisfied with what's handed you? If not, be prepared to take constructive problem-solving action to help assure quality health care for your patients—and quality working conditions for you and other health-care team members.

# 100 Indications for involving outside sources

If you have concerns that your employer can't—or won't—address, what can you do? Actually, several sources can give you the help you need. These outside sources give you a place to turn to when your employer's bureaucracy, indifference, or refusal to share power frustrate your efforts to satisfy your concerns.

What kinds of problems can outside sources help you with? You can seek an outside source's help for any of the following:
• when you want more influence over your salary, benefits, and working conditions
• when you have licensing problems or concerns with standards of care
• when you have a complaint about work-place safety
• when you're concerned about patient-care issues, such as patient rights
• when you need information about civil rights and discriminatory practices
• when you need expert legal counsel.

This entry will explain what kinds of outside sources are available to you and what kinds of assistance each can give. You'll also learn criteria for deciding when to use an outside source.

### Always start with your own employer

Whatever concern or problem you have, always look to your own employer, first, for a solution. For the proper ways to do this, check your institution's policies and rules. For example, the personnel department usually has a procedure you can use to file a grievance about working conditions or other matters. Some institutions have a quality review board to address patient-care issues you're concerned about.

Sometimes your institution won't have the resources or the will to help solve your problem. That's when you may need to go outside.

### Knowing the available outside sources

When dealing with problems that your own institution can't solve, you can appeal to a variety of outside sources for help. They can give you information and guidance on specific problems. (For some problems, you'll find you may need to consult more than one outside source.)

The principal outside sources you can use are:

• government agencies (state and federal)
• labor unions
• professional nursing associations (national, state, and specialty)
• legal agencies.

### How government agencies can help you

An array of federal and state agencies have the legal authority to help you in

> *"Use outside sources when your employer's bureaucracy, indifference, or refusal to share power frustrates your efforts to satisfy your concerns."*

significant ways. As you know, each state has a board of nursing that grants licenses to practice and enforces nurse practice acts (see Entries 1 to 4). Your state board will answer your questions about licensure, and it'll tell you what tasks your nurse practice act allows. Some boards of nursing will also review your complaints about patients'-rights violations (in some states, ombudsmen or consumer protection de-

partments do this).

On the federal level, the U.S. Department of Health and Human Services sets standards for hospitals to receive Medicare and Medicaid reimbursements and research funds. This agency will answer questions you have about whether your institution's meeting federal standards.

Several federal agencies regulate work-place practices and policies. For example, the Equal Employment Opportunity Commission will investigate a complaint you have about discriminatory practices in your institution. The Occupational Safety and Health Administration will investigate complaints about unsafe work-place conditions.

The National Labor Relations Board provides information about collective bargaining practices and oversees union elections where you work. The board also conducts hearings on unfair labor practices. (See Entries 47 to 49.)

Your local district attorney's office will investigate any charges you make regarding criminal violations, from patient abuse to phony Medicare reports, occurring in your institution.

You can expect all these agencies to supply information, explain their own

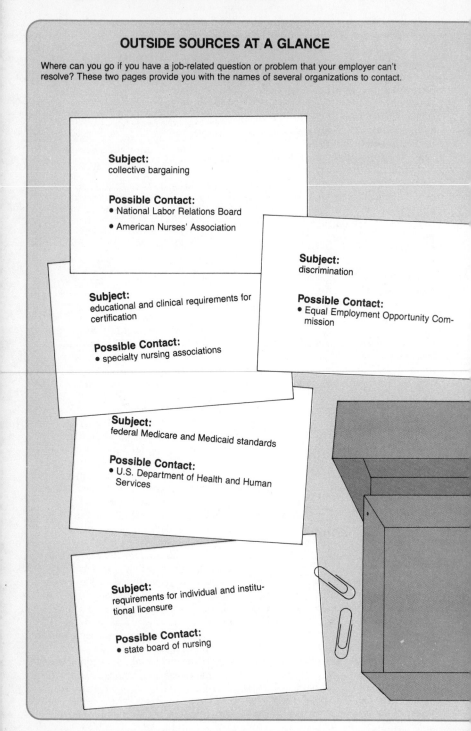

## OUTSIDE SOURCES AT A GLANCE

Where can you go if you have a job-related question or problem that your employer can't resolve? These two pages provide you with the names of several organizations to contact.

**Subject:**
collective bargaining

**Possible Contact:**
- National Labor Relations Board
- American Nurses' Association

**Subject:**
discrimination

**Possible Contact:**
- Equal Employment Opportunity Commission

**Subject:**
educational and clinical requirements for certification

**Possible Contact:**
- specialty nursing associations

**Subject:**
federal Medicare and Medicaid standards

**Possible Contact:**
- U.S. Department of Health and Human Services

**Subject:**
requirements for individual and institutional licensure

**Possible Contact:**
- state board of nursing

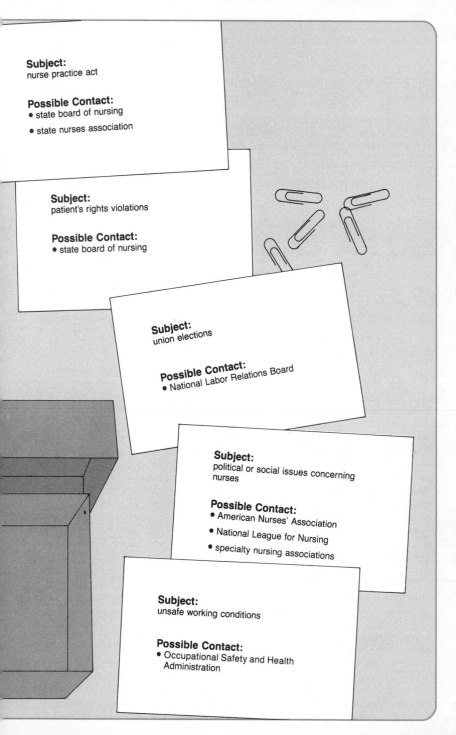

administrative procedures, and explain the law's requirements.

A nongovernment source that nevertheless has enforcement powers is the Joint Commission on the Accreditation of Hospitals (JCAH). (See *Understanding the JCAH,* page 25.) This commission will receive reports or complaints from any nurse who feels the institution where she works has allowed substandard care.

## How labor representation can help you

If you want a greater voice in your institution's policies or an improvement in your economic package, and you don't have a union, consider seeking

---

*"Professional nursing associations help you stay informed about clinical, legal, and ethical issues."*

---

union help. To do so, contact the American Nurses' Association (ANA), or the union that represents nurses at a nearby hospital, to get further information about forming a union (see Entry 47). Some nurses, rather than become affiliated with an established union, prefer to organize their own in-house bargaining unit (see Entry 48). Contact the National Labor Relations Board if you want information on how to do this.

## How professional associations can help you

Professional nursing associations can be very useful outside sources of help. By joining these associations, you'll be able to stay informed about clinical nursing trends as well as legal and ethical issues. You may also receive subscriptions to newsletters and journals as a membership benefit.

These associations give you a voice

in working for change. How? The ANA lobbies Congress—and state nursing associations lobby their state legislatures—to accomplish legislative goals related to nursing. In addition, some state associations serve as collective bargaining agents for nurses, working as their representative in labor negotiations with hospital administrations.

Specialty nursing associations—such as the Association of Operating Room Nurses—represent nurses who practice clinical specialties. In some states, specialty associations have set up boards to certify nurses in the specialty. These boards can tell you about specialty educational and clinical requirements. (See Entry 53.)

Still other professional associations represent nurses' views on national, political, and social issues. For example, nurses concerned about environmental safety have banded together to form Nurses for Environmental Health Watch.

## How legal assistance can help you

Whenever you need legal advice, seek an attorney's counsel. Of course, the most critical need for an attorney arises when a patient sues you for malpractice. Your professional liability insurance company should provide you with an attorney then, but if you don't have insurance or you're unhappy with your defense, you'll have to hire your own attorney (see Entry 42). You can also use an attorney to represent you in hearings before state or federal government agencies, such as a license suspension hearing before your state board of nursing. Your local bar association can often refer you to attorneys who are experienced in medical or labor law.

## A final word

To gain improvements in your professional status and working conditions, and to ensure proper patient care, your first step is always to try to work with your employer. If these efforts fail, however, an outside source of help may be a workable alternative. Of course, reporting your employer to an outside agency may make you uncomfortable. But if serious patient-care issues are involved, your professional (and sometimes legal) duty to your patient may require you to take this action.

## Selected References

Alexander, Edythe L. *Nursing Administration in the Hospital Health Care System,* 2nd ed. St. Louis: C.V. Mosby Co., 1978.

Althaus, Joan N., et al. *Nursing Decentralization: The El Camino Experience.* Rockville, Md.: Aspen Systems Corp., 1981.

Bailey, June T., and Claus, Karen E. *Decision Making in Nursing: Tools for Change.* St. Louis: C.V. Mosby Co., 1975.

Beyers, Marjorie, and Phillips, Carole. *Nursing Management for Patient Care,* 2nd ed. Boston: Little, Brown & Co., 1979.

Bowman, R.A., and Culpepper, R.C. "Power: Rx for Change," *American Journal of Nursing* 74:1053-56, June 1974.

Donovan, Helen M. *Nursing Service Administration: Managing the Enterprise.* St. Louis: C.V. Mosby Co., 1975.

Edwards, Barbara J., and Brilhart, John K. *Communications in Nursing Practice.* St. Louis: C.V. Mosby Co., 1981.

Ganong, Warren L., and Ganong, Joan M. *Nursing Management,* 2nd ed. Rockville, Md.: Aspen Systems Corp., 1980.

Gillies, Dee A. *Nursing Management: A Systems Approach.* Philadelphia: W.B. Saunders Co., 1982.

Hayne, A., and Warren-Bailey, Z. *Nursing Administration of Critical Care.* Rockville, Md.: Aspen Systems Corp., 1982.

Johnson, G.V., and Tingey, S. "Matrix Organization: Blueprint of Nursing Care Organization for the 80s," *Hospital and Health Services Administration* 21:27-37, Winter 1976.

Kalisch, Beatrice J., and Kalisch, Philip A. *Politics of Nursing.* New York: J.B. Lippincott Co., 1981.

Langford, Teddy. *Managing and Being Managed: Preparation for Professional Nursing Practice.* Englewood Cliffs, N.J.: Prentice-Hall, 1981.

O'Brien, Maureen. *Communications and Relationships in Nursing,* 2nd ed. St. Louis: C.V. Mosby Co., 1978.

Rowland, H., and Rowland, B. *Nursing Administration Handbook.* Rockville, Md.: Aspen Systems Corp., 1980.

Smith, Leslie E. "Turning Negative Behavior Around: Realistic Ways to Motivate People Who Cause You Problems," *NursingLife* 3(2):17-23, March/April 1983.

Stevens, Barbara J. *First-Line Patient Care Management,* 2nd ed. Rockville, Md.: Aspen Systems Corp., 1982.

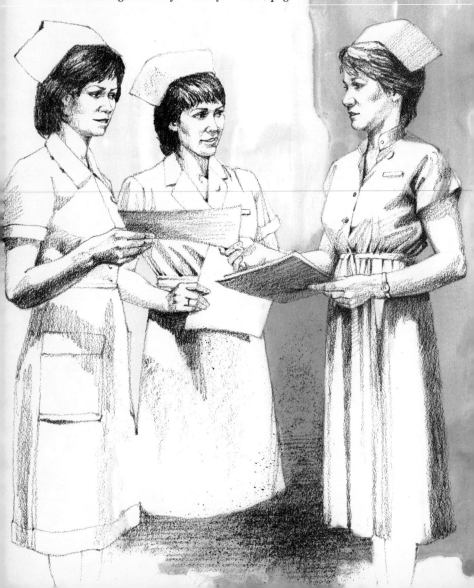

# 16

# Help for the New Manager

## Introduction

Congratulations! You've just been promoted. Of course, you're delighted that your superiors have recognized your abilities and your potential. They've surely considered the quality of your education, your clinical expertise, your communication skills, and your initiative, and decided that you're right for the job. But you're concerned, too. You wonder if you're really equipped to handle the responsibilities and challenges that come with being a nurse manager. You know that being a manager isn't an easy job! You've seen a number of capable nurses struggle to succeed in this new role. But you're eager to give your new responsibilities a try.

Well, here's good news: With some basic preparation, some foresight, and an awareness of the legal and professional aspects of being a nurse manager, you can be as effective a manager as you were a staff nurse. When problems arise, you can rely on many of the skills you developed as a staff nurse, particularly your problem-solving and communication skills. But you also need to develop *problem-preventing* skills that will help your unit run smoothly and efficiently.

And you will have problems. Some of them may have serious legal as well as professional ramifications. For example, what will you do if several nurses call in sick on a holiday weekend? Or imagine that a staff nurse leaves an infant off a cardiac and apnea monitor. The mistake is detected and corrected quickly—but you must discipline the nurse who made it and recommend appropriate inservice education for her. How will you handle the situation? Here's another tough problem: A doctor confronts you about baby John's parents, who are dissatisfied with the care that your nurses gave him on the 3 p.m. to 11 p.m. shift. They're not just dissatisfied—they're *mad.* You, not the nurse who cared for the child, must meet with the doctor and the parents. What will you say to them?

This chapter tells you how to resolve problems like these and prevent similar problems from happening. And it helps you put your legal and professional responsibilities as a manager in perspective.

### What the new manager needs to know

The entries in this chapter discuss a variety of important concerns. You'll find that, along with practical suggestions for resolving management problems, each entry incorporates guidelines for identifying their legal and professional significance.

Patient classification systems are a

primary concern of the new manager. If you understand the philosophy behind them and use them properly, these systems can help you manage effectively and improve the quality of nursing care on your unit. In Entry 101, "Understanding patient classification systems," you'll learn about the advantages and disadvantages of the various types of patient classification systems. This entry also clarifies your responsibility—and your staff's—for implementing an appropriate classification system effectively.

> *"Remember to encourage your staff to share with you ideas they may have on improving the unit's functioning."*

Staffing, of course, is another major concern for the nurse manager. Entry 102, "Understanding staffing patterns," offers some fresh suggestions for planning, implementing, and evaluating your unit's staffing needs.

Your next steps in taking charge are evaluating the patient-care delivery system in use on your unit and considering whether any changes would improve patient care. Entry 103, "Understanding patient-care delivery systems," explores the advantages and disadvantages of four patient-care delivery systems. You'll also learn the steps necessary to implement and maintain each system and to evaluate its effectiveness.

### Establishing productive relationships

Once you've put your unit's basic operational mechanisms in gear, you'll have time—and you'll need it!—for establishing productive relationships with your staff. You can probably foresee certain interpersonal problems

connected with your promotion. Staff reactions are bound to differ—and some will be negative. Entry 104, "When you're promoted," discusses the kinds of immediate reactions, lingering feelings, and possible problems that you can anticipate in staff members who were once your peers. The entry presents a five-faceted practical approach to effectively integrating yourself into your new nurse-manager role.

As you probably know, competent delegation to subordinates can significantly increase your effectiveness as a manager. Entry 105, "The art of delegating," explores the problems some managers have with delegating—and shows you how to become adept at this important managerial technique.

Entry 106, "Making staff assignments effectively," emphasizes your responsibility for assigning staff only on the basis of their legally and professionally accepted scope of practice. This entry stresses the risks involved in assigning staff on any other basis— for example, assigning an LPN, because she's available and an RN isn't, to do a task only an RN should do. Making assignments this way invites problems with giving good patient care—and invites legal action, too, if a patient's injured while in the care of an improperly assigned staff member.

Entry 107, "How to discipline effectively," discusses various leadership styles and the current trend toward increased staff participation in leadership responsibilities. An informative, step-by-step guide to effective discipline, this entry will increase your confidence in situations when you must discipline staff members.

As a manager, you'll probably experience periods when you simply don't have enough time to do all you should. If this happens too frequently to suit you, some advice on how to make the most of your time can help. Entry 108, "Effective time management," will tell you how to use your time efficiently and how to evaluate and improve your staff's use of time.

Because staff morale profoundly affects both productivity and quality of care on the unit, you're responsible for making sure that morale on your unit remains high. Entry 109, "Motivation and morale: Keys to successful management," describes morale-building techniques and proven ways of motivating staff. The entry also provides strategies for diagnosing and treating problems with morale and motivation.

Once you're on good terms with your staff and familiar with their attitudes and capabilities, you can begin to consider ways to help them grow and be even more productive. One way to do this is by promoting staff members' autonomy—their ability to function independently. Entry 110, "Promoting autonomy within your staff," tells you how to use nursing diagnosis and the nursing process as tools to develop your staff's autonomy and increase their professional accountability.

## A final word

Most staff nurses who are promoted to management positions become highly effective nurse managers. But the transformation doesn't happen overnight. It takes place gradually as a nurse manager acquires the necessary skills, applies them to the management of her unit's activities, and learns from her successes and mistakes.

Through trial and error, you'll discover which management techniques work—and don't work—for you. Don't be discouraged when, occasionally, your best efforts fail. This happens to every good manager once in a while. Just discontinue the unproductive activity and try something else you think may work; you're sure to find something that's right for your staff and you. Remember to encourage your staff to share with you ideas they may have on improving the unit's functioning.

Being a nurse manager means more than just keeping the unit running well. It also means striving to fulfill your own and your staff's fullest professional potential.

# 101 Understanding patient classification systems

As you probably know, a patient classification system is a method of grouping patients on a unit according to how much nursing care they need. To determine this, you must assess each patient's needs, using indicators such as daily living activities, treatments, medications, teaching time, and psychosocial factors. Then you place the patient in the appropriate patient-care classification. Once you've done this for all patients on the unit, you can use one of two systems—the prototype evaluation system or the factor evaluation system—to determine the number of staff nurses you need.

Why is patient classification used? One reason is that evaluating the care your patients need can help document the need for additional professional staff on your unit. But perhaps the main reason is to help hold down rising health-care costs.

During the past 30 years or so, as health-care costs have risen, hospital administrators have continually evaluated how to use their resources most efficiently. Because their most expensive resource is personnel—specifically *nursing* personnel—they've zeroed in on cost-effective ways of providing nursing care.

In 1956, Johns Hopkins University Hospital approached this problem by developing a three-tiered system for classifying patients according to the amount of nursing time they required. Since then, patient classification systems have been widely accepted. Health-care institutions have continued to develop new and better systems, and in 1980, the Joint Commission on Accreditation of Hospitals (JCAH) began requiring that institutions base their master staffing plans on patient

GLOSSARY

## KEY TERMS IN THIS ENTRY

**factor evaluation** • A way of classifying patients by calculating the amount and type of care each patient needs.

**prototype evaluation** • A way of classifying patients by using a form that describes typical characteristics of several groups of patients.

classification systems.

Patient classification also provides a method for documenting the relationships among the care a patient needs, the quality of care he receives, and the cost of the care he receives. As you probably know, private and public third-party payers require this information.

### Understanding common types of systems

Two types of classification systems exist: prototype evaluation and factor evaluation. With a *prototype evaluation* system, you use a form that describes typical characteristics of patients in each of several classifications. After reading these descriptions, you match your patient with the appropriate category. This type of system is quick and easy to use. However, it has some disadvantages. First, the classification process must be highly subjective, because the classification descriptions are broad and poorly defined. Second, the system can be manipulated to show an apparent need for additional staff. Finally, most prototype systems don't allow time for dealing with a patient's psychosocial needs or for teaching a patient about his condition.

With the *factor evaluation* system, you use a checklist that assigns numeric values to many possible patient-care needs. After you identify the specific needs that apply to your patient,

you add up the corresponding values. When you have this sum, you look at a conversion chart to find your patient's classification. This type of system provides a more objective means of classifying patients, and it also allows time for meeting a patient's psychosocial needs. However, it takes more time to use, and is more cumbersome, than the prototype evaluation system.

### Understanding classification's benefits

A patient classification system allows a nurse manager to use her nursing staff efficiently and effectively. How? By predicting the number of nurses she'll need to meet patient-care requirements and by providing a productivity goal for the nursing unit. She can make accurate staffing assignments, monitor monthly productivity, plan long-term staffing and budgets, and discuss her unit's plans and problems knowledgeably with hospital administrators.

A patient classification system also makes staffing less complicated for the nurse manager. That means she has more time to manage employees and provide patient care. In fact, a classification system that's begun as a way to plan staffing can gradually become a quality assessment tool. For example, it can help a nurse manager discover that certain tasks her nurses perform should be assigned to other personnel or departments. Or it can help her identify inefficient use of staff or facilities.

If the system's used to ensure an adequate staff, then each nurse will be responsible for a fairly distributed portion of the workload and will have sufficient time to provide the required patient care. Obviously, staff morale improves when each nurse knows what's expected of her and is given sufficient time to accomplish it (see Entry 109).

Overall, a patient classification system helps improve the quality of care. That's because it helps ensure that:
• nurses get the proper amount of time to provide care

• nurses have a guide to implementing the nursing process—particularly assessment and care-plan implementation

• patient care is of consistently high quality. How does a patient classification system ensure this? By providing the means for auditing that care.

### Problems with classification

Problems with patient classification systems can stem from nurses' perceptions of them. Some nurses view classification as a time-consuming mathematical exercise that takes them away from their patients. Many staff nurses feel that using their own professional judgment is better than using a classification system. Other nurses say that no system can accurately measure their time and the value of their care.

Still other nurses criticize patient classification systems because, they say, the systems can't predict staffing needs in an unanticipated crisis, or can't guarantee an adequate supply of nurses to meet patient-care demands. Perhaps, other nurses counter, these aren't realistic expectations of any system.

Insufficient funds or a chronic shortage of nurses can hinder implementing and maintaining any system. To work properly, a patient classification system requires constant monitoring by the first-line manager—in particular, to prevent manipulation that could indicate a false need for increased numbers of nurses. The management team must be committed to the system, or else it *can* become a meaningless, time-consuming paper exercise.

Problems often arise because a manager doesn't explain the system fully. The staff nurses may therefore view it simply as "something to keep management happy." Or they may see it as a means of increasing their work load, particularly if they feel that the expectations the system produces aren't realistic, because they're based on averages and don't account for day-to-day variations in patient needs.

For a patient classification system to work, management must be committed to using it. This includes understanding staff concerns and trying to resolve them.

### Understanding the legal aspects

A classification system can provide legal protection for a hospital—or proof of liability. Why? Because both systems require documentation of how much patient care is needed and how much is delivered. If a hospital uses a classification system but doesn't have the staff to make it work properly, it can actually document its own liability. As a nurse manager, remember this when you document the amount of care your patients require. Your hospital and you are responsible for delivering it.

### A final word

Because they provide the only reliable way to estimate staffing needs, patient classification systems are here to stay. And third-party payers and hospital boards will continue to require nursing departments to prove they're using their staff efficiently.

Whether you're a staff nurse or a manager, you have a responsibility for helping your system work. Take the initiative to understand the system, and make a professional commitment to use it. Encourage your colleagues or subordinates to use the system correctly and help prevent manipulation. When appropriate, suggest ways of improving it, and serve on committees that formally evaluate it. Remember, the system will work if *you* help make it work.

# 102 Understanding staffing patterns

Can you name a policy at work that has a more dramatic day-to-day impact on your life than staffing patterns? Consider this: Staffing patterns determine what weekdays you and your unit's staff

GLOSSARY

## KEY TERMS IN THIS ENTRY

**flexible staffing patterns** • Work schedules that vary—for example, 10- and 12-hour shifts, shorter workweeks, and special weekend schedules.

**traditional staffing patterns** • Work schedules that follow 8-hour shifts, 7 days a week, including evening and night shifts.

work, what holidays and weekends you work, what hours and shifts you work, and how many patients you're responsible for when you work. In a 1981 *RN* magazine poll of 13,000 nurses, approximately 69% said they considered adequate staffing patterns a crucial job issue. Among nurses in their first year of practice, that figure jumped to approximately 80%. So how institutions are staffed deeply affects not only nurses' professional practice, but their personal lives as well.

Staffing patterns that show little regard for your (and your staff's) concerns and interests prevent all of you from satisfactorily balancing your work obligations and your home life. At work, for example, understaffing can lead to an unreasonable work pace and keep you from giving quality patient care (see Entries 19 and 99). At home, the fatigue and stress that poor staffing patterns cause can prevent full enjoyment of your time with your family and friends.

The increasing popularity of agency nursing, which offers flexible working hours, indicates the importance nurses attach to staffing patterns. (For more information about agency nursing, see Entry 10.) Many nurses turn down full-time positions, giving up certain employment benefits, to work through agencies and be able to choose their own work hours. Why? Because of dissatisfaction with their institutions' traditional staffing patterns. These

institutions typically schedule nurses in 8-hour shifts, 7 days a week. Two thirds of these shifts, of course, are the evening and night shifts, which are difficult to staff because they're incompatible with the standard 9-to-5 schedule most other professionals enjoy. And many nurses must also work weekends and holidays—another source of discontent. This traditional staffing pattern can cause fatigue and even burnout (see Entry 68), leading to high staff turnover rates. Those nurses who remain on the job must sometimes work overtime and double shifts—under even more intense stress. Problems with traditional staffing patterns place burdens on employers, too, who must spend additional funds for recruitment and orientation and for temporary supplemental nursing staff.

## Understanding flexible staffing patterns

Recently, recognizing the problems that traditional staffing patterns can cause, some health-care institutions have begun using *flexible staffing patterns*. These include 10- and 12-hour shifts, shorter workweeks, and special weekend scheduling. When staffing patterns are flexible, everyone—nurses, patients, and employers—can benefit. Perhaps most important, these benefits can mean better patient care. For example, because flexible staffing patterns reduce nurse turnover rates, continuity of care improves. And fewer nursing errors occur because nurses' fatigue is reduced and so is employers' need for temporary supplemental staff—whose unfamiliarity with the employers' policies and methods, as you know, can cause errors. Finally, flexible staffing patterns give you more time to plan, so your patients benefit from careful preparation and coordination of their care.

## Considering nurse : patient ratios

Health-care institutions have also begun to appreciate another aspect of staffing patterns—nurse:patient ratios. To determine appropriate nurse:patient ratios, employers have developed *patient classification systems* (see Entry 101) to measure the amount of nursing care each patient requires. When this information is converted into the actual number of RNs, LPNs/LVNs, and nursing assistants needed to provide care for patients in specific classifications, employers can develop staffing patterns that match patient-care needs with the corresponding number and mix of nursing personnel.

### Does your unit need a new staffing pattern?

Every staffing pattern has problems. And some nurses prefer traditional 8-hour shift staffing patterns because they

---

*"How institutions are staffed deeply affects not only nurses' professional practice but their personal life-style as well."*

---

don't want to work longer hours. So before you conclude that your unit needs a different staffing pattern, consider these guidelines:

• *Determine if your current staffing system needs changing.* To do this, collect data on its advantages and disadvantages. Survey all staff (if possible, include former staff members) for their opinions about staffing and scheduling problems. Find out if they feel that rotating shifts and weekend assignments are distributed fairly. Do some nurses frequently work consecutive shifts? How much time off do they have between shifts? Does the staffing pattern allow nurses to predict future days off? Does it provide flexibility for time-off requests and sick calls?

• *Check the status of such job-satisfaction indicators* as turnover rates and absenteeism rates.

• *Tabulate the amount of resources used to maintain the current staffing pattern.* Resources include the number of full-time and part-time positions budgeted for the unit as well as the time and money spent managing for supplemental staff, such as agency nurses.

• *Calculate your nursing staff's average "down time" during the year.* To do this, figure the average vacation time, number of paid holidays, and number of paid sick days a typical nurse on your staff uses during the year. This will probably add up to four or five weeks. Multiply this number by the number of RNs, then LPNs/LVNs, and then nursing assistants on your staff to *determine the number of weeks in a year when your staff will be short at least one RN, LPN/LVN, or nursing assistant.* For example, 5 weeks times 10 RNs equals 50 weeks. This calculation also shows, of course, the average productive time—the time when they're present and working—of the staff on your unit. These calculations will be of considerable value when you're assessing the effectiveness of your unit's present staffing pattern.

• *Document your unit's use of supplemental staffing agencies* and float personnel to maintain the present staffing pattern.

• *Find out how your staffing alternatives are restricted* by laws, departmental policies, and union contracts.

• *Remember that patients' needs take priority over all other considerations.* Is your unit's present staffing pattern facilitating high-quality patient care? If it is, maybe you shouldn't consider changing it.

### How to change a staffing pattern

Once you've accumulated the information you need to assess your unit's staffing pattern, carefully consider what you've learned. Does it indicate that the staffing pattern's unpopular—maybe unfair? If it does, you may be able to get the pattern changed by presenting your conclusions to your nurse manager, along with recommendations for solutions (and the rationale behind your recommendations). (See *Comparing Staffing Patterns*.)

When you recommend a new staffing pattern, use the same criteria that you used to identify the present pattern's problems. These criteria include the

costs to maintain the new schedule and the expected benefits in recruitment and in retaining staff. Remember, however, that you won't be able to guarantee your recommendations will result in improvement. Only after the new staffing pattern's implemented will you be able to measure its results.

To implement a new staffing pattern,

## COMPARING STAFFING PATTERNS

| STAFFING PATTERN | HOW PATTERN WORKS |
|---|---|
| 10-hour shift | • Nurse works four 10-hour shifts a week (for example, 8 a.m. to 6 p.m.)<br>• One 8-hour shift (for example, 4 p.m. to 12) to ensure coverage in 24-hour period—overlaps 10-hour shifts |
| 12-hour shift (first version) | • Nurse works three 12-hour shifts one week and four 12-hour shifts the following week<br>• Nurse receives 4 hours of overtime pay |
| 12-hour shift (second version) | • Nurse works four 8-hour shifts one week, 12-hour shifts on the weekend, and three 8-hour shifts the following week, with the 2nd weekend off<br>• Nurse receives 8 hours of overtime pay for 12-hour weekend shifts |
| Baylor plan | • Involves two groups of nurses: one group works 12-hour shifts every weekend; other group works 8-hour shifts every weekday<br>• The weekend day shift receives 32 hours of pay for 24 hours of work; the weekend night shift receives 40 hours of pay for 24 hours of work |

adopt a pilot plan—a trial plan that you'll test over a specific period of time. Confine the new staffing pattern to a small group, at first, to provide a comparison with the old pattern and to keep close control of how well the new one's working. Be sure you tell all the staff about the changes before you implement them. Emphasize that the pilot plan is a trial effort. Encourage everyone to give the new staffing pattern a fair trial, and invite them to make suggestions for improvement. As part of your new staffing pattern, develop contingency plans to counter absenteeism and any other predictable setbacks that could affect the new staffing pattern's success.

| ADVANTAGES | DISADVANTAGES |
|---|---|
| • Allows nurse 1 extra day off each week<br>• Provides unit with additional personnel for 2 hours during shift overlaps<br>• Improves patient-care continuity | • Increases institution's short-term costs<br>• Requires nurse managers to devise schedules giving staff 3 days off each week<br>• Requires scheduling one 8-hour shift because two nonoverlapping 10-hour shifts leave 4 hours of workday uncovered<br>• Lengthens work day |
| • Allows nurse 3 extra days off in a 2-week period<br>• Eliminates third shift<br>• Improves patient-care continuity | • Increases institution's costs for overtime pay<br>• Requires nurse managers to devise schedules giving staff the extra days off (2 extra days the 1st week, and 1 extra day the next week)<br>• Lengthens work day |
| • Allows nurse 1 extra day off each 2-week period<br>• Eliminates third shift<br>• Improves patient-care continuity | • Increases institution's costs for overtime pay<br>• Requires nurse managers to devise schedules to cover extra days off<br>• Lengthens work day |
| • Provides incentive for nurses to work weekends<br>• Provides incentive for nurses who want weekends off<br>• Eliminates third shift on weekends | • Increases personnel costs<br>• Decreases patient-care continuity because of weekday/weekend split |

**A final word**
For too long, health-care institutions planned staffing patterns without regard to the schedules' effects on nurses' jobs and life-styles. But now, acknowledging the connection between job satisfaction and staffing patterns, many institutions are encouraging innovative staffing-pattern changes. If you believe your unit's staffing pattern must be changed, take the initiative.

Remember, no single staffing pattern will satisfy everyone. Matching your staff's and your patients' needs requires a willingness to compromise. For example, although many nurses want to work 10-hour shifts, some can't—because of family commitments, or for other reasons. When conflicts develop over staffing patterns, they must be resolved quickly, before they produce discord, and patient-care needs should always take priority. After all, a staffing pattern that's convenient for nurses can't be considered successful unless it also serves patients' needs. And an effective staffing pattern must also meet your institution's needs. Be sure to keep these requirements in mind when you're recommending innovative changes.

# 103 Understanding patient-care delivery systems

If you're like most nurses, how much you (and your staff) enjoy working is strongly affected by the kind of patient-care delivery system your institution uses. Why? Because the system you work under influences:
• your work load
• your opportunity to give quality care
• your ability to implement health teaching and discharge planning
• your institution's and your unit's in-service education policies
• your access to resource persons

• your unit's staffing patterns.

As you know, health-care institutions can choose from four basic systems to deliver patient care: the case system, the functional (task-oriented) system, the team system, and the primary nursing system (see *Selecting a Patient-Care Delivery System,* pages 632 and 633); sometimes a combination of primary and team nursing proves effective. These four systems differ in several important ways. Because of this, your degree of job satisfaction can suffer if you're not comfortable with your institution's choice.

What happens when a patient-care delivery system conflicts with your training or personal nursing philosophy? Here's an illustrative example: Barbara Clayton, RN, newly graduated with a bachelor's degree, accepted a job on a 40-bed orthopedic unit where functional nursing was the delivery system used. Assigned as a medication nurse, Barbara worked hard to fit into the system. But she found this difficult because the system conflicted with the holistic philosophy of direct patient care that she learned at school. In spite of this, however, she at first felt that her oft-repeated service as the medicine and treatment nurse on the day shift and the charge nurse on night shift was giving her valuable training and improving her skills. But after several months on the job, she realized she'd become more concerned with dispensing medications than with assessing her patients' need for medication, and with checking I.V. drip rates than with patient teaching and discharge planning. She soon realized that her head nurse and nurse manager, who she'd thought *were* doing patient teaching and discharge planning, weren't. In fact, they seemed more removed from these concerns than *she* was!

Before long, Barbara grew very uncomfortable with what she perceived as the delivery system's impersonal nature. When she realized that the delivery system didn't match her expectations of how a nurse should give care, she found another job where the patient-care delivery system was more compatible with her own ideas of nursing practice.

Besides nursing staff turnover because of job dissatisfaction, other indications of an inefficient patient-care delivery system include insufficient patient-care continuity and persistent patient complaints about lack of attention. An indication of a failing delivery system is nurse managers who spend

> *"Your degree of job satisfaction can suffer if you're not comfortable with your institution's patient-care delivery system."*

more time juggling staffing patterns than providing needed supervision and inservice education to improve the quality of patient care.

### Assessing the system you're using now

To assess whether you should recommend changing your present patient-care delivery system, follow these guidelines:

● *Evaluate your institution's nursing philosophy, authority, structure, and decision-making processes.* Do these favor the probable success of one system over the others? For example, to implement primary nursing, your institution would have to encourage the kind of decentralized decision-making among nurses that primary nursing requires. (See *Selecting a Patient-Care Delivery System*, pages 632 and 633.)

● *Find out how many nurses your institution employs* in its various units, as well as its mix of educational and experience levels. You need a sufficient number of properly educated nurses to implement certain systems. For example, if a 30-bed adolescent unit has a few RNs, several LPNs or LVNs, and a half dozen aides, this staffing capability allows use of only the functional or team systems.

● *Assess your institution's adaptability and flexibility.* Are the nursing, medical, and administrative staffs generally receptive to new ideas and innovative solutions to problems?

● *Consider the patient population.* Is the present system for delivery of care in use because the patient population requires it? Would another delivery system provide the care this population needs? For example, if you work in a 20-bed cancer unit where discharge planning and individualized continuity of care are emphasized, and primary nursing is the patient-care delivery system now in use, you probably shouldn't consider changing to another system. Why? Because primary nursing fits the philosophy of care in your unit.

### Avoiding pitfalls when implementing patient-care delivery systems

Certain pitfalls exist that can undermine your best intentions when you at-

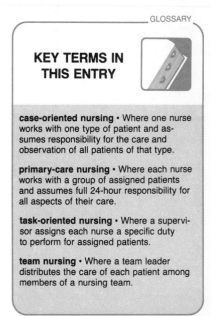

GLOSSARY

## KEY TERMS IN THIS ENTRY

**case-oriented nursing** • Where one nurse works with one type of patient and assumes responsibility for the care and observation of all patients of that type.

**primary-care nursing** • Where each nurse works with a group of assigned patients and assumes full 24-hour responsibility for all aspects of their care.

**task-oriented nursing** • Where a supervisor assigns each nurse a specific duty to perform for assigned patients.

**team nursing** • Where a team leader distributes the care of each patient among members of a nursing team.

## SELECTING A PATIENT-CARE DELIVERY SYSTEM

Which patient-care delivery system should you select to use on your unit? Your choice depends on your circumstances. Ask your hospital administrator which system the hospital prefers. The information below describes each system.

| DELIVERY SYSTEM | DESCRIPTION | ACCOUNTABILITY FOR PATIENT CARE |
|---|---|---|
| Case-oriented nursing | • Based on holistic philosophy of nursing<br>• Nurse is responsible for care and observation of specific patients<br>• Uses 1-to-1 nurse : patient ratio | • Nurse manager's responsibility |
| Task-oriented nursing | • Based on task-oriented philosophy of nursing<br>• Nurse performs specific nursing tasks according to charge nurse's schedule | • Charge nurse's responsibility |
| Team nursing | • Based on group philosophy of nursing<br>• Six or seven professional and nonprofessional personnel work as a team—supervised by a team leader | • Team nurse leader's responsibility |
| Primary-care nursing | • Based on comprehensive, personal philosophy of nursing<br>• Nurse is responsible for all aspects of care—from assessing patient's condition to coordinating his care—for specific patients<br>• Uses 1-to-1 nurse : patient ratio and case-method assignments | • Nurse manager's responsibility |

tempt to implement a new patient-care delivery system. To avoid these pitfalls, follow these recommendations:

• *Include the staff in planning,* whether you're improving an existing delivery system or changing the system entirely. Inform everyone of the system's methods and goals. The surest route to system failure is excluding your subordinates in the planning phase.

• *Develop job descriptions for all nursing positions before the system's implemented.* You can amend the job descriptions later if necessary, but you must have them in place before the system gets underway. They provide the required structure and direction for both the staff and the managers.

• *Plan evaluations and nursing audits* to diagnose problems quickly and manage them effectively.

• *Strive to create a system that enhances nurses' job satisfaction.* For example, provide rewards for competent performance, and show confidence in the staff's independent decision-making skills.

• *Evaluate the delivery system contin-*

| NURSE MANAGER'S ROLE | ADVANTAGES | DISADVANTAGES |
|---|---|---|
| • Recruits self-directed nurses<br>• Provides resource network for staff nurses<br>• Directs inservice education | • Improves nurse's responsiveness to patient's changing needs<br>• Improves continuity of care<br>• May increase nurse's job satisfaction | • Increases personnel costs |
| • Manages communications problems<br>• Motivates staff (because of limited dimensions of jobs) | • Reduces personnel costs<br>• Supports cost controls | • Fragments nursing care<br>• May decrease job satisfaction<br>• Decreases personal contact with patient<br>• Limits continuity of care |
| • Recruits nurses with leadership ability<br>• Serves as a resource person<br>• Helps plan inservice education | • Supports comprehensive care<br>• May increase job satisfaction<br>• Increases cost effectiveness | • Decreases personal contact with patient<br>• Limits continuity of care |
| • Allows staff appropriate independence<br>• Recruits more educated and sophisticated staff<br>• Serves as resource person | • May increase job satisfaction<br>• Improves continuity of care<br>• Allows independent decision making<br>• Supports direct nurse : patient communication<br>• Encourages discharge planning<br>• Improves quality of care<br>• May increase cost effectiveness when comparing nurses aides' and LPNs' "down time" | • Increases personnel costs initially<br>• Requires properly trained nurses to carry out system's principles<br>• Restricts opportunity for evening and night shift nurses to participate |

*ually* for effectiveness and efficiency. Devise ways to measure and monitor the system's cost.

• *Make sure you staff the delivery system adequately.* Understaffing will harm any system's chance of success. Here's an example: Nurses for a 14-bed intensive-care nursery planned and developed a primary nursing delivery system. The nurses felt so enthusiastic and confident that they decided to proceed with the new system even though the administration approved staffing that omitted two evening and two night nursing positions. After a 6-month period, the staff abandoned the new system. What happened? You can probably guess: the severe understaffing forced the nurses to work longer hours and sometimes double shifts. The excessive work pace simply left them exhausted. The system might have been successful if the nurses had insisted that each shift be staffed adequately before the new system was implemented.

### A final word
The patient-care delivery system you

use on your unit is closely linked to your staff's degree of job satisfaction. Take the time now to examine both. If your staff seems happy, the delivery system probably isn't a problem. What if they're unhappy? The delivery system may be contributing to the problem. In this situation, you have two choices: You can try to change the system, or you may have to change staff. Whatever you do, never lose sight of your constant goal as a nurse manager: to provide the highest quality patient care.

# 104 When you're promoted

If you just found out you've been promoted to head nurse or manager in your unit, of course you feel proud and happy. But if you're like most nurses, you're probably also concerned about making the transition from staff to management.

This transition can be challenging—especially because supervising your friends and former co-workers can be difficult at first. You can make this transition more smoothly if you identify

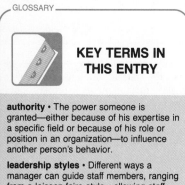

GLOSSARY

**KEY TERMS IN THIS ENTRY**

**authority** • The power someone is granted—either because of his expertise in a specific field or because of his role or position in an organization—to influence another person's behavior.

**leadership styles** • Different ways a manager can guide staff members, ranging from a laissez-faire style—allowing staff members freedom to make decisions—to an authoritative style.

problems early and find ways to deal with them effectively.

## Understanding your co-workers' initial reactions

When your supervisors announce your promotion, many of your co-workers will wish you well. But don't be surprised if some have a quite different reaction to your success.

For example, think about the co-workers who applied for the same position. They probably won't completely share your happiness. In fact, some of them may be jealous and resentful. Other co-workers may simply be apprehensive: will your promotion affect their relationship with you? They may not be sure how they should act toward you now.

Don't let reactions like these discourage you. Your co-workers need time to get used to the idea that you'll be their manager. If you perform effectively over the first few months, you'll win their acceptance.

## Starting out as a manager

Try to settle into your new position slowly—don't try to take on the world at once. One of the first things you may want to do is talk with any staff members who also applied for your position. Give them a chance to tell you how they feel about your promotion. This allows you to evaluate how well they'll accept you as a leader. (See *Challenge for the New Leader*, page 639, and *How to Lead as Well as Manage*.) If you suspect that a staff member's feelings of jealousy or resentment may interfere with her work, discuss your concerns with *your* supervisor. You don't want someone on the staff who'll consistently undermine your efforts.

Of course, you don't want to be too hasty in concluding that your former co-workers won't cooperate with you now that you're their manager. Their early reactions may not indicate how they'll feel after a month or two. They'll need a settling-in period, too!

If a staff member wants to know why

## HOW TO LEAD AS WELL AS MANAGE

How can a manager get the most from her employees with the least amount of effort? By being a good leader as well as a good manager. A manager can become a good leader by practicing the six P's—possibility thinking, political sense, prior achievement, poise, pliability, and principles.

 **Possibility thinking** is, simply, looking for opportunities in every situation and in every person. If you'll concentrate on isolating each of your subordinates' strengths, you can use them with maximum effectiveness.

 **Political sense** entails matching personalities with the tasks you assign, and redirecting anyone whose personality threatens your group's effectiveness. Try to assign subordinates to projects they're personally interested in to avoid "slugs," whose lack of interest can slow down the whole group.

 **Prior achievement** can be your biggest motivator. To gain subordinates' confidence, relate their previous successes to the goals you're asking them to achieve now. If you've achieved similar goals yourself in the past, tell your subordinates about the sense of accomplishment you felt.

 **Poise** is the ability to handle yourself well in all situations. To increase your leadership, practice controlling your emotions, making speeches, and freeing yourself from prejudices that stifle appropriate responses. The confidence you exude will gain your subordinates' respect.

 **Pliability** is the ability to adapt to change. You can improve your pliability by increasing your communication with your subordinates, encouraging them to help you in problem solving, and listening to their ideas and suggestions with an open mind.

 **Principles** are your definition of what's right and wrong in your organization. Identify your principles, and set your staff's goals according to those principles. Without clear-cut principles, you're sunk before you start.

Adapted with permission from Mary E. Tramel and Helen Reynolds, *Executive Leadership: How to Get It and Make It Work* (Englewood Cliffs, N.J.: Prentice-Hall, Inc., 1981).

she wasn't selected for the promotion, ask your supervisor to set up a conference with her. Your supervisor should explain this decision, because she made it. In fact, because you're so new to management, you should probably refer most personnel questions to an experienced manager until you feel confident that you can answer them knowledgeably.

You may want to ask all of your staff members about changes they'd recommend in the unit's health-care delivery. Prepare a form of specific questions for them to answer. Then you can compare their thoughts with yours. You also may find your staff's answers useful when you formulate their annual goals and objectives.

### Dealing with your initial impulses

When you start your new job, you'll probably feel terrific. Having achieved a personal and professional goal, you'll be bursting with energy and enthusiasm. But for a while, until you get your feet firmly on the ground, try to avoid telling your staff about your management plans. Here's why. When a nurse becomes a supervisor of a unit where she's worked for a few years, she typically has grand ideas about how to improve things. Of course, ideas for improvement are fine. But don't share them with your staff until you've had time to evaluate how realistic they are. You may even decide, after a while, that some of your early ideas aren't as good as you thought they were—that something else will work better.

As a manager considering changes on the unit, you also need to identify who has the power to implement changes. You don't want to promise something you can't deliver.

## Coping with new skills and relationships

When you get over your initial euphoria at being promoted, reality will begin to sink in. You'll probably feel unsure of yourself until you learn and develop the new skills you need. This is a typical reaction when new nurse managers realize they can't use their clinical skills to achieve their new jobs' goals. These feelings of insecurity may also be complicated by feelings of loneliness. Obviously, your professional relationships with your former co-workers will change. And you may notice differences developing in your per-

## CONSIDERING A PROMOTION

Imagine you're offered a promotion. Your first reaction is probably to accept it with few questions asked. But before you do, stop and ask yourself, "Do I really want this job? Do I want to give up the work I'm doing now? Do I want to do the work the new job entails?"

Even though you've wanted the promotion for years, a little soul-searching at the last minute may uncover realistic reasons for refusing it. You may have recently discovered that you don't like administrative work. Or this may be a poor time in your life to accept more responsibilities, even if the hours and pay are better. In such situations, the decision to refuse the promotion is fairly easy.

Sometimes the decision is much harder because the offer of a promotion arouses inner conflicts you don't understand. You may have a "feeling" you don't want the promotion, but you can't figure out why. In many cases, such conflicts indicate an unconscious fear of success. If you're offered a promotion and you feel uneasy, try to talk to someone about your uneasiness. He doesn't have to be a professional counselor. Even a friend can help, because

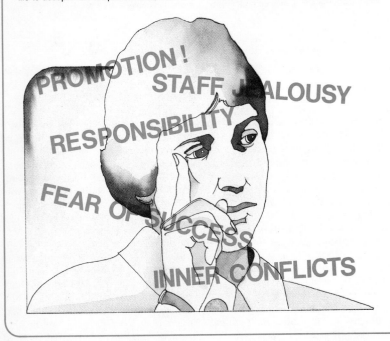

sonal relationships with them as well. This is normal, although it'll make you feel uncomfortable at first. For example, old friends may not be as relaxed when you're around. You may even find that conversations stop when you enter a room. Don't fight it by trying to be the "old buddy" staff nurse they knew. You can't manage them *and* maintain that role. As a nurse manager, you certainly don't want to find yourself in positions where your authority's compromised or your staff try to take advantage of you.

If you want to maintain a close friendship with someone you're supervising now, talk with her about the need to separate personal and professional relationships. Make sure she understands that your decisions on the job don't reflect any favoritism.

You *can* be a good manager and keep your staff-nurse friends. But you may also find, as time goes on, that you're making new friends among your fellow managers. Remember that these changing and developing relationships contribute to your professional growth.

## Adjusting to your new routine

Because of your new responsibilities, your daily routine will be different, too. You'll do a lot more paperwork, so you'll need an office. A makeshift one will do—as long as it's private and close to your clinical area.

Your new routine may also include some clinical duties—for instance, you may be expected to relieve staff members at lunch. Find out right away if your position requires clinical work; misunderstandings over such matters can breed discontent among staff members.

You may need to adjust your schedule so you have time to talk with the staff. For example, you may find that by going to work early two or three times a week, you'll have time to talk with the night-shift staff and with the nurses arriving for the day shift. To talk to the evening shift nurses, you can stay at work later on the other days. Use this "extra" time to chat and show concern for the staff and their work.

You may decide to stop joining the staff for breaks and lunches. Remember, they need time away from their manager. On rough days, they may need to vent their frustrations to each other. If you're with them, they may not feel comfortable doing this, or they may look to you to solve problems they should solve themselves. And you'll probably find that you're more com-

you need a listener more than a counselor.

If you talk about your feelings, you may uncover another unconscious fear—the fear that others won't like you after you're promoted. This fear may be a projection of your own feelings. Someone who wants success and promotions may envy people who've already achieved success. If you're such a person, you may have had these feelings all your life—toward your parents and teachers as a child, and now toward your own supervisors.

When a person like this finally gets a chance to be a supervisor, he tends to project his own hostility and envy onto others. He thinks, "Now everybody's going to hate me." If you have that fear, try to analyze your feelings toward authority figures. If you've felt envious and hostile toward them, you may indeed project those feelings onto your friends. Being aware of that tendency will help you cope with those feelings if you decide to accept the promotion. It'll help you grow, too.

A third reason why people fear promotions: Becoming a supervisor unconsciously stirs up identity problems. This is particularly common in women. Despite the women's rights movement, our society still holds a stereotype that being a "boss" requires masculine attributes. For that reason, many women offered a promotion find themselves in conflict: how can they be successful managers without losing their femininity? Because this fear is unconscious and not rational, it can develop in any profession—even in the nursing profession, where most managers are women.

Try to uncover your own feelings *before* you decide to accept a promotion, and you'll have a greater chance of enjoying it.

# WHEN YOUR FRIEND'S PROMOTED AND YOU'RE NOT

If you and your friend apply for the same promotion and she gets it, you'll face a problem that's both professional and personal. You'll have to deal with the fact that you didn't get something you thought you deserved. And you'll also have to deal with an old friend in a new relationship. Here are some questions you'll probably have, and some helpful answers:

• *Why wasn't I promoted?* Of course, you'll want to know why you didn't get the position. The best way to get an answer is to ask the person who made the decision. Make an appointment with this person. Try to make the meeting constructive by requesting specific reasons why you weren't given the job. After the meeting, set goals for strengthening your skills so that, when the next promotion opportunity arises, you'll be ready for the challenge.

• *How can I deal with the jealousy and resentment I feel?* You smile and congratulate your friend, but chances are you resent the fact that she was promoted over you. Try to examine your feelings and attitudes a week or two after the news of her promo-

tion. If you still feel jealous and resentful, talk to your friend. Tell her how you feel, so you and she can try to work it out together.

• *What about our friendship?* The fact that the two of you are friends doesn't have to change, but the character of your relationship will. Have a down-to-earth talk with your friend to establish some standards for your relationship. Both of you should understand that, at work, your professional relationship will have to take precedence. If you want to remain friends, don't expect favoritism or ask for it. If you do, you'll be putting your friend in a tough situation that could destroy your friendship.

• *Should I transfer to another unit?* If your feelings about the promotion are affecting your attitude toward your work, you should consider a transfer. After all, you don't want a career disappointment to affect your clinical performance. But bear in mind that a transfer won't solve your entire problem. You still must try to assess your disappointment honestly, and get over it quickly.

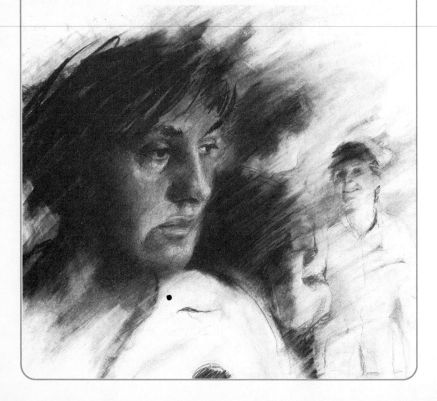

fortable at lunch with your new friends in management. Then, when *you* need to vent your frustrations, you can do so with *your* colleagues. You'll seldom want to show frustration in front of your staff.

## Supervising the staff

As a manager, you must ensure that everyone does her work correctly and follows your institution's and unit's policies. This can create a distance between you and your staff nurses. Why?

Because you can't reprimand or discipline someone one minute and be her buddy the next.

Although you must enforce official policies and procedures, you shouldn't use them to cover your insecurities. Certain new managers fail to trust their own judgment about the merits of new ideas. These managers retain old policies as a form of security and act more like "enforcers" than leaders. Don't become the unit dictator, enforcing policies without regard to staff input or

---

ADVICE

## CHALLENGE FOR THE NEW LEADER

*I'm the newly appointed head nurse of a 68-bed medical/ surgical unit in a suburban hospital, and I'm having a problem that other head nurses have probably also encountered. I'm talking about the problem of informal "leaders"—staff members who assume an unofficial leadership.*

*In my case, I was brought in from the outside and now find that two old-timers are challenging my authority. One's an LPN who's worked on this floor for almost 10 years. The other's a seasoned staff nurse who, I hear, had hoped to become head nurse. These two women question my decisions and judgment, encourage others to be lax in implementing my policies, and generally undermine my authority. I know I should be in full control of the situation, but I feel threatened by these women. How can I assert my leadership and meet the challenge of my authority?—RN, Neb.*

You're new on the job, and you come from the outside. You are bound to arouse some resentment.

You're also dealing with the threat of change. Management specialists have found that any staff will resist a major change. Established workers equate change with some form of loss—whether the facts support their feeling or not. Unsettled, and threatened by the change, some staff members will attempt to support and strengthen the remnants of the old, preexisting organization.

*What's the resolution?* It's never easy to satisfy "old staff," but here are a few suggestions:

• Try to see your appointment through the eyes of your staff members. Once you understand their point of view, their concern, anger, and hostility will be less threatening.
• Include the would-be leaders in the new changes. If you want to win them over, ask for their suggestions. And by all means, praise any good suggestions (and use them if you can).
• Ask yourself if there are other stress factors in the situation which may be provoking additional dissension. For example: Is there a staff shortage?
• Discuss the situation at length with all of those involved. Be direct and open. Talking it out is still the best way to let off steam, and to put the problem into a more sensible, less emotional perspective. Once the problem has been aired, your informal leaders won't have their secret, tense environment in which to operate. They'll back down or back away.

And if the staff sees your ability to handle conflict and tension with authority and common sense, it will begin to have confidence in you and to acknowledge your role as head nurse. Your staff will react to you as boss because you're being the boss—in a thoughtful, well-balanced sense of the word.

---

This letter was taken from the files of *Nursing* magazine.

special circumstances. Dictating how things are to be done (your way) can discourage team spirit and staff enthusiasm. If staff members approach you with ideas for changes on the unit, use your managerial skills and listen to their suggestions. If an idea has merit, consider implementing it even if a contradictory policy is already spelled out. Remember, in many instances, policies can be changed and are changed when the need is evident.

### A final word
Now that you're a manager evaluating the work of your staff, don't forget to take time to evaluate yourself. You need to monitor your own performance and identify areas for growth. After 6 months in your new job, schedule a conference with your supervisor to discuss your role and performance.

Remember, managing—especially managing friends and former co-workers—isn't right for everyone. You may eventually decide that nursing administration isn't what you want to do. But for now, give yourself a chance to settle into your exciting new role. As you learn your responsibilities and grow more confident, you'll probably find that your friends and former co-workers accept you as their leader—and that you like your job.

# 105 The art of delegating

As a nurse manager, you're responsible and accountable for the nursing care provided on your unit, as well as for the unit's functioning. But as you know, you sometimes need help to get all your work done. That's why you must delegate.

### What is delegating?
Delegating is asking someone to perform a task that's one of *your* responsibilities. This differs from assigning, which is designating someone to perform a task that's one of *her* responsibilities.

Delegating is also a key to your success as a manager. Many nurse managers—particularly recently promoted ones—believe that they must do their staff's work as well as their own supervisory duties. Some managers even believe that delegating is a sign of weakness and disorganization. In fact, the opposite is true: delegating is a sign of being secure and being organized. To delegate effectively, your first task is simply to recognize that you can't do everything yourself. Decide that you'll trust your staff to assess their patients' nursing-care needs, set priorities, and develop care plans. Then, decide which of your own activities you must do, and which ones you can delegate.

### Benefits of delegating
A nurse manager who doesn't take the time to orient staff or help them grow will never be able to delegate effectively. And that means problems for her, the patients, and the staff. When you delegate effectively, making sure that the best person does the job, you help make your unit's nursing care more cost-effective, and you save time. In the short run, of course, you may need to spend extra time to orient your staff to the delegating methods you'll be using and to the new tasks they may be asked to do. But you'll find that this time is well spent. Delegating will help free you from having to perform tasks you don't have time to do, and it will facilitate your staff's professional growth.

### What are the barriers to delegating?
Probably the most universally recognized barrier to effective delegation is simply *fear*. Either a manager may be afraid to delegate, or a staff member may be afraid to accept the delegated responsibility.

Some nurse managers are afraid to delegate because they either don't know their staff or don't trust them. These nurses worry that staff members will make mistakes that reflect badly on their managers. Other nurse managers don't delegate because they fear the staff member will do the job too well, perhaps even better than they could. When such a nurse does delegate, usually she supervises too closely and undermines her purpose in delegating. The staff member she's delegated to probably thinks: "If she's going to check on me every 10 minutes, I'll let her do this herself!"

Some nurses don't delegate because they fear they'll lose control. This fear is unfounded. Delegating doesn't mean

---

> *"A nurse manager who doesn't take the time to help those under her grow will never be able to delegate effectively."*

---

giving up control. In fact, the nurse who delegates decides how much control she'll retain. She may tell a staff member anything from "Take action; you don't need to discuss this with me" to "Look into the problem, tell me the facts, and I'll make the decision."

Whatever its causes, you can overcome the fear of delegating. Here are some tips:

• Get to know your staff members and their individual abilities.

• Keep the lines of communication open, so you can help solve problems your staff members may have with delegated responsibilities.

• Keep in mind that when a staff member performs a delegated task well, this reflects positively on you.

Sometimes a staff member may not accept a task because she's afraid of failing, of making a mistake, or of ac-

cepting responsibility. As her manager, you need to ask yourself whether these fears may be well founded. For example, if a staff member doesn't have the necessary skill or knowledge to perform a task you're delegating to her, can she—or can't she—count on you to help her learn the task? Or maybe she thinks that if she accepts the task and makes a mistake, you'll blow it out of proportion. Obviously, you need to reassure her that you're delegating in good faith and will accept her best effort to do the delegated task.

Sometimes, of course, a staff member prevents effective delegation. For example, your effort to delegate a task to a staff member who's unwilling to accept responsibility and make decisions is pretty certain to fail.

To avoid establishing barriers to effective delegating, review your behavior when you delegated in the past. How did you deal with less-than-positive results? Then set up goals for yourself. Talk with your staff and try to identify the cause of their reluctance to accept delegated responsibility. For staff who are interested, help them set goals for accepting delegated responsibilities.

Occasionally, the situation itself prevents delegating. For example, in a crisis, you obviously can't delegate a complex task to an untrained staff member.

### Learning how to delegate

First, analyze your job and identify the tasks that you can probably delegate. Usually you can delegate routine tasks,

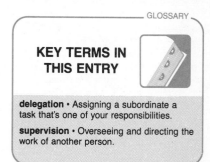

GLOSSARY

## KEY TERMS IN THIS ENTRY

**delegation** • Assigning a subordinate a task that's one of your responsibilities.

**supervision** • Overseeing and directing the work of another person.

## WHO CAN DO WHAT? DELEGATING TO RNs and LPNs or LVNs

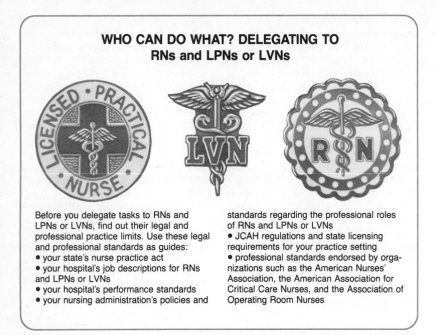

Before you delegate tasks to RNs and LPNs or LVNs, find out their legal and professional practice limits. Use these legal and professional standards as guides:
- your state's nurse practice act
- your hospital's job descriptions for RNs and LPNs or LVNs
- your hospital's performance standards
- your nursing administration's policies and standards regarding the professional roles of RNs and LPNs or LVNs
- JCAH regulations and state licensing requirements for your practice setting
- professional standards endorsed by organizations such as the American Nurses' Association, the American Association for Critical Care Nurses, and the Association of Operating Room Nurses

tasks required during an emergency, and tasks that must be done when you're not present in the unit.

Next, decide to whom you'll delegate specific tasks. This decision is crucial to your success in delegating. You must know the skills, abilities, and interests of your staff members before you can delegate effectively. If you delegate a task to a staff member who doesn't know how to do it, *you must be available to assist and support her.* Otherwise, the outcome may not be what you wanted.

Knowing the skills, abilities, and interests of your staff will also help you decide if you need to check on their work. For example, if you know that a nursing assistant has just learned to take vital signs, you might ask her to perform this task, but you'd verify her findings. (Explain to your staff that you need to evaluate their abilities so you can plan inservice help to close gaps in knowledge and skills, and so you can make assignments most appropriately.) Of course, if you know a nursing assistant is competent and has been taking vital signs for 6 months, you'll usually accept her findings.

To delegate properly, you must ensure that:
- the staff member you delegate to accepts responsibility for doing the task
- you grant her sufficient authority to complete the task
- you and she both understand, and agree on, the expected results.

### A final word

Your success at delegating depends largely on your attitude. You must be willing to encourage independence among your staff. A staff member won't perform a task exactly as you would, but as long as the results are acceptable, don't redo it. (Remember, supervising too closely or redoing delegated tasks will frustrate staff members and may make them unwilling to accept other tasks.) When a staff member makes a mistake, don't take away her authority to do the task. Instead, use the incident as an opportunity to teach her how to do the task properly and avoid making the same mistake in the future. Above all, *reward good work.*

# 106 Making staff assignments effectively

One of the most difficult aspects of nursing management is making assignments for professional and nonprofessional staff. If you're a new manager, you may wonder what the fuss is all about. After all, isn't making an assignment just telling someone to perform a task that falls within the scope of her responsibilities?

Unfortunately, the answer is no. Making assignments is much more difficult than just giving people orders. When you assign tasks to your staff, you must thoroughly understand RNs', LPNs'/LVNs', and nurse's aides' proper scopes of responsibility. And you must *consistently* make assignments based on this understanding. Remember, a nurse practicing within the legal scope of her responsibilities (see Entry 1) must also give care that meets applicable professional standards for the tasks she's performing (see Entry 2). To ensure that her nurses are assigned on the basis of their legal scope of practice, their training, and their ability to give patients the care they need, a nurse manager should use a set of *written standards* for making assignments. (See *Using Hospital Standards to Make Nonprofessional Staff Assignments*, page 645). These standards usually combine standards sponsored by the Joint Committee on Accreditation of Hospitals (JCAH) with staff-prepared unit standards.

Of course, job descriptions created for RNs, LPNs/LVNs, and aides provide general guidelines for making staff assignments. These job descriptions reflect:

• regulations of state licensing agencies and the JCAH

• recommendations of professional organizations (such as ANA, AACN, and AORN)

• ways in which nursing administration distinguishes among the roles of RNs, LPNs/LVNs, and aides in day-to-day situations.

But these guidelines don't state exactly what tasks RNs, LPNs/LVNs, and aides can perform. This is why a written set of unit standards for making assignments is so important.

Here are eight JCAH-sponsored standards for making staff assignments that provide safe, effective care:

• Assignments must be consistent with staff members' legal and professional ability to perform them.

• Assignments must be consistent with patients' medical care plans.

• RNs must plan, supervise, and evaluate all patients' care. If an LPN or LVN is assigned to a patient's care, an RN must also be assigned—in writing—to that patient. She doesn't have to provide all the patient's care, but she must be assigned to work with the LPN or LVN.

• An RN must assess a patient prior to assigning him to non-RN staff.

• Staff assignments should take infection control measures into account. For example, if an RN's assigned to one or more patients with highly infectious diseases, then the rest of her patients should be assigned on the basis of low cross-infection risk.

• An RN must retain responsibility for patients cared for by students, private-duty nurses, and agency-provided staff.

• Continuity of patient care must be

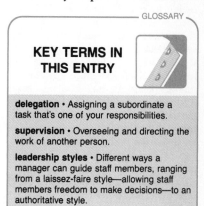

GLOSSARY

**KEY TERMS IN THIS ENTRY**

**delegation** • Assigning a subordinate a task that's one of your responsibilities.

**supervision** • Overseeing and directing the work of another person.

**leadership styles** • Different ways a manager can guide staff members, ranging from a laissez-faire style—allowing staff members freedom to make decisions—to an authoritative style.

ensured, so nurses can develop in-depth knowledge of their patients.

• The unit's geographic layout must provide for nursing staff's proximity to patients.

These standards can serve as a basis for your unit's written standards for making staff assignments. For best results, staff and management should meet and work together to create a set of standards that everyone's comfortable with.

## Avoiding common pitfalls in assigning staff

As a nurse manager responsible for making staff assignments, be careful to steer clear of pitfalls that can cause role confusion among your staff and create working relationships characterized by

> *"Avoid making assignments that reflect staff availability instead of capability."*

hostility, mistrust, and jealousy. Here are some of the most common pitfalls:

• *Letting friendships affect the assignments you make.* As a manager, you must separate your professional relationships from personal ones. Always assign RNs, LPNs or LVNs, and aides according to their professional capabilities and legal responsibilities. Never let friendship affect your judgment. Assigning an LPN who's a friend to perform an RN's responsibility is not only inappropriate, it may also be illegal. And it'll probably cause anger among the staff. The situation may be complicated further if another manager, or an RN, tries to limit your friend's duties. Obviously, the solution is to assign tasks on a consistently professional basis, regardless of your personal feelings about certain staff members.

• *Assigning tasks based only on staff members' demonstrated skills—*

whether or not those skills are supported by appropriate education, training, or licensure. You've probably heard a nurse manager say something like this: "Mary's an excellent LPN. She can do everything an RN can do, except give I.V. meds and defibrillate." What does this attitude indicate? That the manager feels the only distinction between LPNs and RNs is an ability or willingness to perform a series of tasks. A statement like this can mislead you, if you're a new manager. Should you make your assignments this way, too? The answer to this question is unequivocally *no*. You shouldn't base your assignments on whether an RN or an LPN has the skill to hang an I.V., to administer I.V. medications, or to discontinue a subclavian catheter. Instead, you must assign your staff on the basis of whether legal and professional standards permit them to perform the tasks that patients need done.

• *Relying solely on job descriptions.* If you work in an institution where the formal definitions of RN, LPN or LVN, and aide responsibilities appear in their job descriptions, work with your nursing administration to draft *specific* expectations for staff members' functions. (Remember, the purpose of a job description is to *generally* define duties and responsibilities. Job descriptions don't give specific details about what a worker may or may not do.) Be sure these details appear in your unit's or department's written standards for assigning staff—and in other protocols where they're appropriate.

• *Making inconsistent assignments that confuse staff about their roles.* Avoid making assignments that reflect staff *availability* instead of staff *capability.* Just because an LPN is handy, you shouldn't assign her to do the work of an RN you don't have available for an assignment. As mentioned above, this practice is not only inappropriate—it's often (depending on what you ask the LPN to do) *illegal.*

Suppose that on the 11 p.m. to 7 a.m. shift on weekends and holidays, when

## USING HOSPITAL STANDARDS TO MAKE NONPROFESSIONAL STAFF ASSIGNMENTS

If you supervise LPNs or LVNs, or NAs, reread your hospital's performance standards for these staff members. This will help you avoid confusion concerning their responsibilities. Use the hospital's performance standards as a guide when you assign tasks. These standards, of course, will vary from one hospital to another. Here's a sampling of standards a typical hospital might use for nonprofessional staff performing nursing functions:

PERFORMANCE STANDARDS

HOSPITAL POLICIES

**LPNs should:**
• add to Kardex problem list and goal columns after discussing the entries with a coassigned RN and receiving her authorization.
• perform routine observations of the patient's major body systems once every shift, have observations validated by a coassigned RN, and chart them properly on the assessment flow sheet and nursing progress notes.
• conduct routine patient education as outlined in hospital nursing programs or as specified in the RN's care plan.
• provide information to doctors on request.
• accept verbal orders to continue or change a doctor's orders *after* a coassigned RN validates the verbal order.

**LPNs and NAs should:**
• attend one patient-care conference and one discharge-planning conference per month.
• add to Kardex-care plan once per shift after a coassigned RN authorizes the addition.
• document the patient's physical care on the nursing care flow sheet and the bedside intake and output sheet, according to established guidelines. (A coassigned RN will incorporate information from the nonprofessional staff into the nursing progress notes.)

fewer RNs are on duty, you allow LPNs to perform tasks that exceed their legal and professional scope of practice. And then, in the middle of the week on the 7 a.m. to 3 p.m. shift, when many RNs are on duty, you don't permit LPNs to perform those same tasks. Understandably, your staff will resent your inconsistency and feel confused about their roles on the unit. And of course, if a patient's injured by an LPN you've inappropriately assigned, you could be in legal hot water (see Chapter 6).

Inconsistent assignment practices can create "political" problems for you, too. If other nurse managers besides you make assignments without following written standards, opposing factions may develop among staff members. When this happens, LPNs/LVNs who want to do *more* align themselves with managers who'll give them

---

> *"The only proper way to make assignments is to base them on the appropriate written standards."*

---

greater (even if inappropriate) responsibilities, and LPNs who *don't* want to take on more sophisticated tasks align themselves with managers who give them less responsibility. The latter practice may be safer legally—but it's still not a good way to use the staff. The result of this division of staff ranks can be belligerent attitudes and lack of cooperation, failure (and even refusal) to complete work assignments, and—a natural sequel—poor patient care. The *only* proper way to make assignments is to base them on the appropriate written standards.

## Developing assignment skills

Usually, when you're promoted to nurse manager, your institution's nursing ad-

ministration will help you learn how to make assignments and supervise your staff. But your training shouldn't end there. Your nursing administration should hold regular meetings to ensure that all nurse managers understand and use the appropriate standards for staff assignments. At these meetings, you should be able to review assignment procedures in light of written standards. These meetings should also help you improve and update your overall leadership capabilities. If your institution doesn't have regular meetings where managers can talk face-to-face with higher-level administrators, request that it start them.

Then, at your monthly meetings with staff, you can address potential or actual problems of role confusion and uncertainty about assignments. Invite staff members to raise questions and discuss problems. Be sure your staff understands that you must resolve problems like these by interpreting your institution's written standards.

To establish a procedure for your staff to report violations of staff-assignment standards, encourage them to directly and confidentially report to you details of what happened and what should have been done to comply with the standards for assignment. Be sure that names, dates, shifts, and patient-care circumstances are reported, so you can follow up violations effectively. When you receive such reports, follow them up *immediately*. This will signal your staff that you're committed to making assignments based on appropriate legal and professional standards.

### A final word

As a manager, you must make staff assignments correctly and consistently. This involves a mutual understanding, between you and your staff, of legal and professional responsibilities. When you make assignments *only* on this basis, you help minimize potential role confusion. And you help your staff, your institution, and yourself by ensuring good care and avoiding liability.

# 107 How to discipline effectively

Today, as you may know, one of the biggest concerns among managers in industry is diminished employee productivity. Unfortunately, this phenomenon isn't limited to manufacturing companies. It's occurring in organizations that provide services, as well, including health-care institutions—where productivity is measured in terms of the delivery of quality health care. Experts attribute this decrease in productivity to a number of factors, all connected by a common thread—management.

A manager's primary responsibility is to train and manage subordinates so they're encouraged to feel committed to the organization they work for. Studies have shown that managers who lack interest, commitment, or strong ability to manage and train their subordinates can cause disillusionment and decreased productivity among them.

To manage effectively, you must commit yourself to a particular leadership style, give your staff ongoing instruction about the values, procedures, and norms practiced at your institution, and *establish and maintain discipline on your unit.*

## Understanding the purposes of discipline
Discipline may be described as behavior that complies with certain rules of conduct. But from a manager's point of view, the term refers to actions needed to bring a person into compliance with those rules. The primary purpose of discipline is not to punish past behavior but to ensure quality performance in the future. To achieve this goal, any disciplinary action you take against a staff member should:
* promote recognition of her role as a member of the health team
* create and maintain working conditions that promote productivity and job satisfaction
* encourage cohesive and cooperative work relationships among subordinates
* clarify her job responsibilities
* demonstrate the merits of self-control.

## Using preventive discipline
You can sometimes avoid taking direct disciplinary action with subordinates if you learn to exercise preventive discipline effectively. Preventive discipline involves three techniques that give your staff a clear understanding of your expectations of them. The techniques also convey the means by which your staff can meet those expectations. The three techniques are:
* The performance appraisal, your annual (or semi-annual), formal assessment of a staff member's value to the organization. (See *Avoiding Simplistic Performance Evaluations,* page 650.) During the appraisal, you can help her identify goals and develop a plan for professional growth. For example, if she identifies a goal of becoming assistant head nurse, you can suggest a plan of action to help her accomplish this. Her adherence to this plan is a kind of discipline that will benefit both

GLOSSARY

## KEY TERMS IN THIS ENTRY

**corrective discipline** • Action a supervisor takes to stop a subordinate's improper behavior.

**leadership styles** • Different ways a manager can guide staff members, ranging from a laissez-faire style—allowing staff members freedom to make decisions—to an authoritative style.

**preventive discipline** • Discipline that involves three techniques—performance appraisals, coaching, and counseling—to give subordinates a clear understanding of a supervisor's expectations.

## IS THE NURSE THE ONLY ONE AT FAULT?

Suppose a nurse in your unit has violated hospital policy. Before you decide how you should discipline her, investigate the problem thoroughly and identify all of the contributing factors. Don't be too quick to assume that the nurse was completely at fault. Either you or your institution's policies may have played a part. These lists can help you view the nurse's behavior objectively and discipline her fairly.

**DOES YOUR INSTITUTION:**
- interpret its purpose inconsistently?
- provide unsound employment policies?
- impose unfair labor practices on employees?
- provide inadequate facilities or equipment?
- follow insufficient hiring practices?
- describe nurses' roles and responsibilities inaccurately?
- train nurses improperly?
- fail to support managers' decisions?

**AS A NURSE MANAGER, DO YOU:**
- use an inappropriate leadership style? For example, you may be using a laissez-faire style when one particular nurse needs more direction from you.
- fail to resolve conflicts quickly and effectively?
- lack assertiveness?
- lack effective managerial skills? Does each nurse understand her responsibilities and the responsibilities of her co-workers?
- lack flexibility in dealing with your staff?
- play favorites with your staff, or single some staff members out for excessive criticism?

of you. To encourage her, you might suggest that she attend seminars, obtain weekly coaching, and assume new charge duties as her head nurse delegates them.

- **Coaching,** your ongoing, informal commentary on staff members' work performance. Coaching includes feedback, advice, corrective suggestions, and reinforcement about specific aspects of the job. For example, you might say, "Rounds are to be made at least hourly on all patients during the night," or "You followed the admission procedure perfectly."

- **Counseling,** your attention to a staff member's personal problem that's impeding her job performance. The degree and depth of your involvement in this type of situation will vary widely. Most often, you're responsible for telling the staff member to discontinue her unacceptable behavior, and for counseling to bring about improvement. Of course, you shouldn't get heavily involved in a long-term counseling relationship.

### Using corrective discipline

Certain unacceptable actions of your staff members—for example, mistreatment of patients, frequent medication errors, breach of sterile technique, unexcused absence, lying, stealing, sleeping on the job, inaccurate record-keeping, or a surly attitude—require corrective discipline. Corrective discipline involves an action that you take to stop a staff member's improper behavior. It represents a demand from the organization that the employee change the behavior. (Note: As you're probably aware, some unacceptable nursing actions are also illegal—and may require that you make a report to the authorities. See Chapters 1 through 6.) But keep in mind the fact that the staff member isn't always solely responsible for her behavior. You, as a nurse manager, and your institution's policies can sometimes contribute. Before you take any disciplinary action, consider all the possible causes of the problem (see *Is the Nurse the Only One at Fault?*). Once you've pinpointed the cause, you can implement a fair and effective solution. Consider the following:

*To correct your institution's failings.* Managers at every level are responsible for knowing their institutions' policies

and practices and promoting needed changes. As a matter of fact, this is one of the major transitions that staff who are promoted to management must make. Here's how to effectively influence your institution's policies and practices:
• Interpret and emphasize your institution's goals to your staff.
• Insist on, and enforce, fair policies and practices.
• Investigate and suggest upgrading of facilities and equipment.
• Write accurate job descriptions.
• Seek and support educational opportunities for yourself and your employees.
• Provide instruction for staff members.

*To correct your own failings.* Your staff members look to you for guidance and support. But you can only assist them if you clearly understand your responsibilities and carry them out objectively and professionally. To strengthen your managerial skills, to increase your self-confidence, and to help others respect and trust you, follow these guidelines:
• Familiarize yourself with conflict management.
• Encourage formation of collegial support systems, so that the staff share their concerns with each other and help one another solve problems.
• Be responsive and flexible so that you can deal individually with each staff member's problems as they arise.
• Deal with your staff fairly and consistently, so they know what to expect from you.
• Be assertive (see Entry 69).

*To correct individual staff members' failings.* As a manager, you're responsible for motivating your subordinates and for guiding their career growth. To demonstrate strong leadership and effective management, follow these guidelines:
• Teach, train, and generally keep your staff well-informed about developments and opportunities in nursing.
• Counsel staff members when neces-

sary, or arrange for them to receive counseling services.
• Confront staff members with their problem behavior.
• Correct staff members when their behavior is unacceptable.
• When conflicts are unresolvable, transfer staff members to more appropriate assignments.
• Terminate staff members when necessary.

## A step-by-step guide to disciplining subordinates

Disciplining a staff member isn't easy. The actions you take must be carefully thought out so the outcome is positive, not negative.

Lack of discipline or ineffective discipline can produce in your staff a state of mind characterized by low morale, reduced self-respect, and serious job dissatisfaction. This, in turn, leads to work of diminished quality, possibly affecting your unit's quality of care. But too much or too stringent discipline can also have a negative effect: an overdisciplined staff member may either rebel or comply to the point of complete passivity—fearing (or refusing) to exercise her professional judgment, creativity, and initiative.

Effective discipline doesn't result in a negative outcome. Instead, it can increase a staff member's self-respect and self-confidence, and it can strengthen her trust in you and your institution.

To discipline a staff member effectively, follow these guidelines:
• Gather all the facts. Familiarize yourself with the staff member's behavior, and review your institution's policies, state licensure laws (see Entry 3), and the nurses' professional code. Then check through the unit's employment records: did similar situations happen before? How were those employees handled?
• Determine your position with regard to the staff member's unacceptable behavior. Know your feelings, the support you can offer the staff member, and the nature and extent of the backup you'll

## AVOIDING SIMPLISTIC PERFORMANCE EVALUATIONS

Before you write a performance evaluation, remember that you face a major pitfall—oversimplification. It takes many forms. Are you any one of the following?

- The *lenient supervisor* sees everyone through rose-colored glasses.

- The *top sergeant* takes a tough-minded approach and rates every employee's overall performance a notch or two below what it merits.

- The *sunshine supervisor* rates an employee's overall performance high if one behavior seemed particularly good.

- The *single-event supervisor* bases the whole evaluation on some memorable event, good or bad.

- The *short-memory supervisor* bases a whole year's evaluation on whatever happened yesterday.

Avoid oversimplifying by setting specific standards and goals every time you evaluate an employee, and by documenting the employee's performance throughout the year.

get from administration.

- Arrange to meet with the staff member in private and without interruptions. Allow ample time, and have all the necessary background material readily available. Be sure the disciplinary actions you're considering are consistent with your institution's policies.
- When the two of you meet, be attentive, consistent, fair, and professional during your discussion. State your po-

sition. Be concise and specific—for example, "Your lateness must stop."

- Actively listen to your staff member's explanation of what caused her unacceptable behavior. Be flexible enough to allow for extenuating and unusual circumstances.
- Together, review the facts of what happened to make sure the picture is complete. Then work with the staff member, using problem-solving techniques, to decide on actions she'll take to correct her behavior.
- To end the session, make sure the staff member clearly understands your expectations of her—and the consequences if she fails to meet those expectations.
- Document your meeting, including details of the plan the two of you developed to correct the problem. Both of you should sign the document.
- In your interactions with her after your meeting, demonstrate that you expect improvement in the staff member's behavior. Your confident attitude will benefit everyone.
- Record changes that you observe in the staff member's behavior. Write down specific incidents following your meeting that represent either positive or negative responses to your disciplinary action.
- If the staff member's behavior improves, continue to coach and encourage her. If it doesn't, consider transfer or termination.

### A final word

The disciplinary actions you take with your staff should be consistent with your institution's policies, with your personal and professional values, and with the particular leadership style you've established. Remember—when you consistently maintain high standards for your nursing staff's behavior, you demonstrate your commitment to the profession, your respect for patients, and your investment in helping your staff grow professionally. As a nurse manager, you can't afford to do anything less.

# 108 Effective time management

Admit it: Couldn't you—like all of us—meet more of your top-priority objectives if you used your time more effectively? Even with all you accomplish during your busy workday, you could probably be even more productive if you managed your time better—right? Here's help. This entry explains practical techniques for managing your time and offers tips on how to avoid common on-the-job time-wasters.

## Using time-management techniques

To use your time effectively and efficiently, you must plan. "Planning is bringing the future into the present so you can do something about it now," according to time management expert Alan Lakein.

Planning is pretty easy to describe. It's establishing goals and identifying objectives to achieve those goals. You need goals, so you identify short- and long-term goals and assign priorities to them. This way, you know what order to follow in accomplishing them. Establishing your priorities enables you to focus your attention and energy for a maximum timesaving effect.

Several common and successful time-management techniques can help you keep your attention focused on your goals. Use these techniques to get a better grasp on your time:

● *Write a daily to-do list.* Each day, compose a list of all the tasks you must perform. Give each listed item a priority. For example, designate a task you consider critically important an A priority. Use a B priority for moderately important tasks and a C priority for minimally important tasks.

To use your time most effectively, concentrate first on your A-priority tasks. Resist the temptation to do C-priority tasks first—in many instances, these are fairly straightforward, easily accomplished tasks that promise a quick return for your effort. You'll feel satisfied crossing C-priority tasks off your to-do list, but they don't really help you achieve your most important goals. And remember, when you work on C-priority tasks, you're using valuable time you might more profitably spend completing tasks with A-priorities.

A to-do list helps you use your time wisely, especially during busy days and slack days. When you find yourself with a few extra minutes, tackle an A-priority task. If you don't have time to complete the A-priority task, you can at least do a portion of it. By taking this portion-at-a-time approach, you're breaking down a difficult A-priority task into smaller, more manageable tasks.

As a written illustration of your priorities, a to-do list will help keep you from becoming sidetracked.

● *Establish deadlines.* Deadlines provide you with target dates and help you avoid delays. Deadlines become particularly important when you're working toward a goal that involves achieving many interim objectives.

● *Concentrate on one task at a time.* By concentrating on one task, you can complete that task in a minimal amount of time with a minimal amount of aggravation. This is particularly true when you must suddenly deal with a

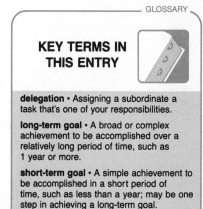

GLOSSARY

### KEY TERMS IN THIS ENTRY

**delegation** • Assigning a subordinate a task that's one of your responsibilities.

**long-term goal** • A broad or complex achievement to be accomplished over a relatively long period of time, such as 1 year or more.

**short-term goal** • A simple achievement to be accomplished in a short period of time, such as less than a year; may be one step in achieving a long-term goal.

potential crisis—which automatically becomes an A-priority. For example, suppose gastric drainage is escaping from a Salem sump tube's vent lumen. The nurse taking care of the patient can't alleviate the problem and asks you for help. As you try to stop the drainage, you focus on what you're doing, not on your other to-do-list tasks. If you don't concentrate on the task at hand, you may miss important clues that would enable you to solve the present problem more quickly.

• *Avoid distractions.* Distractions interrupt your concentration and rob you of precious time. For example, nurses' stations are notoriously noisy and busy. If the noise there distracts you while you're trying to do your charting, find a quiet place for the task. You'll probably discover that you can chart more accurately and quickly when you're not distracted.

• *Delegate tasks* (see Entry 105). Delegating takes time initially, because you must know your staff's skills, knowledge, and interests well. But delegating tasks can help you use your time effectively, so it's worth your initial effort. When you delegate, make sure you clearly assign responsibility, grant authority, and create accountability. You and the staff member you delegate to must understand the desired outcome and the deadline. Decide, too, how frequently you'll assess a staff member's progress in completing a delegated task.

• *Avoid postponements.* Putting off doing a task until the last minute can waste time *and* increase your stress level. As you probably know, working under severe stress can increase your mental and physical fatigue (see Entry 68). You might take twice as long to complete a task when you're tired than when you're rested. Similarly, when you're asked to complete a task that's an A-priority task for your supervisor but a C-priority task for you, don't waste

## HOW TO PREVENT TIME-WASTING MEETINGS

As you know, properly structured meetings can produce profitable results. But unstructured meetings are notorious time-wasters. Before you attend a meeting, ask why you've been invited. Can you really contribute to the discussion with your experience or interest in the topic? If you're thinking about calling a meeting, ask yourself if it's really needed. Can you accomplish what you want in a simpler way?

If you decide you need to call a meeting, follow this advice to save time:

• Prepare an agenda. Knowing what will be discussed allows the participants to prepare for the meeting by gathering documents or doing research. In your agenda memo, state the starting and ending time of the meeting and list the agenda items according to the priority of subject matter.

• Invite only people who have the knowledge and authority to make decisions about the meeting's topic. Resist the temptation to invite other people because you think they'd like to come or because inviting them seems politically advantageous. These situations can have negative instead of positive effects, when the participants find out the meeting is wasting their time because it doesn't directly concern them.

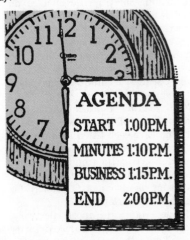

AGENDA

START 1:00 P.M.

MINUTES 1:10 P.M.

BUSINESS 1:15 P.M.

END 2:00 P.M.

time complaining. Perform the task as competently and as soon as you can.

• *Make appointments.* Arrange appointments to meet with people who are helping you get your work done or achieve your goals. Appointments let each of you know the meeting's purpose. (See *How to Prevent Time-Wasting Meetings.*) Then you can set aside the necessary time and come prepared. For example, if you want to talk to your head nurse about your performance appraisal—especially about your goals for the next year—schedule an appointment with her. Tell her what you want to talk about. Both of you can bring any documents you need for your discussion.

• *Don't answer the telephone.* A ringing telephone's a distracting temptation! Let the unit's secretary answer the phone, unless she's extremely busy. If you do answer, most often the call won't be for you, so you'll have to find the person or the information the caller wants. This may not be especially difficult to do—but it will consume some of your time.

• *Keep a daily time log.* As one time-use expert has said, "The misuse of time seldom involves an isolated incident—it's usually part of a well-established pattern of behavior."

To help you identify time-wasting activities, keep a time log and review it regularly to see how you spend your time. You don't need an elaborate journal, just a written log of the tasks you perform during the day. Fill in the log at regular intervals, such as every 15 minutes, for a week. Although you don't need to keep a time log for any specific period, the longer you keep it, the more data you'll have to help you identify time-wasting activity more easily.

## Banishing time-wasting activities

These activities eat away at your valuable time, forcing delays in your deadlines and more stress on you. Here's a list of the most common nursing time-wasters and some tips on how you can reduce their time-wasting effects:

• *Interruptions.* A day free from interruptions doesn't exist. In fact, most interruptions are part of your job. You can't avoid some interruptions, such as a family's requests for information. If you've identified your goals, you can get back on track after any interruption. How? By asking yourself, "What's the best use of my time right now?" That will help you refocus your efforts and energies toward your goals, after you've dealt with the interruption.

• *Crises.* You can't avoid crises, but you can keep them to a minimum by planning (for example, dealing with a doctor assertively now, to avoid a possible crisis later) and by using time-management techniques. When crises

---

*"When you delegate, make sure you clearly assign responsibility...and create accountability."*

---

do arise, don't panic. Use your skills to confront one task at a time.

Once a crisis has passed, don't forget how you reacted. Learn from each crisis. Analyze it and ask yourself: "How and why did the crisis happen? How did I handle it? What can I do to prevent it or a similar crisis from occurring?" Remember, every crisis you can prevent means more time for you.

• *Socializing with co-workers.* Socializing at work is pleasant, yes—but it wastes considerable chunks of your time. Keep socializing to a minimum. When co-workers want to socialize, politely tell them that you must continue your work. Otherwise, you'll come to a day's end and find that you haven't accomplished your goals.

• *Misidentifying the problem.* Fostering a problem-solving climate is an excellent time-management technique that you, as a nurse manager, can initiate. By encouraging your staff to solve their own problems, you'll help them to become more independent. But problem solving can become a serious time-waster. How? By attempting to solve a problem without clearly identifying it first. For example, suppose a doctor comes hurrying out of a patient's room and almost runs into you. He's fuming about the patient's intake and output record. He asks you if it's correct. You say yes—then he's off mumbling about people not knowing what's going on with this patient's intake and output.

How would you react? If you decide he's mad at you, or he's been rude to you, you could spend 10 or 15 minutes complaining to your colleagues about his behavior. This time might be entirely wasted if he actually was mad at the medical residents for the way they wrote the order for fluid replacement for this patient. You could avoid wasting this time, of course, by asking the doctor what the problem is and if you can be of help. Moral: Look before you leap—to erroneous conclusions.

• *Excessive paperwork.* If you're like most nurses, you consider excessive paperwork one of the most significant time wasters you face. Paperwork is necessary, of course, to ensure documentation and continuity of care. You can't avoid paperwork, so don't postpone it. Do it, and don't waste time complaining. When you must enter the same information on several different forms, try to combine the paperwork to get it done faster. And anytime you have a suggestion to alleviate paperwork, confer with your co-workers and supervisors.

• *Inability to say no.* Learn to say no logically, rationally, and tactfully. When you're asked to accept an additional delegated responsibility or to work an extra shift, consider your (and your patients') priorities. If you say yes, will you be able to achieve your day's goals according to the priorities you've established? If your answer's no, and you decide to refuse the extra work, don't feel guilty.

**A final word**
Effective time-management techniques will never become obsolete. If anything, they'll become even more important as you strive to achieve your own goals and those you've established with your staff. Remember, knowing time-management techniques isn't enough. You must put them to work.

Time-management techniques prove that you can control your time and your life. If you don't use them, you're missing out on achieving goals that are otherwise within your grasp.

# 109 Motivation and morale: Keys to successful management

What's your nursing staff's common purpose? Of course, it's giving quality patient care. As a nurse manager, your purpose is to get your staff's care up to that standard as quickly as possible (if it's not there already), and then to ensure they continue to meet that standard. Your keys to success are *motivation* and *morale*.

If you could be present at every nursing intervention that takes place on your unit, you could personally direct your staff to give consistently high-quality care. But, of course, you can't do this. Instead, you must depend on your staff members' shared commitment to the goal of quality care that you've set for them. To develop that commitment, you need to *motivate* your staff, using strategies and actions that will increase their enthusiasm for achieving the goal. And you need to promote their *morale*—the sense of shared responsibility and job satisfaction that reflects your motivating efforts. Then you can feel secure about the quality of care your staff provides, whether you're on the scene for a nursing intervention or not.

## What motivates people?

A couple of hundred years ago, motivation was a fairly simple matter. That's because, in that period when most people produced and sold their own goods, a direct link existed between a person's effort and his reward. Usually, the harder he worked, the more he produced to sell and the more money he made. Each person could decide for himself how much to produce.

Of course, the Industrial Revolution changed all that. More and more, people stopped working for themselves and started working for business organizations. Here managers, not workers, were the ones who set production goals. In this setting, the link between individual effort and individual reward virtually disappeared. To compensate for the loss of individual incentive to produce, and to motivate workers to meet organizations' production goals, managers developed new rewards. These included higher pay, fringe benefits, better working conditions, and shorter hours. Up to the present time, managers have relied mainly on these motivating factors to help them achieve their production goals.

## What motivates nurses?

Recently, researchers have studied less tangible rewards' usefulness in motivating workers, including hospital nursing staffs. One such researcher, Arthur Brief, has identified four "rewards" that a nurse will respond to with increased motivation and job satisfaction. They are:
- the chance to use a variety of professional skills
- the opportunity to perform a meaningful role in a project
- the freedom to choose *how* to do a task
- the chance to learn how well she did the task.

You can adapt your knowledge of these rewards' effectiveness to your staff members' individual circumstances. How? By structuring their work to include these rewards whenever possible.

Of course, as you probably know, these aren't the only factors that affect a nurse's motivation and morale. Here are some others:
- Taking time to consider the types of tasks you ask her to perform is important, too. The best way to prevent a demotivating conflict between a nurse's expectations of what her work will be like and her actual duties is to explain those duties before you hire her. Then, keep her fully informed of changes in the work you expect her to do (see Entry 62).
- Helping staff members develop new skills will also improve their job performance—and satisfaction.
- Including staff members in your decision-making efforts can greatly enhance their sense of importance on the unit. Of course, you won't ask for their input every time you make a decision. But when their support or knowledge can possibly help you, and particularly when your decision will directly affect their nursing care, you should let them share in your decision-making process.

### A case in point

Imagine you're the head nurse on the pediatric unit. You've put a lot of effort into developing a new program to help parents understand their children's treatments. To save your staff nurses' time when teaching parents, you've prepared pamphlets explaining treatments children receive on your unit.

## USING CRITICISM AS A MOTIVATING FACTOR

As a nurse manager, you're responsible for evaluating your subordinates' job performance—probably your least favorite responsibility. But remember, criticism can demotivate or motivate, depending on how you present it. To make your criticism more motivating, try following these suggestions:

• Tell your subordinate you're confident she can improve.

• Avoid arguments by criticizing behavior, not attitude: The criticism "You're lazy" is debatable; "You've forgotten to chart medications" isn't.

• Criticize behavior as soon as it occurs. If your subordinate's aware of her mistake, early criticism will relieve her anxiety.

• Criticize one behavior at a time. Demanding several changes at once will overwhelm your subordinate.

• Make sure your subordinate understands your criticism and your expectations.

• Concentrate on solutions, not causes. Asking "What do you suggest to improve your charting?" works better than "Why are you having so much trouble?"

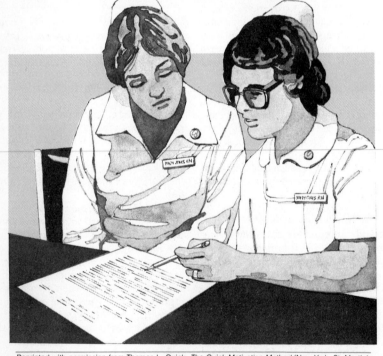

Reprinted with permission from Thomas L. Quick, *The Quick Motivation Method* (New York: St. Martin's Press, 1980).

When you present the program at a staff meeting, most of your nurses seem enthusiastic. But 3 weeks later, you notice that only two pamphlets have been used. Obviously, your staff isn't motivated enough to participate in the new program. What can you do?

You can motivate your staff and save your program. Here's how:

*Assess the situation.* First, you need to consider possible reasons why the program has flopped. Ask yourself these questions:

• Can your parent education program be implemented effectively in your unit? Or must something on the unit be changed to facilitate the program? Consider such changes as restructuring staff assignments to specifically include parent teaching, designating a specific quiet place for staff to teach parents, and structuring a specific time for teaching—for example, a child's naptime or when a child is in the play room.

• Is the information in the pamphlets really helpful, or are changes indicated?

• Has a recent change in the unit made your program obsolete?

• Have other programs failed because of a similar lack of staff motivation?

*Diagnose the cause of your program's failure.* You can zero in on the cause by holding open, nondefensive meetings with staff members. At these meetings, share your perceptions of the problem and allow staff members to state their feelings. Once you and your staff understand each other, you can take steps *together* to resolve the problem.

Assume that in your staff meetings, you discover three main problems:

• Your nurses find that the pamphlets are often irrelevant for specific patient needs.

• They see the pamphlets as an indication that you consider their parent teaching methods inadequate.

• They don't realize that you prepared the pamphlets to save them time and to help the less experienced staff members.

*Solve the problems.* If you allow your staff nurses to develop individual interest and involvement in the program, you can be reasonably sure they'll assume responsibility for its success. And

---

## USING I-MESSAGES

How do you get a staff member who causes problems to *solve* them? Try using "I-messages."

I-messages tell the listener how the speaker feels. To be complete, an I-message must also contain two other components: brief descriptions of the unacceptable behavior and its effects. (I-messages containing only feelings—such as "I'm upset with you" or "I'm really disappointed"—leave the listener bewildered.)

Imagine you're on the receiving end of the following I-message from your supervisor: "When I see you're absent from our nursing grand rounds, I feel strongly that we'll be less effective because we don't have the benefit of your experience and knowledge."

You wouldn't be especially pleased to receive this message (no one ever likes hearing that his behavior is unacceptable to another). But you'd probably be more willing to modify your behavior than if you'd been told what to do, warned, put down, blamed, or lectured. An I-message is a plea for help to the person giving you a problem, and such an appeal is hard to ignore.

Of course, an I-message isn't always immediately successful. After all, the behavior you want to change (to meet your needs) is the behavior the other person chose to meet her needs. No matter how tactful your I-message is, the listener may become anxious, defensive, hurt, apologetic, or resistant when she realizes you want her to change. In such a situation, hammering away with more I-messages is generally useless. Instead, shift to active listening. This shows that you understand and accept (not necessarily agree with, of course) the other person's feelings, defenses, and reasons. Also, she's then more willing to understand and accept your position. Your willingness to listen helps dissipate the other person's hurt, embarrassment, anger, or regret and paves the way for possible change. In some situations, active listening may lead you to change your own attitude—from finding the other person's behavior unacceptable to seeing it as acceptable.

---

Adapted with permission from Thomas Gordon, *L.E.T. Leadership Effectiveness Training* (Wyden Books, 1977).

## TEACHING NURSES TO WRITE NURSING DIAGNOSES

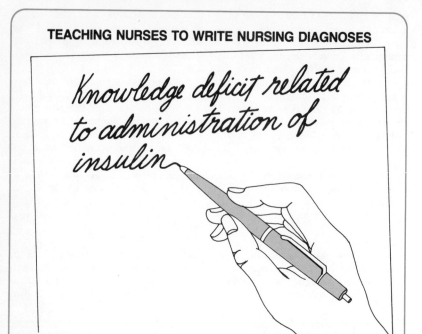

*Knowledge deficit related to administration of insulin*

As you know, the language of the officially recognized nursing diagnoses takes some getting used to. If you think your staff would feel more comfortable using their own words, you can teach them how to write their own nursing diagnoses.

Like the officially published diagnoses, any diagnosis a staff member writes must have two parts: a description of the patient's unhealthy state or behavior, and an identification of the unhealthy condition's cause. The parts should be connected by the words *related to.*

Here are some points your staff should keep in mind when writing nursing diagnoses:

• Nursing diagnoses should concern only patient conditions that require nursing intervention. If a staff member uncovers a condition that requires medical intervention, she should inform the patient's doctor. For example, the nurse should not write "Diabetes mellitus"—this is a medical diagnosis. But if she finds that the patient doesn't understand how and when to administer insulin, she can write "Knowledge deficit related to administration of insulin." Caution your staff that they must never intervene beyond the scope of nursing practice.

• Both parts of the nursing diagnosis must

be changeable, as the patient's status changes. If either one of the parts is irrevocable, nursing intervention can't help. For example, the nurse should not write "Impaired gas exchange related to COPD." She can't treat COPD but she can treat the causes of impaired gas exchange. She should write "Impaired gas exchange related to poor positive breathing patterns, fatigue, and anxiety."

• Nursing diagnoses needn't be restricted to a patient's existing problems. The staff can write a nursing diagnosis for a patient's potential problem, as well. For example, the nurse can write that the patient who has suffered a recent CVA has a "Potential for impairment of skin integrity related to sensory deficit and immobility." In such a situation, the nurse can then initiate treatment to *prevent* skin breakdown.

As your nurses practice writing nursing diagnoses, point out statements that may require further data collection for verification and for determination of cause. And help your staff understand that what represents an unhealthy response in one patient's diagnosis may turn up as the cause in another. The nurse's goal is always to treat the cause of the patient's problem and bring about positive change in the patient's unhealthy condition.

the more you allow them to get involved in improving the program, the greater their commitment will be. So now that you've identified the problems, first explain that preparing the pamphlets was *not* an indication that you thought your staff's parent-teaching efforts inadequate. (If it *was*, see *Using Criticism as a Motivating Factor*, page 656.) Then, encourage staff members to offer constructive changes. For example, ask them how they'd change the pamphlets—or the entire program, so that it addresses the specific needs of all the unit's patients. Most of the staff members will probably welcome the chance to contribute to your decision-making process. Try some of their suggestions, evaluate the results with them, and let them suggest new approaches if needed. As time goes on, you'll probably have a working program *and* a well-motivated staff whose morale is high.

Of course, no matter how open you are with your staff, some members just won't contribute. Perhaps they feel threatened by the additional responsibility you're asking them to assume. Such a reaction by a few nurses is normal. Don't let it deter you. (See *Using I-messages*, page 657.)

You might want to limit participation in the program to those members who contribute to restructuring it. This makes participating in the program a reward for helping create it. You might also want to encourage nurses who aren't participating to suggest other programs for the unit.

Of course, this hypothetical example is just one illustration of how a nurse manager can use motivating and morale-building techniques. You'll find that the open-communication approach pays long-term dividends. Once your staff knows they can talk freely with you, you're likely to have their active cooperation when you want to try other changes on the unit.

### A final word
As a nurse manager, your job is to en-

sure quality patient care. One way you do this is to motivate your nursing staff and to maintain their morale. Remember these pointers:
- Give your staff a chance to use a wide range of nursing skills.
- Assign your nurses to meaningful roles in projects.
- Whenever possible, allow them to choose how to do their assigned tasks.
- Evaluate their work, and offer suggestions for doing it better.
- Most of all, work with your staff to create an atmosphere of open communication and innovative nursing practice. This will produce benefits for all: you'll have a well-motivated staff and the benefit of their ideas for improvements. They'll have higher morale and increased job satisfaction. Most important, your patients will have better care.

---

# 110 Promoting autonomy within your staff

For nursing to be fully recognized and respected as a profession, nurses must strongly assert their capability of functioning autonomously. Today, many forces are at work restricting this capability, including:
- employment agencies' restrictive policies
- certain nurse managers' militaristic attitudes
- doctors' paternalistic (or worse, autocratic) attitudes toward nurses
- some educators' emphasis on the nurse's traditional (some say handmaiden) role.

Of course, many nurses have been trained to rely on the medical community and their nursing superiors for direction in providing patient care. So they don't necessarily have the knowledge or skills to function indepen-

GLOSSARY

## KEY TERMS IN THIS ENTRY

**nursing diagnosis** • Descriptive interpretations—accepted by the National Group on the Classification of Nursing Diagnosis—of collected and categorized information indicating the problems or needs of a patient that nursing care can affect.

**nursing process** • An organizational framework for nursing practice, encompassing all the major steps a nurse takes when caring for a patient.

**nursing theory** • The set of accepted principles that help a nurse analyze nursing practice.

dently. This is where you, as a nurse manager, can make a major contribution to your staff's professional growth—*and* to your profession as a whole. How? By acting to promote autonomy among your nursing staff.

Breaking the bonds of nursing's traditional dependent role won't be easy. (See Entry 85.) *You* know that nurses have the capacity to function independently, but patients, doctors, and administrators need proof. They're all concerned about maintaining patient-care quality—but they're also concerned that independently functioning nurses may cause nursing costs to rise.

Consider how a typical patient views his nursing care. He can't separate what a nurse is doing on a dependent basis from what she's doing independently. He assumes that his doctor directs all his care, including nursing services. So he probably won't be sympathetic to nursing's drive toward autonomy if higher costs are likely to result. He's bound to ask, if he's ever confronted with a hospitalization bill that separates nursing costs from room and board, "Did I really need a nurse to perform the nursing care I received? Or could someone who's paid less have taken just as good care of me?"

Convincing patients, doctors, and administrators that nurses who practice autonomously provide good patient care—and more of it—is the job you and your staff can do *by demonstrating the benefits every day.* This entry shows you how to educate your staff (with emphasis on nursing diagnosis and the nursing process) and motivate them to attain real nursing autonomy. Along the way, they'll also gain increased respect from their health-care colleagues.

## Spearheading autonomy: The nursing process and nursing diagnosis

Autonomy in nursing means nursing practice that's independent, self-directed, and subject to its own rules and regulations. That sounds fine in theory, doesn't it? Like something worth working for. But actually, it's here now. Many nurses don't realize that they have a significant amount of autonomy already. (See *How Autonomous Are You?*, pages 664-666.) For example, the nursing diagnosis and the nursing process, by helping to identify problems that nurses can deal with independently, also help define nursing as an autonomous profession. Together, these techniques provide documented proof of nursing's contribution to patients' recovery.

Consider this hypothetical example: Charlie Baker, age 53, was diagnosed as having squamous cell carcinoma of the tongue and was treated by hemiglossectomy, lymph node dissection, and adjunctive radiation therapy. Obviously, much of the care that nurses provided Charlie throughout his hospitalization involved medical therapy. But because Charlie's nurses also acted autonomously, they were able to provide an extra dimension of care—*nursing care* that clearly made a difference in Charlie's health and acceptance of his altered self-image. Here's what happened:

Through careful assessment and interpretation, Charlie's nurses discovered that he viewed his inability to enjoy eating as his biggest problem.

According to Charlie, "Some stuff tastes funny, some has no taste, and everything's dry as dust." As the nurses gathered data, they were able to arrive at a *nursing diagnosis* because Charlie's problem was amenable to nursing therapies. (If Charlie had required diet therapy, such as enteral hyperalimentation, or medical therapy, such as parenteral hyperalimentation, the nurses' functions would have depended on the respective dietetic or medical diagnoses.)

The nursing diagnosis—"Alteration in nutrition, less than body requirements, related to deficit in moisturizing and tasting foods"—described Charlie's involuntary, negative, physical response to the surgical and radiation therapies that had damaged his taste buds and impaired his salivary glands. His nurses applied the nursing process to assess the problem and to implement a plan that would help Charlie halt losing weight and begin gaining weight. Charlie's nurses helped him attain these goals with a simple, but highly effective, plan. They searched for foods Charlie could taste enough to enjoy, and that would provide him with adequate protein, vitamins, carbohydrates, and fats to meet his caloric needs. And they used a saliva substitute to moisten Charlie's food so he could chew and swallow.

Once they'd determined the foods Charlie could eat, his nurses wrote orders to the dietary and nursing departments for Charlie to have six meals a day with socialization. Family, friends, and staff sat and talked with Charlie during meals, giving him support and encouragement to help him adapt to his new eating habits.

Fluids, of course, were important in the nurses' plan for Charlie. Charlie avoided milk because it tasted salty to him. So the nurses' order called for more fluids with a high nutritional content. The increased fluid intake helped him swallow his food more easily, and it also improved his bowel and urinary function.

So while his doctors autonomously treated Charlie's disease, his nurses autonomously treated his unhealthful response to the disease process and its medical therapy. Charlie had reluctantly submitted to medical therapy because he wanted to stay alive. But he cooperated readily with his nurses. Why? Because their nursing therapy was helping him enjoy his life more.

## Implementing nursing diagnosis and the nursing process

For you to successfully implement nursing diagnosis and the nursing process on your unit, and to establish a truly autonomous nursing staff, two elements must be present. First you, as nurse manager, must be committed to helping your staff grow toward an autonomous nursing practice. You must

*"Your attitudes about autonomy bear directly on the way your nurses perceive their roles."*

see yourself as a coordinator, collaborator, and consultant, rather than as an autocratic authority figure. Second, you must have administrative support.

As you know, your attitudes have a direct bearing on the way your nurses perceive their roles. If you demonstrate enthusiasm and confidence in using nursing diagnosis and the nursing process, you'll motivate even hesitant nurses to at least give the method a try. You can also use your knowledge and enthusiasm to convince the hospital administration that the new approach will enhance patient care. Remember, you'll need administrative backing to obtain the time, money, and tools you need to train your nurses. (Of course, if your staff nurses are already using nursing diagnosis and the nursing process, they're well started on the road

## ACCEPTED NURSING DIAGNOSES

Although you may write your own nursing diagnoses, whenever possible you should refer to and use this official list of nursing diagnoses, accepted at the Fifth National Conference for Classification of Nursing Diagnosis, held in St. Louis, April 13-17, 1982:

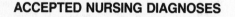

Activity Intolerance
Airway Clearance, Ineffective
Anxiety
Bowel Elimination, Alterations in: Constipation
Bowel Elimination, Alterations in: Diarrhea
Bowel Elimination, Alterations in: Incontinence
Breathing Patterns, Ineffective
Cardiac Output, Alterations in: Decreased
Comfort, Alterations in: Pain
Communication, Impaired Verbal
Coping, Family: Potential for Growth
Coping, Ineffective Family: Compromised
Coping, Ineffective Family: Disabling
Coping, Ineffective Individual
Diversional Activity, Deficit
Family Processes, Alterations
Fear
Fluid Volume, Alterations in: Excess
Fluid Volume Deficit, Actual
Fluid Volume Deficit, Potential
Gas Exchange, Impaired
Grieving, Anticipatory
Grieving, Dysfunctional
Health Maintenance Management, Impaired
Injury, Potential for
Knowledge Deficit (specify)
Mobility, Impaired Physical
Noncompliance (specify)
Nutrition, Alterations in: Less Than Body Requirements
Nutrition, Alterations in: More Than Body Requirements
Nutrition, Alterations in: Potential for More Than Body Requirements
Oral Mucous Membrane, Alterations in

Parenting, Alterations in: Actual
Parenting, Alterations in: Potential
Powerlessness
Rape-Trauma Syndrome
Self-care Deficit (specify level)
Self-concept, Disturbance in
Sensory Perceptual Alterations
Sexual Dysfunction
Skin Integrity, Impairment of: Actual
Skin Integrity, Impairment of: Potential
Sleep Pattern Disturbance
Social Isolation
Spiritual Distress
Thought Processes, Alterations in
Tissue Perfusion, Alteration in
Urinary Elimination, Alteration in Patterns
Violence, Potential for

**Diagnoses to be developed**

Agressive Coping Mode
Aggressive Responsive State
Cognitive Dissonance
Consciousness, Altered Levels of
Decision-making, Impaired/Ineffective
Dependent Coping Mode
Depleted Health Potential
Impulse Dominated State
Impulsive Coping Mode
Manipulative Coping Mode
Memory Deficit
Rational Anger State
Role Disturbance
Self-exaltation State
Self-harm
Social Network Support, Alteration in
Subtle Obstructive Mode
Victim Abuse Syndrome

to nursing autonomy. Review this entry for ways to strengthen your unit's commitment to this goal.)

To begin your staff training program, review and read about and *work with* nursing diagnosis and the nursing process. Do this until you're really comfortable with both techniques. In the meantime, post descriptive literature on unit bulletin boards so that staff can browse through it at their leisure, without pressure to do so. Take the time now to evaluate your staff's present understanding of the two techniques and opinion of their value. If they understand nursing diagnosis, do they believe in its usefulness? Do they understand how the two techniques fit together? Recognizing the value of nursing diagnosis and the nursing process is your staff's vital first step toward autonomy. Why? Because nurses who are comfortable with their work and value it will rarely compromise it. You need that kind of quality work from your staff to prove to others that nursing autonomy is worth promoting.

When you feel ready, actively teach your nurses to use the nursing process. You can begin by spending a few minutes each day with your nurses, either individually or collectively, to discuss problems that their patients have shared with them. If they can't name any specific patient problems, encourage them to identify their patients' strengths and weaknesses. If a patient's weakness is affecting his response to his care, point out to the nurses that this patient probably has an unmet need—a *problem* that they can respond to as nurses and help resolve.

Warn your nurses against trying to resolve patients' problems before identifying them accurately. Advise gathering complete data about a patient's problem by using information already available from his chart and by talking further with him, with his family, with his doctor, and with other health professionals involved in his care.

The next stage involves examining specific patient problems to determine *whose* problems they really are. Suppose a patient's unable to sleep at night. Consider that this problem may require intervention with the staff rather than with the patient. For example, maybe the noise level on the unit is higher than he can tolerate. But what if you determine that this patient's sleeplessness is caused by his fear of dying? Then, as you know, you should decide on a nursing intervention plan. For example, encouraging the patient to discuss his fears and work through them, and perhaps arranging for a pastoral visit, may help resolve the patient's problem.

Once your staff is comfortable with identifying and assessing patient problems and their causes, you should introduce nursing diagnosis. You can do this formally, by posting the official diagnoses that all should use (see *Accepted Nursing Diagnoses*). Or you can encourage nurses to begin by creating their own nursing diagnoses, so that they're not put off by the official language. (See *Teaching Nurses to Write Nursing Diagnoses,* page 658.)

Teaching nurses to use nursing diagnosis and to correlate it with the nursing process will probably require a good deal of your time and effort, especially if your nurses have been traditionally rewarded for *giving* care rather than *planning* it. After all, many nurses consider their workday full already, with carrying out doctors' orders and following policies and procedures to the letter. Nurses such as these may think that adding new functions to their schedules will take time away from other tasks. You may need to demonstrate use of nursing diagnosis and the nursing process for an extended period of time on the unit before your staff—and administration— are able to realize that these functions actually save time *and* promote better patient care.

## Accepting accountability for autonomous actions

As nurses assert the right to determine their own actions, they must be willing

# HOW AUTONOMOUS ARE YOU?

Do you view yourself as an autonomous nurse? To find out, take this test. Rate your response to each statement below. Then, total your score using the directions that follow

| | 1 Strongly Disagree | 2 Disagree | 3 Undecided | 4 Agree | 5 Strongly Agree |
|---|---|---|---|---|---|
| 1. I feel patients should plan their own activities. | | | | | |
| 2. I've fulfilled my responsibility when I report a condition to a doctor. | | | | | |
| 3. I'd feel free to try new approaches to patients' care without the "permission" of an administrative nurse. | | | | | |
| 4. I feel free to recommend nonprescription medication. | | | | | |
| 5. If I requested a psychiatric consult for a patient, I'd feel out of bounds. | | | | | |
| 6. I believe a patient has a right to have all his questions answered for him. | | | | | |
| 7. If I'm not satisfied with the doctor's action, I'd pursue the issue. | | | | | |
| 8. I'm the best person in the hospital to be the patient's advocate if he disagrees with the doctor. | | | | | |
| 9. If a patient is allowed to keep a lot of personal items, it becomes more trouble than it's worth. | | | | | |
| 10. I don't answer too many of the patient's questions because the doctor may have another plan in mind. | | | | | |
| 11. I feel the doctor is far better trained to make decisions than I am. | | | | | |
| 12. I'd never call a patient's family after discharge. | | | | | |
| 13. Patients shouldn't have any responsibility in a hospital. | | | | | |
| 14. Patients should be permitted to go off their units and elsewhere in the hospital. | | | | | |
| 15. If a patient asks why his medication is changed, I'd refer him to his doctor. | | | | | |
| 16. If a policy change affects patient care, I want to understand why the change is necessary. | | | | | |
| 17. Patients should be encouraged to show their feelings. | | | | | |
| 18. I should be able to go into private practice (like a doctor's) if I wish. | | | | | |

the test. You can obtain separate scores indicating your overall degree of nursing autonomy (Subscale 1), your commitment to asserting patients' rights (Subscale 2), and your degree of rejection of traditional role limitations (Subscale 3).

| | Strongly Disagree 1 | Disagree 2 | Undecided 3 | Agree 4 | Strongly Agree 5 |
|---|---|---|---|---|---|
| 19. I feel patients should be told the medications they're taking. | | | | | |
| 20. I should have a right to know why a change is necessary before it's accepted. | | | | | |
| 21. Patients should be told their diagnosis. | | | | | |
| 22. If I make conversation with the patient, there's no need to explain procedures and treatments before they're started. | | | | | |
| 23. I generally know more about the patient than the doctor does. | | | | | |
| 24. Patients in a hospital have a right to select the type of care they wish. | | | | | |
| 25. If I disagree with the doctor, I keep it to myself. | | | | | |
| 26. I feel the patient has the right to expect me, as a nurse, to effectively use my time in improving my skills by taking advantage of educational opportunities offered. | | | | | |
| 27. I'd feel comfortable authorizing a patient to leave the unit to go to another part of the hospital. | | | | | |
| 28. The patient has a right to expect me to regard his personal needs as having priority over mine. | | | | | |
| 29. I feel the patient has a right to refuse care. | | | | | |
| 30. It should be the doctor who decides if the patient can administer his own drugs. | | | | | |
| 31. I'd never refuse to carry out a doctor's order. | | | | | |
| 32. I feel patients should be informed about what constitutes quality health care. | | | | | |
| 33. The patient has a right to expect me to accept his social/cultural code and to consider its influence on his way of life. | | | | | |
| 34. Patients should be permitted to wear what they want. | | | | | |
| 35. I'd never interact with a patient on a first-name basis. | | | | | |
| 36. I rarely give in to patient pressure. | | | | | |

*(continued)*

## HOW AUTONOMOUS ARE YOU? *(continued)*

| | Strongly Disagree (1) | Disagree (2) | Undecided (3) | Agree (4) | Strongly Agree (5) |
|---|---|---|---|---|---|
| 37. Nurses should be held solely legally responsible for their own actions and shouldn't expect to come under the umbrella of the doctor or hospital in a malpractice suit. | | | | | |
| 38. Doctors must decide what nurses can and cannot do in the delivery of health care. | | | | | |
| 39. It's the nurse's prerogative to decide whether or not to wear a uniform. | | | | | |
| 40. I'd give the patient his diagnosis if he asks. | | | | | |
| 41. It should be the nurse's decision when to talk to the terminally ill patient about his condition. | | | | | |
| 42. I think it's my responsibility to initiate public health referrals on patients. | | | | | |
| 43. I feel I should suggest to patients, family, and doctors any community resources I know are available. | | | | | |
| 44. Patients can expect me to speak up for them. | | | | | |
| 45. I'd never ask a patient about his or her sexual life. | | | | | |
| 46. I'd talk very little to patients about their pasts. | | | | | |
| 47. I rarely ask a patient a personal question. | | | | | |

To score Subscale 1 (nursing autonomy):
- Add the scores for these statements: 1, 2, 3, 4, 8, 14, 18, 23, 24, 27, 34, 37, 39, 40, 41, and 42.
- Subtract this total from 90.
- Add the remainder to the total score for these statements: 5, 9, 10, 11, 12, 15, 30, 36, 38, 45, and 46.

To score Subscale 2 (patients' rights):
- Add the scores for these statements: 6, 16, 17, 19, 20, 21, 26, 28, 29, 32, 33, 34, 43, and 44.
- Subtract the total from 84.

To score Subscale 3 (rejection of traditional role limitations):
- Subtract your score for statement 7 from 6.
- Add the remainder to the total score for these statements: 2, 5, 10, 11, 13, 22, 25, 31, 35, 45, 46, and 47.

Now, compare your score with the scores of 700 nurses surveyed. Mean scores for subscale 1 ranged from 73.9 to 102.1; for subscale 2, from 53.8 to 61.3; and for subscale 3, from 45.8 to 56.1. The higher your score, the more autonomous you are.

Adapted with permission from Loren Pankratz, Ph.D. psychologist, Veterans Administration Medical Center, Portland, Ore.

to be held accountable for the results of those actions.

Today, nurses who assert their autonomy do more than carry out tasks. They diagnose conditions and plan appropriate interventions, and they accept responsibility for the outcome of their care. For example, suppose you write a nursing diagnosis for an immobile patient as "Alteration in tissue perfusion related to immobility." Once you've made this nursing diagnosis, you assume responsibility for planning and carrying out therapies to improve the tissue perfusion, such as turning the patient every 2 hours. Consequently, you also become accountable for the therapeutic outcome—whether or not your intervention improved the patient's tissue perfusion.

Some nurses fear the legal implications of increased professional accountability. But if your decision-making and nursing interventions stem from sound nursing knowledge, you should be able to assume increased accountability with confidence.

## A final word

Through autonomy, nurses today are independently defining their body of knowledge, determining their mode of practice, and promoting their right to provide specialized health care. Using the nursing process and nursing diagnosis is the spearhead of that effort. These techniques help nurses zero in on specific patient problems they can address with their *nursing* expertise. Through autonomy, the nursing profession finally will become fully self-governing.

## Selected References

Althaus, J.N., et al. "Nurse Staffing in a Decentralized Organization," Part 1. *Journal of Nursing Administration* 12:34-39, March 1982.

Bragg, T.L. "Motivation and Dissatisfaction," *Nursing Management* 13:20-22, August 1982.

Brief, A.P. "Turnover among Hospital Nurses: A Suggested Model," *Journal of Nursing Administration*, 6:55-57, October 1976.

Clark, E. "The Demise of the Traditional 5-40 Workweek," *American Journal of Nursing* 81:1138-41, June 1981.

Eusanio, P.L. "Effective Scheduling—the Foundation for Quality Care," *Journal of Nursing Administration* 8:12-17, January 1978.

Giovannetti, P. "Understanding Patient Classification Systems," *Journal of Nursing Administration* 9:4-8, February 1979.

Kellman, Donna. "The Ten-Hour Schedule," *Nursing Management* 14(2):58-62, February 1983.

Kenwood, N.J., and Martens, L.C. "Morale Problems: A Structured Group Approach," *Nursing Management* 13:37-39, July 1982.

Lakein, Alan. *How to Get Control of Your Time and Your Life.* New York: New American Library, 1974.

McConnell, E.A. "Delegation—Myth or Reality?" *Supervisor Nurse* 10:20-21, October 1979.

McIntyre, R. "What to Do When You Feel Overwhelmed by Added Responsibility," *NursingLife* 1:66-69, July/August 1981.

Metcalf, M.L. "The 12-Hour Weekend Plan—Does the Nursing Staff Really Like It?" *Journal of Nursing Administration* 12(10):16-19, October 1982.

Mundinger, Mary O. *Autonomy in Nursing.* Rockville, Md.: Aspen Systems Corp., 1980.

Shubin, S. "Promotion and Friendship—Can You Mix Them?" *NursingLife* 1:30-35, November/December 1981.

Stevens, Barbara J. "Assigning, Staffing, and Scheduling," in *The Nurse as Executive*, 2nd ed. Rockville, Md.: Aspen Systems Corp., 1980.

Vik, A.G., and MacKay, R.C. "How Does the 12-Hour Shift Affect Patient Care?" *Journal of Nursing Administration* 12:11-14, January 1982.

Wandelt, M.A., et al. "Why Nurses Leave Nursing and What Can Be Done About It," *American Journal of Nursing* 81:72-77, January 1981.

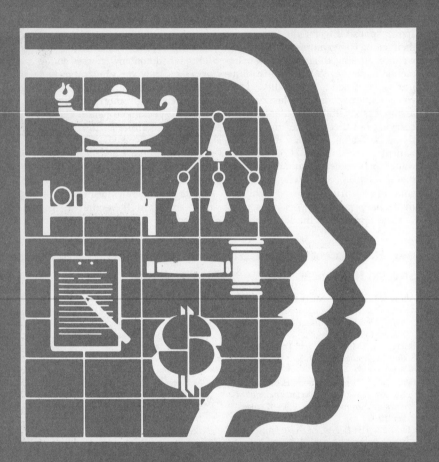

# Fact
# Finder

A legal and professional ready-reference guide for nurses

## BASIC HUMAN RIGHTS

The Bill of Rights and Amendment XIV of the Constitution of the United States define the basic human rights that all persons under all circumstances, including hospitalization, are entitled to. These rights are as follows:

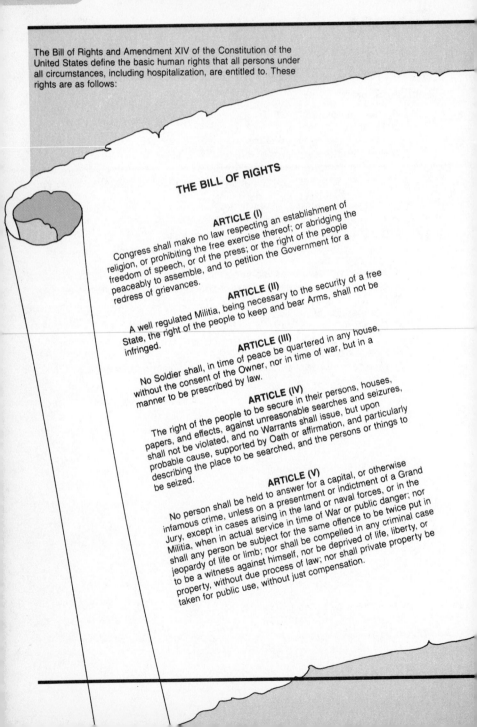

# THE BILL OF RIGHTS

## ARTICLE (I)

Congress shall make no law respecting an establishment of religion, or prohibiting the free exercise thereof; or abridging the freedom of speech, or of the press; or the right of the people peaceably to assemble, and to petition the Government for a redress of grievances.

## ARTICLE (II)

A well regulated Militia, being necessary to the security of a free State, the right of the people to keep and bear Arms, shall not be infringed.

## ARTICLE (III)

No Soldier shall, in time of peace be quartered in any house, without the consent of the Owner, nor in time of war, but in a manner to be prescribed by law.

## ARTICLE (IV)

The right of the people to be secure in their persons, houses, papers, and effects, against unreasonable searches and seizures, shall not be violated, and no Warrants shall issue, but upon probable cause, supported by Oath or affirmation, and particularly describing the place to be searched, and the persons or things to be seized.

## ARTICLE (V)

No person shall be held to answer for a capital, or otherwise infamous crime, unless on a presentment or indictment of a Grand Jury, except in cases arising in the land or naval forces, or in the Militia, when in actual service in time of War or public danger; nor shall any person be subject for the same offence to be twice put in jeopardy of life or limb; nor shall be compelled in any criminal case to be a witness against himself, nor be deprived of life, liberty, or property, without due process of law; nor shall private property be taken for public use, without just compensation.

### ARTICLE (VI)

In all criminal prosecutions, the accused shall enjoy the right to a speedy and public trial, by an impartial jury of the State and district wherein the crime shall have been committed, which district shall have been previously ascertained by law, and to be informed of the nature and cause of the accusation; to be confronted with the witnesses against him; to have compulsory process for obtaining witnesses in his favor, and to have the Assistance of Counsel for his defence.

### ARTICLE (VII)

In Suits at common law, where the value in controversy shall exceed twenty dollars, the right of trial by jury shall be preserved, and no fact tried by a jury shall be otherwise re-examined in any Court of the United States, than according to the rules of the common law.

### ARTICLE (VIII)

Excessive bail shall not be required, nor excessive fines imposed, nor cruel and unusual punishments inflicted.

### ARTICLE (IX)

The enumeration in the Constitution, of certain rights, shall not be construed to deny or disparage others retained by the people.

### ARTICLE (X)

The powers not delegated to the United States by the Constitution, nor prohibited by it to the States, are reserved to the States respectively, or to the people.

### ARTICLE (Amendment) XIV

Section I. All persons born or naturalized in the United States, and subject to the jurisdiction thereof, are citizens of the United States and of the State wherein they reside. No State shall make or enforce any law which shall abridge the privileges or immunities of citizens of the United States; nor shall any State deprive any person of life, liberty, or property, without due process of law; nor deny to any person within its jurisdiction the equal protection of the laws.

## Nursing's Role in Patient's Rights

The National League for Nursing believes nurses are responsible for upholding these rights of patients:

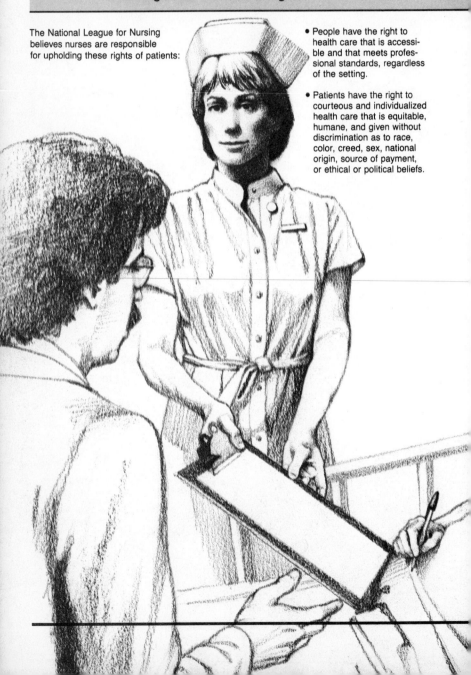

- People have the right to health care that is accessible and that meets professional standards, regardless of the setting.

- Patients have the right to courteous and individualized health care that is equitable, humane, and given without discrimination as to race, color, creed, sex, national origin, source of payment, or ethical or political beliefs.

- Patients have the right to information about their diagnosis, prognosis, and treatment—including alternatives to care and risks involved—in terms they and their families can readily understand, so that they can give their informed consent.

- Patients have the legal right to informed participation in all decisions concerning their health care.

- Patients have the right to information about the qualifications, names, and titles of personnel responsible for providing their health care.

- Patients have the right to refuse observation by those not directly involved in their care.

- Patients have the right to privacy during interview, examination, and treatment.

- Patients have the right to privacy in communicating and visiting with persons of their choice.

- Patients have the right to refuse treatments, medications, or participation in research and experimentation, without punitive action being taken against them.

- Patients have the right to coordination and continuity of health care.

- Patients have the right to appropriate instruction or education from health care personnel so that they can achieve an optimal level of wellness and an understanding of their basic health needs.

- Patients have the right to confidentiality of all records (except as otherwise provided for by law or third-party payer contracts) and all communications, written or oral, between patients and health care providers.

- Patients have the right of access to all health records pertaining to them, the right to challenge and to have their records corrected for accuracy, and the right to transfer of all such records in the case of continuing care.

- Patients have the right to information on the charges for services, including the right to challenge these.

- Above all, patients have the right to be fully informed as to all their rights in all health care settings.

The National League for Nursing urges its membership, through action and example, to demonstrate that the profession of nursing is committed to the concepts of patient's rights.

Reprinted with permission of the National League for Nursing.

(continued)

**PATIENT'S BILLS OF RIGHTS** *(continued)*

## A Model Patient's Bill of Rights

The American Civil Liberties Union has developed this patient's bill of rights as a model for any health institution wishing to develop its own.

*Preamble:* As you enter this health care facility, it is our duty to remind you that your health care is a cooperative effort between you as a patient and the doctors and hospital staff. During your stay a patients' rights advocate will be available to you. The duty of the advocate is to assist you in all the decisions you must make and in all situations in which your health and welfare are at stake. The advocate's first responsibility is to help you understand the role of all who will be working with you, and to help you understand what your rights as a patient are. Your advocate can be reached at any time of the day by dialing _____. The following is a list of your rights as a patient. Your advocate's duty is to see to it that you are afforded these rights. You should call your advocate whenever you have any questions or concerns about any of these rights.

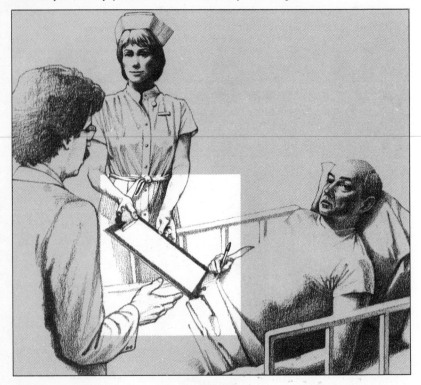

- The patient has a legal right to informed participation in all decisions involving his/her health care program.

- We recognize the right of all potential patients to know what research and experi-mental protocols are being used in our facility and what alternatives are available in the community.

- The patient has a legal right to privacy regarding the source of payment for treat-ment and care. This right in-cludes access to the highest degree of care with-out regard to the source of payment for that treatment and care.

- We recognize the right of a

potential patient to complete and accurate information concerning medical care and procedures.

- The patient has a legal right to prompt attention, especially in an emergency situation.

- The patient has a legal right to a clear, concise explanation in layperson's terms of all proposed procedures, including the possibilities of any risk of mortality or serious side effects, problems related to recuperation, and probability of success, and will not be subjected to any procedure without his/her voluntary, competent and understanding consent. The specifics of such consent shall be set out in a written consent form, signed by the patient.

- The patient has a legal right to a clear, complete, and accurate evaluation of his/her condition and prognosis without treatment before being asked to consent to any test or procedure.

- We recognize the right of the patient to know the identity and professional status of all those providing service. All personnel have been instructed to introduce themselves, state their status, and explain their role in the health care of the patient. Part of this right is the right of the patient to know the identity of the physician responsible for his/her care.

- We recognize the right of any patient who does not speak English to have access to an interpreter.

- The patient has a right to all the information contained in his/her medical record while in the health care facility, and to examine the record on request.

- We recognize the right of a patient to discuss his/her condition with a consultant specialist, at the patient's request and expense.

- The patient has a legal right not to have any test or procedure, designed for educational purposes rather than his/her direct personal benefit, performed on him/her.

- The patient has a legal right to refuse any particular drug, test, procedure, or treatment.

- The patient has a legal right to privacy of both person and information with respect to: the hospital staff, other doctors, residents, interns and medical students, researchers, nurses, other hospital personnel, and other patients.

- We recognize the patient's right of access to people outside the health care facility by means of visitors and the telephone. Parents may stay with their children and relatives with terminally ill patients 24 hours a day.

- The patient has a legal right to leave the health care facility regardless of his/her physical condition or financial status, although the patient may be requested to sign a release stating that he/she is leaving against the medical judgment of his/her doctor or the hospital.

- The patient has a right not to be transferred to another facility unless he/she has received a complete explanation of the desirability of and need for the transfer. If the patient does not agree to transfer, the patient has the right to a consultant's opinion on the desirability of transfer.

- A patient has a right to be notified of his/her impending discharge at least one day before it is accomplished, to insist on a consultation by an expert on the desirability of discharge, and to have a person of the patient's choice notified in advance.

- The patient has a right, regardless of the source of payment, to examine and receive an itemized and detailed explanation of the total bill for services rendered in the facility.

- The patient has a right to competent counseling from the hospital staff to help in obtaining financial assistance from public or private sources to meet the expense of services received in the institution.

- The patient has a right to timely prior notice of the termination of his/her eligibility for reimbursement by any third-party payor for the expense of hospital care.

- At the termination of his/her stay at the health care facility we recognize the right of a patient to a complete copy of the information contained in his/her medical record.

- We recognize the right of all patients to have 24-hour-a-day access to a patient's rights advocate, who may act on behalf of the patient to assert or protect the rights set out in this document.

# UNDERSTANDING TYPES OF LAW

## PUBLIC LAW

Public law deals with an individual's relationship to the state. As the chart below indicates, the legal aspects of that relationship may concern matters of constitutional, administrative, or criminal law.

| CONSTITUTIONAL LAW | ADMINISTRATIVE LAW | CRIMINAL LAW |
|---|---|---|
| **FEDERAL**<br>• U.S. Constitution<br>• Civil Rights Act | **FEDERAL**<br>• Food, Drug, and Cosmetic Act<br>• Social Security Act (Medicare/Medicaid)<br>• National Labor Relations Act | **FEDERAL**<br>• Comprehensive Drug Abuse Prevention and Control Act (Controlled Substance Acts)<br>• Kidnapping |
| **STATE**<br>• State constitution | **STATE**<br>• Nurse Practice Act<br>• Medical Practice Act<br>• Pharmacy Act<br>• Workmen's Compensation laws<br>• State Labor Relations Act<br>• Employment Security Act | **STATE**<br>• Criminal code that defines murder, manslaughter, criminal negligence, rape, fraud, illegal possession of drugs (and other controlled substances), theft, assault, battery |

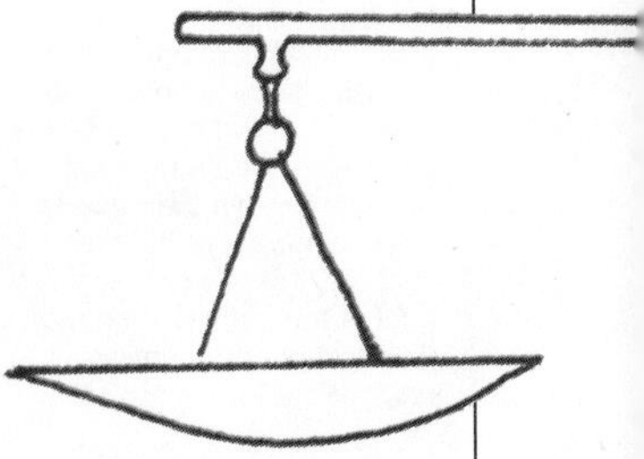

## PRIVATE (CIVIL) LAW

Private law deals with the relationships between individuals. As the chart below indicates, the legal aspect of these relationships divides into matters that concern contract law, torts, or protective/reporting law. Note that protective/reporting laws are sometimes considered criminal law, depending on how the state has classified them.

| CONTRACT LAWS | TORTS | PROTECTIVE/ REPORTING LAWS |
|---|---|---|
| **FEDERAL**<br><br>• None | **FEDERAL**<br><br>• Federal Torts Claims Act (to allow claims against the state) | **FEDERAL**<br><br>• Child Abuse Prevention and Treatment Act<br>• Privacy Act of 1974 |
| **STATE**<br><br>• Employment contracts<br>• Business contracts with clients<br>• Contracts with allied groups<br>• Uniform Commercial Code | **STATE**<br><br>• State Torts Claims Act (to allow claims against the state)<br>• Negligence (common law claim)<br>• Malpractice statute (professional liability)<br>• Assault<br>• Battery<br>• False imprisonment<br>• Invasion of privacy<br>• Libel | **STATE**<br><br>• Age of consent statutes for medical treatment, drugs, sexually transmitted disease<br>• Privileged communications statute<br>• Abortion statute<br>• Good Samaritan Act<br>• Child abuse/neglect statute<br>• Elderly abuse statute<br>• Domestic violence statute<br>• Involuntary hospitalization statute<br>• Living will legislation |

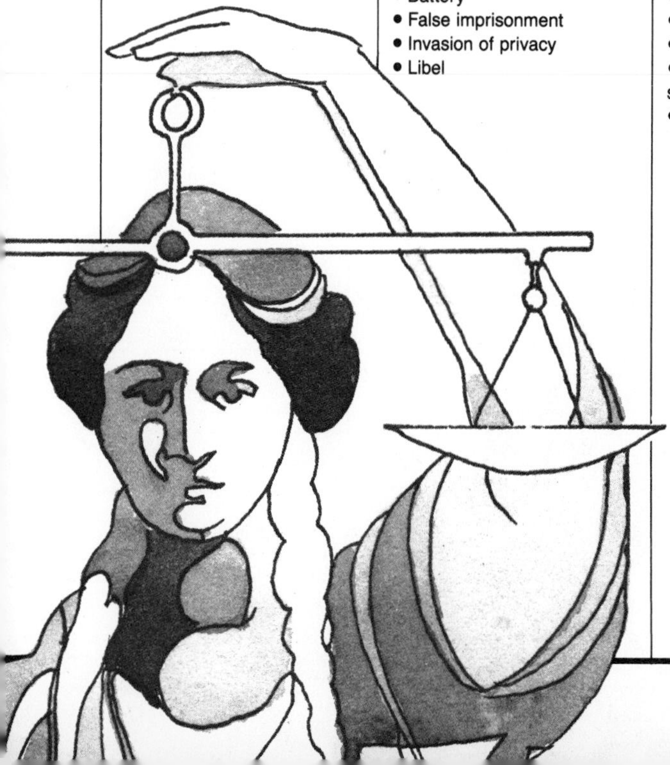

# D

## TORTS AND THEIR DEFENSES

A tort is any private or civil wrong (excluding wrongs occurring within a contractual relationship), to a person or property, for which the injured party can claim damages in a court of law. Your attorney's plan for defending you in a tort action would depend on whether the wrong you allegedly committed was intentional or unintentional and the nature of that wrong. This chart lists the types of defenses possible for each type of tort.

| | | NATURE OF TORT |
|---|---|---|
| UNINTENTIONAL | | Negligence |
| INTENTIONAL | | Assault |
| | | Libel (written defamation) |
| | | Slander (spoken defamation) |
| | | Battery |
| | | False imprisonment |
| | | Invasion of privacy (injury to person's feelings) |

| ELEMENTS PLAINTIFF MUST PROVE | POSSIBLE DEFENSES |
|---|---|
| • defendant owed duty to plaintiff<br>• breach of duty occurred<br>• breach of duty caused injury<br>• defendant owes plaintiff compensatory damages (for prima facie case) | • plaintiff's comparative negligence<br>• plaintiff's assumption of the risk<br>• unavoidable accident<br>• nonemployment emergency (covered by Good Samaritan Act) |
| • defendant's intent<br>• plaintiff's fear (immediate) of harmful or offensive touching | • plaintiff's consent<br>• privilege* (in situations requiring self-defense, defense of others, preventing plaintiff's self-inflicted harm) |
| • defamatory statement written by defendant and communicated to third party (no damages need be proven) | • truth of statement<br>• privilege:<br>absolute: judges/attorney/witnesses/juries during legal proceeding; consent of plaintiff<br>partial: employment references; reports to regulatory boards |
| • damages caused by a defamatory statement communicated by defendant to third party (generally damages need be proven except in these four cases: when the defendant accuses the plaintiff of a crime; when the defendant accuses the plaintiff of having a loathsome disease; when the defendant uses words that affect the plaintiff's profession or business; when the defendant calls a woman unchaste.) | see Libel |
| • defendant's intent<br>• occurrence of harmful or offensive touching<br>• absence of plaintiff's consent | see Assault |
| • unlawful restraint of plaintiff's personal liberty or<br>• unlawful detention of plaintiff | • privilege*<br>• statute that allows restraint or detention of:<br>mentally ill or dangerous persons<br>persons with communicable disease |
| • Invasion of a personal interest caused by defendant's behavior (facts must be presented so that defendant's behavior can be categorized under one of four recognized causes of action) | • plaintiff's consent<br>• your privilege under:<br>disclosure statute<br>judicial mandate (subpoena) |

*This defense is qualified: only reasonable force—that which is necessary under the circumstances—is allowed.

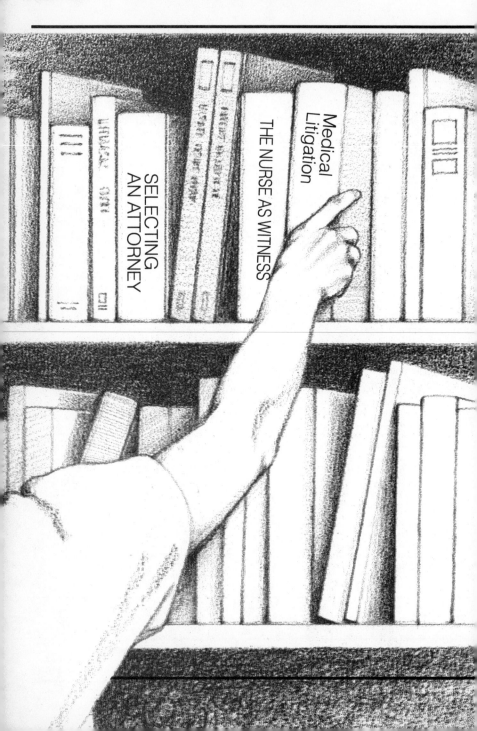

How do you look up a law (statute or regulation) or court case? First, go to your county court-house law library or local law school library with your legal citation in hand. If you're looking for an overview or summary of a law or court case, look up your citation in a standard legal reference, such as a legal encyclopedia *(Corpus Juris Secundum)* or a legal text *(Restatements of Law)*.

If you want to locate a complete text of the law or case, you must first have a full citation, such as the ones shown here.

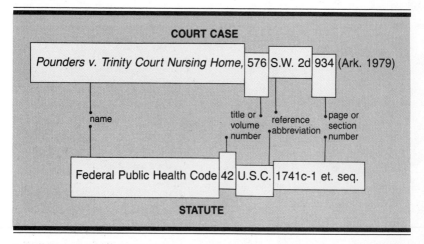

A full citation includes the name of the law or court case and a series of identifying numbers and letters. If you're missing some or all of the identifying numbers and letters, you'll need to look up the law or case name in the index of one of the legal references listed on page 681.

Once you get the full citation, you'll need to know how to interpret it. The letters in the series of identifying numbers and letters are an abbreviation for the legal reference that contains the law or case. For example, "L.W." stands for *United States Law Week*. (To find out what the abbreviation in your citation stands for, see the list of common legal references on page 683.)

The number that precedes the abbreviation indicates either a volume number or title classification within the legal reference. A title classification is a body of laws or cases on a particular subject, such as malpractice. A title can be one book or many books, depending on the amount of cases that bear on the titles.

If you're dealing with a law, one set of numbers follows the abbreviation. They indicate the section within the reference volume or title in which you'll find the law.

If you're dealing with a court case, two sets of numbers follow the abbreviation. The first set indicates the page where you'll find the case. The second set, in parentheses, indicates the year of the decision.

Sometimes, a court case on the state level will have two complete series of identifying numbers. The first series is the *official citation*, indicating where the case can be found in that state's set of court case decisions. The second series is the *unofficial citation*, indicating where the case can be found in a commercially published set of court case decisions grouped by region. These regional sets are explained in the listing on page 681. Interpreting this second series of numbers and letters works exactly the same way that interpreting the first series works. If the case citation only quotes the regional (commercial) listing, then the state court that heard the case, such as the Pennsylvania Commonwealth Court, is included in the parentheses with the date of the case.

*(continued)*

**HOW TO INTERPRET LEGAL CITATIONS** *(continued)*

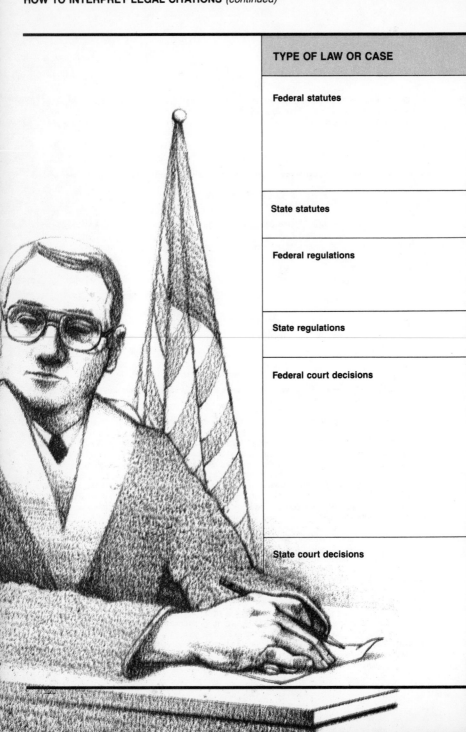

| TYPE OF LAW OR CASE |
| --- |
| Federal statutes |
| State statutes |
| Federal regulations |
| State regulations |
| Federal court decisions |
| State court decisions |

| LEGAL REFERENCE | ABBREVIATION |
|---|---|
| *United States Law Week*<br>(contains chronologic list of recently enacted statutes) | L.W. |
| *United States Statutes at Large*<br>(contains chronologic lists of all statutes enacted during a single legislative session) | STAT. or STAT. AT L. |
| *United States Code*<br>(contains all statutes arranged by title) | U.S.C. |
| All states publish state statutes in official state sets | Standard state abbreviations |
| *Code of Federal Regulations*<br>(contains federal regulations arranged by title) | C.F.R. |
| *The Federal Register*<br>(contains updates to the C.F.R.) | F.R. |
| All states publish state regulations in offical state sets | Standard state abbreviations |
| *United States Law Week*<br>(contains recently issued unofficial Supreme Court decisions) | L.W. |
| *United States Reports*<br>(contains official federal court decisions) | U.S. |
| *Supreme Court Reporter*<br>(contains official Supreme Court decisions) | S. Ct. |
| *Lawyers Edition, United States Supreme Court*<br>(contains official Supreme Court decisions) | L. Ed. |
| *Federal Reporter*<br>(contains court of appeals decisions) | F. |
| *Federal Supplement Series*<br>(contains Federal District Court of Appeals decisions) | F. Supp. |
| About two thirds of the states publish state court decisions in official state sets | Standard state abbreviations |
| All states are included in the commercially published National Reporter System, which groups state court decisions by region:<br>*North Eastern Reporter*<br>*Atlantic Reporter*<br>*South Eastern Reporter*<br>*Southern Reporter*<br>*North Western Reporter*<br>*South Western Reporter*<br>*Pacific Reporter* | <br><br>N.E.<br>A.<br>S.E.<br>So.<br>N.W.<br>S.W.<br>P. |

When you accept a job, you'll probably have the opportunity to negotiate a job contract. To get the best contract terms possible, use the guidelines that follow. If necessary, delete or modify those sections of the guidelines that don't address your needs or goals. For example, instead of bargaining for time off that includes vacation, sick days, holidays, and educational leave, you might negotiate for 60 paid working days off that you could use at your own discretion.

Keep in mind that negotiating requires give and take. So don't be disappointed if you don't get all that you wanted in your first written contract. Each time you negotiate, you'll get better at it and, perhaps, gain additional benefits.

This agreement is entered into this _____ day of _____ ____ by and between the _____(hospital, clinic, or individual physician) hereinafter referred to as the employer and _____ (name of individual nurse) hereinafter referred to as the employee.

Witnesseth:
Whereas it is the desire of the parties to this Agreement to promote mutual cooperation and understanding in the interest of maintaining quality patient care and to formulate rules to govern the relationship between them, now therefore, the parties agree as follows:

## SUGGESTED CONTRACT LANGUAGE

## BASIS FOR JUSTIFICATION

### ARTICLE I
#### Duties, Responsibilities, and Authority

The duties, responsibility, and authority of the nurse position shall be as follows: _____

Include job title, job description, and lines of authority.

### ARTICLE II
#### Salary

The employer will pay _____salary per month or _____per year.

In some work settings a probationary period may be required and the salary is less during this period. The probationary period would be negotiable unless within a civil service structure.

A yearly increase (increment) should be negotiated with payment started automatically on the anniversary date of employment each year. This would be over and above the cost-of-living increase negotiable when the contract is reopened.

### ARTICLE III
#### Hours of Work and Premium Pay

Time and one half shall be paid for all work in excess of 8 hours per day or 40 hours per week.

The negotiated salary is usually based upon a 40-hour workweek. It is contemplated that nurses will frequently work additional hours.

If contemplating innumerable hours of overtime and taking calls (nurse practitioners, etc.), negotiate a more substantial salary in lieu of all overtime and special on-call benefits.

| SUGGESTED CONTRACT LANGUAGE | BASIS FOR JUSTIFICATION |
|---|---|

### ARTICLE IV
#### Vacation

Vacation with pay will be at the rate of _____ working days per month and cumulative up to _____working days. Vacations will be scheduled only after consultation with and approval of the employee.

The goal would be to negotiate one month's vacation per year, not including holidays.

### ARTICLE V
#### Holidays

Holidays with pay will include the following:
1.
2.
3.
4.
5.
6.
7.
8.
9.
10.
11.
12.

The number of holidays vary, usually from 8 to 12. Some contracts now specify the employee's birthday.

If the employee has elected to include Article III—overtime for holidays should be negotiated. Nurses in some instances are realizing double pay for holidays.

(continued)

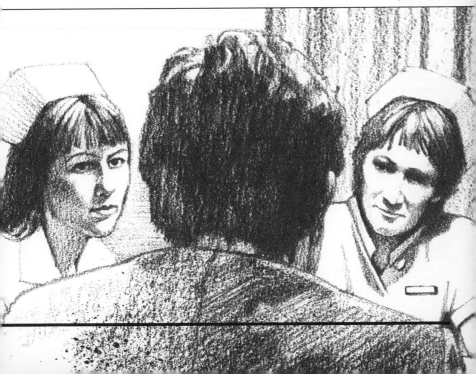

**AMERICAN NURSES' ASSOCIATION GUIDELINES
FOR THE INDIVIDUAL NURSE CONTRACT** *(continued)*

**SUGGESTED CONTRACT LANGUAGE       BASIS FOR JUSTIFICATION**

### ARTICLE VI
Nursing Education

The parties recognize the need for the employee to participate in continuing education programs.

The term education or educational as used in this article shall incude, but not be limited to, workshops, seminars, conferences, clinics, and other professional activities.

Any educational program required by the employer will be funded by the employer.

The employee may request attendance in an educational program or course of instruction, and the employer will approve such request if the following conditions are met:

    a. The educational program or course of instruction is related to the employee's job and will improve the professional skills to meet the needs of the employee.

    b. Attendance in the educational program or course of instruction will not unreasonably disrupt the normal operations of the employer.

Depending upon the circumstances, a specific number of days for educational leave may be negotiated per year. If flexibility is desired, use the articles without including a specific number of days.

To tighten the effectiveness of educational leave, the following addition may be made:

"In the event the employer is unable in good faith to grant the educational leave request the employer will set forth in writing the reasons for the denial."

    b. may be used as an excuse by the employer, but conversely may make the article more acceptable.

### ARTICLE VII
Sabbatical Leave

The employer will grant sabbatical leave to the employee after seven years' service with the employer as a registered professional nurse. Such leave shall not extend beyond one year.

In reviewing a request for sabbatical leave, the employer will consider and may approve on the following basis:

    a. The nature and length of professional educational course work, research, or other professional activity which the employee plans to undertake during the sabbatical leave.

    b. Whether the employee's absence during the leave will adversely affect providing essential services.

Employee while on sabbatical leave will be paid an amount equal to one half of the compensation which the employee was receiving at commencement of leave. The payments shall be made in regular monthly installments.

For your information, there is a precedent established for sabbatical leave in a group contract covering 620 nurses in Hawaii.

All university contracts should cover sabbatical as well.

    b. is again debatable but may be necessary.

| SUGGESTED CONTRACT LANGUAGE | BASIS FOR JUSTIFICATION |
|---|---|

Prior to the start of a sabbatical leave the employee and employer will enter into a supplement to this agreement which shall provide for the following:

   a. The employee will agree to return to work upon expiration of the sabbatical leave.

   b. Upon return from the sabbatical leave the employee will agree to work in the appropriate department for a period of two continuous years.

   c. The employee will be guaranteed return to the same or equivalent position at the expiration of the sabbatical leave.

   d. Upon the employee's return the salary rate will be the same as at the time of leave, and the increment date will be advanced equivalent to the duration of the leave.

d. Salary upon return is negotiable but should never be less than when sabbatical started.

The employee will not be deprived of any accumulated vacation allowance or sick leave credit but shall not accrue vacation allowance or sick leave credits during the leave period.

## ARTICLE VIII
### Other benefits

The employee shall be eligible to participate in the following employee benefit plans:

   1.
   2.
   3.

A reminder to check other benefit plans and include in the contract. As a substitute, a clause may be used stating "This agreement shall not be construed or applied in any manner to impair or diminish any existing rights, privileges, or benefits which would otherwise be available to the employee."

## ARTICLE IX
### Sick Leave

The employee will be entitled to sick leave with pay on the basis of _____working days for each month of continuous employment cumulative to _____working days.

Sick leave will be allowed for medical, dental, optical, and optometrical appointments which cannot be scheduled during off-duty time.

Sick leave is usually accrued at one day per month. The accumulation of leave varies greatly. An accumulation of several months becomes valuable.

Sick leave can now be used for maternity leave. Maternity leave has not been discussed, as the woman's equal rights under EEOC Guidelines delineate she use maternity leave at her own discretion with consultation from her personal physician. The employee's return to her position is guaranteed. Employers can no longer establish regulations discriminatory against the pregnant woman.

*(continued)*

# AMERICAN NURSES' ASSOCIATION GUIDELINES
# FOR THE INDIVIDUAL NURSE CONTRACT *(continued)*

| SUGGESTED CONTRACT LANGUAGE | BASIS FOR JUSTIFICATION |
|---|---|

### ARTICLE X
#### Leave of Absence for Death in the Family

The employee will be allowed three working days as funeral leave with pay which will not be deducted from any other leave to which the employee may be entitled. Funeral leaves will be granted on such days as designated by the employee provided they fall within a reasonable period of time after a death in the immediate family.

The meaning of family is a negotiable item.

Alternative or in addition to would be an article titled Personal Leave. The employee could use _____days per year at her own discretion for personal business.

### ARTICLE XI
#### Health Benefits

Existing medical coverage plans vary to an unbelievable degree. In state, city, and county employment, nurses are usually covered by the civil service benefits applied to all employees in that system.

The applicant must investigate what exists and if the programs are inadequate, and she must negotiate for individual coverage.

Retirement plans also vary. In many instances, in the private sector you must be employed for 2 years before being eligible to participate, with little or no vesting for 5 to 15 years. Many nurses match employer's funds monthly for a better retirement program.

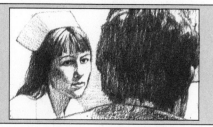

### ARTICLE XII
#### Transportation

Mileage for the use of personal automobiles will be computed from the employee's first call or from her official work station to her return to that station.

Mileage runs 15 to 20¢ per mile ordinarily. There are existing contracts that cover a car allowance if the car is used daily and heavily. This allowance, in some instances, is $50 per month.

The IRS allows 20¢ per mile. If the full 20¢ cannot be negotiated, the remainder can be claimed as an income tax deduction if records are adequate.

| SUGGESTED CONTRACT LANGUAGE | BASIS FOR JUSTIFICATION |

## ARTICLE XIII
### The Grievance Procedure

It is the intention of the parties that an employee grievance, which arises out of alleged violation, misinterpretation, or misapplication of this agreement, shall be resolved in accordance with provisions set forth herein.

Definition of a grievance: The term "grievance," as used in this agreement, shall mean a complaint filed by the employee alleging a violation, misinterpretation, or misapplication of a specific provision of this agreement occurring after its effective date. A grievance shall, whenever possible, be discussed and settled informally between the employee and her immediate supervisor. The employee may, if she desires, be assisted by a representative of her nurses' association.

Formal steps:

Step 1:
If the matter is not satisfactorily settled on an informal basis, the employee may institute a formal grievance by setting forth in writing the nature of the complaint, the specific term or provision of the agreement allegedly violated, and the remedy sought.

The grievance shall be presented to the appropriate employer representative in writing within 14 days after the occurrence of the alleged violation.

After the presentation of the grievance, the employee and the nurses association representative shall be offered an opportunity to meet with the appropriate employer representative in an attempt to settle the grievance. The decision of the employer representative shall be in writing and shall be transmitted to the employee within 14 days after receipt of the written grievance unless extended by mutual consent.

Step 2:
Arbitration
If the matter is not satisfactorily settled at Step 1 and the employee desires to proceed with arbitration, the employee shall serve written notice on the employer of the desire to arbitrate within 5 days of receipt of the written decision of the employer under Step 1.

In state civil service, a grievance procedure probably already exists.

If an additional step from "appropriate employer representative" to the administrator is needed, it should be included as Step 2, and arbitration would become Step 3.

*(continued)*

## AMERICAN NURSES' ASSOCIATION GUIDELINES
## FOR THE INDIVIDUAL NURSE CONTRACT *(continued)*

| SUGGESTED CONTRACT LANGUAGE | BASIS FOR JUSTIFICATION |
|---|---|

Selection of an arbitrator shall be by agreement if possible or, if the parties cannot so agree within 5 days, from a list of five arbitrators obtained by request to the Federal Mediation and Conciliation Service with the parties alternately striking names until only one name remains.

An arbitrator can also be obtained through the American Arbitration Association, but an administrative fee is charged.

The award of the arbitrator shall be accepted as final and binding. There shall be no appeal from the arbitrator's decision by either party if such decision is within the scope of the arbitrator's authority as described below:

   a. The arbitrator shall not have the power to add to, subtract from, disregard, alter, or modify any of the terms of this agreement.

   b. His power shall be limited to deciding whether the employer has violated any of the terms of this agreement. It is understood that any matter that is not specifically set forth in this agreement shall not be subject to arbitration.

   c. In any case of discipline or discharge where the arbitrator finds that such discipline or discharge was improper, the arbitrator may set aside, reduce, or modify the action taken by the employer. If the penalty is set aside, reduced, or otherwise changed, the arbitrator may award back pay to compensate the employee wholly or partially for any wages or other benefits lost because of the penalty.

The fees and expenses of the arbitrator shall be shared equally by the employer and the employee.

### ARTICLE XIV
Evaluation

Written evaluations of the employee's performance will be presented at _____ intervals. A copy of the evaluation will be given to the employee, and a conference will be held with the employee regarding the evaluation. If the employee does not accept the evaluation as written, the employee's exceptions to the evaluation shall be attached to and made a part of the evaluation.

## SUGGESTED CONTRACT LANGUAGE       BASIS FOR JUSTIFICATION

### ARTICLE XV
Resignation or Termination

In the event there is a need for the employee to resign, one month's prior written notice will be given to the employer.

Termination or other discipline of the employee shall be only for just cause. One month's prior written notice of termination will be given. Termination or other discipline of the employee is subject to the grievance procedure herein.

If termination is attempted by the employer without just cause, the nurse may prefer to ensure several months' payment of salary in lieu of use of the grievance procedure; i.e., the nurse will be paid through termination date of contract.

A specific time could be negotiated: 3 months, 6 months, or 1 year. The state nurses association can be used for consultation.

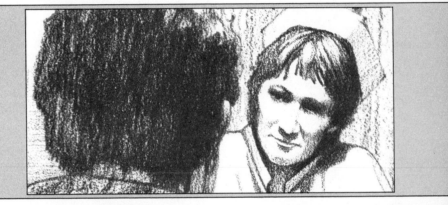

### ARTICLE XVI
Duration

The contract shall remain in full force and effect 1 year from the date first written above and shall be automatically renewed on a year-to-year basis thereafter. Each such 1-year period will be a new duration period with a new effective date.

Either party may serve upon the other party a written notice of intention to amend or terminate this agreement. The notice must be served at least 60 days before the first anniversary date of the agreement or any anniversary date thereafter and must state the nature of the amendment sought.

The parties will meet with respect to the requested amendments within 30 days of receipt of said notice.

It is not wise to negotiate for too long a period of time, with the economy as unpredictable as it is. A contract for a one-year period is sufficient. It is to the employee's advantage to renegotiate each year.

These guidelines are a product of a joint effort by the American Nurses' Association Economic and General Welfare Department and the Council of Nurse Practitioners in the Nursing of Children.

# G

## REQUIREMENTS FOR A VALID WILL

Here are the 50 states' requirements for preparing legally acceptable wills. As a nurse, you won't often deal with patients who are preparing their wills. And when this does happen, your function's likely to be limited to signing as a witness (see Entry 20).

| | Age when a person can make a will disposing of real property | Age when a person can make a will disposing of personal property | Number of persons required to witness a will | Oral (holographic) wills recognized |
|---|---|---|---|---|
| Alabama | 21 | 18 | 2 | No |
| Alaska | 19 | 19 | 2 | Yes |
| Arizona | 18 | 18 | 2 | Yes |
| Arkansas | 18 | 18 | 2 | Yes |
| California | 18 | 18 | 2 | Yes |
| Colorado | 18 | 18 | 2 | Yes |
| Connecticut | 18 | 18 | 2 | No |
| Delaware | 18 | 18 | 2 | No |
| D.C. | 18 | 18 | 2 | No |
| Florida | 18 | 18 | 2 | No |
| Georgia | 14 | 14 | 2 | No |
| Hawaii | 18 | 18 | 2 | Yes |
| Idaho | 18 | 18 | 2 | Yes |
| Illinois | 18 | 18 | 2 | No |
| Indiana | 18 | 18 | 2 | No |
| Iowa | 19 | 19 | 2 | No |
| Kansas | 18 | 18 | 2 | No |
| Kentucky | 18 | 18 | 2 | Yes |
| Louisiana | 16 | 16 | 2 | Yes |
| Maine | 18 | 18 | 3 | No |
| Maryland | 18 | 18 | 2 | No |
| Massachusetts | 18 | 18 | 3 | No |
| Michigan | 18 | 18 | 2 | No |
| Minnesota | 18 | 18 | 2 | No |
| Mississippi | 18 | 18 | 2 | Yes |
| Missouri | 18 | 18 | 2 | No |
| Montana | 18 | 18 | 2 | Yes |
| Nebraska | 18 | 18 | 2 | Yes |
| Nevada | 18 | 18 | 2 | Yes |
| New Hampshire | 18 | 18 | 3 | No |
| New Jersey | 18 | 18 | 2 | No |
| New Mexico | 18 | 18 | 2 | No |
| New York | 18 | 18 | 2 | No |
| North Carolina | 18 | 18 | 2 | Yes |

| | Age when a person can make a will disposing of real property | Age when a person can make a will disposing of personal property | Number of persons required to witness a will | Oral (holographic) wills recognized |
|---|---|---|---|---|
| North Dakota | 18 | 18 | 2 | Yes |
| Ohio | 18 | 18 | 2 | No |
| Oklahoma | 18 | 18 | 2 | Yes |
| Oregon | 18 | 18 | 2 | No |
| Pennsylvania | 18 | 18 | 2 | Yes |
| Rhode Island | 18 | 18 | 2 | No |
| South Carolina | 18 | 18 | 3 | No |
| South Dakota | 18 | 18 | 2 | Yes |
| Tennessee | 18 | 18 | 2 | Yes |
| Texas | 18 | 18 | 2 | Yes |
| Utah | 18 | 18 | 2 | Yes |
| Vermont | 18 | 18 | 3 | No |
| Virginia | 18 | 18 | 2 | Yes |
| Washington | 18 | 18 | 2 | No |
| West Virginia | 18 | 18 | 2 | Yes |
| Wisconsin | 18 | 18 | 2 | No |
| Wyoming | 21 | 21 | 2 | Yes |

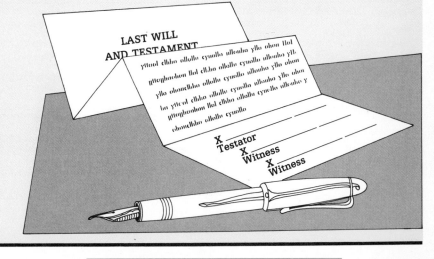

# CHILD ABUSE STATUTES

| STATE | CITATION | APPLIES TO |
|---|---|---|
| Alabama | Ala. Code Tit. 26, Section 26-14-1 (1975) | Hospitals, clinics, sanitariums, doctors, physicians, surgeons, medical examiners, coroners, dentists, osteopaths, optometrists, chiropractors, podiatrists, nurses, school teachers and officials, peace officers, law enforcement officials, pharmacists, social workers, day-care workers or employees, mental health professionals, any other person called on to render aid or medical assistance to any child, or any person. |
| Alaska | Alaska Stat. Sections 47.17.010 to 47.17.070 (1971) | Practitioners of healing arts, school teachers, social workers, peace officers and officers of the division of corrections, administrative officers of institutions, or any other person. |
| Arizona | Ariz. Rev. Stat. Ann. Section 13-842.01 (1976) | Physician, hospital intern or resident, surgeon, dentist, osteopath, chiropractor, podiatrist, medical examiner, nurse, psychologist, school personnel, social worker, peace officer, or any other person responsible for the care of children. |
| Arkansas | Ark. Stat. Ann. Sections 42.807-42.818 (1975) | Physician, surgeon, coroner, dentist, osteopath, resident, intern, registered nurse, hospital personnel (engaged in admission, examination, care, or treatment), teacher, school official, social service worker, day-care center worker, or any other child or foster-care worker, mental health professional, peace officer, law enforcement official, and any other person. |
| California | Cal. Penal Code Sections 11161.5 to 11161.7 | Physician; surgeon; dentist; resident; intern; podiatrist; chiropractor; marriage, family, or child counselor; psychologist; religious practitioner; registered nurse employed by public health agency, school, or school district; superintendent or supervisor of child welfare; certified pupil personnel employee of public or private school system; principal or teacher; licensed day-care worker; administrator of summer day camp or child-care center; social worker; peace officer; probation officer. |
| Colorado | Colo. Rev. Stat. Ann. Sections 19-10-101 through 19-10-115 (1975) | Physician or surgeon including physicians in training, child health associate, medical examiner or coroner, dentist, osteopath, optometrist, chiropractor, chiropodist or podiatrist, registered nurse, licensed practical nurse, hospital personnel engaged in admission, care, or treatment, Christian Science practitioner, school official or employee, social worker, worker in a family-care home or child-care center, mental health professional, any other person. |

| AGE LIMIT | REPORT TO | IMMUNITY PROVISION | PHYSICIAN-PATIENT PRIVILEGE ELIMINATED | NATURE OF OFFENSE FOR NOT REPORTING |
|---|---|---|---|---|
| 18 | Duly constituted authority—chief of police, sheriff, Department of Pensions and Security or its designee, but not an agency involved in the acts or omissions of reported child abuse or neglect. | Yes | Yes | Misdemeanor |
| 16 | Department of Health and Welfare, peace officer. | Yes | Yes | None |
| 18 | Municipal or county peace officer or protective services of state Department of Economic Security. | Yes | Yes | Misdemeanor |
| 18 | Person in charge of institution or his designated agent who shall report. District or state Social Services Division of the Department of Social and Rehabilitative Services. | Yes | Yes | Misdemeanor. Civil liability for damages proximately caused by failure to report |
| 18 | Local police authority, juvenile probation department, county welfare department, county health department. | Yes | No | None |
| "Child" | Local law enforcement agency or the county or district department of social services. Receiving agency is to report to central registry. | Yes | Yes | Class 2 petty offense. Civil liability for damages proximately caused by failure to report |

*(continued)*

## CHILD ABUSE STATUTES *(continued)*

| STATE | CITATION | APPLIES TO |
|---|---|---|
| Connecticut | Conn. Gen. Stat. Rev. Section 17-38a (1973) | Physician, nurse, medical examiner, dentist, psychologist, school teacher, principal, guidance counselor, social worker, police officer, clergyman, coroner, osteopath, optometrist, chiropractor, podiatrist, any person paid to care for children, or mental health professional. |
| Delaware | Del. Code Ann. Tit. 16 Sections 1001 to 1008 (Supp. 1972) | Physician; any person in healing arts, medicine, osteopathy, or dentistry; intern; resident; nurse; school employee; social worker; psychologist; medical examiner, or any other person. |
| Florida | Fla. Stat. Ann. Sections 827.01 to 827.09 (1977) | Physician, dentist, podiatrist, optometrist, intern, resident, nurse, teacher, social worker, employee of a public or private facility serving children. |
| Georgia | Ga. Code Ann. Sections 74-109 to 74-11 (1977) | Social workers, teachers, school administrators, child-care personnel, day-care personnel, law enforcement personnel, any other person. |
| Hawaii | Hawaii Rev. Stat. Sections 350-1 to 350-5 (1968), as amended, (Supp. 7) | Doctor of medicine, osteopathy, dentistry, or any of the other healing arts; registered nurse; school teacher; social worker; medical examiner; and any other person. |
| Idaho | Idaho Code Sections 16-1619 through 16-1629 (1976) | Physician, resident, intern, nurse, coroner, school teacher, day-care personnel, social worker, any other person. |
| Illinois | Ill. Ann. Stat. Ch. 23 Sections 2051-2061 (1975) | Physician, hospital, surgeon, dentist, osteopath, chiropractor, podiatrist, Christian Science practitioner, coroner, school teacher, school administrator, truant officer, social worker, social services administrator, registered nurse, licensed practical nurse, director or staff assistant of a nursery school or a child day-care center, law enforcement officer, or personnel of the Illinois Department of Public Aid. |
| Indiana | Ind. Ann. Stat. Sections 12-3-4.1-1 to 12-3-4.1-6 (1973) | Any person. |
| Iowa | Iowa Code Ann. Sections 235A.1 to 235A.24 | Health practitioner, social worker, certified psychologist, certified school employee, employee of a licensed day-care facility, member of the staff of a mental health center, peace officer, any other person. |

| AGE LIMIT | REPORT TO | IMMUNITY PROVISION | PHYSICIAN-PATIENT PRIVILEGE ELIMINATED | NATURE OF OFFENSE FOR NOT REPORTING |
|---|---|---|---|---|
| 18 | State Commission of Social Services or local police department. | Yes | Yes | Misdemeanor |
| * | Division of Social Services of Department of Health and Social Services. | Yes | Yes | Misdemeanor |
| 17 | Person in charge of institution, Department of Health and Rehabilitative Services. | Yes | Yes | Misdemeanor of 2nd degree |
| 18 | Person in charge of institution, county health officer, child welfare agency designated by Department of Human Resources, and police authority. | Yes | No | Misdemeanor |
| 18 | Person in charge of medical facility, Department of Social Services and Housing. | Yes | Yes | None |
| 18 | Law enforcement agency, person in charge of the institution or designee. Law enforcement officials are to report to Department of Health and Welfare. | Yes | Yes | None |
| "Child" | Department of Child and Family Services, local law enforcement agency. | Yes | Yes | None |
| "Child" | County department of public welfare, law enforcement agency. | Yes | Yes | Misdemeanor |
| 18 | Department of Social Services, law enforcement agency. | Yes | Yes | Misdemeanor. Civil liability for damages proximately caused by failure to report |

* 18 or mentally retarded

(continued)

698

| STATE | CITATION | APPLIES TO |
|-------|----------|------------|
| **Kansas** | Kan. Stat. Ann. 38-716 to 38-756 | Persons licensed to practice healing arts, dentistry, optometrist, engaged in postgraduate training programs approved by the state board of healing arts, certified psychologists, Christian Science practitioners, licensed social workers, every licensed professional nurse or licensed practical nurse, teacher, school administrator or other employee of a school, chief administrative officer of a medical-care facility, every person licensed by the secretary of health and environment to provide child-care services or employees of the person so licensed at the place where the child-care services are being provided to the child, or any law enforcement officer. |
| **Kentucky** | Ky. Rev. Stat. Ann. Sec. 199.335 (1964) as amended 1970, 1972, 1974 | Physician, osteopathic physician, nurse, teacher, school administrator, social worker, coroner, medical examiner, and any other person. |
| **Louisiana** | La. R.S. 14:403 (1964) as amended 1970, 1974, 1975, and 1977 | Any person, physicians, interns, residents, nurses, hospital staff members, teachers, social workers, other persons or agencies having responsibility for care of children. |
| **Maine** | Me. Rev. Stat. Ann. Tit. 22 Sections 3853-3860 (1975) as amended 1977 | Any medical physician, resident, intern, medical examiner, dentist, osteopathic physician, chiropractor, podiatrist, registered or licensed practical nurse, Christian Science practitioner, teacher, school official, social worker, homemaker, home health aide, medical or social service worker for families and children, psychologist, child-care personnel, mental health professional, or law enforcement official. |
| **Maryland** | Md. Ann. Code Art. 27, Sec. 35A-(1977) | Every health practitioner, educator, social worker, or law enforcement officer who contacts, examines, attends, or treats a child. |
| **Massachusetts** | Mass. Ann. c. 119 Section 51A (1973) as amended 1975 and 1977 | Physician, medical intern, medical examiner, dentist, nurse (public or private), school teacher, educational administrator, guidance or family counselor, probation officer, social worker or policeman. Any other person may report. |
| **Michigan** | Mich. Statutes Ann. Section 25.248 (1)-(Mich. Comp. Law Section 722.621) (1975) | Physician, coroner, dentist, medical examiner, nurse, audiologist, certified social worker, social worker, technician, school administrator, counselor or teacher, law enforcement officer, duly regulated child-care provider. |

| AGE LIMIT | REPORT TO | IMMUNITY PROVISION | PHYSICIAN-PATIENT PRIVILEGE ELIMINATED | NATURE OF OFFENSE FOR NOT REPORTING |
|---|---|---|---|---|
| "Child" | District court of county in which such examination or attendance is made, treatment is given, school is located, or such abuse or neglect is extant; or the Department of Social and Rehabilitation Services. | Yes | Yes | Misdemeanor |
| 18 | Person in charge of institution, Department of Human Resources. | Yes | Yes | None |
| 18 | Parish child welfare unit, parish agency responsible for protection of juveniles, local or state law enforcement agency. | Yes | Yes | Misdemeanor |
| 18 | Person in charge of institution, Department of Health and Welfare. | No | Yes | Civil violation |
| 18 | Local department of social services, appropriate law enforcement agency. | Yes | No | None |
| 18 | Person in charge of institution, Department of Public Welfare, attorney for county, and medical examiner if death occurs. | Yes | Yes | Misdemeanor |
| 18 | Department of Social Services, person in charge of institution. | Yes | Yes | Civil liability for damages proximately caused by failure to report |

*(continued)*

**CHILD ABUSE STATUTES** *(continued)*

| STATE | CITATION | APPLIES TO |
|---|---|---|
| **Minnesota** | Minn. Stat. Ann. Section 626.556 (1975) | Professional or his delegate engaged in practice of the healing arts, social services, hospital administration, psychological or psychiatric treatment, child care, education, or law enforcement. Any person may report. |
| **Mississippi** | Miss. Code Ann. Sections 43-24-1, 43-24-7, 43-21-11, 43-23-9, 43-23-3 (1977) | Licensed doctor of medicine, dentist, intern, resident, registered nurse, psychologist, teacher, social worker, school principal, child-care giver, minister, any law enforcement officer, and all other persons. |
| **Missouri** | Mo. Ann. Stat. Sections 210.110 to 210.165 (1975) | Physician, medical examiner, coroner, dentist, chiropractor, optometrist, podiatrist, resident, intern, nurse, hospital and clinic personnel, health practitioner, psychologist, mental health professional, social worker, day-care center worker or other child-care worker, juvenile officer, probation or parole officer, teacher, principal or other school official, minister, Christian Science practitioner, peace officer, law enforcement official, other person with responsibility for the care of children. Any other person may report. |
| **Montana** | Mont. Rev. Code Ann. Sections 10-1300 to 10-1322 (1974) as amended (1977) | Physician, nurse, teacher, social worker, attorney, law enforcement officer, any other person. |
| **Nebraska** | Neb. Rev. Stat. Supp. Sections 28-1501 to 28-1508 (1975) | Physician, medical institution, nurse, school employee, social worker, any other person. |
| **Nevada** | Nevada Rev. Stat. Sections 200.501 through 200.508 | Physician, dentist, chiropractor, optometrist, resident or intern licensed in Nevada; superintendent, manager, or other person in charge of a hospital or similar institution; professional or practical nurse, physician assistant, psychologist, emergency medical technician, or ambulance attendant licensed or certified to practice in Nevada; attorney, social worker, school authority, or teacher; every person who maintains or is employed by a licensed child-care facility or children's camp. |
| **New Hampshire** | New Hampshire Rev. Stat. Ann. Sections 169.37 to 169.45 (1975) as amended 1975 | Physician, surgeon, county medical referee, psychiatrist, resident, intern, dentist, osteopath, optometrist, chiropractor, psychologist, therapist, registered nurse, hospital personnel, Christian Science practitioner, teacher, school official, school nurse, school counselor, social worker, day-care worker, any other child- or foster-care worker, law enforcement official, priest, minister, or rabbi, or any other person. |

| AGE LIMIT | REPORT TO | IMMUNITY PROVISION | PHYSICIAN-PATIENT PRIVILEGE ELIMINATED | NATURE OF OFFENSE FOR NOT REPORTING |
|---|---|---|---|---|
| "Child" | Local welfare agency, police department; deaths to medical examiner or coroner who will notify the local welfare agency or police department. | Yes | Yes | Misdemeanor |
| 18 | County welfare department which will thereafter make a referral to the person designated by the judge of the county youth court or family court. | Yes | Yes | None |
| 18 | Person in charge of institution, Missouri Division of Family Service; deaths to medical examiner or coroner who will report to the police, peace officer, prosecuting juvenile officer, Missouri Division of Family Services. | Yes | Yes | Misdemeanor |
| 18 | Department of Social and Rehabilitation Services, local affiliate, county attorney where child resides. | No | Yes | None |
| * | Department of Public Welfare, police department, town marshal, office of sheriff. | No | No | None |
| 18 | Local office of Welfare Division of Department of Human Resources, any county agency authorized by juvenile courts to receive reports, any police department or sheriff's office. | Yes | Yes | Gross misdemeanor (Could interpret to cover failure to report.) |
| 18 | Bureau of Child and Family Services, Division of Welfare, Department of Health and Welfare. | Yes | Yes | Misdemeanor |

*18, or incompetent or disabled persons, or age 6 or younger left unattended in a motor vehicle

(continued)

## CHILD ABUSE STATUTES *(continued)*

| STATE | CITATION | APPLIES TO |
|-------|----------|------------|
| **New Jersey** | New Jersey Rev. Stat. Ann. Sections 9:6-8.1 to 9:6-8.7 (1974) | Any person. |
| **New Mexico** | N.M. Stat. Ann. Sections 13-14-14.1 to 13-14-14.2 (1973) | Physician, resident, intern, law enforcement officer, registered nurse, visiting nurse, school teacher, social worker, any other person. |
| **New York** | N.Y. Soc. Service Law Sections 411 to 428 (1973) | Physician, surgeon, medical examiner, coroner, dentist, osteopath, optometrist, resident, intern, registered nurse, Christian Science practitioner, hospital personnel, social services worker, school official, day-care center director, peace officer, mental health professional, and any other person. |
| **North Carolina** | N.C. Cent. Stat. Sections 110-117 to 110-119 (1977) | Physician or administrator of a hospital, clinic, or other medical facility to which children are brought. |
| **North Dakota** | N.D. Cent. Code Sections 50-25.1-01 to 50-25.1-14 (1975) as amended, 1977 | Physician, nurse, dentist, optometrist, medical examiner or coroner, any other medical or mental health professional, school teacher or administrator, school counselor, social worker, day-care center or any other child-care worker, police, law enforcement officer, and any other person. |
| **Ohio** | Ohio Rev. Code Ann. Section 2151-42.1 (1977) | Attorney; physician, intern, resident, dentist, podiatrist, or practitioner of a limited branch of medicine or surgery as defined in section 4731.15 of the revised code; registered or licensed practical nurse, visiting nurse, or other health-care professional; licensed psychologist, speech pathologist, or audiologist; coroner; administrator or employee of a child day-care center; administrator or employee of a certified child-care agency or other public or private child services agency; school teacher or school authority; social worker; or person rendering spiritual treatment through prayer in accordance with the tenets of a well-recognized religion. |
| **Oklahoma** | Okla. Stat. Ann. Tit. 21 Sections 845-848 (1965), as amended 1977 | Physicians, surgeons, dentists, osteopathic physicians, residents, interns, every other person. |

| AGE LIMIT | REPORT TO | IMMUNITY PROVISION | PHYSICIAN-PATIENT PRIVILEGE ELIMINATED | NATURE OF OFFENSE FOR NOT REPORTING |
|---|---|---|---|---|
| 18 | Bureau of Child Services, Division of Youth and Family Services. | Yes | | Misdemeanor |
| 18 | County social services office of the Health and Social Services Department in the county of child's residence or probation services office in judicial district of child's residence. | Yes | Yes | Misdemeanor |
| * | Statewide Central Register of Child Abuse and Maltreatment, local child protective service, person in charge of institution. | Yes | Yes | Class A misdemeanor. Civil liability for damages proximately caused by failure to report |
| 18 | Director of social services of county where child resides, parents, other caretakers. | No | No | None |
| 18 | Division of Community Services of the Social Service Board of North Dakota. | Yes | Yes | Class B misdemeanor |
| 18 | Person in charge of institution, Children Services Board or county department of welfare exercising the children services function, or municipal or county police officer in county of child's residence or where abuse or neglect occurred. | Yes | No | None |
| 18 | County office of the Department of Institutions, Social and Rehabilitative Services where injury occurred. | Yes | Yes | Misdemeanor |

* Abused, 16; maltreated, 18

## CHILD ABUSE STATUTES *(continued)*

| STATE | CITATION | APPLIES TO |
|---|---|---|
| **Oregon** | Ore. Rev. Stat. Sections 418.740 to 418.775 (1975) | Public or private official, physician, intern, resident, or dentist; school employee; licensed practical or registered nurse; employee of department of human resources, county health department, community mental health program; county juvenile department; licensed child-caring agency; peace officer; psychologist; clergyman; social worker; optometrist; chiropractor; certified provider of day care or foster care; attorney; law enforcement agency; police department; sheriff's office; or county juvenile department. |
| **Pennsylvania** | Pa. Stat. Ann. Tit. 11 Sections 2201 to 2224 (1975) | Any person who in the course of their employment, occupation, or practice of their profession contacts children; licensed physician; medical examiner; coroner; dentist; osteopath; optometrist; chiropractor; podiatrist; intern; registered nurse or licensed practical nurse; hospital personnel engaged in the admission, examination, care or treatment of persons; a Christian Science practitioner; school administrator; school teacher; school nurse; social services worker; day-care center worker or any other child-care or foster-care worker; mental health professional; or peace officer or law enforcement official. |
| **Rhode Island** | R.I. Gen. Laws Ann. Sections 40-11-1 to 40-11-17 (1976) | Physicians, and any person. |
| **South Carolina** | S.C. Code Ann. Sections 20-9-10 to 20-9-70 (1962) as amended 1972, 1974, 1976 | Practitioner of healing arts, resident, intern, registered nurse, visiting nurse, school teacher, social worker, any other person. |
| **South Dakota** | S.D. Compiled. Laws Ann. Sections 26-10-11, 26-10-15 (1964) as amended 1973, 1976 | Physician, surgeon, dentist, doctor of osteopathy, chiropractor, optometrist, podiatrist, psychologist, social worker, hospital intern or resident, law enforcement officer, teacher, school counselor, school official, nurse, or coroner. |
| **Tennessee** | Tenn. Code Ann. Sections 37-1201, 37-1212 (1973) as amended 1975 | Any person. |

| AGE LIMIT | REPORT TO | IMMUNITY PROVISION | PHYSICIAN-PATIENT PRIVILEGE ELIMINATED | NATURE OF OFFENSE FOR NOT REPORTING |
|---|---|---|---|---|
| 18 | Local office of Children's Services Division, law enforcement agency. | Yes | No | Misdemeanor |
| 18 | Person in charge of institution or agency, Department of Public Welfare of the Commonwealth of Pennsylvania. | Yes | Yes | First failure to report is a summary offense, subsequent failure to report is a misdemeanor of the 3rd degree |
| 18 | Director of Social and Rehabilitative Services, law enforcement agency. | Yes | Yes | None |
| 18 | County department of social services, county sheriff's office, chief county law enforcement officer. | Yes | Yes | Misdemeanor |
| 18 | Person in charge of institution. | Yes | Yes | Class I misdemeanor |
| * | Judge with juvenile jurisdiction, Tennessee Department of Human Resources, office of sheriff, law enforcement official where child resides, person in charge of institution. | Yes | Yes | Misdemeanor |

*18, reasonably presumed to be under 18

(continued)

## CHILD ABUSE STATUTES (continued)

| STATE | CITATION | APPLIES TO |
|---|---|---|
| Texas | Tex. Family Code Ann. Sections 34.01 to 34.06 (1975) | Any person. |
| Utah | Utah Code Ann. Sections 55-16-1 to 55-16-6 (1975) | Any person. |
| Vermont | Vt. Stat. Ann. Sections 1351 to 1355 (1974) as amended 1975, 1976 and 1977 | Physician, surgeon, osteopath, chiropractor, or physician assistant licensed or registered; resident physician, intern, or any hospital administrator; psychologist, school teacher, day-care worker, school principal or school guidance counselor; mental health professional, social worker, probation officer, clergyman, or any other person. |
| Virginia | Va. Code Ann. Sections 63.1-248.1 to 63.1-248.17 (1975) | Persons licensed to practice healing arts; residents; interns; nurses; social workers; probation officers; teachers; persons employed in a public or private school, kindergarten, or nursery; persons providing child care for pay on a regular basis; Christian Science practitioner; mental health professional or law enforcement officer. Any person may report. |
| Washington | Wash. Rev. Code Ann. Sections 26.44.010 to 26.44.900 (1975) | Practitioner, professional school personnel, nurse, social worker, psychologist, pharmacist, employee of social or health services. Any person may report. |
| Wisconsin | Wis. Stat. Ann. Section 48.981 (1974) | Physician, surgeon, nurse, hospital administrator, dentist, social worker, school administrator. |
| West Virginia | West Va. Code Ann. Sections 49-6A. 1 to 49-6A-10 (1977) | Medical, dental, mental health professional; Christian Science practitioner; religious healer; school teacher or other school personnel; social service worker; child-care or foster-care worker; peace officer, or law enforcement official. Any other person may report. |
| Wyoming | Wyo. Stat. Ann. Sections 14-28.1 to 14-28.13 (1974) | Physician, surgeon, dentist, osteopath, chiropractor, podiatrist, intern, resident, nurse, druggist, pharmacist, laboratory technician, school teacher or administrator, social worker, any other person. |
| District of Columbia | D.C. Code Ann. Sections 2-161 to 2-169 (1977) | Physician, psychologist, medical examiner, dentist, chiropractor, registered nurse, licensed practical nurse, person involved in the care and treatment of patients, law enforcement officer, school official, teacher, social service worker, day-care worker, and mental health professional. Any person may report. |

| AGE LIMIT | REPORT TO | IMMUNITY PROVISION | PHYSICIAN-PATIENT PRIVILEGE ELIMINATED | NATURE OF OFFENSE FOR NOT REPORTING |
|---|---|---|---|---|
| * | State Department of Public Welfare, agency designated by court to protect children, local or state law enforcement agency. | Yes | Yes | Class B misdemeanor |
| 18 | Local city police, county sheriff's office, office of the Division of Family Services, person in charge of institution. | Yes | Yes | Misdemeanor |
| ** | Commissioner of Social and Rehabilitative Services. | Yes | No | Misdemeanor |
| 18 | Person in charge of institution or department, Department of Welfare of the county or city where child resides or abuse or neglect occurred; juvenile and domestic relations district court if an employee of the Department of Welfare is the one suspected of abusing the child. | Yes | Yes | Misdemeanor |
| † | Law enforcement agency, Department of Social and Health Services. | Yes | No | Misdemeanor |
| †† | County child welfare agency, sheriff, city police department. | Yes | †† | Misdemeanor |
| 18 | Local state department of child protective services agency; report deaths to medical examiner or coroner. | Yes | Yes | Misdemeanor |
| 19 | Person in charge of institution, Department of Health and Social Services, Division of Public Assistance and Social Services. | Yes | Yes | None |
| 18 | Person in charge of institution, Metropolitan Police Department of the District of Columbia, Child Protective Services Division of the Department of Human Resources. | Yes | Yes | Misdemeanor |

* 18 who has not been married
** Under age of majority
†18, any mentally retarded person

††See Section 325.21

## ALABAMA • Title 46
**Professional Nursing**
None.
**Practical Nursing**
None.

## ALASKA • Title 8
**Professional Nursing**
The practice of professional nursing means the performance for compensation of any act in the observation, care and counsel of the ill, injured or infirm, or in the maintenance of health or in prevention of illness of others, or in the supervision and teaching of other personnel, or in the administration of medications and treatments as prescribed by a licensed physician or dentist; requiring substantial specialized judgment and skill and based on knowledge and application of the principles of biological, physical and social sciences. The foregoing shall not be deemed to include acts of diagnosis or prescription or therapeutic or corrective measures.
**Practical Nursing**
The practice of practical nursing means the performance for compensation of selected acts in the care or prevention of illness, and in the care of the ill, injured or infirm under the direction of a licensed professional nurse of a licensed physician or a licensed dentist; and not requiring the substantial specialized skill, judgment and knowledge required in professional nursing.

## ARIZONA • Title 32
**Professional Nursing**
"Professional Nursing" means the performance... of professional services requiring the application of the biological, physical or social sciences and nursing skills in the care of the sick, in the prevention of disease or in the conservation of health.
**Practical Nursing**
"Practical Nursing" means the performance of such services requiring those technical skills... performed under the direction of a licensed physician or registered professional nurse, requiring a knowledge of nursing procedures but not requiring the professional knowledge and skill required for professional nursing.

## ARKANSAS • Title 72
**Professional Nursing**
The practice of nursing is defined as follows: A person practices nursing... who... (a) performs any professional service requiring the application of principles of nursing based on biologic, physical and social sciences, such as responsible supervision of a patient requiring skill in observation of symptoms and reactions and the accurate recording of the facts, and carrying out of treatments and medications as prescribed by a licensed physician, and the application of such nursing procedures as involve understanding of cause and effect in order to safeguard the life and health of a patient and others;...
**Practical Nursing**
Similar to Arizona definition.

## CALIFORNIA • Business and Professions Code
**Professional Nursing**
The practice of nursing... is the performing of professional services requiring technical skill and special knowledge based on the principles of scientific medicine,... practiced in conjunction with curative or preventive medicine prescribed by a licensed physician and the application of such nursing procedures as involve understanding of cause and effect in order to safeguard life and health of a patient and others.
**Practical Nursing**
None.

## COLORADO • Chapter 12
**Professional Nursing**
Similar to Alaska definition.
**Practical Nursing**
Similar to Alaska definition.

## CONNECTICUT • Title 19
**Professional Nursing**
The practice of nursing is defined as follows:
(a) The performing... under the direction
of a licensed physician, of any professional
service requiring special education, knowledge
and skill in nursing care of those mentally or
physically ill and in the prevention of illness;...
**Practical Nursing**
Similar to Arizona definition.

## DELAWARE • Title 24
**Professional Nursing**
None.
**Practical Nursing**
Similar to Arizona definition.

## DISTRICT OF COLUMBIA • Title 2
**Professional Nursing**
None.
**Practical Nursing**
None.

## FLORIDA • Chapter 464
**Professional Nursing**
See Alaska definition.
**Practical Nursing**
The practice of practical nursing shall mean
the performance of nursing acts in the care of
the ill, injured or infirm under the direction
of a licensed physician or by a licensed dentist,
or a registered professional nurse; provided,
however, that all such acts do not require
the specialized skill, judgment and knowledge
required in professional nursing.

## GEORGIA • Section 84
**Professional Nursing**
None.
**Practical Nursing**
Practical nursing is the care of subacute,
convalescent and chronic patients in their own
homes or in institutions, or... working under
the direction of a licensed physician or
registered professional nurse.

*(continued)*

## STATE-BY-STATE DEFINITIONS
## OF NURSING PRACTICE *(continued)*

### HAWAII • Title 25
**Professional Nursing**
See Alaska definition.
**Practical Nursing**
See Alaska definition.

### IDAHO • Title 54-1401
**Professional Nursing**
Similar to Arizona definition.
**Practical Nursing**
Similar to Georgia definition.

### ILLINOIS • Chapter 3
**Professional Nursing**
Similar to Arizona definition.
**Practical Nursing**
"Practical Nursing" means the performance under the direction of a licensed physician, dentist or registered professional nurse of such simple nursing procedures as may be required in the care of a patient and the conservation of health.

### INDIANA • Section 25
**Professional Nursing**
Similar to Arizona definition.
**Practical Nursing**
Similar to Georgia definition.

### IOWA • Title 8
**Professional Nursing**
Practice of nursing is a performance of any professional services requiring the application of principles of biological, physical and social sciences and nursing skills in the observation of symptoms, reactions and the accurate recording of facts and carrying out of treatments and medication prescribed by licensed physicians in the care of the sick, in the prevention of disease or the conservation of health.
**Practical Nursing**
Similar to Georgia definition.

### KANSAS • Section 17-2707
**Professional Nursing**
Similar to Iowa definition.
**Practical Nursing**
Similar to Georgia definition.

## KENTUCKY • Title 26
**Professional Nursing**
Similar to Arizona definition.
**Practical Nursing**
Similar to Arizona definition.

## LOUISIANA • Title 37
**Professional Nursing**
Similar to Arkansas definition.
**Practical Nursing**
Practical nursing is the performance of such nursing service as is prescribed by a licensed physician, requiring a knowledge of similar nursing procedures but not requiring professional knowledge and skills required for professional nursing.

## MAINE • Title 32
**Professional Nursing**
The practice of professional nursing means the performance for compensation of any of the services which necessitate the specialized knowledge, judgment and skill required for the application of nursing as based upon principles of biological, physical and social sciences in the (a) observation and care of the ill, injured or infirm; (b) maintenance of health or prevention of illness of others; (c) supervision and teaching of other personnel; (d) administration of medications and treatments as prescribed by a licensed physician or dentist.
**Practical Nursing**
Similar to Georgia definition.

## MARYLAND • Section 7
**Professional Nursing**
None.
**Practical Nursing**
None.

## MASSACHUSETTS • Chapter 13
**Professional Nursing**
Professional nursing shall mean the performance for compensation of any of those services in observing and caring for the ill, injured and infirm, in applying counsel and procedures to safeguard life and health, in administering treatment or medication prescribed by a physician or dentist, or in teaching or supervising others, which are commonly performed by registered nurses and which require specialized knowledge and skill such as are taught and acquired under the established curriculum in a school for nurses duly approved in accordance with this chapter.
**Practical Nursing**
Practical nursing shall mean the performance... of any of those services in observing and caring for the ill, injured or infirm, in applying counsel and procedures to safeguard life and health, in administering treatment or medication prescribed by a physician or dentist, or in teaching or supervising others, which are commonly performed by licensed practical nurses and which require specialized knowledge and skills such as are taught and acquired under the established curriculum in a school for practical nurses duly approved in accordance with this chapter.

## MICHIGAN • Chapter 325
**Professional Nursing**
Similar to Arkansas definition.
**Practical Nursing**
Similar to Arizona definition.

## MINNESOTA • Part I, Section 15-0424
**Professional Nursing**
The practice of professional nursing means the performance for compensation or personal profit of a professional service in the care of those mentally or physically ill or in the prevention of illness or in the supervision of others engaged in caring for the ill or prevention of illness which requires special education, knowledge and skill such as that ordinarily expected of an individual who has completed a course of instruction.
**Practical Nursing**
Similar to Arizona definition.

*(continued)*

**STATE-BY-STATE DEFINITIONS
OF NURSING PRACTICE** *(continued)*

### MISSISSIPPI • Title 73-15-1
**Professional Nursing**
A Registered Professional Nurse is one who possesses a blend of intellectual attainments, attitudes and manual skills based on the principles of scientific medicine... practiced in conjunction with curative or preventive medicines.
**Practical Nursing**
A Practical Nurse... (cares for) selected convalescent and subacutely or chronically ill patients. He or she may be expected to assist the professional nurse in a team relationship;... to give limited household assistance when necessary;... works only under the direct orders of a licensed physician or the supervision of a registered professional nurse.

### MISSOURI • Title 22
**Professional Nursing**
Similar to Arizona definition.
**Practical Nursing**
Similar to Georgia definition.

### MONTANA • Title 62
**Professional Nursing**
Similar to Arizona definition.
**Practical Nursing**
Practical nursing includes the care of selected convalescent, subacutely and chronically ill patients... assisting the professional nurse in a team relationship, especially in the care of those more acutely ill. The practical nurse provides nursing service in institutions, and in private homes where she is prepared to give household assistance when necessary.
She may be employed by a private individual, a hospital or a health agency. The practical nurse works under the direct supervision of a registered nurse where such supervision is possible and obtainable, and similarly, under the direct supervision of a doctor.

### NEBRASKA • Chapter 33
**Professional Nursing**
Similar to Arizona definition.
**Practical Nursing**
Practical nursing shall mean the performance of services and nursing skills in the care of the sick, in the prevention of disease, or in the conservation of health, not involving the specialized education, knowledge and skill required in professional nursing.

### NEVADA • Title 54
**Professional Nursing**
Similar to Arizona definition.
**Practical Nursing**
Similar to Arizona definition.

### NEW HAMPSHIRE • Title 30
**Professional Nursing**
Similar to Arkansas definition.
**Practical Nursing**
Similar to Georgia definition.

### NEW JERSEY • Section 45
**Professional Nursing**
Similar to Arkansas definition.
**Practical Nursing**
Similar to Arizona definition.

### NEW MEXICO • Chapter 61
**Professional Nursing**
Similar to Arizona definition.
**Practical Nursing**
Similar to Georgia definition.

## NEW YORK • Section 6500
**Professional Nursing**
Similar to Arkansas definition.
**Practical Nursing**
Similar to Arizona definition.

## NORTH CAROLINA • Division 12
**Professional Nursing**
Similar to Arkansas definition.
**Practical Nursing**
None.

## NORTH DAKOTA • Chapter 43
**Professional Nursing**
"Professional Nursing" shall mean one of the services for the care of the sick, for the prevention of illness and for the promotion of health which is carried on under medical direction. Nursing is designed to provide physical, mental and emotional care for the patient; to care for his immediate environments; to carry out treatment prescribed by the physician; to teach the patient and his family the nursing care which they may have to perform; to give general health instruction, to supervise auxiliary workers, to coordinate the services of other workers contributing to patient and family care and to participate in research related to health.
**Practical Nursing**
None.

## OHIO • Title 47
**Professional Nursing**
The practice of professional nursing is a performance of any professional service requiring the application of principles of nursing based on biological, physical and social sciences, such as responsible supervision of a patient requiring skill in observation of symptoms and reactions and the accurate recording of same, and execution of treatments and medications as prescribed by a licensed physician, and the application of such nursing procedures as involve understanding of cause and effect in order to safeguard life and health, and the instruction, supervision of nurses, and the administration of nursing services in institutions and health agencies.
**Practical Nursing**
Practical nursing is... to perform nursing services and the care of the sick, in rehabilitation, and in the prevention of illness under the supervision of a licensed physician or a registered nurse.

## OKLAHOMA • Title 59
**Professional Nursing**
Similar to Arizona definition.
**Practical Nursing**
Licensed practical nurse shall mean a person trained to care for selected subacute, convalescent and chronic patients, and to assist the professional nurse in a team relationship, especially in the care of those more acutely ill. She may be employed by the lay public, hospitals and agencies. A licensed practical nurse works only under the direct orders of a licensed physician or the supervision of a registered nurse.

## OREGON • Title 52
**Professional Nursing**
The practice of professional nursing is the performance for compensation of any act, requiring substantial specialized judgment and skill and based on knowledge and application of the principles of biological, physical and social science, in the observation, care and counsel of the ill, injured or infirm, or in the maintenance of health or prevention of illness of others, or in the supervision and teaching of principles and technics of nursing to other personnel involved in the nursing care of patients, or the administration of medications and treatments, whether the piercing of tissues is involved or not, as prescribed by a person authorized to practice medicine or surgery, osteopathy or dentistry in Oregon. This section does not authorize a licensed professional nurse to perform acts of diagnosis or prescription of therapeutic or corrective measures.
**Practical Nursing**
Similar to Arizona definition.

## PENNSYLVANIA • Title 35
**Professional Nursing**
Similar to Arizona definition.
**Practical Nursing**
Similar to Arizona definition.

## RHODE ISLAND • Chapter 5-34
**Professional Nursing**
Similar to Arizona definition.
**Practical Nursing**
Similar to Georgia definition.

*(continued)*

STATE-BY-STATE DEFINITIONS
OF NURSING PRACTICE *(continued)*

## SOUTH CAROLINA • Section 40
**Professional Nursing**
None.
**Practical Nursing**
None.

## SOUTH DAKOTA • Title 36
**Professional Nursing**
The practice of professional nursing means the performance for compensation of such acts within the field of nursing as require substantial specialized skill, knowledge or training, or knowledge and application of the principles of physical, biological or social science, or the supervision of less skilled nursing service workers.
**Practical Nursing**
The practice of practical nursing means the performance... of any acts within the field of nursing that do not require the degree of skill, knowledge or training involved in professional nursing.

## TENNESSEE • Section 63-1-107
**Professional Nursing**
The practice of professional nursing is defined as the performance of any service:
   a. rendered pursuant to a consensual agreement.
   b. requiring the application of the principles based upon the biologic, physical and social sciences in the supervision of a patient involving:
   1. The observations of symptoms and reactions
   2. The accurate recordation of facts
   3. The fulfillment of legal orders of a duly licensed physician concerning treatments and medications with an understanding of cause and effect
   4. The accurate application of procedures and technics with an understanding of cause and effect and
   5. The additional safeguarding of the physical and mental care of the patient by the employment of any nonremedial means, including, but not limiting, the health direction and education of the patient.
**Practical Nursing**
Similar to Alaska and Georgia definitions.

## TEXAS • Article 4520
**Professional Nursing**
None.
**Practical Nursing**
None.

## UTAH • Title 58
**Professional Nursing**
Similar to Arkansas definition.
**Practical Nursing**
Similar to Arizona definition.

## VERMONT • Title 26
**Professional Nursing**
None.
**Practical Nursing**
"Practical Nursing" or "the practice of practical nursing" means the performance of services requiring the specialized knowledge, skill and judgment necessary for carrying out selected aspects of the designated nursing regimen at the direction of a licensed registered professional nurse, licensed physician or licensed dentist in:
   a. Health teaching and health counseling
   b. Provision of care which is supportive or restorative to life and well-being directly to the patient or through supervision of nursing assistants, or
   c. Execution of a medical regimen at the direction of a licensed physician or licensed dentist who need not be physically present.

## VIRGINIA • Title 54
**Professional Nursing**
Similar to Arkansas definition.
**Practical Nursing**
Similar to Arizona definition.

## WASHINGTON • Chapter 18.88 RCN
**Professional Nursing**
None.
**Practical Nursing**
Similar to Arizona definition.

## WEST VIRGINIA • Chapter 30
**Professional Nursing**
Similar to Arkansas definition.
**Practical Nursing**
Similar to Arizona definition.

## WISCONSIN • Title 3
### Professional Nursing
The practice of professional nursing... means the performance... of any act in the observation or care of the ill, injured or infirm, or for the maintenance of health or prevention of illness of others, which act requires substantial nursing skill, knowledge or training, or application of nursing principles based on biological, physical and social sciences, such as the supervision of a patient, the observation and recording of symptoms and reactions, the execution of procedures and technics in the treatment of the sick under the general or special supervision or direction of a physician, the execution of general nursing procedures and technics and the supervision and direction of trained practical nurses and less skilled assistants.
### Practical Nursing
(Practical nursing means the performance of) simple procedures in the physical care of the patient, and... such other procedures as may be directed by the attending physician.

## WYOMING • Title 33
### Professional Nursing
The practice of professional nursing means the performance... of any act in the care of the ill or injured, or administration of medications and performance of treatments as prescribed by a licensed physician or dentist, or in the prevention of disease of others, requiring substantial specialized skill, training or knowledge and application of the principles of physical, biological and social sciences, or supervision of less skilled workers in the field.
### Practical Nursing
The practice of practical nursing means the performance... of any act in the care of the ill, injured or infirm, or in the prevention of disease and in carrying out medical orders as prescribed by a licensed physician or dentist, requiring knowledge of simple nursing procedures, but not requiring the degree of specialized skill essential for professional nursing, and to give assistance to the professional nurse in the care of the ill, injured or infirm. Provided, however, they shall not administer narcotics, and shall only administer simple oral medication except under the direction of a registered nurse, doctor or dentist.

# NURSE PRACTICE ACTS: GROUNDS FOR LICENSE DENIAL, REVOCATION, OR SUSPENSION

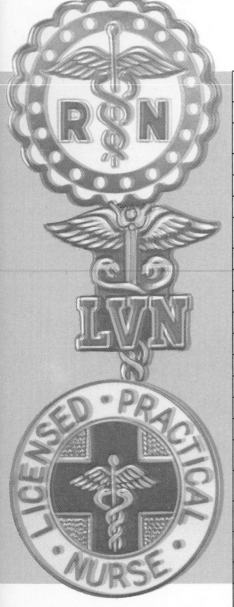

| | |
|---|---|
| Obtaining or attempting to obtain nursing license by fraud or deceit | |
| Impersonating a licensed nurse | |
| Denial, suspension, revocation of license in another jurisdiction | |
| Conviction of felony | |
| Conviction of crime involving moral turpitude | |
| Habitual intoxication or drug addiction | |
| Possessing, selling, distributing controlled substances | |
| Negligence | |
| Violating patient privacy | |
| Falsifying patient records | |
| Mental/physical unfitness | |
| Involvement in criminal abortion | |
| Unprofessional conduct | |
| Professional incompetence | |
| Violating any provision of nurse practice act | |
| False, misleading, deceptive advertising | |
| Failing to report persons who violate nurse practice act | |
| Failing to report suspected child abuse or neglect | |
| Practicing while knowingly infected with contagious disease | |
| Failing to obtain U.S. citizenship during time allotted | |
| Practicing beyond scope of nursing | |
| Discriminating against patients on grounds of age, race, sex | |

| | Alabama Title 34 | Alaska Title 8 | Arizona Title 32 | Arkansas Title 72 | California Business and Professions Code | Colorado Chapter 12 | Connecticut Title 20 | Delaware Title 24 | District of Columbia Title 2 | Florida Chapter 455 |
|---|---|---|---|---|---|---|---|---|---|---|
| | ● | ● | ● | ● | ● | ● | ● | ● | ● | ● |
| | | ● | | | ● | | | ● | ● | ● |
| | | | ● | | ● | ● | | ● | ● | ● |
| | ● | ● | ● | ● | ● | ● | ● | ● | ● | ● |
| | ● | ● | | ● | ● | ● | ● | | | |
| | | ● | ● | ● | ● | ● | ● | ● | ● | ● |
| | | | | | | | | | | ● |
| | | ● | | ● | ● | ● | ● | ● | ● | |
| | | | | | | ● | | ● | | |
| | | | | | | ● | | | | |
| | ● | ● | | ● | | ● | ● | | ● | ● |
| | | | ● | | ● | | | | | |
| | ● | ● | ● | ● | ● | | | | ● | ● |
| | ● | ● | | | ● | | | | | |
| | ● | ● | ● | ● | ● | ● | | | ● | ● |
| | | | | | | | | | | ● |
| | | | | | ● | | | | | ● |
| | | | | | | | | | | |
| | | | | | | | | | | |
| | | | | | | | | | | |
| | | | | | | | | | | |
| | | | | | | | | | | |
| | | | | | | | | | | |

(continued)

## NURSE PRACTICE ACTS: GROUNDS FOR
## LICENSE DENIAL, REVOCATION, OR SUSPENSION (continued)

| | Georgia Section 84 | Hawaii Title 25 | Idaho Title 54 | Illinois Chapter 111 | Indiana Section 25 | |
|---|---|---|---|---|---|---|
| Obtaining or attempting to obtain nursing license by fraud or deceit | ● | ● | ● | ● | ● | |
| Impersonating a licensed nurse | ● | ● | ● | | ● | |
| Denial, suspension, revocation of license in another jurisdiction | ● | | ● | | | |
| Conviction of felony | ● | | ● | ● | ● | |
| Conviction of crime involving moral turpitude | ● | ● | | ● | | |
| Habitual intoxication or drug addiction | | ● | ● | ● | ● | |
| Possessing, selling, distributing controlled substances | | | | | | |
| Negligence | ● | ● | ● | ● | | |
| Violating patient privacy | | | | | | |
| Falsifying patient records | | | | | | |
| Mental/physical unfitness | ● | ● | ● | | ● | |
| Involvement in criminal abortion | | | | | | |
| Unprofessional conduct | ● | ● | ● | ● | | |
| Professional incompetence | ● | | | | ● | |
| Violating any provision of nurse practice act | ● | ● | ● | ● | ● | |
| False, misleading, deceptive advertising | | | | | | |
| Failing to report persons who violate nurse practice act | | | | | | |
| Failing to report suspected child abuse or neglect | | | | ● | | |
| Practicing while knowingly infected with contagious disease | | | ● | | | |
| Failing to obtain U.S. citizenship during time allotted | | | | | | |
| Practicing beyond scope of nursing | | | | | | |
| Discriminating against patients on grounds of age, race, sex | | | | | | |

| | Iowa Title 8 | Kansas Section 65 | Kentucky Title 26 | Louisiana Title 37 | Maine Title 32 | Maryland Title 22 | Massachusetts Chapter 13 | Michigan Chapter 325 | Minnesota Part I, Section 148.171 | Mississippi Title 73 |
|---|---|---|---|---|---|---|---|---|---|---|
| | ● | ● | ● | ● | ● | ● | ● | ● | ● | ● |
| | ● | | | | | ● | ● | ● | | ● |
| | | | ● | | | ● | | ● | | ● |
| | ● | ● | ● | ● | ● | ● | ● | ● | ● | ● |
| | | | ● | | | ● | ● | | ● | ● |
| | ● | ● | | ● | ● | ● | | ● | ● | ● |
| | | | | | | | | | | |
| | | ● | ● | ● | ● | ● | | ● | ● | ● |
| | | | | | | | | | | |
| | | | | | | ● | | | | |
| | | ● | | ● | ● | | ● | ● | | |
| | | | | | | | | | | |
| | | ● | | | | ● | ● | ● | | ● |
| | ● | | | | | ● | ● | | ● | ● |
| | ● | ● | ● | ● | ● | ● | ● | ● | ● | ● |
| | ● | | | | | | | | | |
| | | | | | | | | | | |
| | | | | | | | | | | |
| | | | | | | | | | | |
| | | | | | | | | | | |
| | | | | | | | | | | |
| | | | | | | | | | | |

(continued)

# NURSE PRACTICE ACTS: GROUNDS FOR
## LICENSE DENIAL, REVOCATION, OR SUSPENSION *(continued)*

| | Missouri Title 22 | Montana Title 37 | Nebraska Title 71 | Nevada Title 54 | New Hampshire Title 30 |
|---|---|---|---|---|---|
| Obtaining or attempting to obtain nursing license by fraud or deceit | ● | ● | ● | ● | ● |
| Impersonating a licensed nurse | ● | | | ● | |
| Denial, suspension, revocation of license in another jurisdiction | ● | | | | ● |
| Conviction of felony | ● | | ● | ● | ● |
| Conviction of crime involving moral turpitude | ● | | | ● | |
| Habitual intoxication or drug addiction | ● | ● | ● | ● | ● |
| Possessing, selling, distributing controlled substances | | | | | |
| Negligence | ● | ● | ● | ● | ● |
| Violating patient privacy | | | | | |
| Falsifying patient records | | | | | |
| Mental/physical unfitness | ● | ● | ● | ● | ● |
| Involvement in criminal abortion | | | | ● | |
| Unprofessional conduct | | ● | ● | ● | ● |
| Professional incompetence | | ● | | ● | ● |
| Violating any provision of nurse practice act | ● | ● | ● | ● | ● |
| False, misleading, deceptive advertising | ● | | | | ● |
| Failing to report persons who violate nurse practice act | | | | | |
| Failing to report suspected child abuse or neglect | | | | | |
| Practicing while knowingly infected with contagious disease | | | | | |
| Failing to obtain U.S. citizenship during time allotted | | | | | |
| Practicing beyond scope of nursing | | | | ● | |
| Discriminating against patients on grounds of age, race, sex | | | | | |

| | New Jersey Section 45 | New Mexico Chapter 61 | New York Education Law | North Carolina Division 12 | North Dakota Title 43 | Ohio Title 47 | Oklahoma Title 59 | Oregon Title 52 | Pennsylvania Title 63 | Rhode Island Chapter 5 |
|---|---|---|---|---|---|---|---|---|---|---|
| | ● | ● | ● | ● | ● | ● | ● | ● | ● | ● |
| | ● | ● | ● | ● | | ● | ● | ● | ● | |
| | ● | | ● | | ● | | | ● | | |
| | ● | ● | ● | ● | ● | ● | ● | ● | ● | |
| | ● | | ● | | ● | ● | ● | ● | ● | ● |
| | ● | ● | ● | | | ● | ● | ● | ● | ● |
| | | | | | | | | | | |
| | ● | | ● | ● | ● | ● | ● | ● | ● | ● |
| | | | | | | | | | | |
| | | | | | | | | | | |
| | ● | ● | ● | ● | ● | ● | ● | ● | | ● |
| | | | | | | | | | | |
| | ● | ● | ● | ● | ● | | ● | ● | ● | ● |
| | ● | ● | ● | ● | | ● | ● | | | |
| | ● | ● | ● | ● | ● | ● | ● | ● | ● | ● |
| | | | | | | | | | | |
| | | | | | | | | | | |
| | | | | | | | | | | |
| | | | | | | | | | ● | |
| | | | | | | | | | ● | |
| | | | | | | | | | | |
| | | | ● | | | | | | | |

(continued)

## NURSE PRACTICE ACTS: GROUNDS FOR
## LICENSE DENIAL, REVOCATION, OR SUSPENSION (continued)

| | South Carolina Section 40 | South Dakota Title 36 | Tennessee Section 63 | Texas Article 4513 | Utah Title 58 | |
|---|---|---|---|---|---|---|
| Obtaining or attempting to obtain nursing license by fraud or deceit | ● | ● | ● | ● | ● | |
| Impersonating a licensed nurse | ● | ● | | ● | | |
| Denial, suspension, revocation of license in another jurisdiction | ● | ● | | ● | ● | |
| Conviction of felony | ● | | ● | ● | | |
| Conviction of crime involving moral turpitude | ● | | | ● | | |
| Habitual intoxication or drug addiction | ● | ● | ● | ● | ● | |
| Possessing, selling, distributing controlled substances | | | | | | |
| Negligence | ● | ● | ● | | ● | |
| Violating patient privacy | | | | | | |
| Falsifying patient records | | | | | | |
| Mental/physical unfitness | ● | | ● | ● | ● | |
| Involvement in criminal abortion | | | | | | |
| Unprofessional conduct | ● | | ● | ● | ● | |
| Professional incompetence | ● | | ● | | | |
| Violating any provision of nurse practice act | | ● | ● | ● | ● | |
| False, misleading, deceptive advertising | | | | | | |
| Failing to report persons who violate nurse practice act | | | | | | |
| Failing to report suspected child abuse or neglect | | | | | | |
| Practicing while knowingly infected with contagious disease | | | | | | |
| Failing to obtain U.S. citizenship during time allotted | | | | | | |
| Practicing beyond scope of nursing | | ● | | | | |
| Discriminating against patients on grounds of age, race, sex | | | | | | |

| | Vermont Title 26 | Virginia Title 54 | Washington Chapter 18 | West Virginia Chapter 30 | Wisconsin Title 3 | Wyoming Title 33 |
|---|---|---|---|---|---|---|
| | ● | ● | ● | ● | ● | ● |
| | ● | | ● | ● | ● | ● |
| | | | ● | | | ● |
| | ● | ● | | ● | ● | ● |
| | | | ● | | | |
| | | ● | ● | ● | ● | ● |
| | | | | | | |
| | ● | ● | ● | ● | | ● |
| | | | | | | |
| | | | | | | |
| | ● | ● | ● | ● | ● | ● |
| | | | | | | |
| | ● | ● | ● | ● | ● | ● |
| | ● | ● | ● | ● | | |
| | ● | ● | ● | ● | | ● |
| | | | | | | |
| | | | | | | |
| | | | | | | |
| | | | | | | |
| | | | | | | |
| | | | | | | |
| | | | | | | |

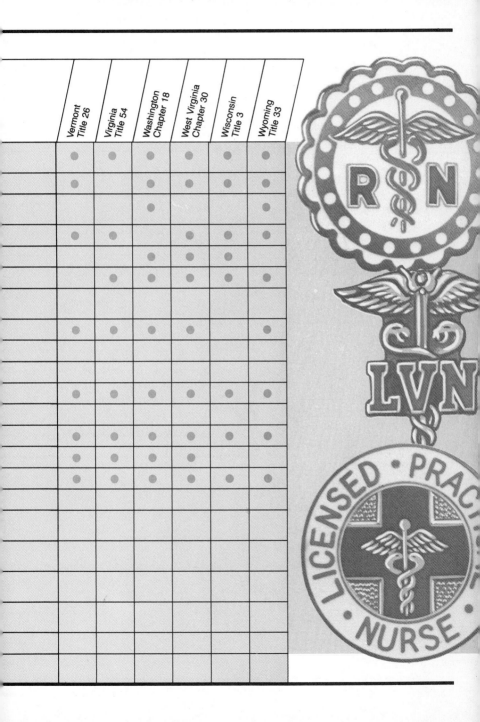

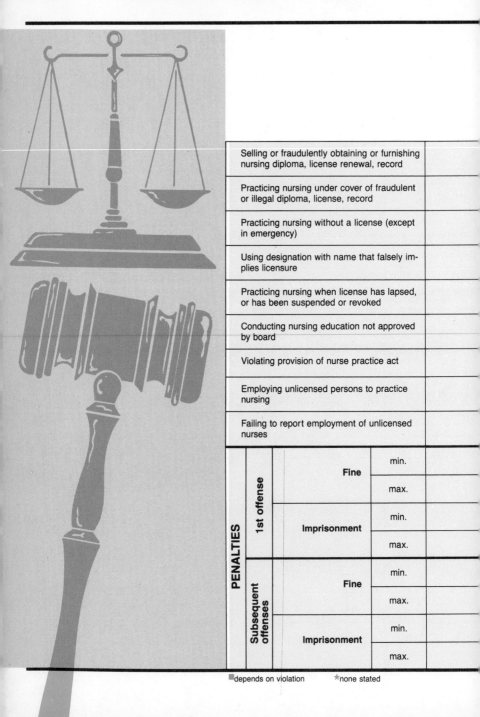

| | | | | |
|---|---|---|---|---|
| Selling or fraudulently obtaining or furnishing nursing diploma, license renewal, record | | | | |
| Practicing nursing under cover of fraudulent or illegal diploma, license, record | | | | |
| Practicing nursing without a license (except in emergency) | | | | |
| Using designation with name that falsely implies licensure | | | | |
| Practicing nursing when license has lapsed, or has been suspended or revoked | | | | |
| Conducting nursing education not approved by board | | | | |
| Violating provision of nurse practice act | | | | |
| Employing unlicensed persons to practice nursing | | | | |
| Failing to report employment of unlicensed nurses | | | | |

| PENALTIES | 1st offense | Fine | min. | |
| | | | max. | |
| | | Imprisonment | min. | |
| | | | max. | |
| | Subsequent offenses | Fine | min. | |
| | | | max. | |
| | | Imprisonment | min. | |
| | | | max. | |

■depends on violation     ★none stated

| | Alabama Title 34 | Alaska Title 8 | Arizona Title 32 | Arkansas Title 72 | California Business and Professions Code | Colorado Chapter 12 | Connecticut Title 20 | Delaware Title 24 | District of Columbia Title 2 | Florida Chapter 455 |
|---|---|---|---|---|---|---|---|---|---|---|
| | ● | ● | | ● | ● | ● | ● | ● | ● | |
| | ● | ● | | ● | ● | | ● | ● | ● | |
| | ● | ● | ● | ● | ● | ● | ● | ● | ● | ● |
| | ● | ● | ● | ● | ● | ● | ● | ● | ● | |
| | ● | ● | | ● | ● | ● | ● | ● | ● | ● |
| | ● | ● | ● | ● | | | | ● | | |
| | ● | ● | ● | ● | ● | | ● | ● | ● | |
| | | | | | | | | | | ● |
| | | | | | | | | | | |
| | | $10 | | $25 | | | | | | |
| | $100 | $500 | ■ | $500 | $2500 | $500 | $500 | $500 | $300 | |
| | | 10 days | | | | | | | | |
| | | 1 yr | | 30 days | 6 mos | 90 days | 6 mos | 1 yr | 90 days | |
| | $100 | $10 | | $25 | $2,500 | $500 | | | | |
| | $200 | $500 | ■ | $500 | | | $500 | $500 | $300 | |
| | | 10 days | | | | | | | | |
| | 1 yr | 1 yr | | 30 days | 6 mos | 90 days | 6 mos | 1 yr | 90 days | |

(continued)

## NURSE PRACTICE ACTS: MISDEMEANORS SUBJECT TO PENALTY *(continued)*

| | Georgia Section 84 | Hawaii Title 25 | Idaho Title 54 | Illinois Chapter 111 | Indiana Section 25 |
|---|:---:|:---:|:---:|:---:|:---:|
| Selling or fraudulently obtaining or furnishing nursing diploma, license renewal, record | ● | ● | ● | ● | ● |
| Practicing nursing under cover of fraudulent or illegal diploma, license, record | ● | ● | | ● | ● |
| Practicing nursing without a license (except in emergency) | ● | ● | ● | ● | ● |
| Using designation with name that falsely implies licensure | ● | ● | ● | ● | ● |
| Practicing nursing when license has lapsed, or has been suspended or revoked | ● | ● | | ● | ● |
| Conducting nursing education not approved by board | ● | ● | | ● | ● |
| Violating provision of nurse practice act | ● | ● | ● | ● | ● |
| Employing unlicensed persons to practice nursing | | | ● | | |
| Failing to report employment of unlicensed nurses | | | | | |

| PENALTIES | | | | Georgia Section 84 | Hawaii Title 25 | Idaho Title 54 | Illinois Chapter 111 | Indiana Section 25 |
|---|---|---|---|---|---|---|---|---|
| **1st offense** | **Fine** | | min. | | | | | |
| | | | max. | | $500 | $300 | ■ | ■ |
| | **Imprisonment** | | min. | | | | | |
| | | | max. | | | 6 mos | | |
| **Subsequent offenses** | **Fine** | | min. | | | | | |
| | | | max. | | $1,000 | $300 | ■ | ■ |
| | **Imprisonment** | | min. | | | | | |
| | | | max. | | 1 yr | 6 mos | | |

■ depends on violation     ★ none stated

| | Iowa Title 8 | Kansas Section 65 | Kentucky Title 26 | Louisiana Title 37 | Maine Title 32 | Maryland Title 22 | Massachusetts Chapter 13 | Michigan Chapter 325 | Minnesota Part I, Section 148.171 | Mississippi Title 73 |
|---|---|---|---|---|---|---|---|---|---|---|
| | ● | ● | ● | ● | ● | ● | ● | ● | ● | ● |
| | ● | ● | | ● | ● | ● | ● | ● | ● | ● |
| | ● | ● | | ● | ● | ● | ● | ● | ● | ● |
| | ● | ● | | ● | ● | ● | ● | ● | ● | ● |
| | ● | ● | | ● | ● | ● | ● | ● | ● | ● |
| | | | | | ● | | | ● | ● | ● |
| | ● | ● | ● | ● | ● | ● | ● | ● | ● | ● |
| | | | | | | ● | ● | ● | | ● |
| | | | | | | ● | | | | |
| | | | | $10 | $100 | | | | | $100 |
| | ■ | ★ | ■ | $100 | $500 | $100 | ■ | $500 | ★ | $1,000 |
| | | | | | 30 days | | | | | 1 yr |
| | | | | 30 days | 6 mos | | | 6 mos | | |
| | | | | $100 | $100 | | | | | $100 |
| | ■ | ★ | ■ | $300 | $500 | $500 | ■ | $500 | ★ | $1,000 |
| | | | | | 30 days | | | | | 1 yr |
| | | | | 60 days | 6 mos | 6 mos | | 6 mos | | |

(continued)

## NURSE PRACTICE ACTS: MISDEMEANORS SUBJECT TO PENALTY *(continued)*

| | Missouri Title 22 | Montana Title 37 | Nebraska Title 71 | Nevada Title 54 | New Hampshire Title 30 |
|---|---|---|---|---|---|
| Selling or fraudulently obtaining or furnishing nursing diploma, license renewal, record | ● | ● | ● | ● | ● |
| Practicing nursing under cover of fraudulent or illegal diploma, license, record | ● | ● | ● | ● | ● |
| Practicing nursing without a license (except in emergency) | ● | ● | ● | ● | ● |
| Using designation with name that falsely implies licensure | ● | ● | ● | ● | ● |
| Practicing nursing when license has lapsed, or has been suspended or revoked | ● | ● | ● | ● | ● |
| Conducting nursing education not approved by board | ● | ● | ● | | ● |
| Violating provision of nurse practice act | ● | ● | ● | ● | ● |
| Employing unlicensed persons to practice nursing | | | | | |
| Failing to report employment of unlicensed nurses | | | | | |

| PENALTIES | | | | | Missouri Title 22 | Montana Title 37 | Nebraska Title 71 | Nevada Title 54 | New Hampshire Title 30 |
|---|---|---|---|---|---|---|---|---|---|
| 1st offense | Fine | min. | | | | $100 | | | |
| | | max. | | ■ | | | ■ | ■ | ■ |
| | Imprisonment | min. | | | | | | | |
| | | max. | | | | | | | |
| Subsequent offenses | Fine | min. | | | | | | | |
| | | max. | | ■ | | $300 | ■ | ■ | ■ |
| | Imprisonment | min. | | | | | | | |
| | | max. | | | | 6 mos | | | |

■ depends on violation   ★ none stated

| | New Jersey Section 45 | New Mexico Chapter 61 | New York Education Law | North Carolina Division 12 | North Dakota Title 43 | Ohio Title 47 | Oklahoma Title 59 | Oregon Title 52 | Pennsylvania Title 63 | Rhode Island Chapter 5 |
|---|---|---|---|---|---|---|---|---|---|---|
| | ● | ● | ● | ● | ● | ● | | ● | ● | ● |
| | ● | ● | ● | ● | ● | ● | | ● | ● | ● |
| | ● | ● | ● | ● | ● | ● | | ● | ● | ● |
| | ● | ● | ● | | | ● | | ● | ● | ● |
| | ● | ● | ● | | | ● | | ● | ● | ● |
| | ● | | | ● | ● | | | | | ● |
| | ● | ● | ● | | | ● | ● | ● | ● | ● |
| | | ● | | ● | | | | ● | | |
| | | | | | | | | | | |
| | | | | | | $100 | $50 | | $50 | $300 |
| | $200 | $1,000 | ■ | ■ | ■ | $500 | $100 | ★ | | |
| | | | | | | | | | | |
| | | 1 yr | | | | 90 days | | | | |
| | | | | | | $100 | $100 per violation | | $100 | $500 |
| | $500 per violation | $1,000 | ■ | ■ | ■ | $500 | | ★ | $200 | |
| | | | | | | | | | | |
| | | 1 yr | | | | 90 days | | | 30 days | 1 yr |

(continued)

## NURSE PRACTICE ACTS: MISDEMEANORS SUBJECT TO PENALTY *(continued)*

| | South Carolina Section 40 | South Dakota Title 36 | Tennessee Section 63 | Texas Article 4513 | Utah Title 58 |
|---|---|---|---|---|---|
| Selling or fraudulently obtaining or furnishing nursing diploma, license renewal, record | | ● | ● | ● | ● |
| Practicing nursing under cover of fraudulent or illegal diploma, license, record | | ● | ● | ● | ● |
| Practicing nursing without a license (except in emergency) | | ● | ● | ● | ● |
| Using designation with name that falsely implies licensure | | ● | ● | ● | ● |
| Practicing nursing when license has lapsed, or has been suspended or revoked | | ● | ● | ● | ● |
| Conducting nursing education not approved by board | | | ● | | ● |
| Violating provision of nurse practice act | ● | ● | ● | ● | ● |
| Employing unlicensed persons to practice nursing | | | | | |
| Failing to report employment of unlicensed nurses | | | | | |

| PENALTIES | | | | South Carolina Section 40 | South Dakota Title 36 | Tennessee Section 63 | Texas Article 4513 | Utah Title 58 |
|---|---|---|---|---|---|---|---|---|
| 1st offense | Fine | min. | | ★ | ★ | | $50 | $50 |
| | | max. | | | | | $100 | $500 |
| | Imprisonment | min. | | | | | | ■ |
| | | max. | | | | 11 mos 29 days | 30 days | |
| Subsequent offenses | Fine | min. | | ★ | ★ | | $50 | $50 |
| | | max. | | | | | $100 | $500 |
| | Imprisonment | min. | | | | | | ■ |
| | | max. | | | | 11 mos 29 days | 30 days | |

■ depends on violation     ★ none stated

| | Vermont Title 26 | Virginia Title 54 | Washington Chapter 18 | West Virginia Chapter 30 | Wisconsin Title 3 | Wyoming Title 33 |
|---|---|---|---|---|---|---|
| | ● | ● | ● | ● | | |
| | ● | ● | ● | ● | | |
| | ● | ● | ● | ● | | |
| | ● | ● | ● | ● | | |
| | ● | ● | ● | ● | | |
| | ● | ● | | ● | | |
| | ● | ● | ● | ● | ● | ● |
| | ● | | | | | |
| | | | | | | |
| | | | | $25 | | |
| | $1,000 | ■ | ■ | $100 | ★ | ★ |
| | | | | | | |
| | 6 mos | | | | | |
| | | | | $25 | | |
| | $1,000 | ■ | ■ | $100 | ★ | ★ |
| | | | | | | |
| | 6 mos | | | | | |

L

Unlike the nurse practice acts in the United States, most Canadian provincial nurse practice acts don't define registered nursing practice; they just describe qualifications for becoming a registered nurse (RN) and grounds for RN license denial, revocation, or suspension. Two provinces, Newfoundland and Prince Edward Island, *do* define the term "registered nurse." Their definition is "any person who is possessed of the qualifications required by this Act, and who is authorized to offer service for the care of the sick and to give care intended for the prevention of disease and to receive remuneration therefor, and who is a member in good standing of the [provincial] association."

The Yukon Territory has no RN licensing body. To practice there, an RN must be registered with one of the 10 provincial nurses associations or with the Northwest Territories' nurses association. All these associations require annual licensure renewal (as specified in the provincial nurse practice acts).

# RN

| **Qualifications for RN licensure** |
| --- |
| Graduation from high school or equivalent |
| Enrollment in an approved nursing program |
| Graduation from an approved nursing program |
| Proper academic qualifications |
| Prescribed amount of clinical experience |
| Passing the registered nurse examination |
| Paying registration fee |
| Good character |
| Fluency in English or French |
| Age 21 or older |
| **Grounds for RN license denial, revocation, or suspension** |
| Dishonesty |
| Professional misconduct |
| Professional incompetence |
| Physical or mental incompetence |
| Addiction to drugs or alcohol |
| Breaching the nurse practice act |
| Indictment for, or conviction of, a criminal act |
| Failure to pay registration fee |
| Fraud or misrepresentation in obtaining license |
| Fraudulent use of the initials or title "RN" |

| **Penalty for fraudulent use of the initials or title "RN"** | Fine |
| --- | --- |
| | Jail sentence |

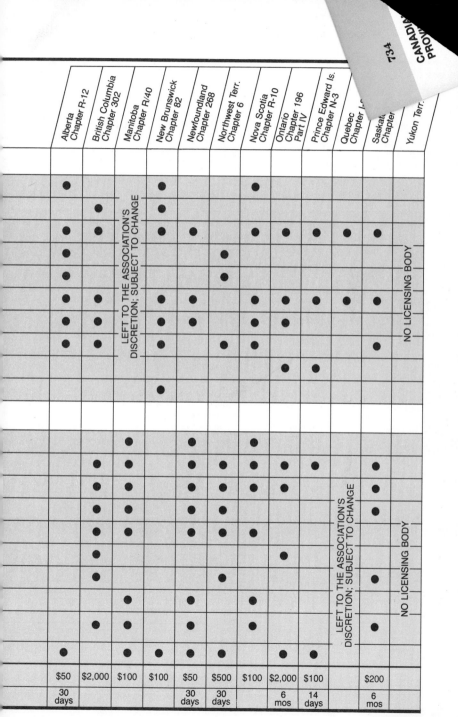

(continued)

Of the provinces that recognize registered nursing assistants, only one, Saskatchewan, actually defines the term in its nurse practice act. It says a nursing assistant is "a person who is trained to care for convalescent, subacutely ill and chronically ill patients, and to assist nurses in the care of acutely ill patients, and who is certified as a nursing assistant..."

Newfoundland, the Northwest Territories, and the Yukon Territory have no licensing bodies for nursing assistants or practical nurses. To practice there, an NA or LPN must be registered with one of the associations in the provinces that do have NA or LPN licensing boards. All such associations require annual licensure renewal (as specified in the provincial nurse practice acts).

# NA or LPN

| | | |
|---|---|---|
| **Qualifications for NA or LPN licensure** | | |
| Graduation from approved NA or LPN program | | |
| Prescribed amount of clinical experience | | |
| Passing NA or LPN examination | | |
| Paying registration fee | | |
| Good character | | |
| Fluency in English or French | | |
| Age 21 or older | | |
| **Grounds for NA or LPN license denial, revocation, or suspension** | | |
| Dishonesty | | |
| Professional misconduct | | |
| Professional incompetence | | |
| Physical or mental incompetence | | |
| Addiction to drugs or alcohol | | |
| Conviction for a criminal act | | |
| Failure to pay registration fee | | |
| Fraud or misrepresentation in obtaining license | | |
| Fraudulent use of the initials or title "NA" or "LPN" | | |
| **Penalty for fraudulent use of the initials or title "NA" or "LPN"** | Fine | |
| | Jail sentence | |

| Alberta Chapter N-13 | British Columbia Chapter 300 | Manitoba Chapter P100 | New Brunswick Chapter 60 | Newfoundland | Northwest Terr. | Nova Scotia Chapter R-10 | Ontario Chapter 196 Part IV | Prince Edward Is. | Quebec | Saskatchewan Chapter R-12.1 | Yukon Terr. |
|---|---|---|---|---|---|---|---|---|---|---|---|
| RNA | LPN | LPN | RNA |  |  | RNA | RNA | RNA | RNA | CNA |  |
| • |  | • | • | NO LICENSING BODY | NO LICENSING BODY | LEFT TO THE ASSOCIATION'S DISCRETION; SUBJECT TO CHANGE | • | LEFT TO THE ASSOCIATION'S DISCRETION; SUBJECT TO CHANGE | LEFT TO THE ASSOCIATION'S DISCRETION; SUBJECT TO CHANGE | • | NO LICENSING BODY |
|  |  | • |  |  |  |  |  |  |  |  |  |
|  |  | • |  |  |  |  | • |  |  | • |  |
| • | • | • |  |  |  |  | • |  |  |  |  |
| • |  |  | • |  |  |  |  |  |  | • |  |
|  |  |  |  |  |  |  | • |  |  |  |  |
|  |  | • |  |  |  |  |  |  |  |  |  |
|  |  | • |  | NO LICENSING BODY | NO LICENSING BODY |  |  | LEFT TO THE ASSOCIATION'S DISCRETION; SUBJECT TO CHANGE | LEFT TO THE ASSOCIATION'S DISCRETION; SUBJECT TO CHANGE |  | NO LICENSING BODY |
|  |  | • |  |  |  |  | • |  |  | • |  |
|  |  | • |  |  |  |  | • |  |  | • |  |
|  |  | • |  |  |  |  |  |  |  | • |  |
|  |  | • |  |  |  |  |  |  |  |  |  |
|  |  |  |  |  |  |  |  |  |  |  |  |
| • |  |  |  |  |  |  |  |  |  | • |  |
|  |  | • |  |  |  |  |  |  |  | • |  |
| • | • | • | • |  |  | • | • |  |  | • |  |
| $500 | $100 | $100 | $100 |  |  | $100 | $2,000 |  |  | $50 |  |
|  |  |  |  |  |  | 6 mos |  |  |  | 3 mos |  |

## American Nurses' Association's
## Resolutions on Entry into Practice

### RESOLUTION 56:
### Identification and titling of establishment of two categories of nursing practice

*Whereas,* ANA for the past 13 years has upheld the position that the "minimum preparation for beginning professional practice at the present time should be baccalaureate degree education in nursing," and the "minimum preparation for beginning technical nursing practice at the present time should be associate degree education in nursing,"

*Therefore be it resolved that:* ANA ensure that two categories of nursing practice be clearly identified and titled by 1980.

*And be it further resolved that:* By 1985 minimum preparation for entry into professional nursing practice is the baccalaureate degree in nursing,

*And be it further resolved that:* ANA, through appropriate structural units, work closely with SNAs and other nursing organizations to identify the two defined categories of nursing practice,

*And be it further resolved that:* National guidelines for implementation be identified and reported back to ANA membership by 1980.

### RESOLUTION 57:
### Establishing a mechanism for deriving competency statements for two categories of nursing practice

*Whereas,* ANA for the past 13 years has upheld the position that the "minimum preparation for beginning professional practice at the present time should be baccalaureate degree education in nursing," and the "minimum preparation for beginning technical nursing practice at the present time should be associate degree education in nursing," and

*Whereas,* Nursing groups throughout the country have developed, or are in the process of developing competency statements of two categories of nursing practice, and

*Whereas,* There is a need for statements to clearly differentiate the competencies for associate and baccalaureate degree prepared nurses,

*Therefore be it resolved that:* ANA establish a mechanism for deriving a comprehensive statement of compentencies for two categories of nursing practice by 1980.

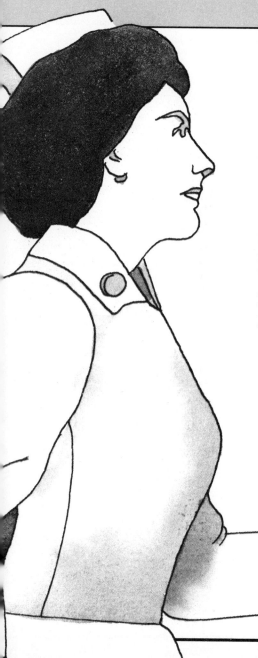

### RESOLUTION 58:
### Increasing accessibility of career mobility programs in nursing

*Whereas,* Since 1965 ANA has supported the position that all nurses obtain educational preparation in colleges and universities, and

*Whereas,* The Commission on Nursing Education has developed standards to ensure quality educational programs, and

*Whereas,* The overwhelming majority of registered nurses currently do not hold a baccalaureate degree in nursing and vocational nurses do not hold an associate degree, and

*Whereas,* Future employment of nurses undoubtedly will be based on academic preparation as well as licensure, and

*Whereas,* There are limited educational opportunities for large numbers of nondegreed nurses in many geographic areas, and

*Whereas,* Flexible and nontraditional programs in nursing education can be developed while ensuring academic integrity,

*Therefore be it resolved that:* ANA actively support increased accessibility to high quality career mobility programs which utilize flexible approaches for individuals seeking academic degrees in nursing.

Reprinted with permission of the American Nurses' Association

*(continued)*

**POSITION STATEMENTS ON ENTRY INTO PRACTICE** *(continued)*

## NLN's Position Statement on Nursing Roles— Scope and Preparation

The quality of nursing and health care has been a concern of the National League for Nursing since its inception in 1952. In view of this concern, NLN has constantly striven to improve the quality of the nursing education programs that provide the manpower necessary to meet society's needs for nursing care.

Democratic society being always in flux, a number of changes in the demographic, economic, social, cultural, and political environments are affecting the delivery of nursing and health care. Consumers' awareness about and expectations of health care continue to grow as knowledge about health is more and more widely disseminated through popular channels. The League has constantly sought not only to identify these changes, but also to incorporate appropriate responses to them within its goals and programs.

A striking and continuing shift has occurred in the responsibility for health care provision. Activities once exclusively medical are now considered to lie within the province of nursing as well; nursing, in turn, has relinquished certain of its responsibilities to other health-care providers.

The social forces impinging upon nursing place demands for greater responsibility and accountability on both the profession and the individual practitioner. Increased sharing by nurses of accountability for the quality and cost of health care compels greater concern not only for the education of graduates of nursing programs—that they be adequately prepared to make independent decisions based on sound knowledge and experience—but also for their appropriate utilization within the health-care system.

In light of these changes, the NLN reaffirms its goal of improving the standards for quality nursing education, nursing service, and health-care delivery.

Nursing as an occupation, in the broadest sense, covers a wide range of activities that may be viewed as a continuum beginning with simple nurturing tasks, progressing through increasingly complex responsibilities, and culminating in critical decision-making activities. To meet the reality of this wide range of responsibilities and activities, a corresponding range of nursing practice roles is required; these have come to be referred to as vocational, technical, and professional nursing practice.

For each nursing role, adequate preservice preparation must be required. Since professional nurses are expected to provide the leadership for all nursing personnel, they need a broad background of knowledge and of clinical skills that will equip them to make the independent judgments and critical decisions necessary in a complex health-care delivery system.

Given the need for such a broad background in the arts and sciences, as well as in nursing, professional nursing practice requires the minimum of a baccalaureate degree with a major in nursing. Preparation for technical nursing practice requires an associate degree or a diploma in nursing. Preparation for vocational nursing requires a certificate or diploma in vocational/practical nursing.

Therefore, to meet the varied needs of the public, the National League for Nursing supports the education of nurses in programs that differ in purposes and lengths and that prepare for varying kinds of practice entailing different degrees of responsibility.

Moreover, to meet society's needs and the changing personal career goals of nurses, opportunities should be provided for individuals to progress within the nursing field. A clear definition of the purposes and a general agreement on the content of each nursing program will facilitate educational mobility for graduates.

More nurses with graduate preparation (i.e., master's and doctoral degrees) are required to provide leadership in nursing service, nursing education, and nursing research. In turn, greater numbers of baccalaureate graduates are required—not only by the increased complexity and scope of care, but also as a base for progression into graduate programs for the eventual assumption of leadership positions.

Community involvement in planning the development of nursing programs is essential to assure the appropriate mix of nursing personnel to meet the needs of each community.

## AACN's Position Statement on Entry into Practice

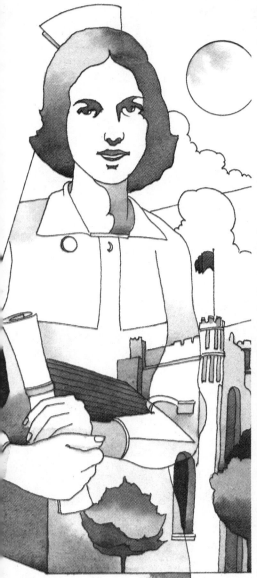

AACN supports the consumer's right to optimum health care in all settings. The registered nurse is committed to ensuring that all patients receive optimal care. This nurses' practice is based on the following:
- Individual professional accountability
- Thorough knowledge of the interrelatedness of body systems and the dynamic nature of the life process
- Recognition and appreciation of the individual's wholeness, uniqueness, and significant social and environmental relationships
- Appreciation of the collaborative role of all members of the health-care team.

Therefore, be it resolved that the minimal preparation for entry into professional nursing practice should be the baccalaureate degree in nursing;

Be it further resolved that registered nurses not currently holding a baccalaureate degree in nursing be granted professional status;

Problems exist which hinder the registered nurse in achieving a baccalaureate degree in nursing. Therefore, be it resolved that AACN pursue, in conjunction with appropriate nursing and legislative organizations, solutions to the problems which include but are not limited to: (a) lowered self-esteem resulting from required repetition of previously mastered nursing experiences, (b) altered life styles due to the time commitment necessary to complete the baccalaureate degree in nursing and to accomplish daily preparation for classes, (c) expenses related to pursuit of the baccalaureate degree in nursing, (d) geographical inaccessibility and insufficient number of baccalaureate degree nursing programs, (e) limited nontraditional baccalaureate degree programs, (f) lack of standard criteria in assigning academic credit for previously completed course work, clinical experience, and challenge examinations, (g) conflicting work and school schedules;

Based upon a recognition and thorough understanding of these problems which exist for many of its members, be it further resolved that AACN continually address the problems and incorporate mechanisms into organizational activities that will assist the AACN member without a baccalaureate degree in nursing to attain said degree.

Reprinted with permission of the American Association of Critical Care Nurses

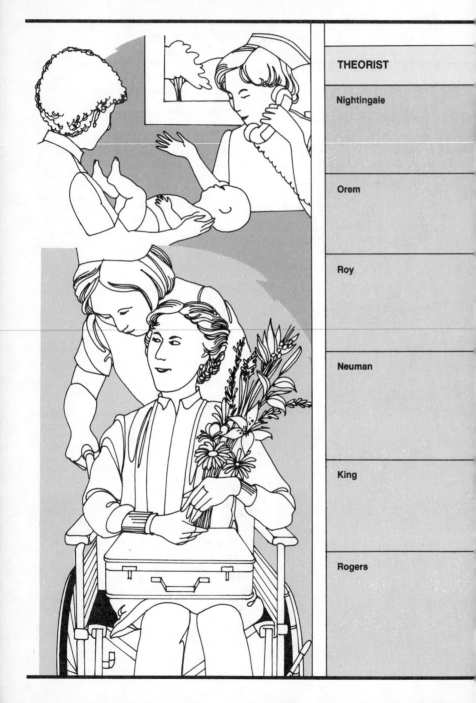

| THEORIST |
|---|
| Nightingale |
| Orem |
| Roy |
| Neuman |
| King |
| Rogers |

| MAIN CONCEPTS | NURSING APPLICATION |
|---|---|
| • Dominant theme: relationship of patient-nurse-environment<br>• Emphasis on physical, rather than psycho-social, environment<br>• Acceptance of nursing as a noncurative science | • Provide the best possible physical and psychological environment for patient, including factors such as fresh air, warmth, cleanliness, rest, and proper nutrition |
| • Dominant theme: restoring patient self-care capabilities<br>• Emphasis on physical well-being | • Assist patient to achieve level of self-care compatible with his health status by determining patient's self-care deficits and by planning system of therapeutic self-care with the patient |
| • Dominant theme: man's continual interaction with and adaptation to his ever-changing environment; adaptation occurs through four modes: physiologic needs, self-concept, role function (purpose in life), and interdependence | • Assess patient's adaptive abilities to each mode<br>• Where deficits occur, manipulate the influencing factors to help the patient adapt; factors are: focal stimuli (causes of behavior), contextual stimuli (contributing factors), and residual stimuli (effects not verified) |
| • Dominant theme: division of man's total framework into two main components: stress and his reaction to stress | • Assess the stressors (any problem or condition that penetrates man's normal line of defense) in four main aspects of patient's life: physiologic, psychologic, sociocultural, and developmental<br>• Help strengthen patient's defenses through preventative, symptomatic, and reconstitution interventions |
| • Dominant theme: man and his social systems, perceptions, interpersonal relationships, and health<br>• Man responds to his environment as a reacting being, time-oriented being, and social being | • Act, react, and interact with patient to assess his social system, perceptions, interpersonal relationships, and health<br>• Ideally, intervene through transaction—the active involvement of both nurse and patient to restore the patient's health |
| • Dominant theme: man and environment as irreducible systems integral to each other, and continually and innovatively evolving<br>• Building blocks: energy fields, universe of open systems, pattern and organization, four-dimensionality<br>• Principles of homeodynamics (describe nature and direction of unitary human development): resonancy, helicy, integrality | • Apply principles of homeodynamics to assess man's evolving manifestations of the human field<br>• Intervene to help patient strengthen the integrity of his human field, and to repattern his human and environmental fields to attain maximum health potential |

## American Nurses' Association Code For Nurses

The Code for Nurses is based upon belief about the nature of individuals, nursing, health, and society. Recipients and providers of nursing services are viewed as individuals and groups who possess basic rights and responsibilities, and whose values and circumstances command respect at all times. Nursing encompasses the promotion and restoration of health, the prevention of illness, and the alleviation of suffering. *The statements of the Code and their interpretation provide guidance for conduct and relationships in carrying out nursing responsibilities consistent with the ethical obligations of the profession and quality in nursing care.*

• The nurse provides services with respect for human dignity and the uniqueness of the client unrestricted by considerations of social or economic status, personal attributes, or the nature of health problems.

• The nurse safeguards the client's right to privacy by judiciously protecting information of a confidential nature.

• The nurse acts to safeguard the client and the public when health care and safety are affected by the incompetent, unethical, or illegal practice of any person.

• The nurse assumes responsibility and accountability for individual nursing judgments and actions.

• The nurse maintains competence in nursing.

• The nurse exercises informed judgment and uses individual competence and qualifications as criteria in seeking consultation, accepting responsibilities, and delegating nursing activities to others.

• The nurse participates in activities that contribute to the ongoing development of the profession's body of knowledge.

• The nurse participates in the profession's efforts to implement and improve standards of nursing.

• The nurse participates in the profession's efforts to establish and maintain conditions of employment conducive to high-quality nursing care.

• The nurse participates in the profession's effort to protect the public from misinformation and misrepresentation and to maintain the integrity of nursing.

• The nurse collaborates with members of the health professions and other citizens in promoting community and national efforts to meet the health needs of the public.

Reprinted with permission of the American Nurses' Association

(continued)

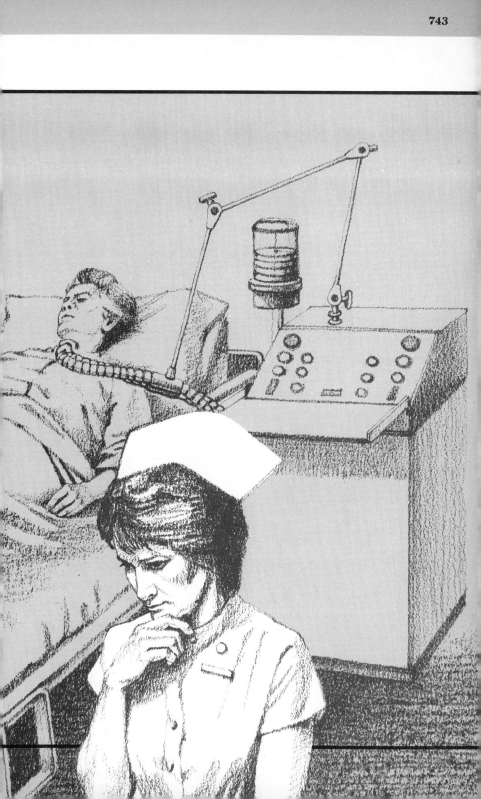

**CODES FOR NURSES** *(continued)*

## Code of Ethics For The Licensed Practical Nurse

- The licensed practical nurse shall practice her profession with integrity.
- The licensed practical nurse shall be loyal—to the physician, to the patient, and to her employer.
- The licensed practical nurse strives to know her limitations and to stay within the bounds of these limitations.
- The licensed practical nurse is sincere in the performance of her duties and generous in rendering service.
- The licensed practical nurse considers no duty too menial if it contributes to the welfare and comfort of her patient.
- The licensed practical nurse accepts only that monetary compensation which is provided for in the contract under which she is employed, and she does not solicit gifts.
- The licensed practical nurse holds in confidence all information entrusted to her.
- The licensed practical nurse shall be a good citizen.
- The licensed practical nurse participates in and shares responsibility for meeting health needs.
- The licensed practical nurse faithfully carries out the orders of the physician or registered nurse under whom she serves.
- The licensed practical nurse refrains from entering into conversation with the patient about personal experiences, personal problems, and personal ailments.
- The licensed practical nurse abstains from administering self-medication, and in event of personal illness, takes only those medications prescribed by a licensed physician.
- The licensed practical nurse respects the dignity of the uniform by never wearing it in a public place.
- The licensed practical nurse respects the religious beliefs of all patients.
- The licensed practical nurse abides by the Golden Rule in her daily relationship with people in all walks of life.
- The licensed practical nurse is a member of The National Federation of Licensed Practical Nurses, Inc., and the state and local membership associations.
- The licensed practical nurse may give credit to a commercial product or service, but does not identify herself with advertising, sales, or promotion.

Reprinted with permission of The National Federation of Licensed Practical Nurses

## International Council Of Nurses Code For Nurses

The fundamental responsibility of the nurse is fourfold: to promote health, to prevent illness, to restore health, and to alleviate suffering.

The need for nursing is universal. Inherent in nursing is respect for life, dignity, and rights of man. It is unrestricted by considerations of nationality, race, creed, color, age, sex, politics, or social status.

Nurses render health services to the individual, the family, and the community, and coordinate their services with those of related groups.

### NURSES AND PEOPLE
The nurse's primary responsibility is to those people who require nursing care.

The nurse, in providing care, respects the beliefs, values, and customs of the individual.

The nurse holds in confidence personal information and uses judgment in sharing this information.

### NURSES AND PRACTICE
The nurse carries personal responsibility for nursing practice and for maintaining competence by continual learning.

The nurse maintains the highest standards of nursing care possible within the reality of a specific situation.

The nurse uses judgment in relation to individual competence when accepting and delegating responsibilities.

The nurse, when acting in a professional capacity, should at all times maintain standards of personal conduct that would reflect credit upon the profession.

### NURSES AND CO-WORKERS
The nurse sustains a cooperative relationship with co-workers in nursing and other fields.

The nurse takes appropriate action to safeguard the individual when his care is endangered by a co-worker or any other person.

### NURSES AND THE PROFESSION
The nurse plays the major role in determining and implementing desirable standards of nursing practice and nursing education.

The nurse is active in developing a core of professional knowledge.

The nurse, acting through the professional organization, participates in establishing and maintaining equitable social and economic working conditions in nursing.

Reprinted with permission of the International Council of Nurses

**NURSES AND SOCIETY**
The nurse shares with other citizens the responsibility for initiating and supporting action to meet the health and social needs of the public.

# P

## DIRECTORY OF PROFESSIONAL ORGANIZATIONS

### INTERNATIONAL

**International Council of Nurses and the Florence Nightingale International Foundation**
P.O. Box 42
1211 Geneva 20, Switzerland

**Pan American Health Organization WHO Regional Office for the Americas**
525 23rd St., N.W.
Washington, D.C. 20037

**People to People Health Foundation (Project Hope)**
Millwood, Va. 22646

**World Health Organization**
Avenue Appia
1211 Geneva 27, Switzerland

### CANADA

#### National Organizations

**Canadian Nurses Association**
50 The Driveway
Ottawa, Ont. K2P 1E2

#### Provincial Professional Associations/Boards of Nursing

**ALBERTA**
**Alberta Association of Registered Nurses**
10256 112th St.
Edmonton, Alta. T5K 1M6

**Alberta Nursing Assistants Registration Board**
10030 107th St., 8th Floor
Edmonton, Alta. T5J 3E4

**BRITISH COLUMBIA**
**Registered Nurses' Association of British Columbia**
2855 Arbutus St.
Vancouver, B.C. V6J 3Y8

**British Columbia Council of Practical Nurses**
3405 Willingdon Ave.
Burnaby, B.C. V5G 3H4

**MANITOBA**
**Manitoba Association of Registered Nurses**
647 Broadway
Winnipeg, Man. R3C 0X2

**Manitoba Association of Licensed Practical Nurses**
1-130 Marion
Winnipeg, Man. R2H 0T4

**NEW BRUNSWICK**
**New Brunswick Association of Registered Nurses**
231 Saunders St.
Fredericton, N.B. E3B 1N6

**Association of New Brunswick Registered Nursing Assistants**
39 Coventry Crescent
Fredericton, N.B. E3B 4P4

**NEWFOUNDLAND**
**Association of Registered Nurses of Newfoundland**
55 Military Rd., P.O. Box 4185
St. John's, N.F. A1C 6A1

**NORTHWEST TERRITORY**
**Northwest Territory Registered Nurses' Association**
Box 2757
Yellowknife, N.W.T. X0E 1H0

**NOVA SCOTIA**
**Registered Nurses' Association of Nova Scotia**
6035 Coburg Rd.
Halifax, N.S. B3H 1Y8

**Nova Scotia Board of Registration for Nursing Assistants**
5614 Fenwick St.
Halifax, N.S. B3H 1P9

**ONTARIO**
**College of Nurses of Ontario**
600 Eglinton Ave. E.
Toronto, Ont. M4P 1P4

**Registered Nurses' Association of Ontario**
33 Price St.
Toronto, Ont. M4W 1Z2

**PRINCE EDWARD ISLAND**
**Association of Nurses of Prince Edward Island**
41 Palmers Lane
Charlottetown, P.E.I. C1A 5V7

**Prince Edward Island Licensed Nursing Assistants Association**
P.O. Box 1253
Charlottetown, P.E.I. C1A 7M8

**QUEBEC**
**Order of Nurses of Quebec**
4200 Dorchester Blvd. W.
Montreal, Que. H3Z 1V4

**Professional Corporation of Nursing Assistants of Quebec**
1980 Sherbrook West, Rm. 920
Montreal, Que. H3H 1E8

**SASKATCHEWAN**
**Saskatchewan Registered Nurses' Association**
2066 Retallack St.
Regina, Sak. S4T 2K2

**YUKON TERRITORY**
There are no associations for nurses in the Yukon.

## UNITED STATES
### National Organizations

**Alpha Tau Delta National Fraternity for Professional Nurses**
489 Serento Circle
Thousand Oaks, Calif. 91360

**American Academy of Ambulatory Nursing Administration**
2901 W. Busch Blvd. Suite 600
Tampa, Fla. 33618

**American Association of Colleges of Nursing**
11 DuPont Circle, Suite 430
Washington, D.C. 20036

**American Association of Critical Care Nurses**
One Civic Plaza
Newport Beach, Calif. 92660

**American Association of Nephrology Nurses and Technicians**
N. Woodbury Rd.
Box 56
Pitman, N.J. 08071

*(continued)*

## DIRECTORY OF PROFESSIONAL ORGANIZATIONS *(continued)*

**American Association of Neurosurgical Nurses**
National Office
625 N. Michigan Ave., Suite 1519
Chicago, Ill. 60611

**American Association of Nurse Anesthetists**
216 Higgins Rd.
Park Ridge, Ill. 60068

**American Association of Occupational Health Nurses, Inc.**
3500 Piedmont Rd., N.E.
Atlanta, Ga. 30305

**American Cancer Society**
777 3rd Ave.
New York, N.Y. 10017

**American College of Nurse-Midwives**
1522 K St., N.W., Suite 1120
Washington, D.C. 20005

**American Heart Association**
7320 Greenville Ave.
Dallas, Tex. 75231

**American Holistic Nurses' Association**
P.O. Box 116
Telluride, Colo. 81435

**American Hospital Association Division of Nursing**
840 N. Lake Shore Dr.
Chicago, Ill. 60611

**American Nurses' Association**
2420 Pershing Rd.
Kansas City, Mo. 64108

**American Public Health Association**
1015 15th St., N.W.
Washington, D.C. 20005

**American Red Cross**
17th & D St., N.W.
Washington, D.C. 20006

**American Society for Nursing Service Administrators, American Hospital Association**
840 N. Lake Shore Dr.
Chicago, Ill. 60611

**American Urological Association Allied**
6845 Lake Shore Dr.
P.O. Box 9397
Raytown, Mo. 64133

**Association for the Care of Children's Health**
3615 Wisconsin Ave., N.W.
Washington, D.C. 20016

**Association of Operating Room Nurses**
10170 E. Mississippi Ave.
Denver, Colo. 80231

**Association of Pediatric Oncology Nurses**
% Lorraine Bivalec
Pacific Medical Center
P.O. Box 7999
San Francisco, Calif. 94120

**Association for Practitioners in Infection Control**
23341 N. Milwaukee Ave.
Half Day, Ill. 60069

**Association of Rehabilitation Nurses**
2506 Gross Point Rd.
Evanston, Ill. 60201

**Emergency Department Nurses Association**
666 N. Lake Shore Dr., Suite 1131
Chicago, Ill. 60611

**Catholic Health Association of the U.S.**
4455 Woodson Rd.
St. Louis, Mo. 63134

**Emergency Department Nurses Association**
666 N. Lake Shore Dr., Suite 1131
Chicago, Ill. 60611

**Federation for Accessible Nursing Education and Licensure**
P.O. Box 22417
Seattle, Wash. 98122
Pres., Lorraine Sherk

**National Association for Practical Nurse Education and Service**
254 W. 31st St.
New York, N.Y. 10001

**National Association of Hispanic Nurses**
4359 Stockdale
San Antonio, Tex. 78233
Pres., Hector Hugo Gonzalez
Sec., Dahlia Rojas

**National Association of Nurse Recruiters**
111 E. Wacker Dr. #600
Chicago, Ill. 60601
Ex. dir., Martha A. DeGraaf
Pres., Gail Capehart Long

**National Association of Orthopaedic Nurses, Inc.**
N. Woodbury Rd.
Box 56
Pitman, N.J. 08071
Pres., Mary Faut Rodts

**National Association of Pediatric Nurse Associates and Practitioners**
N. Woodbury Rd.
Box 56
Pitman, N.J. 08071
Ex. dir., Mavis McGuire
Pres., Sally Walsh

**National Association of School Nurses**
7706 John Hancock Lane
Dayton, Ohio 45459
Pres., Judy Beck
Ex. dir., Peggy Rufner

**National Black Nurses Association, Inc.**
425 Ohio Building
175 S. Main St.
Akron, Ohio 44308

**National Council of State Boards of Nursing**
303 E. Ohio, Suite 2010
Chicago, Ill. 60611

**National Federation of Licensed Practical Nurses, Inc.**
214 S. Driver
P.O. Box 11038
Durham, N.C. 27703

**National Intravenous Therapy Association, Inc.**
87 Blanchard Rd., Suite 4
Cambridge, Mass. 02138

**National League for Nursing**
10 Columbus Circle
New York, N.Y. 10019

**National Nurses Society on Alcoholism**
P.O. Box 7728
Indian Creek Branch
Shawnee Mission, Kan. 66207

**National Student Nurses' Association, Inc.**
10 Columbus Circle
New York, N.Y. 10019

**Nurses Association of the American College of Obstetricians and Gynecologists**
600 Maryland Ave., S.W., Suite 200 E
Washington, D.C. 20024

**Nurses Christian Fellowship**
233 Langdon St.
Madison, Wis. 53703

**Nurses Educational Funds, Inc.**
555 W. 57th St.
New York, N.Y. 10019

**Nurses House, Inc.**
60 E. 42nd St., Rm. 1616
New York, N.Y. 10165

**Oncology Nursing Society**
701 Washington Rd.
Pittsburgh, Pa. 15228

**Sigma Theta Tau**
**National Honor Society of Nursing**
1100 W. Michigan St.
Indianapolis, Ind. 46223

**The Society for Nursing History**
Nursing Education Dept.
Box 150
Teachers College
Columbia University
New York, N.Y. 10027

## Regional

**Midwest Alliance in Nursing**
Rm. 108-BR
Indiana University
1226 W. Michigan St.
Indianapolis, Ind. 46223

**New England Board of Higher Education**
School St.
Wenham, Mass. 01984

**Southern Regional Education Board**
1340 Spring St., N.W.
Atlanta, Ga. 30309

**Western Interstate Commission for Higher Education**
P.O. Drawer P
Boulder, Colo. 80302

## State Professional Associations

**Alabama State Nurses Association**
360 N. Hull St.
Montgomery 36197

**Alaska Nurses Association**
237 E. 3rd Ave.
Anchorage 99501

**Arizona Nurses Association**
4525 N. 12th St.
Phoenix 85014

**Arkansas State Nurses Association**
117 S. Cedar
Little Rock 72205

**California Nurses Association**
1855 Folsom St., Rm. 670
San Francisco 94103

**Colorado Nurses Association**
5453 E. Evans Place
Denver 80222

**Connecticut Nurses Association**
1 Prestige Dr.
Meriden 06450

*(continued)*

## DIRECTORY OF PROFESSIONAL ORGANIZATIONS *(continued)*

**Delaware Nurses Association**
1003 Delaware Ave., Rm. 301
Wilmington 19806

**District of Columbia Nurses Association**
3000 Connecticut Ave., N.W.
Washington 20008

**Florida Nurses Association**
Box 6985
Orlando 32853

**Georgia Nurses Association**
1362 W. Peachtree St., N.W.
Atlanta 30309

**Hawaii Nurses Association**
677 Ala Moana #1014
Honolulu 96813

**Idaho Nurses Association**
1134 N. Orchard #8
Boise 83706

**Illinois Nurses Association**
20 N. Wacker Dr., Suite 2520
Chicago 60606

**Indiana State Nurses Association**
2915 N. High School Rd.
Indianapolis 46224

**Iowa Nurses Association**
215 Shops Bldg.
Des Moines 50309

**Kansas State Nurses Association**
820 Quincy St., Rm. 520
Topeka 66612

**Kentucky Nurses Association**
P.O. Box 8342
Station E
1400 S. 1st St.
Louisville 40208

**Louisiana State Nurses Association**
P.O. Box 837
Metairie 70004

**Maine State Nurses Association**
283 Water St.
P.O. Box 507
Augusta 04330

**Maryland Nurses Association**
5820 Southwestern Blvd.
Baltimore 21227

**Massachusetts Nurses Association**
376 Boylston St.
Boston 02116

**Michigan Nurses Association**
120 Spartan Ave.
East Lansing 48823

**Minnesota Nurses Association**
1821 University Ave., Rm. N-377
St. Paul 55104

**Mississippi Nurses Association**
135 Bounds St., Suite 100
Jackson 39206

**Missouri Nurses Association**
206 E. Dunklin St.
P.O. Box 325
Jefferson City 65102

**Montana Nurses Association**
P.O. Box 5718
2001 11th Ave.
Helena 59604

**Nebraska Nurses Association**
10730 Pacific St., Suite 26
Omaha 68114

**Nevada Nurses Association**
3660 Baker Lane
Reno 89509

**New Hampshire Nurses Association**
48 West St.
Concord 03301

**New Jersey State Nurses Association**
320 W. State St.
Trenton 08618

**New Mexico Nurses Association**
525 San Pedro, N.E., Suite 100
Albuquerque 87108

**New York State Nurses Association**
2113 Western Ave.
Guilderland 12084

**North Carolina Nurses Association**
Box 12025
Raleigh 27605

**North Dakota State Nurses Association**
103½ S. 3rd St.
Bismarck 58501

**Ohio Nurses Association**
4000 E. Main St.
P.O. Box 13169
Columbus 43213

**Oklahoma Nurses Association**
6414 N. Santa Fe, Suite A
Oklahoma City 73116

**Oregon Nurses Association**
9730 S.W. Cascade Blvd., Suite 103
Tigard 97223

**Pennsylvania Nurses Association**
2515 N. Front St.
Harrisburg 17110

**Puerto Rico Board of Nurse Examiners**
800 Roberto H. Todd Ave.
Stop 18, Santurce
Pres., Adelaida M. Sanavitis
Luisa A. de Abadia, ex. dir.
Program of Quality Control of Health
Services

**Rhode Island State Nurses Association**
345 Blackstone Blvd.
H.C. Hall Bldg. (South)
Providence 02906

**South Carolina Nurses Association**
1821 Gadsden St.
Columbia 29201

**South Dakota Nurses Association**
1505 S. Minnesota, Suite 6
Sioux Falls 57105

**Tennessee Nurses Association**
1720 West End Bldg., Suite 400
Nashville 37203

**Texas Nurses Association**
314 Highland Mall Blvd., Suite 504
Austin 78752

**Utah Nurses Association**
1058 E. 9th South
Salt Lake City 84105

**Vermont State Nurses Association**
72 Hungerford Terrace
Burlington 05401

**Virginia Nurses Association**
1311 High Point Ave.
Richmond 23230

**Washington State Nurses Association**
4th & Vine Bldg.
2615 4th Ave., Suite 380
Seattle 98121

**West Virginia Nurses Association**
Union Bldg.
723 Kanawha Blvd., E., Suite 511
Charleston 25301

**Wisconsin Nurses Association**
206 E. Olin Ave.
Madison 53713

**Wyoming Nurses Association**
Majestic Bldg., Rm. 305
1603 Capitol Ave.
Cheyenne 82001

## Boards of Nursing

**Alabama**
**State Board of Nursing**
500 East Blvd., Suite 203
Montgomery 36117

**Alaska**
**Board of Nursing Licensing**
Dept. of Commerce and Economic
Development
Pouch D
Juneau 99811

**Board of Nursing**
142 E. 3rd Ave.
Anchorage 99501

**Arizona**
State Board of Nursing
1645 W. Jefferson, Rm. 254
Phoenix 85007

**Arkansas**
**State Board of Nursing**
4120 W. Markham, Suite 308
Little Rock 77205

**California**
**Board of Registered Nursing**
1020 N. St.
Sacramento 95814

**Board of Vocational Nurse & Psychiatric
Technician Examiners**
1020 N. St.
Sacramento 95814

**Colorado**
**State Board of Nursing**
1525 Sherman St.
Denver 80203

**Connecticut**
**Board of Examiners for Nursing**
79 Elm St.
Hartford 06106

**Delaware**
**Board of Nursing**
Margaret O'Neill Bldg.
Federal & Court Sts.
Dover 19901

**District of Columbia**
**Registered Nurses Examining Board**
614 H St., N.W.
Washington 20001

*(continued)*

# DIRECTORY OF PROFESSIONAL ORGANIZATIONS *(continued)*

**Practical Nurses Examining Board**
614 H St., N.W.
Washington 20001

**Florida**
**Board of Nursing**
111 E. Coastline Dr.
Jacksonville 32202

**Georgia**
**Board of Nursing**
166 Pryor St., S.W.
Atlanta 30303

**Board of Licensed Practical Nurses**
166 Pryor St., S.W.
Atlanta 30303

**Hawaii**
**Board of Nursing**
P.O. Box 3469
Honolulu 96801

**Idaho**
**State Board of Nursing**
Hall of Mirrors
700 W. State, 2nd fl.
Boise 83720

**Illinois**
**Department of Registration & Education**
Nurse Section
320 W. Washington St.
Springfield 62786

**Indiana**
**State Board of Nurses Registration and Nursing Education**
964 N. Pennsylvania
Indianapolis 46204

**Iowa**
**Board of Nursing**
1223 E. Court
Des Moines 50319

**Kansas**
**State Board of Nursing**
P.O. Box 1098
503 Kansas Ave.
Topeka 66601

**Kentucky**
**Board of Nursing Education and Nurse Registration**
4010 Dupont Circle
Louisville 40207

**Louisiana**
**State Board of Nursing**
150 Baronne St.
New Orleans 70112

**Board of Practical Nurse Examiners**
150 Baronne St.
New Orleans 70112

**Maine**
**State Board of Nursing**
295 Water St.
Augusta 04330

**Maryland**
**Board of Examiners of Nurses**
201 W. Preston St.
Baltimore 21201

**Massachusetts**
**Board of Registration in Nursing**
100 Cambridge St., Rm. 1509
Boston 02202

**Michigan**
**Board of Nursing**
P.O. Box 30018
905 Southland
Lansing 48909

**Minnesota**
**Board of Nursing**
717 Delaware St. S.E.
Minneapolis 55414

**Mississippi**
**Board of Nursing**
135 Bounds St., Suite 101
Jackson 39206

**Missouri**
3523 N. Ten Mile Dr.
Box 656
Jefferson City 65102-0656

**Montana**
**Board of Nursing**
Dept. of Commerce
1424 9th Ave.
Helena 59620

**Nebraska**
**State Board of Nursing**
Box 95065
State House Station
Lincoln 68509

**Nevada**
**Board of Nursing**
1135 Terminal Way
Reno 89502

**New Hampshire**
**Board of Nursing Education and Nurse Registration**
105 Loudon Rd.
Concord 03301

**New Jersey**
**Board of Nursing**
1100 Raymond Blvd.
Newark 07102

**New Mexico**
**Board of Nursing**
5301 Central N.E.
Albuquerque 87108

**New York**
**Board for Nursing**
State Education Department
Cultural Education Center
Albany 12230

**North Carolina**
**Board of Nursing**
Box 2129
Raleigh 27602

**North Dakota**
**Board of Nursing**
418 E. Rosser Ave.
Bismarck 58501

**Ohio**
**Board of Nursing Education and Nurse Registration**
65 S. Front St.
Columbus 43215

**Oklahoma**
**Board of Nurse Registration and Nursing Education**
4001 N. Lincoln Blvd., Suite 400
Oklahoma City 73105

**Oregon**
**Board of Nursing**
1400 S.W. 5th Ave.
Portland 97201

**Pennsylvania**
**State Board of Nurse Examiners**
Box 2649
Harrisburg 17120

**Rhode Island**
**Board of Nurse Registration and Nursing Education**
Cannon Health Building
75 Davis St.
Providence 02908

**South Carolina**
**Board of Nursing**
1777 St. Julian Place, Suite 102
Columbia 29204

**South Dakota**
**Board of Nursing**
304 S. Phillips Ave.
Sioux Falls 57102

**Tennessee**
**Board of Nursing**
TDPH State Office Bldg.
Ben Allen Rd.
Nashville 37216

**Texas**
**Board of Nurse Examiners**
1300 E. Anderson Lane, Bldg. C
Austin 78752

**Utah**
**Division of Registration Board of Nursing**
Heber M. Wells Bldg.
160 E. 300 South
P.O. Box 5802
Salt Lake City 84110

**Vermont**
**Board of Nursing**
Pavilion Office Bldg.
109 State St.
Montpelier 05602

**Virginia**
**Board of Nursing**
517 W. Grace St.
P.O. Box 27708
Richmond 23261

**Washington**
**Board of Nursing**
Box 9649
Olympia 98504

**West Virginia**
**Board of Nurse Examiners**
Embleton Bldg.
922 Quarrier St.
Charleston 25301

**Wisconsin**
**Board of Nursing**
P.O. Box 8936
Madison 53708

**Wyoming**
**Board of Nursing**
2223 Warren Ave.
Cheyenne 82002

## HEALTH-CARE WORKERS' JOB TITLES

| | PRIMARY | ALTERNATE |
|---|---|---|
| **A** | **Administration** | |
| | Health administrator | Health officer or commissioner |
| | | Environmental control administrator |
| | | Health agency executive director |
| | | Health care administrator |
| | | Hospital administrator |
| | | Medical care administrator |
| | | Nursing home administrator |
| | | Public health administrator |
| | Health program analyst | Public health analyst |
| | | Public health specialist |
| | Health program representative | Public health advisor |
| | Health systems analyst | Public health representative |
| **C** | **Clinical laboratory services** | |
| | Clinical laboratory scientist | Clinical chemist |
| | | Microbiologist |
| | Clinical laboratory technologist | Medical laboratory technologist |
| | | Medical technologist |
| | | Blood banking technologist |

HEAD NURSE COORDINATOR

SUPERVISOR

EDUCATO

CLINICAL SPECIALIST

| PRIMARY | ALTERNATE |
|---|---|
| | Chemistry technologist |
| | Hematology technologist |
| | Microbiology technologist |
| Clinical laboratory technician | Medical laboratory technician |
| | Medical technician |
| | Cytotechnician |
| | Cytotechnologist |
| Clinical laboratory aide | Laboratory assistant |
| | Certified laboratory assistant |
| | Histologic aide |
| | Histologic technician |
| | Pathology laboratory aide |

**D** **Dentistry and allied services**

| Dentist | Endodontist |
|---|---|
| | Oral pathologist |
| | Oral surgeon |
| | Orthodontist |
| | Pedodontist |
| | Periodontist |
| | Prosthodontist |
| | Public health dentist |
| Dental hygienist | |
| Dental assistant | |
| Dental laboratory technician | Dental laboratory assistant |

**Dietetic and nutritional services**

| Dietitian | Administrative dietitian |
|---|---|
| | Consultant (public health) dietitian |
| | Research dietitian |
| | Teaching dietitian |
| | Therapeutic dietitian |
| Nutritionist | Public health nutritionist |
| Dietary technician | Dietary (food service) assistant |
| | Food service manager |
| | Food service technician |
| Dietary aide | Dietary (food service) worker |
| Food service supervisor | Dietary (food service) worker |

**E** **Environmental health services**

| Environmental scientist | Sanitary sciences specialist |
|---|---|
| | Air pollution meteorologist |
| | Environmental control chemist |
| | Estuarine oceanographer |
| | Groundwater hydrologist |
| | Health physicist |
| | Limnologist |

*(continued)*

## HEALTH-CARE WORKERS' JOB TITLES *(continued)*

| | PRIMARY | ALTERNATE |
|---|---|---|
| **E** *(continued)* | Environmental engineer | Sanitary engineer<br>Air pollution engineer<br>Hospital engineer<br>Industrial hygiene engineer<br>Public health engineer<br>Radiologic health engineer |
| | Environmental technologist | Sanitarian<br>Air pollution specialist<br>Industrial hygienist<br>Radiologic health specialist |
| | Environmental technician | Sanitarian technician<br>Environmental engineering technician<br>Radiologic health technician (monitor) |
| | Environmental aide | Sanitarian aide<br>Environmental engineering aide<br>Sewage plant assistant<br>Waterworks assistant |

**F**    **Food and drug protective services**
Food technologist
Food and drug inspector
Food and drug analyst

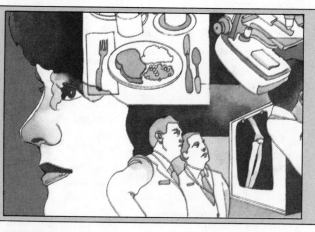

**H**    **Health education**
Health educator

Community health educator
Public health educator
School health educator
School health coordinator

Health education aide

| PRIMARY | ALTERNATE |
|---------|-----------|

### I Information and communication

| Health information specialist | Biomedical communication specialist |
| Health science writer | Medical writer |
| Health technical writer | Medical technical writer<br>Medical editor |
| Medical illustrator | Medical photographer |

### L Library services

Medical librarian
Medical library assistant

| Hospital librarian | Patients' librarian |

### M Medical record services

| Medical record librarian | Medical record specialist<br>Medical record technologist |
| Medical record technician | Medical record assistant |
| Medical record clerk | Medical record aide |

### Medicine and osteopathy

| Physician | Doctor of Medicine—M.D. |
| Osteopathic physician | Doctor of Osteopathy—D.O. |
| Physician or osteopathic physician | Allergist<br>Anesthesiologist<br>Aviation medicine specialist<br>Cardiovascular disease specialist<br>Colon and rectal surgeon (proctologist)<br>Dermatologist<br>Forensic pathologist<br>Gastroenterologist<br>General practitioner<br>Gynecologist<br>Internist<br>Manipulative therapy specialist<br>Neurologic surgeon<br>Neurologist<br>Occupational medicine specialist<br>Obstetrician<br>Ophthalmologist<br>Orthopedic surgeon<br>Otolaryngologist (otorhinolaryngologist)<br>Pathologist<br>Pediatrician<br>Physiatrist (physical medicine<br>   and rehabilitation specialist)<br>Plastic surgeon<br>Preventive medicine specialist<br>Psychiatrist |

*(continued)*

## HEALTH-CARE WORKERS' JOB TITLES *(continued)*

| PRIMARY | ALTERNATE |
|---------|-----------|
| **M** *(continued)* | Public health physician<br>Pulmonary disease specialist<br>Radiologist<br>Surgeon<br>Thoracic surgeon<br>Urologist<br>Intern<br>Resident<br>Fellow |
| **Midwifery**<br>Midwife | Lay midwife<br>Nurse midwife |

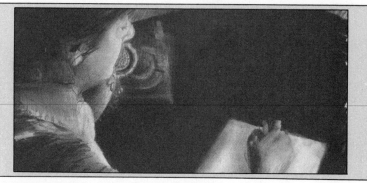

| PRIMARY | ALTERNATE |
|---------|-----------|
| **N** **Natural sciences**<br>Anatomist | Cytologist<br>Embryologist<br>Histologist |
| Botanist | |
| Chemist | Bioanalyst<br>Biochemist<br>Clinical chemist<br>Environmental control chemist |
| Ecologist<br>Entomologist<br>Epidemiologist<br>Geneticist | |
| Hydrologist | Groundwater hydrologist |
| Immunologist | |
| Meteorologist | Air pollution meteorologist |
| Microbiologist | Bacteriologist<br>Mycologist<br>Parasitologist<br>Virologist |

| PRIMARY | ALTERNATE |
|---------|-----------|
| Nutritionist | |
| Oceanographer | Estuarine oceanographer |
| Pathologist | |
| Pharmacologist | Toxicologist |
| Physicist | Health physicist |
| | Biophysicist |
| Physiologist | |
| Sanitary sciences specialist | |
| Zoologist | Limnologist |
| **Nursing and related services** | |
| Nurse | Registered nurse—RN |
| | Graduate nurse |
| | Professional nurse |
| | Hospital nurse |
| | Occupational health (industrial) nurse |
| | Office nurse |
| | Private duty nurse |
| | Public health nurse |
| | School nurse |
| | Nurse anesthetist |
| | Nurse midwife |
| | Obstetrical nurse |
| | Psychiatric nurse |
| | Pediatric nurse |
| | Surgical (operating room) nurse |
| Practical nurse | Licensed practical nurse |
| | Vocational nurse |
| | Licensed vocational nurse |
| Nursing aide | Nursing assistant |
| | Psychiatric (mental health) aide |
| Orderly | Nursing assistant |
| | Psychiatric (mental health) aide |
| Attendant | Nursing assistant |
| | Psychiatric (mental health) aide |
| Home health aide | Home aide—homemaker |
| | Visiting health aide |
| Ward clerk | Floor clerk |

O

| **Occupational therapy** | |
|---------|-----------|
| Occupational therapist | |
| Occupational therapy assistant | Occupational therapy technician |
| Occupational therapy aide | |

*(continued)*

## HEALTH-CARE WORKERS' JOB TITLES *(continued)*

| | PRIMARY | ALTERNATE |
|---|---|---|
| **O** *(continued)* | **Orthotic and prosthetic technology** | |
| | Orthotist | Orthopedic brace maker |
| | Orthotic aide | |
| | Prosthetist | Artificial limb maker |
| | Prosthetic aide | |
| | Restoration technician | |
| **P** | **Pharmacy** | |
| | Pharmacist | Community pharmacist |
| | | Hospital pharmacist |
| | | Industrial pharmacist |
| | | Pharmacy helper |
| | **Physical therapy** | |
| | Physical therapist | |
| | Physical therapy assistant | Physical therapy technician |
| | Physical therapy aide | |
| | **Podiatry** | |
| | Podiatrist | Chiropodist |
| | | Foot orthopedist |
| | | Foot roentgenologist |
| | | Podiatric surgeon |
| | | Pododermatologist |
| **R** | **Radiologic technology** | |
| | Radiologic technologist | X-ray technician |
| | Radiologic technician | Radiation therapy technician |
| **S** | **Social work** | |
| | Clinical social worker | Medical social worker |
| | | Psychiatric social worker |
| | Clinical social work assistant | |
| | Clinical social work aide | Clinical casework aide |
| | **Specialized rehabilitation services** | |
| | Corrective therapist | |
| | Corrective therapy aide | |
| | Educational therapist | |
| | Manual arts therapist | |
| | Music therapist | |
| | Recreation therapist | Therapeutic recreation specialist |
| | Recreation therapy aide | |
| | Homemaking rehabilitation consultant | |

| PRIMARY | ALTERNATE |
| --- | --- |

**Speech pathology and audiology**

| Audiologist | Hearing therapist |
| Speech pathologist | Speech therapist |

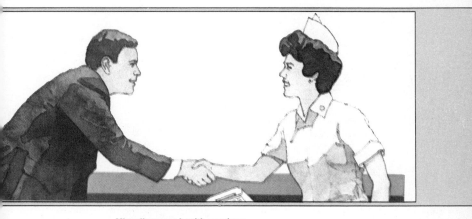

**Miscellaneous health services**

Assistance for physicians:

| Physician's associates | Child health associate |
| | Pediatric associate |
| Physician's assistant | Anesthesiology assistant |
| | Orthopedic assistant |
| Physician's aide | Obstetrical aide |
| | Pediatric aide |
| | Surgical aide |

Emergency health service:
 Medical emergency technician
 Ambulance attendant (aide)

Inhalation therapy:

| Inhalation therapist | Inhalation therapy technician |

 Inhalation therapy aide

Medical machine technology:
 Cardiopulmonary technician
 Electrocardiograph technician
 Electroencephalograph technician

| Other | Biomedical instrument technician |

Nuclear medicine:
 Nuclear medical technologist
 Nuclear medical technician

Other health services:

| Community health aide | Dental health aide |
| | Mental health aide (worker) |
| | School health aide |

What are diagnostic-related groups (DRGs)? They're 470 general medical diagnoses that make up a new patient classification system set up by Medicare. When you care for a Medicare patient, the total amount of money the federal government will pay for the patient's hospital care is based on which DRG the patient falls into. If the hospital bill exceeds this predetermined amount, the hospital must absorb the difference. Hospitals that are able to provide care at a cost below the Medicare amount, however, are rewarded for their efficiency—they can pocket the difference. How do DRGs affect you, the nurse? As is the case for all health team members, DRGs will require you to be extremely cost conscious, providing Medicare patients with the best health care possible within these new financial boundaries.

| DRG NUMBER | MAJOR DIAGNOSTIC CODE* | GENERAL DIAGNOSTIC CLASSIFICATION | DIAGNOSIS |
|---|---|---|---|
| 1 | 1 | ● | Craniotomy age > 17 except for trauma |
| 2 | 1 | ● | Craniotomy for trauma age > 17 |
| 3 | 1 | ● | Craniotomy age < 18 |
| 4 | 1 | ● | Spinal procedures |
| 5 | 1 | ● | Extracranial vascular procedures |
| 6 | 1 | ● | Carpal tunnel release |
| 7 | 1 | ● | Periph + cranial nerve + other nerv syst proc age > 69 and/or dx |
| 8 | 1 | ● | Periph + cranial nerve + other nerv syst proc age < 70 w/o dx 2 |
| 9 | 1 | ◉ | Spinal disorders + injuries |
| 10 | 1 | ◉ | Nervous system neoplasms age > 69 and/or dx 2 |
| 11 | 1 | ◉ | Nervous system neoplasms age < 70 w/o dx 2 |
| 12 | 1 | ◉ | Degenerative nervous system disorders |
| 13 | 1 | ◉ | Multiple sclerosis + cerebellar ataxia |
| 14 | 1 | ◉ | Specific cerebrovascular disorders except TIA |
| 15 | 1 | ◉ | Transient ischemic attacks |
| 16 | 1 | ◉ | Nonspecific cerebrovascular disorders with dx 2 |
| 17 | 1 | ◉ | Nonspecific cerebrovascular disorders w/o dx 2 |
| 18 | 1 | ◉ | Cranial + peripheral nerve disorders age > 69 and/or dx 2 |
| 19 | 1 | ◉ | Cranial + peripheral nerve disorders age < 70 w/o dx 2 |
| 20 | 1 | ◉ | Nervous system infection except viral meningitis |
| 21 | 1 | ◉ | Viral meningitis |
| 22 | 1 | ◉ | Hypertensive encephalopathy |
| 23 | 1 | ◉ | Nontraumatic stupor + coma |
| 24 | 1 | ◉ | Seizure + headache age > 69 and/or dx 2 |
| 25 | 1 | ◉ | Seizure + headache age 18-69 w/o dx 2 |
| 26 | 1 | ◉ | Seizure + headache age 0-17 |

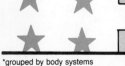

*grouped by body systems     ● surgical     ◉ medical

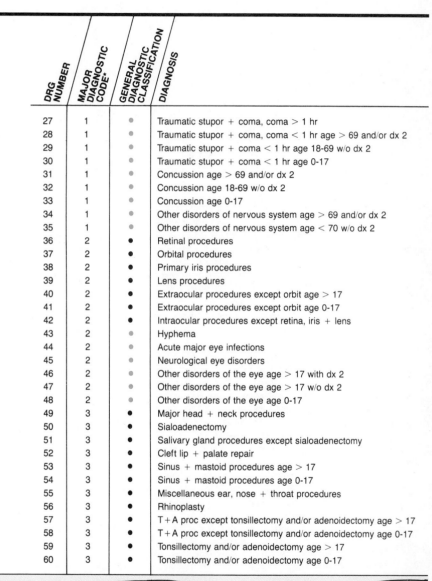

| DRG NUMBER | MAJOR DIAGNOSTIC CODE* | GENERAL DIAGNOSTIC CLASSIFICATION | DIAGNOSIS |
|---|---|---|---|
| 27 | 1 | ◦ | Traumatic stupor + coma, coma > 1 hr |
| 28 | 1 | ◦ | Traumatic stupor + coma, coma < 1 hr age > 69 and/or dx 2 |
| 29 | 1 | ◦ | Traumatic stupor + coma < 1 hr age 18-69 w/o dx 2 |
| 30 | 1 | ◦ | Traumatic stupor + coma < 1 hr age 0-17 |
| 31 | 1 | ◦ | Concussion age > 69 and/or dx 2 |
| 32 | 1 | ◦ | Concussion age 18-69 w/o dx 2 |
| 33 | 1 | ◦ | Concussion age 0-17 |
| 34 | 1 | ◦ | Other disorders of nervous system age > 69 and/or dx 2 |
| 35 | 1 | ◦ | Other disorders of nervous system age < 70 w/o dx 2 |
| 36 | 2 | ● | Retinal procedures |
| 37 | 2 | ● | Orbital procedures |
| 38 | 2 | ● | Primary iris procedures |
| 39 | 2 | ● | Lens procedures |
| 40 | 2 | ● | Extraocular procedures except orbit age > 17 |
| 41 | 2 | ● | Extraocular procedures except orbit age 0-17 |
| 42 | 2 | ● | Intraocular procedures except retina, iris + lens |
| 43 | 2 | ◦ | Hyphema |
| 44 | 2 | ◦ | Acute major eye infections |
| 45 | 2 | ◦ | Neurological eye disorders |
| 46 | 2 | ◦ | Other disorders of the eye age > 17 with dx 2 |
| 47 | 2 | ◦ | Other disorders of the eye age > 17 w/o dx 2 |
| 48 | 2 | ◦ | Other disorders of the eye age 0-17 |
| 49 | 3 | ● | Major head + neck procedures |
| 50 | 3 | ● | Sialoadenectomy |
| 51 | 3 | ● | Salivary gland procedures except sialoadenectomy |
| 52 | 3 | ● | Cleft lip + palate repair |
| 53 | 3 | ● | Sinus + mastoid procedures age > 17 |
| 54 | 3 | ● | Sinus + mastoid procedures age 0-17 |
| 55 | 3 | ● | Miscellaneous ear, nose + throat procedures |
| 56 | 3 | ● | Rhinoplasty |
| 57 | 3 | ● | T + A proc except tonsillectomy and/or adenoidectomy age > 17 |
| 58 | 3 | ● | T + A proc except tonsillectomy and/or adenoidectomy age 0-17 |
| 59 | 3 | ● | Tonsillectomy and/or adenoidectomy age > 17 |
| 60 | 3 | ● | Tonsillectomy and/or adenoidectomy age 0-17 |

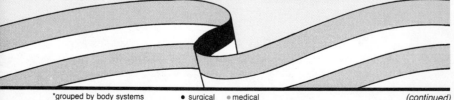

*grouped by body systems     ● surgical   ◦ medical     *(continued)*

**MEDICARE'S PATIENT CLASSIFICATION SYSTEM: DIAGNOSTIC-RELATED GROUPS** *(continued)*

| DRG NUMBER | MAJOR DIAGNOSTIC CODE* | GENERAL DIAGNOSTIC CLASSIFICATION | DIAGNOSIS |
|---|---|---|---|
| 61 | 3 | ● | Myringotomy age > 17 |
| 62 | 3 | ● | Myringotomy age 0-17 |
| 63 | 3 | ● | Other ear, nose + throat O.R. procedures |
| 64 | 3 | ○ | Ear, nose + throat malignancy |
| 65 | 3 | ○ | Dysequilibrium |
| 66 | 3 | ○ | Epistaxis |
| 67 | 3 | ○ | Epiglottitis |
| 68 | 3 | ○ | Otitis media + uri age > 69 and/or dx 2 |
| 69 | 3 | ○ | Otitis media + uri age 18-69 w/o dx 2 |
| 70 | 3 | ○ | Otitis media + uri age 0-17 |
| 71 | 3 | ○ | Laryngotracheitis |
| 72 | 3 | ○ | Nasal trauma + deformity |
| 73 | 3 | ○ | Other ear, nose + throat diagnoses age > 17 |
| 74 | 3 | ○ | Other ear, nose + throat diagnoses age 0-17 |
| 75 | 4 | ● | Major chest procedures |
| 76 | 4 | ● | O.R. proc on the resp system except major chest with dx 2 |
| 77 | 4 | ● | O.R. proc on the resp system except major chest w/o dx 2 |
| 78 | 4 | ○ | Pulmonary embolism |
| 79 | 4 | ○ | Respiratory infections + inflammations age > 69 and/or dx 2 |
| 80 | 4 | ○ | Respiratory infections + inflammations age 18-69 w/o dx 2 |
| 81 | 4 | ○ | Respiratory infections + inflammations age 0-17 |
| 82 | 4 | ○ | Respiratory neoplasms |
| 83 | 4 | ○ | Major chest trauma age > 69 and/or dx 2 |
| 84 | 4 | ○ | Major chest trauma age < 70 w/o dx 2 |
| 85 | 4 | ○ | Pleural effusion age > 69 and/or dx 2 |
| 86 | 4 | ○ | Pleural effusion age > 70 w/o dx 2 |
| 87 | 4 | ○ | Pulmonary edema + respiratory failure |
| 88 | 4 | ○ | Chronic obstructive pulmonary disease |
| 89 | 4 | ○ | Simple pneumonia + pleurisy age > 69 and/or dx 2 |
| 90 | 4 | ○ | Simple pneumonia + pleurisy age 18-69 w/o dx 2 |
| 91 | 4 | ○ | Simple pneumonia + pleurisy age 0-17 |
| 92 | 4 | ○ | Interstitial lung disease age >69 and/or dx 2 |
| 93 | 4 | ○ | Interstitial lung disease age < 70 w/o dx 2 |
| 94 | 4 | ○ | Pneumothorax age > 69 and/or dx 2 |
| 95 | 4 | ○ | Pneumothorax age < 70 w/o dx 2 |

*grouped by body systems     ● surgical     ○ medical

| DRG NUMBER | MAJOR DIAGNOSTIC CODE* | GENERAL DIAGNOSTIC CLASSIFICATION | DIAGNOSIS |
|---|---|---|---|
| 96 | 4 | ◐ | Bronchitis + asthma age > 69 and/or dx 2 |
| 97 | 4 | ◐ | Bronchitis + asthma age 18-69 w/o dx 2 |
| 98 | 4 | ◐ | Bronchitis + asthma age 0-17 |
| 99 | 4 | ◐ | Respiratory signs + symptoms age > 69 and/or dx 2 |
| 100 | 4 | ◐ | Respiratory signs + symptoms age < 70 w/o dx 2 |
| 101 | 4 | ◐ | Other respiratory diagnoses age > 69 and/or dx 2 |
| 102 | 4 | ◐ | Other respiratory diagnoses age < 70 w/o dx 2 |
| 103 | 5 | ● | Heart transplant |
| 104 | 5 | ● | Combined with 105 |
| 105 | 5 | ● | Cardiac valve procedure with pump (w and w/o catheterization) |
| 106 | 5 | ● | Combined with 107 |
| 107 | 5 | ● | Coronary bypass (w and w/o catheterization) |
| 108 | 5 | ● | Cardiothor proc except valve + coronary bypass with pump |
| 109 | 5 | ● | Cardiothoracic procedures w/o pump |
| 110 | 5 | ● | Major reconstructive vascular procedures age > 69 and/or dx 2 |
| 111 | 5 | ● | Major reconstructive vascular procedures age < 70 w/o dx 2 |
| 112 | 5 | ● | Vascular procedures except major reconstruction |
| 113 | 5 | ● | Amputation for circ system disorders except upper limb + toe |
| 114 | 5 | ● | Upper limb + toe amputation for circ system disorders |
| 115 | 5 | ● | Permanent cardiac pacemaker implant with AMI or CHF |
| 116 | 5 | ● | Permanent cardiac pacemaker implant w/o AMI or CHF |
| 117 | 5 | ● | Cardiac pacemaker replace + revis exc pulse gen repl only |
| 118 | 5 | ● | Cardiac pacemaker pulse generator replacement only |
| 119 | 5 | ● | Vein ligation + stripping |
| 120 | 5 | ● | Other O.R. procedures on the circulatory system |
| 121 | 5 | ◐ | Combined with 122 |
| 122 | 5 | ◐ | Circulatory disorders with AMI w and w/o CV comp disch alive |
| 123 | 5 | ◐ | Circulatory disorders with AMI expired |
| 124 | 5 | ◐ | Circulatory disorders exc AMI with card cath, comp dx 1 |
| 125 | 5 | ◐ | Circulatory disorders exc AMI with card cath, uncomp dx 1 |
| 126 | 5 | ◐ | Acute + subacute endocarditis |
| 127 | 5 | ◐ | Heart failure + shock |
| 128 | 5 | ◐ | Deep vein thrombophlebitis |
| 129 | 5 | ◐ | Cardiac arrest |
| 130 | 5 | ◐ | Peripheral vascular disorders age > 69 and/or dx 2 |

*grouped by body systems          ● surgical   ◐ medical                    *(continued)*

## MEDICARE'S PATIENT CLASSIFICATION SYSTEM: DIAGNOSTIC-RELATED GROUPS *(continued)*

| DRG NUMBER | MAJOR DIAGNOSTIC CODE* | GENERAL DIAGNOSTIC CLASSIFICATION | DIAGNOSIS |
|---|---|---|---|
| 131 | 5 | ◐ | Peripheral vascular disorders age < 70 w/o dx 2 |
| 132 | 5 | ◐ | Atherosclerosis age > 69 and/or dx 2 |
| 133 | 5 | ◐ | Atherosclerosis age < 70 w/o dx 2 |
| 134 | 5 | ◐ | Hypertension |
| 135 | 5 | ◐ | Cardiac congenital + valvular disorders age > 69 and/or dx 2 |
| 136 | 5 | ◐ | Cardiac congenital + valvular disorders age 18-69 w/o dx 2 |
| 137 | 5 | ◐ | Cardiac congenital + valvular disorders age 0-17 |
| 138 | 5 | ◐ | Cardiac arrhythmia + conduction disorders age > 69 and/or dx 2 |
| 139 | 5 | ◐ | Cardiac arrhythmia + conduction disorders age < 70 w/o dx 2 |
| 140 | 5 | ◐ | Angina pectoris |
| 141 | 5 | ◐ | Syncope + collapse age > 69 and/or dx 2 |
| 142 | 5 | ◐ | Syncope + collapse age < 70 w/o dx 2 |
| 143 | 5 | ◐ | Chest pain |
| 144 | 5 | ◐ | Other circulatory diagnoses with dx 2 |
| 145 | 5 | ◐ | Other circulatory diagnoses w/o dx 2 |
| 146 | 6 | ● | Rectal resection age > 69 and/or dx 2 |
| 147 | 6 | ● | Rectal resection age < 70 w/o dx 2 |
| 148 | 6 | ● | Major small + large bowel procedures age > 69 and/or dx 2 |
| 149 | 6 | ● | Major small + large bowel procedures age < 70 w/o dx 2 |
| 150 | 6 | ● | Peritoneal adhesiolysis age > 69 and/or dx 2 |
| 151 | 6 | ● | Peritoneal adhesiolysis age < 70 w/o dx 2 |
| 152 | 6 | ● | Minor small + large bowel procedures age > 69 and/or dx 2 |
| 153 | 6 | ● | Minor small + large bowel procedures age < 70 w/o dx 2 |
| 154 | 6 | ● | Stomach, esophageal + duodenal procedures age > 69 and/or dx 2 |
| 155 | 6 | ● | Stomach, esophageal + duodenal procedures age 18-69 w/o dx 2 |
| 156 | 6 | ● | Stomach, esophageal + duodenal procedures age 0-17 |
| 157 | 6 | ● | Anal procedures age > 69 and/or dx 2 |
| 158 | 6 | ● | Anal procedures age < 70 w/o dx 2 |
| 159 | 6 | ● | Hernia procedures except inguinal + femoral age > 69 and/or dx 2 |
| 160 | 6 | ● | Hernia procedures except inguinal + femoral age 18-69 w/o dx 2 |
| 161 | 6 | ● | Inguinal + femoral hernia procedures age > 69 and/or dx 2 |
| 162 | 6 | ● | Inguinal + femoral hernia procedures age 18-60 w/o dx 2 |
| 163 | 6 | ● | Hernia procedures age 0-17 |
| 164 | 6 | ● | Appendectomy with complicated princ diag age > 69 and/or dx 2 |

*grouped by body systems    ● surgical    ◐ medical

| DRG NUMBER | MAJOR DIAGNOSTIC CODE* | GENERAL DIAGNOSTIC CLASSIFICATION | DIAGNOSIS |
|---|---|---|---|
| 165 | 6 | ● | Appendectomy with complicated princ diag age < 70 w/o dx 2 |
| 166 | 6 | ● | Appendectomy w/o complicated princ diag age > 69 and/or dx 2 |
| 167 | 6 | ● | Appendectomy w/o complicated princ diag age < 70 w/o dx 2 |
| 168 | 6 | ● | Procedures on the mouth age > 69 and/or dx 2 |
| 169 | 6 | ● | Procedures on the mouth age < 70 w/o dx 2 |
| 170 | 6 | ● | Other digestive system procedures age > 69 and/or dx 2 |
| 171 | 6 | ● | Other digestive system procedures age < 70 w/o bx 2 |
| 172 | 6 | ○ | Digestive malignancy age > 69 and/or dx 2 |
| 173 | 6 | ○ | Digestive malignancy age < 70 w/o dx 2 |
| 174 | 6 | ○ | G.I. hemorrhage age > 69 and/or dx 2 |
| 175 | 6 | ○ | G.I. hemorrhage age < 70 w/o dx 2 |
| 176 | 6 | ○ | Complicated peptic ulcer |
| 177 | 6 | ○ | Uncomplicated peptic ulcer > 69 and/or dx 2 |
| 178 | 6 | ○ | Uncomplicated peptic ulcer < 70 w/o dx 2 |
| 179 | 6 | ○ | Inflammatory bowel disease |
| 180 | 6 | ○ | G.I. obstruction age > 69 and/or dx 2 |
| 181 | 6 | ○ | G.I. obstruction age > 70 w/o dx 2 |
| 182 | 6 | ○ | Esophagitis, gastroent + misc digest, dis age > 69 and/or dx 2 |
| 183 | 6 | ○ | Esophagitis, gastroent + misc digest, dis age 18-69 w/o dx 2 |
| 184 | 6 | ○ | Esophagitis, gastroenteritis + misc digest, disorders age 0-17 |
| 185 | 6 | ○ | Dental + oral dis exc extractions + restorations age > 17 |
| 186 | 6 | ○ | Dental + oral dis exc extractions + restorations age 0-17 |
| 187 | 6 | ○ | Dental extractions + restorations |
| 188 | 6 | ○ | Other digestive system diagnoses age > 69 and/or dx 2 |
| 189 | 6 | ○ | Other digestive system diagnoses age 18-69 w/o dx 2 |
| 190 | 6 | ○ | Other digestive system diagnoses age 0-17 |
| 191 | 7 | ● | Major pancreas, liver + shunt procedures |
| 192 | 7 | ● | Minor pancreas, liver + shunt procedures |
| 193 | 7 | ● | Biliary tract proc exc tot cholecystectomy age > 69 and/or dx 2 |
| 194 | 7 | ● | Biliary tract proc exc tot cholecystectomy age < 70 w/o dx 2 |
| 195 | 7 | ● | Combined with 197 |
| 196 | 7 | ● | Combined with 198 |
| 197 | 7 | ● | Total cholecystectomy w and w/o C.D.E. age > 69 and/or dx 2 |
| 198 | 7 | ● | Total cholecystectomy w and w/o C.D.E. age < 70 w/o dx 2 |

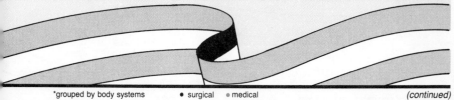

*grouped by body systems    ● surgical   ○ medical    *(continued)*

**MEDICARE'S PATIENT CLASSIFICATION SYSTEM:
DIAGNOSTIC-RELATED GROUPS** *(continued)*

| DRG NUMBER | MAJOR DIAGNOSTIC CODE* | GENERAL DIAGNOSTIC CLASSIFICATION | DIAGNOSIS |
|---|---|---|---|
| 199 | 7 | ● | Hepatobiliary diagnostic procedure for malignancy |
| 200 | 7 | ● | Hepatobiliary diagnostic procedure for nonmalignancy |
| 201 | 7 | ● | Other hepatobiliary or pancreas O.R. procedures |
| 202 | 7 | ○ | Cirrhosis + alcoholic hepatitis |
| 203 | 7 | ○ | Malignancy of hepatobiliary system or pancreas |
| 204 | 7 | ○ | Disorders of pancreas except malignancy |
| 205 | 7 | ○ | Disorders of liver exc malig, cirr, alc hepa age > 69 and/or dx 2 |
| 206 | 7 | ○ | Disorders of liver exc malig, cirr, alc hepa age < 70 w/o dx 2 |
| 207 | 7 | ○ | Disorders of the biliary tract age > 69 and/or dx 2 |
| 208 | 7 | ○ | Disorders of the biliary tract age < 70 w/o dx 2 |
| 209 | 8 | ● | Major joint procedures |
| 210 | 8 | ● | Hip + femur procedures except major joint age > 69 and/or dx 2 |
| 211 | 8 | ● | Hip + femur procedures except major joint age 18-69 w/o dx 2 |
| 212 | 8 | ● | Hip + femur procedures except major joint age 0-17 |
| 213 | 8 | ● | Amputations for musculoskeletal system + conn tissue disorders |
| 214 | 8 | ● | Back + neck procedures age > 69 and/or dx 2 |
| 215 | 8 | ● | Back + neck procedures age < 70 w/o dx 2 |
| 216 | 8 | ● | Biopsies of musculoskeletal system + connective tissue |
| 217 | 8 | ● | Wnd debrid + skn grft exc hand, for muscskeletal + conn tiss dis |
| 218 | 8 | ● | Lower extrem + humer proc exc hip, foot, femur age > 69 and/or dx 2 |
| 219 | 8 | ● | Lower extrem + humer proc exc hip, foot, femur age 18-69 w/o dx 2 |
| 220 | 8 | ● | Lower extrem + humer proc exc hip, foot, femur age 0-17 |
| 221 | 8 | ● | Knee procedures age > 69 and/or dx 2 |
| 222 | 8 | ● | Knee procedures age < 70 w/o dx 2 |
| 223 | 8 | ● | Upper extremity proc exc humerus + hand age > 69 and/or dx 2 |
| 224 | 8 | ● | Upper extremity proc exc humerus + hand age < 70 w/o dx 2 |
| 225 | 8 | ● | Foot procedures |
| 226 | 8 | ● | Soft tissue procedures age > 69 and/or dx 2 |
| 227 | 8 | ● | Soft tissue procedures age < 70 w/o dx 2 |
| 228 | 8 | ● | Ganglion hand procedures |
| 229 | 8 | ● | Hand procedures except ganglion |
| 230 | 8 | ● | Local excision + removal of int fix devices of hip + femur |
| 231 | 8 | ● | Local excision + removal of int fix devices except hip + femur |
| 232 | 8 | ● | Arthroscopy |

*grouped by body systems     ● surgical     ○ medical

| DRG NUMBER | MAJOR DIAGNOSTIC CODE* | GENERAL DIAGNOSTIC CLASSIFICATION | DIAGNOSIS |
|---|---|---|---|
| 233 | 8 | ● | Other musculoskelet sys + conn tiss O.R. proc age > 69 and/or dx |
| 234 | 8 | ● | Other musculoskelet sys + conn tiss O.R. proc age < 70 w/o dx 2 |
| 235 | 8 | ○ | Fractures of femur |
| 236 | 8 | ○ | Fractures of hip + pelvis |
| 237 | 8 | ○ | Sprains, strains, + dislocations of hip, pelvis + thigh |
| 238 | 8 | ○ | Osteomyelitis |
| 239 | 8 | ○ | Pathological fractures + musculoskeletal + conn tiss malignancy |
| 240 | 8 | ○ | Connective tissue disorders age > 69 and/or dx 2 |
| 241 | 8 | ○ | Connective tissue disorders age < 70 w/o dx 2 |
| 242 | 8 | ○ | Septic arthritis |
| 243 | 8 | ○ | Medical back problems |
| 244 | 8 | ○ | Bone diseases + septic arthropathy age > 69 and/or dx 2 |
| 245 | 8 | ○ | Bone diseases + septic arthropathy age < 70 w/o dx 2 |
| 246 | 8 | ○ | Nonspecific arthropathies |
| 247 | 8 | ○ | Signs + symptoms of musculoskeletal system + conn tissue |
| 248 | 8 | ○ | Tendonitis, myositis + bursitis |
| 249 | 8 | ○ | Aftercare, musculoskeletal system + connective tissue |
| 250 | 8 | ○ | Fx, sprns, strns + disl of forearm, hand, foot age > 69 and/or dx 2 |
| 251 | 8 | ○ | Fx, sprns, strns + disl of forearm, hand, foot age 18-69 w/o dx 2 |
| 252 | 8 | ○ | Fx, sprns, strns + disl of forearm, hand, foot age 0-17 |
| 253 | 8 | ○ | Fx, sprns, strns + disl of uparm, lowleg ex foot age > 69 and/or dx |
| 254 | 8 | ○ | Fx, sprns, strns + disl of uparm, lowleg ex foot age 18-69 w/o dx 2 |
| 255 | 8 | ○ | Fx, sprns, strns + disl of uparm, lowleg ex foot age 0-17 |
| 256 | 8 | ○ | Other diagnoses of musculoskeletal system + connective tissue |
| 257 | 9 | ● | Total mastectomy for malignancy age > 69 and/or dx 2 |
| 258 | 9 | ● | Total mastectomy for malignancy age < 70 w/o dx 2 |
| 259 | 9 | ● | Subtotal mastectomy for malignancy age > 69 and/or dx 2 |
| 260 | 9 | ● | Subtotal mastectomy for malignancy age < 70 |
| 261 | 9 | ● | Breast proc for nonmalignancy except biopsy + loc exc |
| 262 | 9 | ● | Breast biopsy + local excision for nonmalignancy |
| 263 | 9 | ● | Skin grafts for skin ulcer or cellulitis age > 69 and/or dx 2 |
| 264 | 9 | ● | Skin grafts for skin ulcer or cellulitis age < 70 w/o dx 2 |
| 265 | 9 | ● | Skin grafts except for skin ulcer or cellulitis with dx 2 |
| 266 | 9 | ● | Skin grafts except for skin ulcer or cellulitis w/o dx 2 |

*grouped by body systems    ● surgical   ○ medical                    *(continued)*

## MEDICARE'S PATIENT CLASSIFICATION SYSTEM:
### DIAGNOSTIC-RELATED GROUPS *(continued)*

| DRG NUMBER | MAJOR DIAGNOSTIC CODE* | GENERAL DIAGNOSTIC CLASSIFICATION | DIAGNOSIS |
|---|---|---|---|
| 267 | 9 | ● | Perianal + pilonidal procedures |
| 268 | 9 | ● | Skin, subcutaneous tissue + breast plastic procedures |
| 269 | 9 | ● | Other skin, subcut tiss + breast O.R. proc age > 69 and/or dx 2 |
| 270 | 9 | ● | Other skin, subcut tiss + breast O.R. proc age < 70 w/o dx 2 |
| 271 | 9 | ◐ | Skin ulcers |
| 272 | 9 | ◐ | Major skin disorders age > 69 and/or dx 2 |
| 273 | 9 | ◐ | Major skin disorders age < 70 w/o dx 2 |
| 274 | 9 | ◐ | Malignant breast disorders age > 69 and/or dx 2 |
| 275 | 9 | ◐ | Malignant breast disorders age < 70 w/o dx 2 |
| 276 | 9 | ◐ | Nonmalignant breast disorders |
| 277 | 9 | ◐ | Cellulitis age > 69 and/or dx 2 |
| 278 | 9 | ◐ | Cellulitis age 18-69 w/o dx 2 |
| 279 | 9 | ◐ | Cellulitis age 0-17 |
| 280 | 9 | ◐ | Trauma to the skin, subcut tiss + breast age > 69 and/or dx 2 |
| 281 | 9 | ◐ | Trauma to the skin, subcut tiss + breast age 18-69 w/o dx 2 |
| 282 | 9 | ◐ | Trauma to the skin, subcut tiss + breast age 0-17 |
| 283 | 9 | ◐ | Minor skin disorders age > 69 and/or dx 2 |
| 284 | 10 | ◐ | Minor skin disorders age < 70 w/o dx 2 |
| 285 | 10 | ● | Amputations for endocrine, nutritional + metabolic disorders |
| 286 | 10 | ● | Adrenal + pituitary procedures |
| 287 | 10 | ● | Skin grafts + wound debride for endoc nutrit + metab disorders |
| 288 | 10 | ● | O.R. procedures for obesity |
| 289 | 10 | ● | Parathyroid procedures |
| 290 | 10 | ● | Thyroid procedures |
| 291 | 10 | ● | Thyroglossal procedures |
| 292 | 10 | ● | Other endocrine, nutrit + metab O.R. proc age > 69 and/or dx 2 |
| 293 | 10 | ● | Other endocrine, nutrit + metab O.R. proc age < 70 w/o dx 2 |
| 294 | 10 | ◐ | Diabetes age > 36 |
| 295 | 10 | ◐ | Diabetes age 0-35 |
| 296 | 10 | ◐ | Nutritional + misc metabolic disorders age > 69 and/or dx 2 |
| 297 | 10 | ◐ | Nutritional + misc metabolic disorders age 18-69 w/o dx 2 |
| 298 | 10 | ◐ | Nutritional + misc metabolic disorders age 0-17 |
| 299 | 10 | ◐ | Inborn errors of metabolism |
| 300 | 10 | ◐ | Endocrine disorders age > 69 and/or dx 2 |

*grouped by body systems   ● surgical   ◐ medical

| DRG NUMBER | MAJOR DIAGNOSTIC CODE* | GENERAL DIAGNOSTIC CLASSIFICATION | DIAGNOSIS |
|---|---|---|---|
| 301 | 10 | ◦ | Endocrine disorders age < 70 w/o dx 2 |
| 302 | 11 | ● | Kidney transplant |
| 303 | 11 | ● | Kidney, ureter + major bladder procedure for neoplasm |
| 304 | 11 | ● | Kidney, ureter + maj bldr proc for nonmalig age > 69 and/or dx 2 |
| 305 | 11 | ● | Kidney, ureter + maj bldr proc for nonmalig age < 70 w/o dx 2 |
| 306 | 11 | ● | Prostatectomy age > 69 and/or dx 2 |
| 307 | 11 | ● | Prostatectomy age <70 w/o dx 2 |
| 308 | 11 | ● | Minor bladder procedures age > 69 and/or dx 2 |
| 309 | 11 | ● | Minor bladder procedures age < 70 w/o dx 2 |
| 310 | 11 | ● | Transurethral procedures age > 69 and/or dx 2 |
| 311 | 11 | ● | Transurethral procedures age < 70 w/o dx 2 |
| 312 | 11 | ● | Urethral procedures, age > 69 and/or dx 2 |
| 313 | 11 | ● | Urethral procedures, age 18-69 w/o dx 2 |
| 314 | 11 | ● | Urethral procedures, age 0-17 |
| 315 | 11 | ● | Other kidney + urinary tract O.R. procedures |
| 316 | 11 | ◦ | Renal failure w/o dialysis |
| 317 | 11 | ◦ | Renal failure with dialysis |
| 318 | 11 | ◦ | Kidney + urinary tract neoplasms age > 69 and/or dx 2 |
| 319 | 11 | ◦ | Kidney + urinary tract neoplasms age < 70 w/o dx 2 |
| 320 | 11 | ◦ | Kidney + urinary tract infections age > 69 and/or dx 2 |
| 321 | 11 | ◦ | Kidney + urinary tract infections age 18-69 w/o dx 2 |
| 322 | 11 | ◦ | Kidney + urinary tract infections age 0-17 |
| 323 | 11 | ◦ | Urinary stones age > 69 and/or dx 2 |
| 324 | 11 | ◦ | Urinary stones age < 70 w/o dx 2 |
| 325 | 11 | ◦ | Kidney + urinary tract signs + symptoms age > 69 and/or dx 2 |
| 326 | 11 | ◦ | Kidney + urinary tract signs + symptoms age 18-69 w/o dx 2 |
| 327 | 11 | ◦ | Kidney + urinary tract signs + symptoms age 0-17 |
| 328 | 11 | ◦ | Urethral stricture age > 69 and/or dx 2 |
| 329 | 11 | ◦ | Urethral stricture age 18-69 w/o dx 2 |
| 330 | 11 | ◦ | Urethral stricture age 0-17 |
| 331 | 11 | ◦ | Other kidney + urinary tract diagnoses age > 69 and/or dx 2 |
| 332 | 11 | ◦ | Other kidney + urinary tract diagnoses age 18-69 w/o dx 2 |
| 333 | 11 | ◦ | Other kidney + urinary tract diagnoses age 0-17 |
| 334 | 12 | ● | Major male pelvic procedures with dx 2 |

*grouped by body systems          ● surgical   ◦ medical                          *(continued)*

## MEDICARE'S PATIENT CLASSIFICATION SYSTEM:
## DIAGNOSTIC-RELATED GROUPS (continued)

| DRG NUMBER | MAJOR DIAGNOSTIC CODE* | GENERAL DIAGNOSTIC CLASSIFICATION | DIAGNOSIS |
|---|---|---|---|
| 335 | 12 | ● | Major male pelvic procedures w/o dx 2 |
| 336 | 12 | ● | Transurethral prostatectomy age > 69 and/or dx 2 |
| 337 | 12 | ● | Transurethral prostatectomy age < 70 w/o dx 2 |
| 338 | 12 | ● | Testes procedures, for malignancy |
| 339 | 12 | ● | Testes procedures, nonmalignant age > 17 |
| 340 | 12 | ● | Testes procedures, nonmalignant age 0-17 |
| 341 | 12 | ● | Penis procedures |
| 342 | 12 | ● | Circumcision age > 17 |
| 343 | 12 | ● | Circumcision age 0-17 |
| 344 | 12 | ● | Other male reproductive system O.R. procedures for malignancy |
| 345 | 12 | ● | Other male reproductive system O.R. proc except for malig |
| 346 | 13 | ● | Malignancy, male reproductive system age > 69 and/or dx 2 |
| 347 | 13 | ● | Malignancy, male reproductive system age < 70 w/o dx 2 |
| 348 | 13 | ● | Benign prostatic hypertrophy age > 69 and/or dx 2 |
| 349 | 13 | ● | Benign prostatic hypertrophy age < 70 w/o dx 2 |
| 350 | 13 | ● | Inflammation of the male reproductive system |
| 351 | 13 | ● | Sterilization, male |
| 352 | 13 | ● | Other male reproductive system diagnoses |
| 353 | 13 | ● | Pelvic evisceration, radical hysterectomy + vulvectomy |
| 354 | 13 | ● | Nonradical hysterectomy age > 69 and/or dx 2 |
| 355 | 13 | ● | Nonradical hysterectomy age < 70 w/o dx 2 |
| 356 | 13 | ● | Female reproductive system reconstructive procedures |
| 357 | 13 | ● | Uterus + adenexa procedures, for malignancy |
| 358 | 13 | ● | Uterus + adenexa proc for nonmalignancy except tubal interrupt |
| 359 | 13 | ● | Tubal interruption for nonmalignancy |
| 360 | 13 | ● | Vagina, cervix + vulva procedures |
| 361 | 13 | ● | Laparoscopy + endoscopy female except tubal interruption |
| 362 | 13 | ● | Laparoscopic tubal interruption |
| 363 | 13 | ● | D+C, conization + radio-implant for malignancy |
| 364 | 13 | ● | D+C, conization except for malignancy |
| 365 | 13 | ● | Other female reproductive system O.R. procedures |
| 366 | 13 | ● | Malignancy, female reproductive system age > 69 and/or dx 2 |
| 367 | 13 | ● | Malignancy, female reproductive system age < 70 w/o dx 2 |
| 368 | 13 | ● | Infections, female reproductive system |

*grouped by body systems          ● surgical    ● medical

| DRG NUMBER | MAJOR DIAGNOSTIC CODE* | GENERAL DIAGNOSTIC CLASSIFICATION | DIAGNOSIS |
|---|---|---|---|
| 369 | 13 | ● | Menstrual + other female reproductive system disorders |
| 370 | 14 | ● | Cesarean section with dx 2 |
| 371 | 14 | ● | Cesarean section w/o dx 2 |
| 372 | 14 | ○ | Vaginal delivery with complicating diagnoses |
| 373 | 14 | ○ | Vaginal delivery w/o complicating diagnoses |
| 374 | 14 | ● | Vaginal delivery with sterilization and/or D + C |
| 375 | 14 | ● | Vaginal delivery with O.R. proc except steril and/or D + C |
| 376 | 14 | ○ | Postpartum diagnoses w/o O.R. procedure |
| 377 | 14 | ● | Postpartum diagnoses with O.R. procedure |
| 378 | 14 | ○ | Ectopic pregnancy |
| 379 | 14 | ○ | Threatened abortion |
| 380 | 14 | ○ | Abortion w/o D + C |
| 381 | 14 | ○ | Abortion with D + C |
| 382 | 14 | ○ | False labor |
| 383 | 14 | ○ | Other antepartum diagnoses with medical complications |
| 384 | 14 | ○ | Other antepartum diagnoses w/o medical complications |
| 385 | 15 | ● | Neonates, died or transferred |
| 386 | 15 | ● | Extreme immaturity, neonate |
| 387 | 15 | ● | Combined with 388 |
| 388 | 15 | ● | Prematurity w and w/o major problems |
| 389 | 15 | ● | Full-term neonate with major problems |
| 390 | 15 | ● | Neonates with other significant problems |
| 391 | 15 | ● | Normal newborns |
| 392 | 16 | ● | Splenectomy age > 17 |
| 393 | 16 | ● | Splenectomy age 0-17 |
| 394 | 16 | ● | Other O.R. procedures of the blood + blood-forming organs |
| 395 | 16 | ○ | Red blood cell disorders age > 17 |
| 396 | 16 | ○ | Red blood cell disorders age 0-17 |
| 397 | 16 | ○ | Coagulation disorders |
| 398 | 16 | ○ | Reticuloendothelial + immunity disorders age > 69 and/or dx 2 |
| 399 | 16 | ○ | Reticuloendothelial + immunity disorders age < 70 w/o dx 2 |
| 400 | 17 | ● | Lymphoma or leukemia with major O.R. procedure |
| 401 | 17 | ● | Lymphoma or leukemia with minor O.R. proc age > 69 and/or dx 2 |
| 402 | 17 | ● | Lymphoma or leukemia with minor O.R. procedure age < 70 w/o dx 2 |

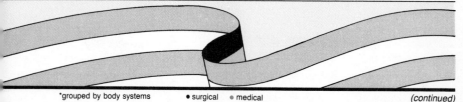

*grouped by body systems    ● surgical  ○ medical    *(continued)*

# MEDICARE'S PATIENT CLASSIFICATION SYSTEM:
## DIAGNOSTIC-RELATED GROUPS *(continued)*

| DRG NUMBER | MAJOR DIAGNOSTIC CODE* | GENERAL DIAGNOSTIC CLASSIFICATION | DIAGNOSIS |
|---|---|---|---|
| 403 | 17 | ● | Lymphoma or leukemia age > 69 and/or dx 2 |
| 404 | 17 | ● | Lymphoma or leukemia age 18-69 w/o dx 2 |
| 405 | 17 | ● | Lymphoma or leukemia age 0-17 |
| 406 | 17 | ● | Myeloprolif disord or poorly diff neoplasm w maj O.R. proc + dx 2 |
| 407 | 17 | ● | Myeloprolif disord or poorly diff neopl w maj O.R. proc w/o dx 2 |
| 408 | 17 | ● | Myeloprolif disord or poorly diff neopl with minor O.R. proc |
| 409 | 17 | ● | Radiotherapy |
| 410 | 17 | ● | Chemotherapy |
| 411 | 17 | ● | History of malignancy w/o endoscopy |
| 412 | 17 | ● | History of malignancy with endoscopy |
| 413 | 17 | ● | Other myeloprolif disord or poorly diff neopl dx age > 69 and/or dx |
| 414 | 17 | ● | Other myeloprolif disord or poorly diff neopl dx age < 70 w/o dx 2 |
| 415 | 18 | ● | O.R. procedure for infections + parasitic diseases |
| 416 | 18 | ● | Septicemia age > 17 |
| 417 | 18 | ● | Septicemia age 0-17 |
| 418 | 18 | ● | Postoperative + posttraumatic infections |
| 419 | 18 | ● | Fever of unknown origin age > 69 and/or dx 2 |
| 420 | 18 | ● | Fever of unknown origin age 18-69 w/o dx 2 |
| 421 | 18 | ● | Viral illness age > 17 |
| 422 | 18 | ● | Viral illness + fever of unknown origin age 0-17 |
| 423 | 18 | ● | Other infectious + parasitic diseases diagnoses |
| 424 | 19 | ● | O.R. procedures with principal diagnosis of mental illness |
| 425 | 19 | ● | Acute adjust react + disturbances of psychosocial dysfunction |
| 426 | 19 | ● | Depressive neuroses |
| 427 | 19 | ● | Neuroses except depressive |
| 428 | 19 | ● | Disorders of personality + impulse control |
| 429 | 19 | ● | Organic disturbances + mental retardation |
| 430 | 19 | ● | Psychoses |
| 431 | 19 | ● | Childhood mental disorders |
| 432 | 19 | ● | Other diagnoses of mental disorders |
| 433 | 20 | ● | Combined 434-438 (discharged AMA not in medpar set) |
| 434 | 20 | ● | Drug dependence |
| 435 | 20 | ● | Drug use except dependence |
| 436 | 20 | ● | Alcohol dependence |

*grouped by body systems   ● surgical   ● medical

| DRG NUMBER | MAJOR DIAGNOSTIC CODE* | GENERAL DIAGNOSTIC CLASSIFICATION | DIAGNOSIS |
|---|---|---|---|
| 437 | 20 | ● | Alcohol use except dependence |
| 438 | 20 | ● | Alcohol + substance-induced organic mental syndrome |
| 439 | 21 | ● | Skin grafts for injuries |
| 440 | 21 | ● | Wound debridements for injuries |
| 441 | 21 | ● | Hand procedures for injuries |
| 442 | 21 | ● | Other O.R. procedures for injuries age > 69 and/or dx 2 |
| 443 | 21 | ● | Other O.R. procedures for injuries age < 70 w/o dx 2 |
| 444 | 21 | ◐ | Multiple trauma age > 69 and/or dx 2 |
| 445 | 21 | ◐ | Multiple trauma age 18-69 w/o dx 2 |
| 446 | 21 | ◐ | Multiple trauma age 0-17 |
| 447 | 21 | ◐ | Allergic reactions age > 17 |
| 448 | 21 | ◐ | Allergic reactions age 0-17 |
| 449 | 21 | ◐ | Toxic effects of drugs age > 69 and/or dx 2 |
| 450 | 21 | ◐ | Toxic effects of drugs age 18-69 w/o dx 2 |
| 451 | 21 | ◐ | Toxic effects of drugs age 0-17 |
| 452 | 21 | ◐ | Complications of treatment age > 69 and/or dx 2 |
| 453 | 21 | ◐ | Complications of treatment age < 70 w/o dx 2 |
| 454 | 21 | ◐ | Other injuries, poisonings + toxic eff diag age > 69 and/or dx 2 |
| 455 | 21 | ◐ | Other injuries, poisonings + toxic eff diag age < 70 w/o dx 2 |
| 456 | 22 | ● | Combined with 457-460 (discharged AMA not in medpar set) |
| 457 | 22 | ● | Extensive burns |
| 458 | 22 | ● | Nonextensive burns with skin grafts |
| 459 | 22 | ● | Nonextensive burns with wound debridement + other O.R. proc |
| 460 | 22 | ● | Nonextensive burns w/o O.R. procedure |
| 461 | 23 | ● | O.R. proc w diagnoses of other contact w hlth services |
| 462 | 23 | ◐ | Rehabilitation |
| 463 | 23 | ● | Signs + symptoms with dx 2 |
| 464 | 23 | ● | Signs + symptoms w/o dx 2 |
| 465 | 23 | ● | Combined with 466 |
| 466 | 23 | ● | Aftercare w and w/o history of malignancy as secondary dx |
| 467 | 23 | ● | Other factors influencing health status |
| 468 | 23 | ● | Unrelated O.R. proc |
| 469 | 23 | ● | PDX invalid as discharge diagnosis |
| 470 | 23 | ● | Ungroupable |

*grouped by body systems   ● surgical   ◐ medical

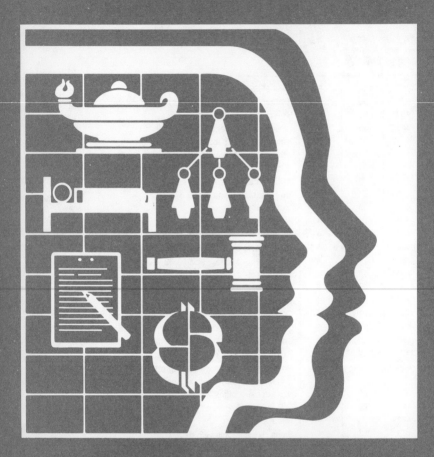

# Glossary
# and Indexes

# Glossary

## A

**abuse of process** • A civil action for damages in which it is alleged that the legal process has been used in a manner not contemplated by law. This action might be brought by a health practitioner attempting to countersue a patient or by a psychiatric patient attempting to demonstrate wrongful confinement.

**academic ladder** • The hierarchy of faculty appointments in a university through which a faculty member must advance from instructor to assistant professor, associate professor, and, finally, to professor.

**accreditation** • Recognition that a school and its nursing program meet high nursing-education standards established by the state board of nursing and accrediting organizations.

**action alternatives** • Any of several possible actions or courses of action chosen by a nurse as part of a goal-oriented nursing-care plan and performed to resolve a problem or to modify the effects a particular problem has on a patient.

**active listening** • Listening that results in a response keyed directly to what the speaker said, so he's encouraged to continue.

**acute stress** • Any emotional, physical, social, or economic change that produces *temporary* physical or mental tension and sometimes may contribute to the onset of illness.

**adaptation model** • A conceptual framework that focuses on the patient as an adaptive system, one in which nursing intervention is required when a deficit develops in the patient's ability to cope with the internal and external demands of the environment. These demands are classified in four groups: physiologic needs, the need for a positive self-concept, the need to perform social roles, and the need to balance dependence and independence. The nurse assesses the patient's maladaptive response and identifies the kind of demand that is causing the problem. Nursing care is planned to promote adaptive responses in order to cope successfully with the current stress on the patient's well-being. This model is frequently used as a conceptual framework for programs of nursing education.

**administrator** • Overseer of the general effectiveness and efficiency of an agency, who is concerned with organization, planning, development, growth, change, operations, budgets, and evaluation.

**admissible** • During a trial, information presented that's authentic, relevant, and reliable to be considered in reaching a decision; nurses' notes are usually admissible if the information in them hasn't been altered.

**admission interview** • The initial history-taking interview when a person is admitted to the hospital.

**adult** • **1.** One who is fully developed and matured and who has attained the intellectual capacity and the emotional and psychological stability characteristic of a mature person. **2.** A person who has reached full legal age.

**adverse drug effect** • A harmful, unintended reaction to a drug administered at normal dosage.

**affidavit** • A written statement that is sworn to before a notary public or an officer of the court.

**affiliated hospital** • A hospital that is associated to some degree with a medical school or health program.

**affirmative defense** • A denial of guilt or wrongdoing based on new evidence rather than on simple denial of a charge, as a plea of immunity according to a good samaritan law. The defendant bears the burden of proof in an affirmative defense.

**agency** • A relationship between two parties in which the first party authorizes the second to act as agent on behalf of the first. It usually implies a contractual arrangement between two parties managed by a third party, the agent.

**agent** • A party authorized to act on behalf of another and to give the other an account of such actions.

**age of majority** • Either 18 or 21 years, depending on the state or Canadian provincial laws.

**Alcoholics Anonymous (AA)** • An international nonprofit organization, founded in 1935, consisting of abstinent alcoholics whose purpose is to help alcoholics stop drinking and maintain sobriety through group support, shared experiences, and faith in a power greater than themselves.

**alcoholism** • The extreme dependence on excessive amounts of alcohol, associated with a cumulative pattern of deviant behaviors. Alcoholism is a chronic illness with a slow, insidious onset, which may occur at any age. The etiology is unknown, but cultural and psychosocial factors are suspect, and families of alcoholics have a higher incidence of alcoholism. Frequent intoxication has cumulative destructive effects on an individual's family and social life, working life, and physical health. The most frequent medical consequences of alcoholism are central nervous system depression and cirrhosis of the liver. The severity of each of these is increased in the absence of food intake. Alcoholic patients also may suffer from alcoholic gastritis, peripheral neuropathies, auditory hallucinations, and cardiac problems. Abrupt withdrawal of alcohol in addiction causes weakness, sweating, and hyperreflexia. The severe form of alcohol withdrawal is called delirium tremens.

**allowable charge** • The maximum amount that a third party, usually an insurance company, will pay to reimburse a provider for a specific service.

**allowable costs** • Components of an institution's costs that are reimbursable as determined by a payment formula. In general, costs of services not considered to be reasonable or necessary to the proper delivery of health services are excluded from allowable costs.

**AMA** • Against medical advice; refers to when a patient decides to leave a health-care facility when his doctor advises him to stay.

**ambulatory care** • All health services provided on an outpatient basis to those who visit a hospital or other health-care facility and depart after treatment on the same day.

**American Academy of Nursing (AAN)** • The honorary organization of the American Nurses' Association, created to recognize superior achievement in nursing in order to promote advances and excellence in nursing practice and education. A person who is elected to membership is given the title of Fellow of the American Academy of Nursing and may use the abbreviation FAAN as an honorific.

**American Medical Association (AMA)** • A professional association whose membership is made up of approximately half of the total licensed physicians in the United States, including practitioners in all recognized medical specialties as well as general primary care physicians. The AMA is governed by a Board of Trustees and House of Delegates. Trustees and delegates represent various state and local medical associations as well as such government agencies as the Public Health Service and medical departments of the Army, Navy, and Air Force.

**American Nurses' Association (ANA)** • The national professional association of registered nurses in the United States. It was founded in 1896 to improve standards of health and the availability of health care given in order to foster high standards for nursing, to promote the professional development of nurses, and to advance the economic and general welfare of nurses. The ANA is made up of 53 constituent associations from 50 states, the District of Columbia, Guam, and the Virgin Islands, representing more than 900 district associations. Members may join one or more of the five Divisions on Nursing Practice: Community Health; Gerontological; Maternal and Child Health; Medical-Surgical; and Psychiatric and Mental Health Nursing. These Divisions are coordinated by the Congress for Nursing Practice. The Congress evaluates changes in the scope of practice, monitors scientific and educational developments, encourages research, and develops statements that describe ANA policies regarding legislation affecting nursing practice. Other commissions within the Association include the Commission on Nursing Education, the Commission on Nursing Services, the Commission on Nursing Research, and the Economic and General Welfare Commission.

**American Red Cross** • One of more than 120 national organizations that seek to reduce human suffering through various health, safety, and disaster relief programs in affiliation with the International Committee of the Red Cross. The Committee and all Red Cross organizations evolved from the Geneva Convention of 1864, following the example and urging of Swiss humanitarian Jean Henri Dunant, who aided wounded French and Austrian soldiers at the Battle of Solferino in 1859. The American Red Cross has more than 130 million members in about 3,100 chapters throughout the United States. Volunteers constitute the entire staffs of about 1,700 chapters. Other chapters maintain small paid staffs and some professionals but depend largely on volunteers.

**analyzing** • In five-step nursing process: a category of nursing behavior in which the health-care needs of the client are identified and the goals of care are selected. The nurse interprets data, identifies problems involving the client, the client's family, and significant others, establishes priorities among goals, integrates the information, and projects the expected outcomes of nursing activities. Although analyzing follows assessing and precedes planning in the five steps of the nursing process, in practice, analyzing is integral to effective nursing practice at all steps of the process. See also **implementation.**

**annual report** • A publication prepared once a year that lists a public corporation's (or company's) officers and summarizes its financial condition for the past year.

**answer** • The response of a defendant to the complaint of a plaintiff. The answer contains a denial of the plaintiff's allegations and may also contain an affirmative defense or a counterclaim. It is the principal pleading on the part of the defense and is prepared in writing, usually by the defense attorney, and submitted to the court.

**antitrust** • Against the operation, establishment, or maintenance of a monopoly in the manufacture, production, or sale of a commodity, providing of a service, or practice of a profession.

**anxiety** • A state or feeling of uneasiness, agitation, uncertainty, and fear resulting from the anticipation of some threat or danger, usually of intrapsychic rather than external origin, whose source is generally unknown or unrecognized. The condition may result as a rational response to a tension-producing situation, like applying for a job, or from a general concern about life's uncertainties. It is a pathologic condition if it is not based in reality and if it is so severe that it results in the inability to function. Kinds of anxiety include castration anxiety, free-floating anxiety, separation anxiety, situational anxiety.

**appellant** • A party that brings an appeal to an appellate court. Having lost the case in a lower court, the appellant requests the court to reconsider the case.

**appellate court** • A court of law that has the power to review the decision of a lower court. It does not make a new determination of the facts of the case; it reviews only the way in which the law was applied in the case.

**appellee** • A party in an appeal that won the case in a lower court. The appellee argues that the decision of the lower court should not be modified by the appellate court.

**aptitude** • A natural ability, tendency, talent, or capability to learn, understand, or acquire a particular skill; mental alertness.

**aptitude test** • Any of a variety of standardized tests for measuring an individual's ability to learn certain skills.

**arbitration** • A process for settling labor disputes by involving a neutral labor relations expert.

**arbitrator** • An impartial person appointed to resolve a dispute between parties. The arbitrator listens to the evidence as presented by the parties in an informal hearing and attempts to arrive at a resolution acceptable to both parties.

**assault** • An attempt or threat by a person to physically injure another person.

**assertiveness** • A style of communication characterized by confidence.

**assessing** • In five-step nursing process: a category of nursing behavior that includes gathering, verifying, and communicating information relative to the client. The nurse collects information from verbal interactions with the client, the client's family, and significant others; examines standard data sources for information; systematically checks for symptoms and signs; determines the client's ability to perform self-care activities; assesses the client's environment; and identifies reactions of the staff (including the nurse who is performing the assessment) to the client and to the client's family and significant others. To verify the data the nurse confirms the observations and perceptions by gathering additional information; discusses the orders and decisions made by other members of the staff with them, when indicated; and personally evaluates and checks the patient's condition. The nurse reports the information that has been gathered and verified. Although assessing is the first of the five steps of the nursing process, preceding analyzing, in practice assessing is integral to effective nursing practice at all steps of the process. See also **implementation.**

**assessment** • **1.** An evaluation or appraisal of a patient's condition. **2.** The process of gathering data needed to formulate a nursing diagnosis. **3.** In a problem-oriented medical record: an examiner's evaluation of the disease or condition based on the patient's subjective report of the symptoms and course of the illness or condition and the examiner's objective findings, including data obtained through laboratory tests, physical examination, and medical history. See also **nursing assessment, problem-oriented medical record.**

**associate degree in nursing** • An academic degree after satisfactory completion of a 2-year course of study, usually at a community or junior college. The recipient is eligible to take the national licensing examination to become a registered nurse. An associate degree in nursing is not available in Canada.

**associate nurse** • *U.S.* **1.** In primary nursing: a nurse who is responsible for implementing a primary nurse's care plans. **2.** In some states, a registered nurse who holds a diploma from a hospital school of nursing or an associate degree from a 2-year academic school of nursing.

**attending physician** • The physician who is responsible for a particular, usually private, patient. In a university setting, an attending physician often also has teaching responsibilities and holds a faculty appointment. Also called **attending** *(informal).*

**attorney of record** • The attorney whose name appears on the legal records for a specific case, as the agent of a specific client.

**audit** • A methodical examination; to examine

with intent to verify. Nursing audits examine standards of nursing care.

**authority** • The power someone is granted—either because of his expertise in a specific field or because of his role or position in an organization—to influence another person's behavior.

**authorization cards** • Cards employees sign to authorize a union election.

**autopsy** • A postmortem examination of a body to determine the cause of death.

# B

**bachelor of science in nursing (BSN)** • An academic degree awarded upon satisfactory completion of a 4-year course of study in an institution of higher learning. The recipient is eligible to take the national certifying examination to become a registered nurse. A BSN degree is prerequisite to advancement in most systems and institutions that employ nurses. Compare **associate degree in nursing.**

**bargaining agent** • A person or group selected by members of a bargaining unit to represent them in negotiations.

**bargaining unit** • A group of employees who participate in collective bargaining as representatives of all employees.

**barrier nursing** • Nursing care of a patient in isolation, performed to prevent the spread of infection by creating an aseptic barrier around the patient. Gown, mask, and gloves are worn by staff or visitors entering the room; the number of staff entering the room is kept to a minimum, and visitors are limited. Contaminated substances are handled according to strict protocols. Specific techniques vary with the indication for isolation.

**BASIC** • *abbr* Beginners' All-purpose Symbolic Instruction Code, a programming language widely used on personal computers and small business systems.

**battered woman syndrome (BWS)** • Repeated episodes of physical assault on a woman by the man with whom she lives, often resulting in serious physical and psychological damage to the woman. Such violence tends to follow a predictable pattern. The first phase is characterized by the man acting increasingly irritable, edgy, and tense. Verbal abuse, insults, and criticism increase, and shoves or slaps begin. The second phase is the time of the acute, violent activity. As the tension mounts, the woman becomes unable to placate the man, and she may argue or defend herself. The man uses this as the justification for his anger and assaults her, often saying that he is "teaching her a lesson." The third stage is characterized by apology and remorse on the part of the man, with promises of change. The calm continues until tension builds again. The battered woman syndrome occurs at all socioeconomic levels, and one half to three quarters of female assault victims are the victims of an attack by a lover or husband. It is estimated that between one and two million women a year are beaten by their husbands. Men who grew up in homes in which the father abused the mother are more likely to beat their wives than are men who lived in nonviolent homes. Personal and cultural attitudes also affect the incidence of wife-battering.

**battery** • The unauthorized touching of a person by another person, such as when a healthcare professional treats a patient beyond what the patient consented to.

**behavior modification techniques** • Techniques used for eradicating or reducing negative behaviors, or for reinforcing positive behaviors, by adjusting the amount of attention and approval a person receives or by manipulating certain aspects of the person's environment.

**benefits** • Nonsalary forms of compensation an employer provides for employees—for example, medical and dental insurance.

**block charting** • A method of charting in which you detail, in paragraph form, procedures you carried out during a block of time.

**board of health** • An administrative body acting on a municipal, county, state, provincial, or national level. The functions, powers, and responsibilities of boards of health vary with the locales. Each board is generally concerned with the recognition of the health needs of the people and the coordination of projects and resources to meet and identify these needs. Among the tasks of most boards of health are prevention of disease, health education, and implementation of laws pertaining to health.

**borrowed-servant doctrine** • A legal doctrine that courts may apply in cases when an employer "lends" his employee's services to another employer who, under this doctrine, becomes liable for the employee's wrongful conduct.

**brain death** • Generally, the cessation of brain wave activity. The legal definition of this condition varies from state to state. (See *Defining Brain Death,* page 108.)

**breach of contract** • Failing to perform all or part of the contracted duty without justification.

**breach of duty** • The neglect or failure to fulfill in a proper manner the duties of an office, job, or position.

**BSN** • *abbr* **bachelor of science in nursing.**

# C

**Canadian Association of University Schools of Nursing (CAUSN)** • A national Canadian organization of nursing schools affiliated with institutions of higher learning.

**Canadian Nurses Association (CNA)** • The official national organization for the professional registered nurses of Canada who are members of one of the 10 provincial nurses' associations and the Northwest Territories' association. The CNA, a federation of these 11 associations, is supported by contributions of the 140,000 members of the regional associations. The chief objective of the CNA is to promote conditions conducive to the good health of the people and to good patient care.

**Canadian Nurses Association Testing Service (CNATS)** • The organizational affiliate of the Canadian Nurses Association that is concerned with testing the graduates of approved schools of nursing to qualify as registered nurses.

**Canadian Nurses' Foundation (CNF)** • A national Canadian foundation organized to support scholarship in nursing. The CNF awards financial support to nurses undertaking graduate studies in nursing and to nurses planning research in nursing.

**Canadian Public Health Association (CPHA)** • A national Canadian organization concerned with issues in public health and epidemiology. Membership is open to professionals and to others interested in these issues.

**"captain of the ship" doctrine** • A legal doctrine that considers a surgeon responsible for the actions of his assistants when those assistants are under the surgeon's supervision. This doctrine is similar to the borrowed-servant doctrine.

**care of the sick** • In public health nursing: the care of sick patients in their homes, as distinguished from health supervision. Public health nursing agencies are reimbursed for the nursing services rendered by the nurses according to the kind of service rendered, as a sick visit or a health supervision visit. Compare **health supervision.**

**career counselor** • A professional person who's trained to guide others in career decision making.

**career ladder** • See **clinical ladder.**

**career plan** • A person's long-term plan for achieving stated career goals.

**case-oriented nursing** • Where one nurse works with one type of patient and assumes responsibility for the care and observation of all patients of that type.

**catastrophic health insurance** • Health insurance that awards benefits to pay for the cost of severe or lengthy disability or illness. Benefits on some policies are not paid until a specified minimum amount, paid by the insured, is exceeded. Most policies have a limit in total benefits paid, and payment for certain kinds of services may either be precluded or limited to a maximum indemnity.

**causa mortis** • A state of mind in a person approaching death.

**CAUSN** • *abbr* **Canadian Association of University Schools of Nursing.**

**CCRN** • *abbr* Certified Critical-Care Registered Nurse.

**Centers for Disease Control (CDC)** • A federal agency of the United States government that provides facilities and services for the investigation, identification, prevention, and control of disease. It is concerned with all aspects of the epidemiology and the laboratory diagnosis of disease. Immunization programs, quarantine regulations and programs, laboratory standards, and community surveillance for disease are among the activities of the CDC.

**centralized structure** • A type of organization with all departments reporting to one entity, commonly the board of directors, which has complete decision-making authority.

**central processing unit (CPU)** • In data processing: the group of physical components of a computer system containing the logical, arithmetical, and control circuits for the system. Also called hardware.

**certification** • Recognition that a nurse is specially qualified, based on predetermined standards, to provide nursing care in a particular area of nursing practice.

**Certified Nurse-Midwife (CNM)** • According to the American College of Nurse-Midwives: "an individual educated in the two disciplines of nursing and midwifery, who possesses evidence of certification according to the requirements of the American College of Nurse-Midwives." See also **midwife.**

**certified registered nurse anesthetist (CRNA)** • See **nurse anesthetist.**

**certify** • **1.** To guarantee formally that certain requirements have been met based on expert knowledge of significant, pertinent facts. **2.** To attest, by a legal process, that someone is insane. **3.** To attest to the fact of someone's death in writing, usually on a form as required by local authority. **4.** To declare that a person has satisfied certain requirements for membership or acceptance into a professional or other group. See also **certification.**

**CEU** • *abbr* **continuing education unit.**

**chain of command** • The power hierarchy within an organization.

**change agent** • A nurse or health-care professional who works to bring about beneficial change for co-workers or patients.

**child abuse** • The physical, sexual, or emotional maltreatment of a child. It may be overt or covert and often results in permanent physical or psychiatric injury, mental impairment, or, sometimes, death. Child abuse occurs predominantly to children less than age 3 years and is the result of complex factors involving both parents and child, compounded by various stressful environmental circumstances, as poor socioeconomic conditions, inadequate physical and emotional support within the family, and any major life change or crisis, especially those crises arising from marital strife. Parents at high risk for abuse are characterized as having unsatisfied needs, difficulty in forming adequate interpersonal relationships, unrealistic expectations of the child, and a lack of nurturing experience, often involving neglect or abuse in their own childhoods. Predisposing factors among children include the temperament, personality, and activity level of the child; birth order; sensitivity to parental needs; and a need for special physical or emotional care resulting from illness, premature birth, or congenital or genetic abnormalities. Also called battered child syndrome. Compare **child neglect.**

**child neglect** • The failure by parents or guardians to provide the basic needs of a child by physical or emotional deprivation that interferes with normal growth and development or that places the child in jeopardy. Compare **child abuse.**

**child welfare** • Any service sponsored by the community or special organizations that provide for the physical, social, or psychological care of children in need of it.

**chronic care** • A pattern of medical and nursing care that focuses on long-term care of people with chronic diseases or conditions, either at home or in a medical facility. It includes care specific to the problem, as well as other measures to encourage self-care, to promote health, and to prevent loss of function.

**chronic stress** • Any emotional, physical, social, or economic change that produces *persistent* physical or mental tension that, if not relieved, produces exhaustion and is likely to contribute to the onset of illness.

**circumstantial evidence** • Testimony based on inference or hearsay rather than actual personal knowledge or observation of the facts in question.

**civil defense laws** • That body of statutory law that is invoked when the jurisdiction is under attack, as in a state of war.

**Civilian Health and Medical Programs for Uniformed Services (CHAMPUS)** • A healthcare insurance system for military dependents and members of the military services when certain kinds of care are not available through the usual military medical service. CHAMPUS is the first, and one of the few, federal third-party reimbursement systems that will pay for care rendered by nurse-midwives and nurse practitioners.

**claims-made policy** • A professional liability insurance policy that covers the holder for the period in which a claim of malpractice is made. The alleged act of malpractice may have occurred at some previous time, but the policy insures the holder when the claim is made.

**client-centered therapy** • A nondirective method of group or individual psychotherapy, originated by Carl Rogers, in which the role of the therapist is to listen to and then reflect or restate without judgment or interpretation the words of the client. The goal of the therapy is personal growth achieved by the client's increased awareness and understanding of his attitudes, feelings, and behavior.

**clinical laboratory** • A laboratory in which tests directly related to the care of patients are performed. Such laboratories use material obtained from patients for testing, as compared with research laboratories where animal and other sources of test material are also used.

**clinical ladder** • A system for recognizing and promoting nurses who demonstrate advanced clinical knowledge and skills.

**clinical research center** • An organization, often associated with a medical school or a teaching hospital, that studies, analyzes, correlates, and describes medical cases. Such centers usually have extensive laboratory facilities and specialized staffs of doctors and medical technicians. Clinical research centers often offer free or inexpensive diagnoses and treatment for patients participating in various research programs and often produce significant new medical information.

**clinical specialist** • A highly specialized nurse whose level of nursing practice can be certified by the American Nurses' Association.

**CNA** • *abbr* Canadian Nurses Association.

**CNATS** • *abbr* Canadian Nurses Association Testing Service.

**CNF** • *abbr* Canadian Nurses' Foundation.

**CNM** • *abbr* certified nurse-midwife.

**CNS** • *abbr* clinical nurse specialist.

**code** • 1. A published body of statutes, as a civil code. 2. A collection of standards and rules of behavior, as a dress code. 3. A symbolic means of representing information for communication or transfer, as a genetic code. 4. *Informal.* A discreet signal used to summon a special team to resuscitate a patient without alarming patients or visitors. See also **no-code order.**

**codes** • 1. A system of assigned terms designed by a medical institution for quick and accurate communication during emergencies or for patient identification. 2. Short values of data used to feed commands to a computerized hospital information system.

**coercion strategy** • A plan for bringing about change in which the initiator forces others to adapt to the change, using his authority over them.

**collective bargaining** • A legal process in which representatives for organized employees negotiate with their employer about such matters as wages, hours, and working conditions.

**collegial relationship** • A professional relationship in which the participants share authority.

**commitment** • **1.** The placement or confinement of an individual in a specialized hospital or other institutional facility. **2.** The legal procedure of admitting a mentally ill person to an institution for psychiatric treatment. The process varies from state to state but usually involves judicial or court action based on medical evidence certifying that the person is mentally ill. See also **certification. 3.** A pledge or contract to fulfill some obligation or agreement, used especially in some forms of psychotherapy or marriage counseling.

**common law** • Law derived from previous court decisions, not from statutes. Also called case law.

**communicable disease** • Any disease transmitted from one person or animal to another, either directly, by contact with excreta or other discharges from the body; indirectly, via substances or inanimate objects, as contaminated drinking glasses, toys, or water; or via vectors, as flies, mosquitoes, ticks, or other insects. To control a communicable disease it is important to identify the organism, prevent its spread to the environment, protect others against contamination, and treat the infected person. Many communicable diseases, by law, must be reported to the health department. Kinds of communicable diseases include those caused by bacteria, chlamydia, fungi, parasites, rickettsiae, and viruses. Also called contagious disease.

**Communicable Disease Center** • Former name of the **Centers for Disease Control.**

**communication** • Any process in which a message containing information is transferred, especially from one person to another, via any of a number of media. Communication may be verbal or nonverbal; it may occur directly, as in a face-to-face conversation or with the observation of a gesture; or it may occur remotely, spanning space and time, as in writing and reading or in making or playing back a recording.

**communication barriers** • Any factors—such as noise, language differences, or emotional preoccupations—that interfere with messages transmitted from one person to another.

**community health nursing** • A field of nursing that is a blend of primary health care and nursing practice with public health nursing. The philosophy of care is based on the belief that care directed to the individual, the family, and the group contributes to the health care of the population as a whole. Participation of all consumers of health care is encouraged in the development of community activities that contribute to the promotion, education, and maintenance of good health. These activities require comprehensive health programs that pay special attention to social and ecological influences and specific populations at risk.

**community medicine** • A branch of medicine that is concerned with the health of the members of a community, municipality, or region.

**community mental health center (CMHC)** • A community-based center that provides comprehensive mental health services. The specific services to be provided are specified in an act of Congress, the Community Mental Health Centers Act; these requirements have been updated periodically. The costs of consultation and educational services, instruction, development, and initial operation of the facility are provided by the federal government. The organization, management, and operation of CMHCs are specified by the Act. Consumer representation in each of these areas is required.

**community nurse practitioner (CNP)** • A nurse who has completed a postbaccalaureate program in community nursing.

**comparative negligence doctrine** • A doctrine by which a court assigns partial responsibility for the defendant's alleged negligence to the plaintiff in the case.

**compensation** • All forms of payment from an employer to an employee, including salary and benefits.

**complaint** • **1.** A pleading by a plaintiff made under oath to initiate a suit. It is a statement of the formal charge and the cause for action against the defendant. For a minor offense, the defendant is tried on the basis of the complaint. A more serious felony prosecution requires an indictment with evidence presented by a state's attorney. **2.** *Informal.* Any ailment, problem, or symptom identified by the client, patient, member of the person's family, or other knowledgeable person. The chief complaint is often the reason that the person has sought health care.

**computerized record system** • A system that stores medical records in the memory bank of a computer.

**confidentiality** • A professional responsibility to keep all privileged information private.

**conflict management** • Directing and using disagreement creatively so its outcome is constructive, rather than destructive.

**consent form** • A document, prepared for a patient's signature, that discloses his proposed treatment in general terms.

**consortium** • Two or more education institutions that combine and coordinate their educational programs.

**constructive conflict** • A disagreement over

such things as goals, methods, or values that stimulates problem solving and is eventually resolved to everyone's satisfaction.

**contact hour** • A unit of measurement that describes 50 minutes of an approved, organized learning experience.

**continuing education** • Formal, organized, educational programs designed to promote the knowledge, skills, and professional attitudes of nurses. The programs are usually short-term and specific; a certificate may be offered for completion of a course and a number of continuing education units (CEUs) may be conferred. Continuing education is required for relicensure in many states.

**continuing education unit (CEU)** • The equivalent of 10 contact hours of participation in an approved continuing education program.

**contract** • A legally binding agreement between two or more people to do, or not do, something.

**contract duties** • Duties defined in an employment contract.

**contract violations** • Actions that break mutually accepted employment rules.

**convalescent home** • See **extended-care facility.**

**cooperation strategy** • A plan for bringing about change in which the initiator influences others to adapt to the change, using open communication and interpersonal skills.

**coping mechanism** • An action taken to temporarily adapt to stress-producing situations.

**coping strategy** • The plan of action a person develops to adapt to temporary stress-producing situations.

**coronary care unit (CCU)** • A specially equipped hospital area designed for the treatment of patients with sudden, life-threatening cardiac conditions. Such units contain resuscitation and monitoring equipment and are staffed by personnel especially trained and skilled in recognizing and immediately responding to cardiac emergencies with cardiopulmonary resuscitation techniques, the administration of antiarrhythmic drugs, and other appropriate therapeutic measures.

**coroner** • A public official who investigates the causes and circumstances of a death occurring within a specific legal jurisdiction or territory, especially a death that may have resulted from unnatural causes. Also called medical examiner.

**corporate liability** • A judicial process by which the court will disregard the usual liability immunity of corporations and corporate officers.

**corrective discipline** • Action a supervisor takes to stop a subordinate's improper behavior.

**cost analysis** • An analysis of the disbursements of a given activity, agency, department, or program.

**cost/benefit ratio** • A ratio that represents the relationship of the cost of an activity to the benefit of its outcome or product.

**cost control** • The process of monitoring and regulating the expenditure of funds by an agency or institution. Budgets, reports, and cost-accounting procedures are performed to achieve cost control. Also known as cost containment.

**cost-effectiveness** • The extent to which an activity is thought to produce tangible benefits in relation to its expense.

**counterclaim** • A claim made by a defendant establishing a cause for action in his favor against the plaintiff. The purpose of a counterclaim is to oppose or detract from the plaintiff's claim or complaint.

**countersignature** • The signature you must obtain from another health professional to verify information, or your signature that verifies another health-care provider's information.

**cover letter** • A letter that a person seeking employment sends, together with his résumé, to a prospective employer. The cover letter states the applicant's interest in applying for a particular job.

**CPHA** • *abbr* the **Canadian Public Health Association.**

**credentialing** • Approval that a continuing education provider receives from various agencies, confirming that the provider's programs meet predetermined educational standards.

**criminal abortion** • The intentional termination of pregnancy under any condition prohibited by law.

**crisis** • An emotionally significant event, an extreme change of status, or an uncertain or crucial time or situation where the outcome will decisively affect a person's future life.

**crisis intervention** • Therapeutic intervention to help resolve a particular and immediate problem. No attempt is made at in-depth analysis. The goal is to restore the person to the level of functioning that existed before the current crisis.

**crisis-intervention unit** • A group trained in emergency medical treatment and in various methods for rendering therapeutic psychiatric assistance to a person or group of persons during a period of crisis. Such networks are found within community hospitals, health-care centers, or as specialized self-contained units, as suicide prevention centers, and operate 24 hours a day.

**CRNA** • *abbr* **certified registered nurse anesthetist.** See **nurse anesthetist.**

**cross-examination** • The questioning of a witness by the attorney for the opposing party.

**CRT** • *abbr* cathode-ray tube, or the display screen on a computer terminal or heart monitor similar to a television screen.

**Current Procedural Terminology (CPT)** • A system developed by the American Medical Association for standardizing the terminology and coding used to describe medical services and procedures.

**custodial care** • Services and care of a nonmedical nature provided on a long-term basis, usually for convalescent and chronically ill individuals. Kinds of custodial care include board, personal assistance.

# D

**damages** • An amount of money a court orders a defendant to pay the plaintiff, in deciding the case in favor of the plaintiff.

**data** • *sing.* **datum** Some pieces of information, especially those that are part of a collection of information to be used in an analysis of a problem, as the diagnosis of a health problem.

**data analysis** • The phase of a research study that includes classifying, coding, and tabulating information needed to perform statistical or qualitative analyses according to the research design and appropriate to the data. Data analysis follows data collection and precedes interpretation or application of the data.

**data base** • A large store or bank of information, especially in a form that can be processed by computer.

**data collection** • **1.** The phase of a research study that includes gathering of information and identification of sampling units as directed by the research design. Data collection precedes data analysis. **2.** In a clinical setting: the gathering of information by observation, interview, examination, and review of records.

**day-care** • A specialized program or facility that provides care for preschool children, usually within a group framework, either as a substitute for or extension of home care, particularly for single parents or for parents who are both employed outside the home. Day-care groups vary in size and function and range from casual neighborhood parent-supervised play groups to formal nursery schools or organized centers run by trained personnel.

**death** • **1.** Apparent death: the cessation of life as indicated by the absence of heartbeat or respiration. **2.** Legal death: the total absence of activity in the brain and the central nervous, cardiovascular, and respiratory systems, as observed and declared by a physician.

**decentralized structure** • A type of organization with each department run by a director who has considerable independent decision-making authority.

**decertification** • The process of voting a union out.

**declared emergency** • The situation when a government official formally identifies a state of emergency.

**decoding** • Deciphering and understanding another person's verbal or nonverbal message.

**default judgment** • A judgment rendered against a defendant because of the defendant's failure to appear in court or to answer the plaintiff's claim within the proper time.

**defendant** • The party that is named in a plaintiff's complaint and against whom the plaintiff's allegations are made. The defendant must respond to the allegations.

**defense mechanism** • An unconscious reaction that offers the self protection from a stressful situation.

**defense of impossibility** • A legal defense that says a violation of a contract was literally impossible to avoid.

**delegation** • Assigning a subordinate a task that's one of your responsibilities.

**delinquency** • **1.** Negligence or failure to fulfill a duty or obligation. **2.** An offense, fault, misdemeanor, or misdeed; a tendency to commit such acts. See also **juvenile delinquency.**

**delinquent** • **1.** Characterized by neglect of duty or violation of law. **2.** One whose behavior is characterized by persistent antisocial, illegal, violent, or criminal acts; a juvenile delinquent.

**dependent nursing function** • A function the nurse performs, with another professional's written order, on the basis of that professional's assessment and judgment, for which that professional is accountable.

**deposition** • A sworn pretrial testimony given by a witness in response to oral or written questions and cross-examination. The deposition is transcribed and may be used for further pretrial investigation. It may also be presented at the trial if the witness cannot be present. Compare **discovery, interrogatories.**

**destructive conflict** • A disagreement over such things as goals, methods, or values that disrupts routine, is counterproductive, and ends in misunderstanding and mutual unhappiness.

**developmental assessment** • Evaluation of a person's physical and psychological development as determined by standardized measurements—for example, of body size and dimensions; by social and psychological functioning; by observations of motor skills; and by tests of intellectual skills and aptitude.

**direct access** • The right of a health-care provider and a patient to interact on a professional basis without interference.

**direct examination** • The first examination of a witness called to the stand by the attorney for the party the witness is representing.

**direct patient care** • Care of a patient provided in person by a member of the staff. Direct patient care may involve any aspects of the health care of a patient, including treatments, counseling, self-care, patient education, and administration of medication.

**disaster** • A sudden event that creates a number of victims with extensive injuries.

**discharge planning** • The formulation of a program by the patient, his family, the health-care team, and appropriate outside agencies to meet physical and psychological needs after the patient leaves the health-care facility.

**discovery** • A pretrial procedure that allows the plaintiff's and defendant's attorneys to examine relevant materials and interrogate all parties to the case.

**dismiss** • To discharge or dispose of an action, suit, or motion trial.

**district** • **1.** A group of patients in an area of a unit in a hospital for whom a head nurse or primary nurse is responsible, usually a subdivision of a ward unit. Patients are customarily assigned to a district on the basis of certain shared needs for nursing care. **2.** The area of a city or town assigned to a public health nurse.

**division** • **1.** An administrative subunit in a hospital, as a division of medical nursing or a division of surgical nursing. **2.** In public health nursing: an area that encompasses several geographical districts.

**DNSc** • *abbr* **Doctor of Nursing Science.**

**doctoral program in nursing** • An educational program of study that offers preparation for a doctoral degree in the field of nursing, designed to prepare nurses for advanced practice and research. Upon successful completion of the course of study, the degree PhD in nursing or DSN (Doctor of Science in Nursing) is awarded.

**Doctor of Medicine (MD)** • See **physician.**

**Doctor of Osteopathy (DO)** • See **physician.**

**doctrine of parens patriae** • A doctrine that appoints the state as legal guardian of a child or incompetent when an individual hasn't been appointed as guardian.

**documentation** • The preparing or assembling of written records.

**drug** • **1.** Any substance taken by mouth, injected into a muscle, the skin, a blood vessel, or a cavity of the body, or applied topically to treat or prevent a disease or condition. Also called medicine. **2.** *Informal.* A narcotic substance.

**drug abuse** • The use of a drug for a nonther-

apeutic effect, especially one for which it was not prescribed or intended. Some of the most commonly abused substances are alcohol, amphetamines, barbiturates, and methaqualone. Drug abuse may lead to organ damage, addiction, and disturbed patterns of behavior. Some illicit drugs, as lysergic acid diethylamide and phencyclidine hydrochloride, have no recognized therapeutic effect. Use of these drugs often incurs criminal penalty in addition to the potential for physical, social, and psychological harm. See also **drug addiction.**

**drug addiction** • A condition characterized by an overwhelming desire to continue taking a drug to which one has become habituated through repeated consumption because it produces a particular effect, usually an alteration of mental activity, attitude, or outlook. Addiction is usually accompanied by a compulsion to obtain the drug, a tendency to increase the dose, a psychological or physical dependence, and detrimental consequences for the individual and society. Common addictive drugs are barbiturates, ethanol, and morphine and other narcotics, especially heroin, which has slightly greater euphorigenic properties than other opium derivatives. See also **alcoholism, drug abuse.**

**Drug Enforcement Administration (DEA)** • An agency of the federal government, empowered to enforce regulations regarding the import or export of narcotic drugs and certain other substances or the traffic of these substances across state lines.

**DSN** • *abbr* Doctor of Science in Nursing.

**duty** • A legal obligation owed by one party to another. Duty may be established by statute or other legal process, as by contract or oath supported by statute, or it may be voluntarily undertaken. Every person has a duty of care to all other people to avoid causing harm or injury by negligence.

**EDNA** • *abbr* **Emergency Department Nurses' Association.**

**edrophonium chloride** • A cholinesterase (parasympathomimetic) agent.

**emancipated minor** • A minor who's legally considered an adult, free from parental care, and completely responsible for his own affairs.

**emergency department** • A section of a health-care facility that is staffed and equipped to provide rapid and varied emergency care, especially for those stricken with sudden and acute illness or those who are the victims of severe trauma.

**Emergency Department Nurses' Association (EDNA)** • A national professional organization of emergency department nurses that defines and promotes emergency nursing practice. The association, headquartered in Chicago, has written and implemented the *Standards of Emergency Nursing Practice.* The association offers a certification examination and awards the designation Certified Emergency Nurse (CEN) to nurses who successfully complete it. EDNA publishes the *Journal of Emergency Nursing (JEN)* and *Continuing Education Core Curriculum of Emergency Nursing Practice.*

**emergency doctrine** • A legal doctrine that assumes a person's consent to medical treatment when the person is in imminent danger and unable to give informed consent to treatment. Emergency doctrine assumes that the person would consent if able to do so.

**Emergency Medical Service (EMS)** • A network of services coordinated to provide aid and medical assistance from primary response to definitive care, involving personnel trained in the rescue, stabilization, transportation, and advanced treatment of trauma or medical emergency patients. Linked by a communications system that operates on both a local and regional level, EMS is usually initiated by a citizen calling to an emergency number. Stages include the first medical response; involvement of ambulance personnel, medium and heavy rescue equipment, and paramedic units, if necessary; and continued care in the hospital with emergency room nurses, emergency room doctors, specialists, and critical-care nurses and physicians. See also **Emergency Medical Technician.**

**Emergency Medical Technician (EMT)** • A person trained in and responsible for the administration of specialized emergency care and the transportation to a medical facility of victims of acute illness or injury. The EMT is trained in basic life support skills, extrication and disentanglement, operation of emergency vehicles, basic anatomy, basic assessment of injury or illness, triage, care for specific injuries and illnesses, environmental emergencies, childbirth, and transport of the patient. EMTs undergo ongoing training in new procedures and must qualify for recertification every 2 years. Kinds of EMTs are Emergency Medical Technician–Advanced Life Support, Emergency Medical Technician–Intravenous, Emergency Medical Technician–Paramedic. See also **Emergency Medical Service.**

**emergency medicine** • A branch of medicine concerned with the diagnosis and treatment of conditions resulting from trauma or sudden illness. The patient's condition is stabilized, and care of the patient is transferred to the primary physician or to a specialist. Emergency medicine requires a broad interdisciplinary training in the physiology and pathology of all the systems of the body.

**emergency nursing** • Nursing care provided to prevent imminent severe damage or death or to avert serious injury. Activities that exemplify emergency nursing care include basic life support, cardiopulmonary resuscitation, control of hemorrhage and burn care.

**emergency theory** • In physiology: a theory stating that when a person is faced with an emergency the adrenal medulla is stimulated by the sympathetic nervous system to release epinephrine, which increases heart rate, raises blood pressure, reduces blood flow to viscera, and mobilizes blood glucose, preparing the body for flight from danger or for the fight to survive.

**employer evaluation instrument** • A form used by an employer to evaluate a prospective employee during the interview and application process.

**employment agency** • An agency that, for a fee, helps place a person in an appropriate job.

**employment interview** • An exploratory meeting between a job applicant and a prospective employer.

**encoding** • Preparing a verbal message—identifying the content of the message, including emotional content, and planning how to articulate it—before transmitting that message to another person.

**euthanasia** • Deliberately bringing about the death of a person who's suffering from an incurable disease or condition, either actively—by administering a lethal drug—or passively—by withholding treatment.

**executing a will** • Carrying out a person's wishes as expressed in his will.

**exit interview** • A formal meeting between an employee and his immediate supervisor, his supervisor's supervisor, or a member of the personnel department, where the employee offers his perspective on the circumstances that prompted his resignation.

**expert witness** • A person who has special knowledge of a subject about which a court requests testimony. Special knowledge may be acquired by experience, education, observation, or study but is not possessed by the average person. An expert witness gives expert testimony or expert evidence. This evidence often serves to educate the court and the jury in the subject under consideration.

**express contract** • A verbal or written agreement between two or more people to do, or not do, something.

**extended-care facility** • An institution devoted to providing medical, nursing, or custodial care for an individual over a prolonged period of time, as during the course of a chronic disease or during the rehabilitation phase after an acute illness. Kinds of extended-care facilities are intermediate-care facility, skilled nursing facility. Also called **convalescent home, nursing home.**

**extended family** • A family group consisting of

the biologic parents, their children, and other family members.

**extraordinary life-support measures** • Resuscitative efforts and therapies done to replace a patient's natural vital functions.

# F

**FAAN** • *abbr* **Fellow of the American Academy of Nursing.**

**factor evaluation** • A way of classifying patients by calculating the amount and type of care each patient needs.

**faculty** • **1.** An ability to do something specific, as learn languages or remember names. **2.** Any mental ability or power, as memory. **3.** A department in an institution of learning or the people who teach in a department of such an institution.

**faculty practice plan** • A medical school system by which faculty members can increase income by practicing their specialty of medicine in a departmental practice in a school-controlled organization. Nursing school faculties are beginning to use this system for retrieval of incomes from service.

**false imprisonment** • The act of confining or restraining a person without his consent for no clinical or legal reason.

**family-centered nursing care** • Nursing care directed toward improving the potential health of a family or any of its members by assessing individual and family health needs and strengths, by identifying problems influencing the health care of the family as a whole as well as those influencing the individual members, by using family resources, by teaching and counseling, and by evaluating progress toward stated goals.

**family health** • An account of the health of the members of the immediate family. Hereditary and familial diseases are especially noted. The family health history is obtained from the patient or family in the initial interview and becomes a part of the permanent record.

**family medicine** • The branch of medicine that is concerned with the diagnosis and treatment of health problems in people of either sex and any age. Practitioners of family medicine are often called family practice physicians, family physicians, or, formerly, general practitioners.

**family nurse practitioner (FNP)** • A nurse practitioner possessing skills necessary for the detection and management of acute self-limiting conditions and management of chronic stable conditions. An FNP provides primary, ambulatory care for families, in collaboration with primary care physicians.

**family physician** • **1.** A medical practitioner of the specialty of family medicine. **2.** A general practitioner. **3.** A family practice physician. See also **family medicine.**

**family practice** • A type of general medical practice concerned with diagnosis and treatment of health problems in people of either sex, of any age.

**FDA** • *abbr* **Food and Drug Administration.**

**Federation Licensing Examination (FLEX)** • The standardized licensing examination for state licensure of physicians. Developed by the Federation of State Medical Boards of the United States, the examination is based on National Board of Medical Examiners test materials.

**fee-for-service** • **1.** A charge made for a professional activity, as for a physical examination. **2.** A system for the payment of professional services in which the practitioner is paid for the particular service rendered, rather than receiving a salary for providing professional services as needed during scheduled hours of work or time on call.

**fellowship** • A grant given to a person for study or training or to allow payment for work on a special project, but not for study toward a degree. It provides a salary and, in some cases, miscellaneous expenses.

**fiduciary relationship** • A legal relationship of confidentiality that exists whenever one person trusts or relies on another—such as a doctor-patient relationship.

**first aid** • The immediate care given to an injured or ill person. It includes self-help and home-care measures if medical assistance isn't readily available. Attention is directed first to the most critical problems: evaluation of the patency of the airway, the presence of bleeding, and the adequacy of cardiac function. The patient is kept warm and as comfortable as possible.

**five-step nursing process** • A nursing process comprising five broad categories of nursing behaviors: assessment, nursing diagnosis, planning, intervention, and evaluation. The nurse gathers information about the patient, formulates nursing diagnoses, develops a plan of care with the patient to meet these diagnoses, implements the plan of care, and evaluates the effects of the intervention. The nurse involves the patient and the patient's family to the greatest extent possible. Implicit in the nursing process is a therapeutic and personal relationship between the nurse, the patient, and the patient's family.

**flexible staffing patterns** • Work schedules that vary—for example, 10- and 12-hour shifts, shorter workweeks, and special weekend schedules.

**flextime, flexitime** • A system of staffing that allows flexible work schedules. A person working 7 hours daily might choose to work from 7 to 3, 10 to 5, or other hours. Use of the system tends to improve morale and decrease turnover.

**FNP** • *abbr* **family nurse practitioner.**

**Food and Drug Administration (FDA)** • A federal agency responsible for the enforcement of federal regulations regarding the manufacture and distribution of food, drugs, and cosmetics.

**forensic medicine** • A branch of medicine that deals with the legal aspects of health care.

**FTC** • *abbr* **Federal Trade Commission.**

**fundamentals of nursing** • The basic principles and practices of nursing as taught in educational programs for nurses, traditionally required in the first semester of the program. The emphasis of this phase of training is on the basic skills of nursing. Currently, nursing educators emphasize the importance of knowledge and understanding of the fundamental needs of man as well as competence in the basic skills as prerequisites to providing comprehensive nursing care.

# G

**Gay Nurses' Alliance (GNA)** • A national organization of homosexual nurses.

**general practitioner (GP)** • A family practice physician. See also **family medicine.**

**geriatrics** • The branch of medicine dealing with the physiology of aging and the diagnosis and treatment of diseases affecting the aged.

**gerontologic nursing** • A type of nursing care, in which a nurse may specialize, that provides specifically for the physical, intellectual, and emotional needs of the elderly.

**graduate medical education** • Formal medical education pursued after receipt of MD or other professional degree in the medical sciences. Graduate medical education is usually obtained as an intern, resident, or fellow, or in continuing medical education programs.

**Graduate Medical Education National Advisory Committee (GMENAC)** • A committee established by order of the Secretary of the Department of Health, Education and Welfare (now the Department of Health and Human Services) to study the manpower issues in health care. The Committee issued its final report in September 1980.

**Graduate Record Examination (GRE)** • An examination administered to graduates of institutions of higher learning. The scores are used as criteria for admission to masters and doctoral programs in many institutions and areas of specialization, including nursing. The examination tests verbal and mathematical aptitudes and abilities.

**grandfather clause** • A waiver that allows a person to continue to practice as a nurse after new qualifications are enacted into law. It further protects the property right of her license but does not confer the equivalent of a bachelor's degree.

**GRE** • *abbr* **Graduate Record Examination.**

**grievance** • A substantial complaint that involves working conditions or contract violations.

**grievance procedure** • Steps employees and employer agree to follow to settle disputes.

**gross negligence** • The flagrant and inexcusable failure to perform a legal duty in reckless disregard of the consequences.

**ground rules** • Rules governing a particular situation that describe legitimate behavior.

**guardian ad litem** • A person appointed by the court to look after a minor's legal interest during certain kinds of litigation.

# H

**"the handmaiden image"** • A term that reflects the outdated view of nurses as the doctors' servants.

**head nurse** • The clinical and administrative leader of the nurses working in a given geographical division of an institution, usually a floor, ward, or unit. The responsibilities of a head nurse may include directing nursing care activities, scheduling of staff, evaluation of nursing personnel, and hiring, firing, or promoting staff nurses. The head nurse may also be responsible for budget preparation and general clinical leadership.

**health assessment** • An evaluation of the health status of an individual by performing a physical examination after obtaining a health history. Various laboratory tests may also be ordered to confirm a clinical impression or to screen for dysfunction. A significant part of the health assessment is counseling and education that may explain aspects of anatomy, physiology, and pathophysiology and that introduces or affirms the general tenets of a healthful way of life. The techniques of the health assessment include: palpation, percussion, auscultation, and inspection, including sight, sound, and smell.

**health-care consumer** • Any actual or potential recipient of health care, as a patient in a hospital, a client in a community mental health center, or a member of a prepaid health maintenance organization.

**health-care industry** • The complex of preventive, remedial, and therapeutic services provided by hospitals and other institutions, nurses, doctors, dentists, government agencies, voluntary agencies, noninstitutional care facilities, pharmaceutical and medical equipment manufacturers, and health insurance companies.

**health certificate** • A statement signed by a health-care provider that attests to the state of a person's health.

**health education** • An educational program directed to the general public that attempts to improve, maintain, and safeguard the health of the community.

**health maintenance** • A program or procedure planned to prevent illness, to maintain maximal function, and to promote health. It is central to health care.

**Health Maintenance Organization (HMO)** • A type of group health-care practice that provides basic and supplemental health maintenance and treatment services to voluntary enrollees who prepay a fixed periodic fee that is set without regard to the amount or kind of services received.

**health professional** • Any person who has completed a course of study in a field of health, as a registered nurse. The person is usually licensed by a governmental agency or certified by a professional organization.

**health provider** • Any individual who provides health services to health-care consumers.

**health screening** • A program designed to evaluate the health status and potential of an individual person. In the process of evaluation, it may be found that a person has a particular disease or condition or is at greater than normal risk of developing a particular disease or condition.

**health supervision** • A visit made by a public health nurse to a patient in his home for the purpose of health teaching, counseling, or monitoring the status of the patient's health, rather than for physical care.

**health systems agency (HSA)** • An agency established under the terms of the National Health Planning and Resources Development Act of 1974. Health planning agencies are intended to provide networks of health planning and resource development services in each of several health service areas established by the Act. Health systems agencies are nonprofit and include private organizations, public regional planning bodies, or local governmental agencies and consumers.

**Hill-Burton Act** • A 1946 amendment to the U.S. Public Health Service Act authorizing grants to states for surveying their hospital and public health center needs and for the planning and construction of additional facilities. Subsequent amendments authorized federal funding for as much as two thirds of the cost of construction projects and broadened the scope of the legislation to include diagnostic and treatment centers, long-term treatment centers, and nursing homes and to aid in modernization of existing hospitals. Also called **Hospital Survey and Construction Act.**

**Hill-Burton programs** • A cluster of programs created by legislation included in the National Health Planning and Resources Development Act of 1974. The programs allow federal monetary assistance for modernization of health facilities, construction of outpatient health centers, construction of inpatient facilities in underserved areas, and the conversion of existing health care facilities for the provision of new health services.

**HMO** • See **Health Maintenance Organization.**

**holistic health care** • A system of comprehensive or total patient care that considers the physical, emotional, social, economic, and spiritual needs of the person; the response to the illness; and the impact of the illness on the person's ability to meet self-care needs. Also called comprehensive care.

**home care** • A health service provided in the client's place of residence for the purpose of promoting, maintaining, or restoring health or minimizing the effects of illness and disability. Service may include such elements as medical, dental, and nursing care, speech and physical therapy, the homemaking services of a home health aide, or the provision of transportation.

**home health agency** • An organization that provides health care in the home. Medicare certification for a home health agency is dependent on the providing of skilled nursing services and of at least one additional therapeutic service.

**hospice** • A system of family-centered care designed to assist the chronically ill person to be comfortable and to maintain a satisfactory lifestyle through the terminal phases of dying. Hospice care is multidisciplinary and includes home visits, professional medical help available on call, teaching and emotional support of the family, and physical care of the client. Some hospice programs provide care in a center as well as in the home.

**hospital information system (HIS)** • A computer-based information system with multi-access units to collect, organize, store, and make available data for problem-solving and decision-making.

**hospital quality assurance program** • A program developed by a hospital committee that monitors the quality of the hospital's diagnostic, therapeutic, prognostic, and other health-care activities.

**Hospital Survey and Construction Act** • See **Hill-Burton Act.**

**house physician** • A physician on call and immediately available in a hospital or other health-care facility.

**human investigations committee** • A committee established in a hospital, school, or university to review applications for research involving human subjects to protect the rights of the people to be studied. Also called **human subjects investigation committee.**

**human subjects investigation committee** • See **human investigations committee.**

# I

**ICCU** • *abbr* **intensive coronary-care unit.**

**-ician** • A combining form meaning a 'specialist in a field': *clinician, pediatrician.*

**ICN** • *abbr* **International Council of Nurses.**

**ICU** • *abbr* **intensive care unit.**

**"ideal nurse"** • A term describing a stereotyped view of nurses as cool, conciliatory, efficient, passive, and indirect in dealing with doctors.

**illegal (criminal) abortion** • Induced termination of a pregnancy under certain circumstances, or at a gestational time, prohibited by law. In Canada, an abortion not approved by a hospital therapeutic abortion committee. Many illegal abortions are performed under medically unsafe conditions.

**immunity from liability** • Exemption of a person or institution, by law, from a legally imposed penalty.

**immunity from suit** • Exemption of a person or institution, by law, from being sued.

**implementation** • **1.** A deliberate action performed to achieve a goal, as carrying out a plan in caring for a patient. **2.** In five-step nursing process: a category of nursing behavior in which the actions necessary for accomplishing the health-care plan are initiated and completed. Implementation includes the performance or assisting in the performance of the client's activities of daily living; counseling and teaching the client or the client's family; giving care to achieve therapeutic goals and to optimize the achievement of health goals by the client; and recording and exchanging information relevant to the client's continued health care. The client may require assistance in performing certain activities of daily living. The nurse helps the client to maintain optimal function, while instituting measures for the client's comfort as necessary. The nurse helps the client and the client's family recognize and manage the emotional and psychological stress of the client's condition. Correct principles, procedures, and techniques of health care are taught, and the client is informed about the current status of his or her health. If necessary, the client or the client's family is referred to a health or social resource in the community. Implementation follows planning and precedes evaluating in the five-step nursing process.

**implied contract** • A verbal or written agree-

ment—inferred rather than expressed—between two or more people to do, or not do, something.

**independent contractor** • A self-employed person who renders services to clients and independently determines how the work will be done.

**independent practice** • The practice of certain aspects of professional nursing that are encompassed by applicable licensure and law and require no supervision or direction from others. Nurses in independent practice may have an office in which they see patients and charge fees for service. In all nursing settings, state practice acts define aspects of nursing practice that are independent and may define those to be done only under supervision or direction of another individual, usually a doctor.

**Index Medicus** • An index published monthly by the National Library of Medicine, which lists articles from medical literature from throughout the world by subject and author. An annual edition, the *Cumulative Index Medicus,* contains all 12 issues of the *Index Medicus.*

**Industrial Medical Association (IMA)** • A professional organization whose members are concerned with the identification, prevention, diagnosis, and treatment of disorders associated with technology and industry.

**ineffective coping behaviors** • Types of behavior, such as denial, that block a person's ability to make competent decisions or to select alternatives for coping with problems.

**informed consent** • Permission obtained from a patient to perform a specific test or procedure, after the patient has been fully informed about the test or procedure.

**injunction** • A court order restraining a person from committing a specific act.

**in loco parentis** • Latin phrase meaning 'in the place of the parent.' The assumption by a person or institution of the parental obligations of caring for a child without adoption.

**inpatient** • **1.** A patient who has been admitted to a hospital or other health-care facility for at least an overnight stay. **2.** Pertaining to the treatment of such a patient or to a health-care facility to which a patient may be admitted for 24-hour care.

**in-service education** • A program of instruction or training that is provided by an agency or institution for its employees. The program is held in the institution or at the agency and is intended to increase the skills and competence of the employees in a specific area.

**institutional licensure** • A proposed procedure in which licensure for almost all health professions would be abandoned and the responsibility for assessing professional competence would fall to the health-care facility where the health professional is employed. Proponents maintain that health needs would be better and more flexibly served. Opponents maintain that knowledge, judgment, and competency are the products of a good basic education in the profession and that educators cannot teach the profession without a set of standardized expectations, as are now provided by government-controlled licensing procedures and certifying examinations.

**institutional review board (IRB)** • A federally approved committee that reviews all research proposals prior to submission of requests for funding to federal government granting agencies.

**integrated care** • Health care that coordinates all aspects of a patient's care as various specialists—such as dietitians, physical therapists, psychologists, doctors, and nurses—provide it.

**intensive care** • Constant, complex, detailed health care as provided in various acute, life-threatening conditions. Special training is necessary to provide intensive care. Also called critical care.

**intensive care unit (ICU)** • A hospital unit in which patients requiring close monitoring and intensive care are housed for as long as needed. An ICU contains highly technical and sophisticated monitoring devices and equipment, and the staff in the unit is educated to give critical care as needed by the patients.

**interdisciplinary (hospital) committee** • A committee of different hospital staff members—including doctors, nurses, and hospital administrators—who coordinate hospital activities to meet the needs of each discipline.

**intermediate care** • A level of medical care for certain chronically ill or disabled individuals in which room and board are provided but skilled nursing care is not.

**intern, interne** • **1.** A physician in the first postgraduate year, learning medical practice under supervision before beginning a residency program. **2.** Any immediate postgraduate trainee in a clinical program. **3.** To work as an intern.

**internal medicine** • The branch of medicine concerned with the study of the physiology and pathology of the internal organs and with the medical diagnosis and treatment of disorders of these organs.

**International Council of Nurses (ICN)** • The oldest international health organization. It is a federation of nurses' associations from 93 nations and was one of the first health organizations to develop strict policies of nondiscrimination based on nationality, race, creed, color, politics, sex, or social status. The objectives of the ICN include promotion of national associations of nurses; improvement of standards of nursing and competence of nurses; improvement of the status of nurses within their countries; and provision of an authoritative international voice for nurses. The

ICN is active in the World Health Organization (WHO), the United Nations Educational, Scientific, and Cultural Organization (UNESCO), and other international organizations.

**International Red Cross Society** • An international philanthropic organization, based in Geneva, concerned primarily with the humane treatment and welfare of the victims of war and calamity and with the neutrality of hospitals and medical personnel in times of war. See also **American Red Cross.**

**internist** • A physician specializing in internal medicine.

**interrogatories** • A series of written questions submitted to a witness or other person having information of interest to the court. The answers are transcribed and are sworn to under oath. Compare **discovery, deposition.**

**intervention** • **1.** Any act performed to prevent harm from occurring to a client or to improve the mental, emotional, or physical function of a client. A physiologic process may be monitored or enhanced, or a pathologic process may be arrested or controlled. **2.** The fourth step of the nursing process. This step includes nursing actions taken to meet patient needs as determined by nursing assessment and diagnosis.

**invalid contract** • Any contract concerning illegal or impossible actions; no legal obligation exists.

**JCAH** • *abbr* Joint Commission on Accreditation of Hospitals.

**job description** • A written statement describing responsibilities of a specific job and the qualifications an applicant for that job should have.

**job placement officer** • An employee of a job placement agency who works with a person seeking a new job.

**job satisfaction** • The gratification a person feels in connection with work-related circumstances and achievements.

**joint appointment** • **1.** A faculty appointment to two institutions within a university or system, as to the schools of nursing and medicine of the same university. **2.** In academic nursing: the appointment of a member of the faculty of a university to a clinical service of an associated service institution. A psychiatric nurse might hold appointment in a university as an assistant professor and might also be a clinical nurse-specialist in a service institution. The practice of joint appointments is said to have begun at Case Western Reserve University, University Hospital.

**Joint Commission on Accreditation of Hospitals (JCAH)** • A private, nongovernmental agency that establishes guidelines for the operation of hospitals and other health-care facilities, conducts accreditation programs and surveys, and encourages the attainment of high standards of institutional medical care. Members include representatives from the American Medical Association, American College of Physicians, and American College of Surgeons.

**joint practice** • **1.** The (usually private) practice of a doctor and a nurse practitioner who work as a team, sharing responsibility for a group of patients. **2.** In inpatient nursing, the practice of making joint decisions about patient care by committees of the doctors and nurses working on a division.

**juvenile delinquency** • Persistent antisocial, illegal, or criminal behavior by children or adolescents to the degree that it cannot be controlled or corrected by the parents, it endangers others in the community, and it becomes the concern of a law enforcement agency. Such behavioral patterns are characterized by aggressiveness, destructiveness, hostility, and cruelty, and occur more frequently in boys than in girls. Causative factors typically involve poor parent-child relationships, especially parental rejection, indifference, and apathy, and unstable family environments where disciplinary methods are lax, erratic, overly strict, or involve harsh physical punishment. Traditional punitive treatments, primarily correctional institutions and reform schools, usually aggravate rather than remedy the situation. More progressive approaches, such as foster-home placement, work and recreational programs, and various community and family counseling services, have been more successful. Behavior therapy and other forms of psychotherapy, often involving the parents as well as the child, are also used as modes of treatment and prevention.

# L

**law** • **1.** In a field of study: a rule, standard, or principle that states a fact or a relationship between factors, as Dalton's law regarding partial pressures of gas or Koch's law regarding the specificity of a pathogen. **2. a.** A rule, principle, or regulation established and promulgated by a government to protect or to restrict the people affected. **b.** The field of study concerned with such laws. **c.** The collected body of the laws of a people, derived from custom and from legislation.

**leadership styles** • Different ways a manager can guide staff members, ranging from a laissez-faire style—allowing staff members freedom to make decisions—to an authoritative style.

**learning** • **1.** The act or process of acquiring knowledge or some skill by means of study,

practice, or experience. **2.** Knowledge, wisdom, or a skill acquired through systematic study or instruction. **3.** In psychology: the modification of behavior through practice, experience, or training.

**legal abortion** • Induced termination of pregnancy by a doctor before the fetus has developed sufficiently to live outside the uterus. The procedure is performed under medically safe conditions prescribed by law.

**legal death** • See **death.**

**levels of care** • A classification of health-care service levels by the kind of care given, the number of people served, and the people providing the care. Kinds of health-care service levels are primary health care, secondary health care, tertiary health care.

**liability** • Legal responsibility for *failure to act,* and so causing harm to another person, or for *actions* that fail to meet standards of care, so causing another person harm.

**liaison** • A nurse who acts as an agent between a patient, the hospital, and the patient's family, and who speaks for the entire health-care team.

**licensed practical nurse (LPN)** • *U.S.* A person trained in basic nursing techniques and direct patient care who practices under the supervision of a registered nurse. The course of training usually lasts 1 year. In Canada an LPN is called a nursing assistant. Also called **licensed vocational nurse** *(U.S.).*

**licensed psychologist** • A person who has earned a Ph.D. in psychology from an accredited graduate school and has completed 2 to 3 years of postgraduate training with special emphasis on the diagnosis and treatment of psychological disorders. Also called clinical psychologist.

**licensed vocational nurse (LVN)** • See **licensed practical nurse.**

**licensure** • The granting of permission by a competent authority (usually a governmental agency) to an organization or individual to engage in a practice or activity that would otherwise be illegal. Kinds of licensure include the issuing of licenses for general hospitals or nursing homes; for health professionals, as physicians; and for the production or distribution of biological products. Licensure is usually granted on the basis of education and examination rather than performance. It is usually permanent, but a periodic fee, demonstration of competence, or continuing education may be required. Licensure may be revoked by the granting agency for incompetence, criminal acts, or other reasons stipulated in the rules governing the specific area of licensure.

**lie detector** • An electronic device or instrument used to detect lying or anxiety in regard to specific questions. A commonly used lie detector is the polygraph recorder, which senses and records pulse, respiratory rate, blood pressure, and perspiration. Some experts hold that certain patterns indicate the presence of anxiety, guilt, or fear, emotions that are likely to occur when the subject is lying.

**litigant** • A party to a lawsuit. See also **defendant, plaintiff.**

**litigate** • To carry on a suit or to contest.

**living will** • A witnessed document indicating a patient's desire to be allowed to die a natural death, rather than be kept alive by heroic, life-sustaining measures.

**locality rule** • Allowance made, when considering evidence in a trial, for the type of community, and its standards, in which the defendant practices his profession.

**long-term goal** • A broad or complex achievement to be accomplished over a relatively long period of time, such as 1 year or more.

**LPN** • *abbr* **licensed practical nurse.**

**LVN** • *abbr* **licensed vocational nurse.** See **licensed practical nurse.**

# M

**M.A.** • *abbr* **Master of Arts.**

**malfeasance** • Performance of an unlawful, wrongful act. Compare **misfeasance, nonfeasance.**

**malpractice** • A professional person's wrongful conduct, improper discharge of professional duties, or failure to meet standards of care—any such actions that result in harm to another person.

**mandatory bargaining issues** • Issues such as wages and working conditions that an employer must address during collective bargaining.

**master's degree program in nursing** • A postgraduate program in a school of nursing, based in a university setting, that grants the degree Master of Science in Nursing (MSN) to successful candidates. Nurses with this degree often work in leadership roles in clinical nursing, as consultants in various settings, and in faculty positions in schools of nursing. Some programs also prepare the nurse to function as a nurse-practitioner in a specific specialty.

**maternity nursing** • Nursing care of women and their families during pregnancy, parturition, and through the first days of the puerperium. Increasingly, postpartum maternity nursing includes the supervision of the mothers' care of their newborns in rooming-in units and may include care of normal newborns in the nursery when they are not with their mothers. Maternity nursing requires extensive instruction of the mothers in the usual behavior and needs of a newborn, expected patterns of growth and development of the infant during the first week, and in details of care needed by the mother during the first weeks after birth. Breast-feeding, bottle-feeding, baby baths, perineal care, nutrition, and danger signs of the puerperium are usually taught by the maternity nurse. Observation for abnormal conditions, as thrombophlebitis, mastitis and other infections, and pre-eclampsia are daily ongoing concerns of the maternity nurse on the postpartum unit. Intrapartum maternity nursing involves the care of mothers in labor and delivery, as well as high-risk technical nursing, emotional support in labor and delivery, and the customary ongoing observation for abnormal signs or symptoms. Often, pregnant women with medical problems associated with pregnancy are cared for on a special high-risk antepartum unit by specially trained maternity nurses.

**matrix structure** • A type of organization based on teams of people from different departments, each team having its own directors who work closely together. The directors have decision-making authority on administrative matters; the teams, on day-to-day working matters.

**MD** • *abbr* **Doctor of Medicine.** See **physician.**

**Medicaid** • A federally funded, state-operated program of medical assistance to people with low incomes; authorized by the Social Security Act.

**Medicaid mill** • *Informal.* A health program or facility that solely or primarily serves persons eligible for Medicaid. Such facilities are found mainly in economically depressed areas where there are few other health services.

**medical center** • **1.** A health-care facility. **2.** A hospital, especially one staffed and equipped to care for many patients and for a large number of kinds of diseases.

**medical model** • The traditional approach to the diagnosis and treatment of illness as practiced by doctors in the western world since the time of Koch and Pasteur. The doctor focuses on the defect, or dysfunction, within the person, using a problem-solving approach. The medical history and the physical examination and diagnostic tests provide the basis for the identification and treatment of a specific illness. The medical model is thus focused on the physical and biological aspects of specific diseases and conditions. Nursing differs from the medical model in that the patient is perceived primarily as a social person relating to the environment; nursing care is formulated on the basis of a nursing assessment that assumes multiple causes for the person's problems.

**medical record** • A written, legal record of every aspect of the patient's care.

**medical release form** • The form an institution

asks a patient to sign when he refuses a particular medical treatment. The form protects both the institution and the health-care professional from liability if the patient's condition worsens because of his refusal.

**medical staff** · All doctors, nurses, and health professionals responsible for providing health care in a hospital or other health-care facility. Medical staff personnel may be full-time or part-time, employed by the facility, or simply affiliated, that is, not employees.

**medical-surgical nursing** · The nursing care of people whose conditions or disorders are treated pharmacologically or surgically.

**Medical Women's International Association (MWIA)** · An international professional organization of women doctors.

**Medicare** · Federally funded national health insurance authorized by the Social Security Act for certain persons age 65 or older.

**medicolegal** · Of or pertaining to both medicine and law. Medicolegal considerations are a significant part of the process of making many patient-care decisions and in determining definitions and policies regarding the treatment of mentally incompetent people and minors, the performance of sterilization or therapeutic abortion, and the care of terminally ill patients. Medicolegal considerations, decisions, definitions, and policies provide the framework for informed consent, professional liability, and many other aspects of health-care practice.

**Mental Health Association (MHA)** · A voluntary, nonprofessional agency dedicated to the improvement of mental health facilities and services in community clinics and hospitals, the recruitment and training of volunteers, and the promotion of mental health legislation. Formerly called the National Association for Mental Health.

**mental health nursing** · See **psychiatric nursing.**

**mental health service** · Any one of a group of government, professional, or lay organizations operating at a community, state, national, or international level to aid in the prevention and treatment of mental disorders. See also **community mental health center.**

**mental status examination** · A diagnostic procedure for determining the mental status of a person. The trained interviewer poses certain questions in a carefully standardized manner and evaluates the verbal responses and behavioral reactions.

**midwife** · 1. In traditional use: a person who assists women in childbirth. 2. According to the International Confederation of Midwives, World Health Organization, and Federation of International Gynecologists and Obstetricians "a person who, having been regularly admitted to a midwifery educational program fully recognized in the country in which it is located, has suc-

cessfully completed the prescribed course of studies in midwifery and has acquired the requisite qualifications to be registered and/or legally licensed to practice midwifery." Among the responsibilities of the midwife are supervision of pregnancy, labor, delivery, and puerperium. The midwife conducts the delivery independently, cares for the newborn, procures medical assistance when necessary, executes emergency measures as required, and may practice in a hospital, clinic, maternity home, or in a woman's home. 3. A lay-midwife. 4. A nurse-midwife or Certified Nurse Midwife.

**minor** · A person not of legal age; beneath the age of majority. Minors usually cannot consent to their own medical treatment unless they are substantially independent from their parents, are married, support themselves, or satisfy other requirements as provided by statute.

**misdemeanor** · An offense that is considered less serious than a felony and carries with it a lesser penalty, usually a fine or imprisonment for less than 1 year.

**misfeasance** · An improper performance of a lawful act, especially in a way that might cause damage or injury. Compare **malfeasance.**

**morale** · The sense of workers' shared responsibility and job satisfaction that reflects the manager's motivating efforts.

**motivation** · The sense of purpose that leads a person to willingly perform a task.

**MS** · *abbr* 1. Master of Science. 2. Master of Surgery.

**MSN** · *abbr* **Master of Science in Nursing.** See **master's degree program in nursing.**

**MT** · *abbr* **Medical Technologist.**

**NAACOG** · *abbr* **Nurses Association of the American College of Obstetrics and Gynecology.**

**NAP-NAP** · *abbr* **National Association of Pediatric Nurse Associates/Practitioners.**

**NAPNES** · *abbr* **National Association for Practical Nurse Education and Services.**

**National Association for Practical Nurse Education and Services (NAPNES)** · A national professional organization concerned with the education of practical nurses and with the services provided by licensed practical nurses.

**National Association of Pediatric Nurse Associates/Practitioners (NAP-NAP)** · A national organization of nurses who are prepared by training or experience to give primary care to pediatric patients. NAP-NAP works in conjunction with the American Academy of Pediatrics.

**National Bureau of Standards (NBS)** · A federal agency in the Department of Commerce that sets accurate measurement standards for commerce, industry, and science in the United States. The NBS compares and coordinates its standards with those of other countries and provides research and technical service to improve computer science, materials technology, building construction, and consumer product safety.

**National Eye Institute (NEI)** • A division of the National Institutes of Health. NEI was established in 1968 to support research in the normal functioning of the human eye and visual system, the pathology of visual disorders, and the rehabilitation of the visually handicapped.

**National Health Service Corps (NHSC)** • A program of the United States Public Health Service (USPHS) in which health-care personnel are placed in areas that are underserved. Nurses, physicians, and dentists serve in rural and urban areas, usually as employees of local health-care agencies. The USPHS pays most of the salary of each corps member.

**National Institute of Child Health and Human Development (NICHHD)** • The Institute in the National Institutes of Health that is concerned with all aspects of the growth, development, and health of the children of the United States.

**National Institutes of Health (NIH)** • An agency within the United States Public Health Service made up of several institutions and constituent divisions, including the Bureau of Health Manpower Education, the National Library of Medicine, the National Cancer Institute, National Institute on Aging, and several research institutes and divisions.

**National League for Nursing (NLN)** • An organization concerned with the improvement of nursing education, nursing service, and the delivery of health care in the United States. Among its many activities are accreditation of nursing programs at all levels, preadmission and achievement tests for nursing students, and compilation of statistical data on nursing manpower and on trends in health-care delivery. It acts as the testing service for the State Board Test Pool Examinations for registered and practical nurse licensure.

**National Male Nurses' Association (NMNA)** • A national organization that promotes the interests and practice of male nurses.

**National Student Nurses' Association (NSNA)** • A national organization of students in the field of nursing. Among its purposes are the improvement of nursing education to improve health care, to aid in the development of the student nurse, and to encourage optimal achievement in the professional role of the nurse and the health care of people.

**NBS** • *abbr* **National Bureau of Standards.**

**N-CAP** • *abbr* **Nurses Coalition for Action in Politics.**

**NCH** • *abbr* **nursing care home.**

**negligent nondisclosure** • The failure to completely inform a patient about his treatment.

**negotiation** • A meeting where an employer and employees confer, discuss, and bargain to reach an agreement.

**NLN** • *abbr* **National League for Nursing.**

**NMNA** • *abbr* **National Male Nurses' Association.**

**no-code order** • A note, written in the patient record and signed by a doctor, instructing staff not to attempt to resuscitate a terminally ill patient if he suffers cardiac or respiratory failure.

**nonfeasance** • A failure to perform a task, duty, or undertaking that one has agreed to perform or that one had a legal duty to perform. Compare **malfeasance, misfeasance.**

**nonverbal cues** • The transmission of information by means other than language, such as behavior, facial expression, and body carriage or position. The message conveyed may conflict with simultaneous verbal information.

**nuclear family** • A family unit consisting of the biologic parents and their children.

**nurse** • **1.** A person educated and licensed in the practice of nursing. The practice of the nurse includes data collection, diagnosis, planning, treatment, and evaluation within the framework of the nurse's singular concern with the person's response to the problem, rather than to the problem itself. The nurse acts to promote, maintain, or restore the health of the person; wellness is the goal. The nurse may be a generalist or a specialist and, as a professional, is ethically and legally accountable for the nursing activites performed and for the actions of others to whom the nurse has delegated responsibility. **2.** To provide nursing care. See also **five-step nursing process, nursing, registered nurse. 3.** To breast-feed an infant.

**nurse anesthetist** • A registered nurse qualified by advanced training in an accredited program in the speciality of nurse anesthetist to manage the anesthetic care of the patient in certain surgical situations.

**nurse clinician** • A nurse who is prepared to identify and diagnose problems of clients by using the expanded knowledge and skills gained by advanced study in a specific area of nursing practice. The specialist may function independently within standing orders or protocols and collaborates with associates to implement a plan of care that is focused on the client.

**Nurse Corps** • The branch within each of the armed services comprised of the nurses within that service, as the Army Nurse Corps. In each of the armed services, the members of the Nurse Corps have the rank, title, responsibilities, and status of officers.

**nurse educator** • A registered nurse whose primary area of interest, competence, and professional practice is the education of nurses.

**nurse practice act** • A law enacted by a state's legislature outlining the legal scope of nursing practice within that state.

**nurse practitioner** • A nurse who, by advanced training and clinical experience in a branch of nursing, as in a master's degree program in nursing, has acquired expert knowledge in a specialized branch of practice.

**nurse's aide** • A person who is employed to carry out basic nonspecialized tasks in the care of a patient, as bathing and feeding, making beds, and transporting patients.

**Nurses' Association of the American College of Obstetrics and Gynecology (NAACOG)** • A national organization of nurses who work in obstetrics and gynecology.

**Nurses' Coalition for Action in Politics (N-CAP)** • An organization that works in association with the American Nurses' Association. It raises funds for political contributions to candidates for public office at the state and national levels.

**nurses' notes** • A means of documenting the nursing care you provide and the patient's response to that care.

**nurse's registry** • An employment agency or listing service for nurses who wish to work in a specific area of nursing, usually for a short period of time or on a per diem basis.

**nurses' station** • An area in a clinic, unit, or ward in a health-care facility that serves as the administrative center for nursing care for a particular group of patients. It is usually centrally located and may be staffed by a ward secretary or clerk who assists with paperwork and the telephone and other communication. Before going on duty, nurses usually meet there to receive daily assignments, to review the patients' charts, and to update the cardex. The nurses' station is equipped appropriately for the care of patients in that area or unit.

**nurse-therapist model** • In psychiatric nursing research: a theoretical framework to clarify the role of the mental-health nurse. Techniques from traditional and contemporary modes of treatment, including transactional analysis and crisis intervention, may be used singly or in various combinations. The nurse therapist chooses the technique or techniques after using the model to examine the nurse-client interaction, the feedback, and the goal of the interaction.

**nursing** • **1.** The professional practice of a nurse. **2.** The process of acting as a nurse, of providing care that encourages and promotes the health of the person being served. **3.** Breast-feeding an infant. See also **nurse.**

**nursing administrator** • A nurse who's responsible for overseeing the efficient management of nursing services.

**nursing assessment** • An identification by a nurse of the needs, preferences, and abilities of a patient. Assessment follows an interview with and observation of a patient by the nurse and considers the symptoms and signs of the condition, the patient's verbal and nonverbal communication, medical and social history, and any other information available. Among the physical aspects assessed are vital signs, skin color and condition, motor and sensory nerve function, nutrition, rest, sleep, activity, elimination, and consciousness. Among the social and emotional factors assessed are religion, occupation, attitude toward hospital and health care, mood, emotional tone, and family ties and responsibilities.

**nursing assistant** • *Canada.* A person trained in basic nursing techniques and direct patient care who practices under the supervision of a registered nurse.

**nursing audit** • A thorough investigation designed to identify, examine, or verify the performance of certain specified aspects of nursing care using established criteria. A concurrent nursing audit is performed during ongoing nursing care. A retrospective nursing audit is performed after discharge from the care facility, using the patient's record. Often, a nursing audit and a medical audit are performed collaboratively, resulting in a joint audit.

**nursing burnout** • The condition of no longer caring about practicing nursing, resulting from chronic, unrelieved, job-related stress. Characterized by physical and emotional exhaustion, sometimes by illness and/or abandonment of a nursing career.

**nursing-care plan** • A plan that is based on a nursing assessment and a nursing diagnosis, devised by a nurse. It has four essential components: the identification of the nursing care problems and a statement of the nursing approach to solve those problems; the statement of the expected benefit to the patient; the statement of the specific actions taken by the nurse that reflect the nursing approach and the achievement of the goals specified; and the evaluation of the patient's response to nursing care and the readjustment of that care as required. The nursing-care plan is begun when the patient is admitted to the health service, and, following the initial nursing assessment, a diagnosis is formulated, and nursing orders are developed. The goal of the process is to ensure that nursing care is consistent with the patient's needs and progress toward self-care. A written nursing-care plan should be a part of every patient's chart; an abbreviated form should be available for quick reference, as in a Rand or cardex file. See also **nursing assessment.**

**nursing diagnosis** • Descriptive interpretations—accepted by the National Group on the Classification of Nursing Diagnosis—of collected and categorized information indicating the problems or needs of a patient that nursing care can affect.

**nursing home** • See **extended-care facility.**

**nursing process** • An organizational framework for nursing practice, encompassing all the major steps a nurse takes when caring for a patient.

**nursing skills** • The cognitive, affective, and psychomotor abilities a nurse uses in delivering nursing care.

**nursing specialty** • A nurse's particular professional field of practice, as surgical, pediatric, obstetric, or psychiatric nursing. Compare **subspecialty.**

**nursing supervisor** • A nurse whose function is the administrative and clinical leadership of the nursing service of a division of a health-care facility, as a nursing supervisor of maternal and infant-care nurses.

**nursing theory** • The set of accepted principles that help a nurse analyze nursing practice.

# O

**occupational therapist** • A person who practices occupational therapy and who may be licensed, registered, certified, or otherwise regulated by law.

**occupational therapy** • A subdivision of physical medicine in which handicapped or convalescing patients are trained in vocational skills and activities of daily life through a program designed to satisfy the specific needs of the patient while providing diversion and exercise.

**Old Age, Survivors, Disability and Health Insurance (OASDHI) program** • A benefit program, administered by the Social Security Administration, that provides cash benefits to workers who are retired or disabled, their dependents, and survivors. This part of the program is commonly referred to as Social Security. The program also provides health insurance benefits for people over 65 and for disabled people under 65. This part of the program is commonly referred to as Medicare. See also **Medicare.**

**ombudsman** • A person who investigates complaints, reports findings, and helps to achieve equitable settlements.

**Oncology Nursing Society (ONS)** • An organization of nurses interested or specialized in nursing of the patient with cancer. The national publication of the ONS is *Oncology Nursing Forum.*

**open shop** • A place of employment where employees may choose whether or not to join a union.

**ordinary negligence** • The inadvertent omission of that care which a reasonably prudent nurse would ordinarily provide under similar circumstances.

**orthopedic nurse** • A nurse whose primary area of interest, competence, and professional practice is in orthopedic nursing.

# P

**patient** • 1. A health-care recipient who is ill or hospitalized. 2. A client in a health-care service.

**patient classification systems** • Ways of grouping patients so that the size of the staff needed to care for them can be estimated accurately.

**patient day (PD)** • A unit in a system of accounting used by health-care facilities and health-care planners. Each day represents a unit of time during which the services of the institution or facility were used by a patient; thus 50 patients in a hospital for 1 day would represent 50 patient days.

**patient overload/staffing shortage** • The situation that occurs when the number of patients exceeds an institution's medical, nursing, and support-staff resources to care for them properly.

**patient record** • A collection of documents that provides a record of each time a person visited or sought treatment and received care or a referral for care from a health-care facility. This confidential record is usually held by the facility, and the information in it is released only to the person, or with the person's written permission. It contains the initial assessment, health history, laboratory reports, and notes by nurses, physicians, and consultants, as well as order sheets, medication sheets, admission records, discharge summaries, and other pertinent data. A problem-oriented medical record also contains a master problem list. The patient record is often a collection of papers held in a folder, but, increasingly, hospitals are computerizing the records after every discharge, making the past record available on visual display terminals. Also called chart *(informal).*

**patient's bill of rights** • A list of patients' rights. The American Hospital Association; health-care institutions; and various medical, nursing, and consumer organizations have prepared such lists, which, in some states, have become law.

**pediatric nurse practitioner (PNP)** • A nurse practitioner who, by advanced study and clinical practice, has gained expert knowledge in the nursing care of infants and children. See also **pediatric nursing.**

**pediatric nursing** • The branch of nursing concerned with the care of infants and children. Pediatric nursing requires knowledge of normal psychomotor, psychosocial, and cognitive growth and development as well as of the health problems and needs of people in this age group. Preventive care and anticipatory guidance are integral to the practice of pediatric nursing. See also **pediatric nurse practitioner.**

**personnel file** • The compilation of an employee's records, including his job application, résumé, continuing-education records, and employment record with that company.

**PharmD** • *abbr* **Doctor of Pharmacy.** One trained to practice in a clinical setting, rather than dispensing medication.

**physical therapist** • A person who is licensed to assist in the examination, testing, and treatment of physically disabled or handicapped people through the use of special exercise, application of heat or cold, use of sonar waves, and other techniques.

**physical therapy** • The treatment of disorders with physical agents and methods, as massage, manipulation, therapeutic exercises, cold, heat (including shortwave, microwave, and ultrasonic diathermy), hydrotherapy, electrical stimulation, and light, to assist in rehabilitating patients and in restoring normal function following an illness or injury. Also called physiotherapy.

**physician** • **1.** A health professional who has earned a degree of Doctor of Medicine (MD) after completion of an approved course of study at an approved medical school and satisfactory completion of National Board Examinations. **2.** A health professional who has earned a degree of Doctor of Osteopathy (DO) by satisfactorily completing a course of education in an approved college of osteopathy.

**physician's assistant (PA)** • A person trained in certain aspects of the practice of medicine to provide assistance to a physician. A physician's assistant is trained by physicians and practices under the direction and supervision and within the legal license of a physician. Training programs vary in length from a few months to 2 years. Health-care experience or academic preparation may be a prerequisite to admission to some programs. Most physician's assistants are prepared for the practice of primary care, but some practice subspecialities, including surgical assisting, dialysis, or radiology. National certification is available to qualified graduates of approved training programs. The national organization is the American Association of Physician's Assistants (AAPA). Also called **physician's associate.**

**physician's associate** • See **physician's assistant.**

**placement service** • An agency that, for a fee, helps place a person in an appropriate job.

**plaintiff** • A person who files a civil lawsuit initiating a legal action. In criminal actions, the prosecution is the plaintiff, acting in behalf of the people of the jurisdiction.

**PNP** • *abbr* **pediatric nurse practitioner.**

**poison control center** • One of a nearly worldwide network of facilities that provide information regarding all aspects of poisoning or intoxication, maintain records of their occurrence, and refer patients to treatment centers.

**policy defense** • Reasons your professional liability insurance company may give—concerning how well you've maintained the policy—for not covering you when you make a claim.

**practicing medicine without a license** • Practicing activities defined under state law in the medical practice act without physician supervision, direction, or control.

**practitioner** • A person qualified to practice in a special professional field, as a nurse practitioner.

**preceptor** • An experienced nurse who assumes responsibility for orienting and training a nurse intern, through actual on-the-job experience.

**preventive discipline** • Discipline that involves three techniques—performance appraisals, coaching, and counseling—to give subordinates a clear understanding of a supervisor's expectations.

**primary-care nursing** • Where each nurse works with a group of assigned patients and assumes full 24-hour responsibility for all aspects of their care.

**primary health care** • A basic level of health care that includes programs directed at the promotion of health, early diagnosis of disease or disability, and prevention of disease. Primary health care is provided in an ambulatory facility to limited numbers of people, often those living in a particular geographic area. In any episode of illness, it is the first patient contact with the health-care system.

**primary nurse** • A nurse who is responsible for the planning, implementation, and evaluation of the nursing care of one or more clients 24 hours a day for the duration of the hospital stay. In primary nursing, nursing care usually includes the development and implementation of a care plan; participation in conferences on the care of a client; collaboration with the client, the health-care team members, and the client's family; referral to community resources; and evaluation of care.

**primary organizer** • The part of the dorsal lip of the blastopore that is self-differentiating and induces the formation of the neural plate that gives rise to the main axis of the embryo.

**primary physician** • **1.** The physician who usually takes care of a person; the physician who first sees a patient for the care of a given health problem. **2.** A family practice physician or general practitioner. See also **family medicine.**

**privileged communication** • A conversation in which the speaker intends the information he's giving to remain private between himself and the listener.

**privilege doctrine** • A doctrine that protects the privacy of persons within a fiduciary relationship, such as a husband and wife, a doctor and patient, or a nurse and patient. During legal proceedings, a court can't force either party to reveal communication that occurred between them unless the party who'd benefit from the protection agrees to it.

**problem-oriented medical record** • A record-keeping system in which you provide information about the patient from the standpoint of what's bothering him.

**problem patient** • A label sometimes applied to a patient on the basis of his inadequate coping capabilities, which lead to inappropriate behaviors that his nurses find irritating and frustrating.

**pro-choice** • The philosophy that a woman has the right to choose either to continue or to terminate her pregnancy.

**professional corporation (PC)** • A corporation formed according to the law of a particular state for the purpose of delivering a professional service.

**professional liability** • A legal concept describing the obligation of a professional person to pay a patient or client for damages caused by the professional's act of omission, commission, or negligence. Professional liability better describes the responsibility of all professionals to their clients than does the concept of malpractice, but the idea of professional liability is central to malpractice.

**professional liability insurance** • A type of liability insurance that protects professional persons against malpractice claims made against them.

**professional network** • In psychiatric nursing: the network of professional resources available to support the psychiatric outpatient in the community. The network may include a therapist, a hospital day-treatment program, social work agency, and other agencies.

**professional nursing** • That level of nursing practice which, according to the American Nurses' Association's entry-level requirement proposal, would require a bachelor's degree.

**professional organization** • An organization created to deal with issues of concern to its members, who share a professional status.

**Professional Standards Review Organization (PSRO)** • An organization formed under Social Security Act Amendments of 1972 to review the services provided under Medicare, Medicaid, and Maternal Child Health programs.

**pro-life** • The philosophy that the unborn fetus has the right to develop to term and to be born.

**proprietary hospital** • A hospital operated as a profit-making organization. Many are owned and operated by physicians primarily for their own patients, but they also accept patients from other physicians. Others are owned by investor groups or large corporations.

**prototype evaluation** • A way of classifying patients by using a form that describes typical characteristics of several groups of patients.

**Provincial Territorial Nurses' Association (PTNA)** • An association of nurses organized at the provincial or territorial level. The Canadian Nurses' Association is a federation of the 11 PTNAs.

**proximate cause** • A legal concept of cause and effect, which says a sequence of natural and continuous events produces an injury that wouldn't have otherwise occurred.

**PSRO** • *abbr* **Professional Standards Review Organization.**

**psychiatric nurse practitioner** • A nurse practitioner who, by advanced study and clinical practice, has gained expert knowledge in the care and prevention of mental disorders. See also **psychiatric nursing.**

**psychiatric nursing** • The branch of nursing concerned with the prevention and cure of mental disorders and their sequelae. It employs theories of human behavior as its scientific framework and requires the use of the self as its art or expression in nursing practice. Some of the activities of the psychiatric nurse include the provision of a safe therapeutic milieu; working with patients, or clients, concerning the real day-to-day problems that they face; identifying and caring for the physical aspects of the patient's problems, including drug reactions; assuming the role of social agent or parent for the patient in various recreational, occupational, and social situations; conducting psychotherapy; and providing leadership and clinical assistance for other nurses and health-care workers. Psychiatric nurses work in many settings; their responsibilities vary with the setting and with the level of expertise, experience, and training of the individual nurse. Also called **mental health nursing.**

**qualified privilege** • A conditional right or immunity granted to the defendant because of the circumstances of a legal case.

**quality of life** • A legal and ethical standard that's determined by relative suffering or pain, not by the degree of disability.

# R

**RCPSC** • *abbr* **Royal College of Physicians and Surgeons of Canada.**

**reality orientation techniques** • Nursing techniques for keeping patients oriented to time, place, and person.

**reality shock** • The transitional jolt many nurses experience when they leave the academic setting and enter actual nursing practice.

**reasonably prudent nurse** • The standard a court uses to judge whether another nurse would have acted similarly to the defendant under similar circumstances.

**Red Cross** • **1.** See **International Red Cross Society. 2.** See **American Red Cross.**

**registered nurse (RN)** • **1.** *United States* A professional nurse who has completed a course of study at a school of nursing accredited by the National League for Nursing and who has taken and passed the State Board Test Pool Examination. A registered nurse may use the initials RN following the signature. RNs are licensed to practice by individual states. **2.** *Canada* A professional nurse who has completed a course of study at an approved school of nursing and who has taken and passed an examination administered by the Canadian Nurses' Association Testing Service. See also **nurse, nursing.**

**Registered Therapist (RT)** • A title awarded by the American Registry of Radiologic Technicians as certification of qualification to act as an X-ray technician.

**registrar** • An administrative officer whose responsibility is to maintain the records of an institution.

**registry** • **1.** An office or agency in which lists of nurses and records pertaining to nurses seeking employment are maintained. **2.** In epidemiology: a listing service for incidence data pertaining to the occurrence of specific diseases or disorders, as a tumor registry.

**rehabilitation center** • A facility providing therapy and training for rehabilitation. The center may offer occupational therapy, physical therapy, vocational training, and such special training as speech therapy.

**resignation** • The formal notification a person gives to terminate his employment.

**res ipsa loquitur** • "The thing speaks for itself." A legal doctrine that applies when the defendant was solely and exclusively in control at the time the plaintiff's injury occurred, so that the injury would *not* have occurred if the defendant had exercised due care. When a court applies this doctrine to a case, the defendant bears the burden of proving that he wasn't negligent.

**respondeat superior** • "Let the master answer." A legal doctrine that makes an employer liable for the consequences of his employee's wrongful conduct while the employee is acting within the scope of his employment.

**résumé** • A written summary of a person's work qualifications and experience, used in applying for jobs.

**resuscitative life-support measures** • Actions taken to reverse an immediate, life-threatening situation; for example, cardiopulmonary resuscitation.

**review committee** • A group of individuals delegated to inspect and report on the quality of health care in a given institution.

**right-of-conscience laws** • A legal equivalent to freedom of thought or of religion.

**right-to-access laws** • Laws that grant a patient the right to see his medical records.

**right-to-die law** • A law that upholds a patient's right to choose death by refusing extraordinary treatment when the patient has no hope of recovery. Also referred to as a *natural death law* or *living-will law.*

**RN** • *abbr* **registered nurse.**

**Royal College of Physicians and Surgeons of Canada (RCPSC)** • A national Canadian organization that recognizes and confers membership on certain qualified physicians and surgeons.

**Rural Clinics Assistance Act** • An act of Congress that permitted the establishment of clinics in certain areas designated rural and underserved, and in some inner cities. The clinics are designed to provide primary care through teams of physicians and nurse practitioners. The act is significant to nursing by being the first federal legislation which allows third-party reimbursement directly to nurses practicing in expanded roles.

# S

**School Nurse Practitioner (SNP)** • A registered nurse qualified by postgraduate study to act as a nurse practitioner in a school.

**scope of practice** • In nursing, the professional nursing activities defined under state or provincial law in each state's (or Canadian province's) nurse practice act.

**secondary health care** • An intermediate level of health care that includes diagnosis and treatment, performed in a hospital having specialized equipment and laboratory facilities.

**service of process** • The delivery of a writ, summons, or complaint to a defendant. The original of the document is shown; a copy is served. Service of process gives reasonable notice to allow the person to appear, testify, and be heard in court.

**settlement** • An agreement made between parties to a suit before a judgment is rendered by a court.

**sexual harassment** • An aggressive, sexually motivated act of physical or verbal violation of a person over whom the aggressor has power. Sexual harassment in the workplace is against the law, since it abridges the victim's right to equal opportunity, privacy, and freedom from assault.

**shift differentials** • Different salary rates paid because of different working conditions or different working hours.

**short-term goal** • A simple achievement to be accomplished in a short period of time, such as less than a year; may be one step in achieving a long-term goal.

**signature code** • A code of letters and/or numbers that you enter into the computer to identify yourself.

**skilled nursing facility (SNF)** • An institution or part of an institution that meets criteria for accreditation established by the sections of the Social Security Act that determine the basis for Medicaid and Medicare reimbursement for skilled nursing care, including rehabilitation and various medical and nursing procedures.

**slow-code order** • A verbal or implicit order from a doctor instructing staff to refrain from resuscitating a terminally ill patient after apparent death, until a point is reached when CPR is unlikely to be successful. *An illegal order.*

**SNA** • *abbr* **1.** State Nurses' Association. **2.** Student Nurses' Association.

**SNF** • *abbr* **skilled nursing facility.**

**SOAP** • An acronym for the format used in problem-oriented record keeping; it represents: *S*ubjective data, *O*bjective data, *A*ssessment data, and *P*lans.

**socialized medicine** • A system for the delivery of health care in which the expense of care is borne by the government.

**Social Security Act** • A federal statute that provides for a national system of old-age assistance, survivors' and old-age insurance benefits, unemployment insurance and compensation, and other public welfare programs, including Medicare and Medicaid.

**Society for Advancement in Nursing (SAIN)** • A group established to advance the nursing profession through higher education.

**source-oriented records** • A record-keeping system in which each professional group within the health-care team keeps separate information on the patient.

**specialization** • Concentration in a specific branch of nursing, or in a particular clinical area, through focused work experience or formal education, or both.

**staff** • **1.** The people who work toward a common goal and are employed or supervised by someone of higher rank, as the nurses in a hospital. **2.** A designation by which a staff nurse is distinguished from a head nurse or other nurse.

**staff development** • In nursing: a process that assists individual nurses in attaining new skills and knowledge, gaining increasing levels of competence, and growing professionally. Various resources outside the agency employing the nurse may be used. The process may include such programs as orientation, in-service education, and continuing education.

**staffing pattern** • In hospital or nursing administration: the number and kinds of staff assigned to the particular units and departments of a hospital. Staffing patterns vary with the unit, department, and shift.

**staff position** • In management theory: a position outside an institution's hierarchy of authority, such as clinical specialist or consultant, counselor, or in-service training or patient education director, as opposed to a line position. A staff person provides a specific service or product and usually reports directly to the administrator or a line supervisor.

**stages of grief** • Five emotional and behavioral stages that a person may experience while in a period of grieving: denial or avoidance, anger, depression, rationalization, and acceptance.

**standard** • **1.** An evaluation that serves as a basis for comparison for evaluating similar phenomena or substances, as a standard for the practice of a profession. **2.** A pharmaceutical preparation or a chemical substance of known quantity, ingredients, and strength that is used to determine the constituents or the strength of another preparation. **3.** Of known value, strength, quality, or ingredients.

**standard death certificate** • A form for a death certificate commonly used throughout the United States. It is the preferred form of the United States Census Bureau.

**standards of care** • In a malpractice lawsuit, those acts performed or omitted that an ordinary, prudent person, in the defendant's position, would have done or not done; a measure by which the defendant's alleged wrongful conduct is compared.

**standing orders** • A written document containing rules, policies, procedures, regulations, and orders for the conduct of patient care in various stipulated clinical situations. The standing orders are usually formulated collectively by the professional members of a department in a hospital or other health-care facility.

**State Board Test Pool Examination** • An examination prepared by the National Council of State Boards of Nursing for testing the competency of a person to perform as a newly licensed registered nurse. Each jurisdiction within the United States and its territories regulates entry into the nursing practice; each requires the candidate to pass the examination. The content is planned to test the candidate's knowledge of the nursing process as applied to the broad areas of nursing practice, including maternal and child health, medical and surgical nursing, and psychiatric nursing. The process includes five steps: assessing, analyzing, planning, implementing, and evaluating. Knowledge, comprehension, application, and analysis of the nursing process are tested as they apply to decision-making situations.

**state medicine** • *Informal.* See **socialized medicine.**

**State Nurses' Association (SNA)** • An association of nurses at the state level. The various State Nurses' Associations are constituent units of the American Nurses' Association.

**state of emergency** • A widespread need for immediate action to counter a threat to the community.

**Statewide Health Coordinating Committee (SHCC)** • A component of the national network of Health Systems Agencies.

**statutes of limitations** • Laws that specify the length of time within which a person may file specific types of lawsuits. The statute of limitations for a medical malpractice case is usually 2 or 3 years.

**statutory law** • A law passed by a federal or state legislature.

**statutory rape** • Sexual intercourse with a female below the age of consent, which varies from state to state.

**stereotyping** • Using subjective judgment to view people with certain characteristics in common as a group, conforming to a standardized mental image.

**steward** • A union representative.

**stress** • Any emotional, physical, social, economic, or other change that produces physical or mental tension and may contribute to the onset of illness; also, the tension itself.

**subspecialty** • A professional and highly specialized field of practice, as nursing in dialysis, or neurology. Compare **specialty.**

**substantive laws** • Laws that define and regulate a person's rights.

**substitutive consent** • Permission obtained from a parent or guardian of a patient who's a minor.

**substitutive judgment** • A legal term indicating the court's substitution of its own judgment for that of a person the court considers unable to make an informed decision, such as an incompetent adult.

**summary judgment** • A judgment requested by any party to a civil action to end the action when it is believed that there is no genuine issue or material fact in dispute.

**summons** • A document issued by a clerk of the court upon the filing of a complaint. A sheriff, marshal, or other appointed person serves the summons, notifying a person that an action has been begun against him. See also **service of process.**

**supervision** • Overseeing and directing the work of another person.

**support group** • People whom a person confides in and draws on for support, either as individuals or in a group setting.

# T

**task-oriented nursing** • Where a supervisor assigns each nurse a specific duty to perform for assigned patients.

**teaching rounds** • The somewhat informal conferences held regularly, often at the beginning of the day. Various members of the department and staff may attend, including nurses, residents, interns, students, attending physicians, and faculty. Specific problems in the care of current patients are discussed.

**team nursing** • Where a team leader distributes the care of each patient among members of a nursing team.

**technical nursing** • That level of nursing practice which, according to the American Nurses' Association's entry-level requirement proposal, would require an associate degree or graduation from a diploma program.

**terminate** • To fulfill all contractual obligations or absolve yourself of the obligation to fulfill them.

**termination process** • The procedure an employer follows to fire an employee.

**territory** • Physical space, aspects of authority, or responsibilities that a person feels belong to him and that he protects.

**testamentary** • Any document, such as a will, which doesn't take effect until after the death of the person who wrote it.

**therapeutic abortion** • Induced termination of pregnancy to preserve the health, safety, or life of the woman.

**therapeutic privilege** • A legal doctrine that permits a doctor, in an emergency situation, to withhold information from the patient if he can prove that disclosing it would adversely affect the patient's health.

**third-party reimbursement** • Reimbursement for services rendered to a person in which an entity other than the giver or receiver of the service is responsible for the payment. Third-party reimbursement for the cost of a subscriber's health care is commonly paid by insurance plans.

**time charting** • A method of charting in which you detail at regular time intervals—for example, every ½ hour—the procedures you carried out at that particular time.

**title** • A section of the Social Security Act that provides for the establishment, funding, and regulation of a service to a specific segment of the population, as Title XIX, which includes medical coverage under Medicaid.

**tort** • A private or civil wrong outside of a contractual relationship.

**traditional staffing patterns** • Work schedules that follow 8-hour shifts, 7 days a week, including evening and night shifts.

**transmission** • Verbal or nonverbal communication with another person.

**turnover rate** • The rate at which a company or institution must replace employees due to resignations and terminations.

# U

**unfair labor practices** • Tactics used by the employer or union that are prohibited by state and federal labor laws.

**Uniform Anatomical Gift Act** • A law, in all 50 states, that allows anyone over age 18 to sign a donor card, willing some or all of his organs after death.

**union shop** • A place of employment where employees must join a union.

**United States Public Health Service (USPHS)** • An agency of the federal government responsible for the control of the arrival from abroad of any people, goods, or substances that may affect the health of U.S. citizens. The agency sets standards for the domestic handling and processing of food and the manufacture of serums, vaccines, cosmetics, and drugs. It supports and performs research, aids localities in times of disaster and epidemics, and provides medical care for certain groups of Americans.

# V

**verbal order** • An order given directly and in person by a doctor to a nurse.

**voluntary bargaining issues** • Issues such as noneconomic fringe benefits that an employer or union may or may not address during collective bargaining.

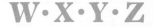

**walking rounds** • Rounds in which the clinician responsible leads a group of junior clinicians on a tour to visit the patients for whom they are collectively responsible. In some hospitals nurses may participate in walking rounds in lieu of or in addition to report.

**workmen's compensation** • Insurance that reimburses an employer for damages he's required to pay when an employee is injured on the job.

**World Health Organization (WHO)** • An agency of the United Nations, affiliated with the Food and Agricultural Organization of the UN, the International Atomic Energy Agency, the International Labor Organization, the Pan American Health Organization, and UNESCO. The WHO is primarily concerned with worldwide or regional health problems, but in emergencies it is authorized to render local assistance on request. Its functions include furnishing technical assistance, stimulating and advancing epidemiologic investigation of diseases, recommending health regulations, promoting cooperation among scientific and professional health groups, and providing information and counsel relating to health matters. Its headquarters are in Geneva, Switzerland.

**writ of habeas corpus** • A constitutional right to a court hearing that any person has when imprisoned or detained for allegedly breaking the law.

**wrongful death statute** • A statute existing in all states that provides that the death of a person can give rise to a cause of legal action brought by the person's beneficiaries in a civil suit against the person whose willful or negligent acts caused the death. Prior to the existence of these statutes, a suit could be brought only if the injured person survived the injury.

**wrongful life action** • A civil suit usually brought against a physician or health facility on the basis of negligence that resulted in the wrongful birth or life of an infant. The parents of the unwanted child seek to obtain payment from the defendant for the medical expenses of pregnancy and delivery, for pain and suffering, and for the education and upbringing of the child. Wrongful life actions have been brought and won in several situations, including malpracticed tubal ligations, vasectomies, and abortions. Failure to diagnose pregnancy in time for abortion and incorrect medical advice leading to the birth of a defective child have also led to malpractice suits for a wrongful life.

# Court-Case Citations
# in *Practices*

## A

**Application of the President and Directors of Georgetown College, Inc.,** 331 F. 2d 1000 (D.C. Cir. 1964); cert. denied, 377 U.S. 978 (1964) *(See Entry 13)*

**Ashley v. Nyack Hospital,** 412 N.Y.S. 2d 388 (App. Div. 1979) *(See Entry 7)*

## B

**Bailie v. Miami Valley Hospital,** 8 Ohio Misc. 193; 221 N.E. 2d 217 (1966) *(See Entry 16)*

**Barber v. Reinking,** 68 Wash. 2d 139; 411 P. 2d 861 (1966) *(See Entries 3, 8, 9)*

**Barber v. Time, Inc.,** 348 Mo. 1199; 159 S.W. 2d 291 (1942) *(See Entry 14)*

**Bazemore v. Savannah Hospital,** 171 Ga. 257; 155 S.E. 194 (1930) *(See Entry 14)*

**Beaudoin v. Watertown Memorial Hospital,** 145 N.W. 2d 166 (Wis. 1966) *(See Entries 14, 40)*

**Bellotti v. Baird I,** 428 U.S. 132 (1976) *(See Entry 26)*

**Bellotti v. Baird II,** 443 U.S. 622 (1979) *(See Entries 14, 26)*

**Big Town Nursing Home v. Newman,** 461 S.W. 2d 195 (Tex. Civ. App. 1970) *(See Entry 16)*

**Booth v. Toronto General Hospital,** (1910) 170 W.R. 118 (Ont. K.B.) *(See Entry 26)*

**Brown v. State,** 56 A.D. 2d 672; 391 N.Y.S. 2d 204 (1977) *(See Entry 23)*

**Buck v. Bell,** 47 S.Ct. 584 (1927) *(See Entry 28)*

**Burdreau v. McDowell,** 256 U.S. 465 (1921) *(See Entry 29)*

**Burke v. Pearson,** 259 S.C. 288; 191 S.E. 2d 721 (1972) *(See Entry 39)*

**Brune v. Belinkoff,** 235 N.E. 2d 793 (Mass. 1968) *(See Entry 39)*

**Byrne v. Boadle,** 159 Eng. Rep. 299 (1863) *(See Entry 40)*

## C

**Cannell v. Medical and Surgical Clinic S.C.,** 315 N.E. 2d 278 (Ill. App. Ct. 1974) *(See Entry 15)*

**Canterbury v. Spence,** 464 F. 2d 772 (D.C. Cir. 1972) *(See Entries 12, 24)*

**Capan v. Divine Providence Hospital,** 270 Pa. Super. 127; 410 A. 2d 1282 (1980) *(See Entry 45)*

**Cardin v. City of Montreal,** 29 D.L.R. 2d 492 (Can. 1961) *(See Entry 40)*

**Carey v. Population Services International,** 431 U.S. 678 (1977) *(See Entries 14, 26)*

**Carr v. St. Paul Fire and Marine Insurance Co.,** 384 F. Supp. 821 (W.D. Ark. 1974) *(See Entry 39)*

**Child v. Vancouver General Hospital,** [1970] 71 W.W.R. 656 (Can. 1969) *(See Entry 39)*

**Cline v. Lund,** 31 Cal. App. 3d 755; 107 Cal. Rptr. 629 (1973) *(See Entries 19, 21)*

**Collins v. Davis,** 44 Misc. 2d 622; 254 N.Y.S. 2d 666 (1964) *(See Entries 13, 28)*

**Collins v. Westlake Community Hospital,** 312 N.E. 2d 614 (Ill. 1974) *(See Chapter 5 Introduction)*

## Colorado State Board of

**Colorado State Board of Nurse Examiners v. Hohu,** 129 Colo. 195; 268 P. 2d 401 (1954) *(See Entry 4)*

**Commissioner of Correction v. Myers,** 399 N.E. 2d 452 (Mass. 1979) *(See Entry 29)*

**Commonwealth v. Gordon,** 431 Pa. 512; 246 A. 2d 325 (1968) *(See Entry 29)*

**Commonwealth v. Storella,** 375 N.E. 2d 348 (Mass. App. Ct. 1978) *(See Entry 29)*

**Commonwealth v. Porn,** 196 Mass. 326; 82 N.E. 31 (1907) *(See Entry 5)*

**Cooper v. National Motor Bearing Co.,** 136 Cal. App. 2d 229; 288 P. 2d 581 (1955) *(See Entries 5, 9)*

**Crowe v. Provost,** 374 S.W. 2d 645 (Tenn. Ct. App. 1963) *(See Entries 39, 42)*

## D

**D. v. D.,** 108 N.J. Super. 149 (1969) *(See Entry 14)*

**Darling v. Charleston Community Memorial Hospital,** 33 Ill. 2d 326; 211 N.E. 2d 253 (1965) *(See Entries 18, 19, 22, 39, 86)*

**Dauling v. Bluefield Sanitarium,** 147 W. Va. 567; 142 S.E. 2d 754 (1965) *(See Entry 39)*

**Davis v. Rodman,** 147 Ark. 385; 227 S.W. 612 (1921) *(See Entry 39)*

**Dembie,** (1963) 21 RFL 46 *(See Entry 14)*

**Dent v. West Virginia,** 129 U.S. 114 (1889) *(See Entries 1, 3)*

**Derrick v. Portland Eye, Ear, Nose and Throat Hospital,** 105 Or. 90 209 P. 344 (1922) *(See Entry 23)*

# T

# U

# V

# W

# X·Y·Z

## Miscellaneous

# Index

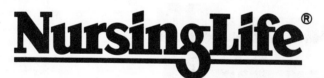

# UNDERSTANDING STATE AND

## PROBATE COURTS
Hear lawsuits involving wills and inheritances.

## CRIMINAL COURTS
Hear criminal lawsuits.

## FAMILY/JUVENILE COURTS
Hear lawsuits involving delinquent or neglected children.

## LOCAL COURTS
Specific courts hear lawsuits according to the types of charges, such as small claims, traffic, and housing.

## LOWER TRIAL COURTS
Hear civil and criminal lawsuits and may hear appeals from probate, criminal, and family/juvenile courts.

## U.S. DISTRICT COURTS
Hear federal criminal and civil lawsuits.

## U.S. COURT OF CLAIMS
Hears lawsuits against the federal government that involve constitutional rights, federal laws or regulations, or government contracts.

## U.S. TAX COURT
Hears lawsuits involving tax disputes.

## U.S. COURT OF APPEALS
Hears appeals from U.S. district courts and the U.S. Tax Court.

## U.S. CUSTOMS COURT
Hears lawsuits involving the U.S. Patent and Trade offices and other federal agencies.

## U.S. COURT OF CUSTOMS AND PATENT APPEALS
Hears appeals from the U.S. Customs Court.